Second Edition

Nutrition across the Life Span

Second Edition

Nutrition across the Life Span

Mary Kay Mitchell
The Ohio State University

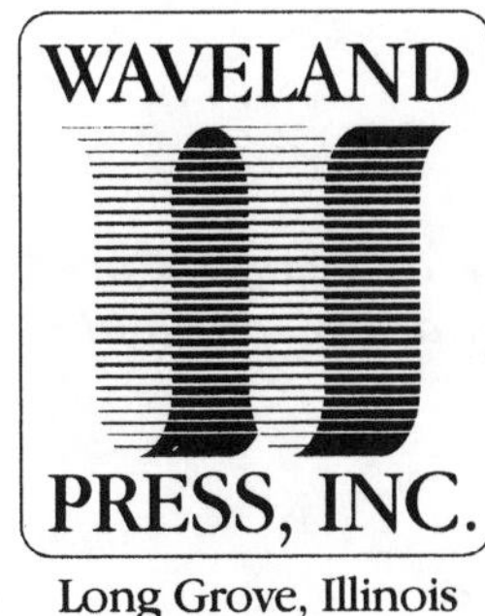

Long Grove, Illinois

For information about this book, contact:
Waveland Press, Inc.
4180 IL Route 83, Suite 101
Long Grove, IL 60047-9580
(847) 634-0081
info@waveland.com
www.waveland.com

Reissued 2008 by Waveland Press, Inc.

10-digit ISBN 1-57766-604-6
13-digit ISBN 978-1-57766-604-2

Printed in the United States of America

7 6 5 4 3 2 1

To Irv, for endless patience, support, humor, and wonderful photographs.
To my family, for their abundant support, patience, and understanding and for making everything worthwhile.

PREFACE

The study of nutrition is both exciting and rewarding. *Nutrition Across the Life Span* is directed toward students and health care professionals who require a more in-depth knowledge of nutritional needs for their work with individuals from embryo to old age. Physiologic and biochemic principles and results of current research are used to build a foundation for exploration of nutrition across the stages of reproduction, growth and development, and maturation and aging. These serve as the basis for consideration of the social, economic, physiologic, and life-style factors that influence nutrition status, food choices, and specific life-stage concerns. Particular attention is paid to using the principles of nutrition in planning and implementing recommendations for dietary change.

ORGANIZATION

As indicated in the *Table of Contents,* the second edition of the book has been reorganized to explore nutrition in reproduction as a basis for studying it sequentially from infancy to old age. Part One, *Foundations,* provides an introduction reviewing energy and nutrient needs and includes important tools such as dietary standards (Dietary Reference Intakes), dietary guidelines, food guides, *Healthy People 2010,* nutrition labeling, and legislation for dietary supplements. Chapter 2 introduces the nutrition assessment skills used in later chapters that address the stages of growth, reproduction, and maturation. The concept of promoting dietary change is explored in Chapter 3. The author, who is new to this edition, draws on her extensive experience in nutrition counseling and education to share principles and guidelines to assist students in understanding factors that influence health and dietary behaviors and considerations to promote change.

Part Two, *Reproduction,* addresses the physiologic changes, nutrition needs and unique concerns of pregnancy, postpartum mothers, and lactation and breast-feeding. Chapter 4 discusses the physiologic and nutritional changes that occur during gestation and postpartum. Chapter 5 addresses nutrition-related factors of age, maternal health status, health conditions, and behaviors that increase the risk of a poor pregnancy outcome. The chapter on lactation and breast-feeding rounds out this unit.

Part Three, *Growth and Development,* contains five chapters that cover the life span from infancy through adolescence. Chapter 7 explores nutrition in normal growth and development during the first year of life, which is followed by a chapter on the nutrition needs and care of high-risk infants. Chapter 9 spans preschool to 12 years and is followed by consideration of nutrition for children with developmental delays and disabilities. Chapter 11, "Nutrition during Adolesence," completes the unit.

Two chapters in Part Four, *The Adult Years,* cover the period from maturation to old age. This unit emphasizes meeting nutrition needs and establishing dietary and activity patterns that promote optimum health and reduction of risk of chronic disease.

The final two chapters, which comprise Part Five, *Special Concerns Across the Life Span*, address nutrition issues associated with eating disorders and physical fitness and performance. These chapters discuss specific issues that influence nutrition status and food-related behaviors across more than one stage of the life span.

FEATURES

Each chapter begins with an outline of topics to be discussed and ends with a list of *Concepts to Remember.* Within the chapters, each major section is preceded by a list of review questions. The outline and the questions give students an idea of the material to be covered in the chapter and, together with *Concepts to Remember,* they provide a useful review tool.

Most chapters are introduced with a *Case Study* that illustrates the importance of nutrition and provides a better perspective for the reader. In each chapter, *Key Terms,* essential to understanding the content, appear in boldface type in the text and are defined in specially designed boxes placed near where the term is first used. Extensive use of tables and illustrations facilitates assimilation of concepts and principles. Most chapters in Parts Two through Five include a *Research Update* box, which provides state-of-the-art information on emerging issues in nutrition as they relate to various stages of the life span.

Following each chapter, an *Application* provides guidelines for using and applying nutrition principles of a particular life span group. For example, in Chapter 4, *Pregnancy,* the *Application* demonstrates the techniques of nutrition assessment and intervention used during pregnancy.

The *Appendices* have been expanded to provide more reference data to support the information presented in the chapters, current data on infant formulas, the CDC growth charts, and additional references for interpretation of anthropometric data, particularly for older adults. A new addition is Appendix G that contains information on cultural food practices.

ACKNOWLEDGEMENTS

I wish to acknowledge the efforts of those individuals who helped with the preparation of the second edition of *Nutrition Across the Life Span.* In particular, thanks to Lois Renker, Jean Mitchell, Susie Wood, and Amy Pearse. Their input was invaluable. Editors Melissa Boyle and Yvonne Alexopoulos provided support and assisted every stage of the revision. Jamie Lyn Thornton performed excellent and careful production work—a special thanks to her for her patience. I am particularly grateful to the many undergraduate and graduate students who made suggestions for change and improvement.

CONTRIBUTORS

Diane L. Habash, PhD, RD, LD
Bionutritionist
General Clinical Research Center
The Ohio State University
Columbus, Ohio

Gail Kaye, PhD, RD, LD
Lecturer
Department of Human Nutrition
The Ohio State University
Columbus, Ohio

Mary Ann Mihok, PhD, RD
Associate Professor of Dietetics
Department of Natural Sciences
Messiah College
Grantham, Pennsylvania

Martha Orabella, MS, RD, LD
Nutrition Consultant
Cincinnati, Ohio

Melody Thompson, MS, RD
Clinical Nutrition Specialist
Ross Pediatric Medical Department
Ross Products Division/Abbott Laboratories
Columbus, Ohio

Kathryn A. Witt, PhD, RD
Associate Professor of Nutrition and Dietetics
Department of Natural Sciences
Messiah College
Grantham, Pennsylvania

REVIEWERS

Rhonda B. Armstrong, RN, MSN
Nursing Instructor
Department of AD Nursing
Hinds Community College
Jackson, Mississippi

Kay Gilbert, PhD, RD
Instructor
Science Department
Truckee Meadows Community College
Reno, Nevada
Consultant and Owner
Gilbert and Gilbert Consultants
Reno/Sparks, Nevada

Lois Peterson Renker, PhD, RD/LD
Associate Professor Emerita
Bowling Green State University
Bowling Green, Ohio
ADA-DEP member

Julie Poh Thurlow, DrPH, RD
Lecturer
Department of Nutritional Sciences
University of Wisconsin
Madison, Wisconsin

CONTENTS

APPENDIXES

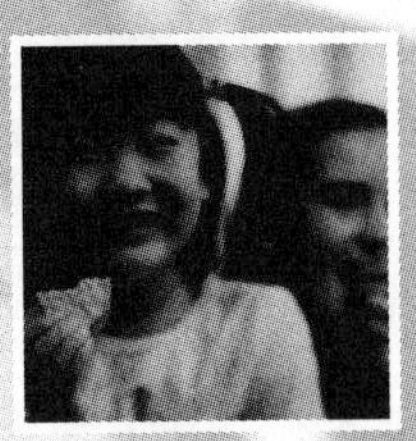

PART ONE

FOUNDATIONS

CHAPTER

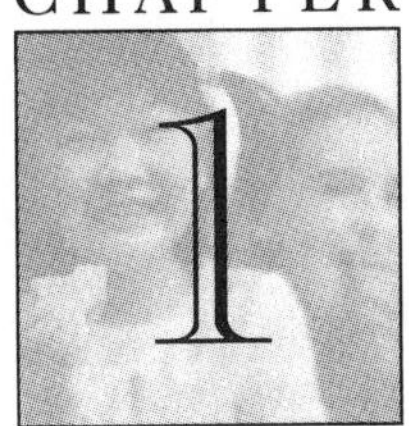

Introduction to Nutrition and the Life Span

Chapter Outline

Nutrition is important at every stage of the life span. In recent years international news reports and fundraising organizations have shown vivid portrayals of the devastation of undernutrition and disease in Third World nations. Severe undernutrition, particularly apparent in infants and young children, contributes to high mortality rates. For youngsters who survive malnutrition, decreases in growth and deficits in physical and mental development are common. Although the observable effects are less dramatic in adults, undernutrition compromises health, endurance, and productivity and increases susceptibility to infection. Marginal food intake places millions of people throughout the world at nutrition risk. These populations are often pushed over the edge to starvation and death by natural disasters of famine, flood, and drought and human conflicts created by economic and political strife.

In North America overt signs of undernutrition are encountered infrequently and classic "deficiency diseases" such as scurvy or beriberi are almost unknown. Here the effects of undernutrition often are subtle, but they still impair the growth and development of infants and children, affect health and performance of adults, and shorten life span. Vulnerable segments of the population are young children, adolescents, pregnant women, older adults, minorities, and those of low socioeconomic status.

In December 2000 the *Guinness Book of Records* reported that the oldest man in the world had passed away in Kansas at the age of 111 years. This is a rather amazing fact because life expectancy at the beginning of the last century was approximately 47 years. Over the twentieth century mortality rates declined dramatically, increasing life expectancy to 76.7 years in 1997. But substantial ethnic and sex differences remain. A white person will typically live approximately 6 years longer than an African-American person, and although the average boy born in 2000 will reach 73 years, his sister will live to be an octogenarian (National Center for Health Statistics [NCHS], 2000). This increase in life expectancy is primarily from decreases in infant mortality and in deaths from infectious diseases. Other contributing factors include the availability of immunizations, improved healthcare and sanitation, and increases in the availability and quality of the food supply.

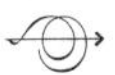

However, it is important to recognize that the three leading causes of death in adults in North America are heart disease, cancer, and stroke. Today there is substantial evidence that the food essential for sustenance and well-being may, depending on the choices people make, contribute to the development and progression of these chronic diseases. Diet-related obesity and dietary factors are associated with diseases of affluence—coronary artery disease, stroke, diabetes mellitus, and some cancers—which are leading causes of mortality and morbidity (NCHS, 1997). Therefore further increases in life expectancy and improvement of the health status of Americans will depend not only on access to adequate quantities of nutritious food, but also on individuals' food choices. Both quality and quantity are important food choices. Unfortunately more and more Americans are "eating out" and a trend in restaurants appears to be to make available or serve much larger portions than dietitians recommend.

On the other hand Americans have become increasingly aware of the importance of nutrition in all aspects of their lives. This is due in part to increased nutrition education and greater media coverage of nutrition research and issues. Foods, diets, and related products form a multibillion-dollar industry that pitches an almost overwhelming array of goods and services to consumers. In 1999 Americans spent $1.7 billion on vitamin and mineral supplements alone (Bloomberg News Service, 2001). Information in marketing and advertising campaigns targeted to people at all stages of the life span ranges from reliable, to questionable, to outright fraudulent. Products advertised run the gamut, from human milk substitutes and "staged" foods for infants to foods and snacks aimed at children who watch television cartoons, fast foods for teenagers, "healthy" foods and dietary supplements, vegetarian diets, quick weight-loss diets for young and middle-aged adults, and programs and products to relieve constipation or heartburn or prolong life for older adults. Thousands upon thousands of products are promoted. Understanding both nutrition needs and the factors that influence food and health behavior is an important tool for making sense of the commercial messages reaching people at all stages of life.

It is assumed that the student using this text has a background in introductory nutrition. This chapter reviews some basic concepts and tools used in nutrition, including energy and nutrient needs, dietary standards and guidelines for food choices, nutrition labeling, national health objectives, and nutrition monitoring. This overview is followed by a brief introduction to the life span, the stages of which will be discussed in detail in future chapters.

NUTRIENT NEEDS

- *What determines energy needs?*
- *Outline the major functions of macronutrients and micronutrients in the body.*
- *What nutrient or other components of foods may have health benefits beyond preventing deficiencies?*

Nutrition is a complex science that involves more than 40 nutrients. Nutrients are substances that are essential for growth and good health. From a practical standpoint nutrients have three general functions in the body: they provide energy, they form structural components of the body, and they regulate body functions. Some nutrients, such as protein, fulfill all three functions. Others, such as vitamins, which function only as regulators, fulfill only one. Traditionally nutrients are divided into the following categories: carbohydrate, lipid, protein, water, vitamin, and mineral.

Energy

The fuel or energy obtained from food is measured in kilocalories or **joules.** The term *calorie* is often substituted for *kilocalorie* in popular literature. In fact the Nutrition Facts Panel required for nutrition labeling lists the energy content of foods in calories (see page 26). Sources of energy to perform body functions are macronutrients. Carbohydrates, proteins, and lipids provide the body 4, 4, and 9 kcal per gram consumed, respectively. Alcohol, which supplies approximately 7 kcal/g, is also a substantial source of energy in the diets of some Americans. It is not considered a nutrient, however, because it has no required function. The macronutrients provide energy for building body compounds, performing muscular movements, promoting nerve transmission, and maintaining ion balance. To maintain body weight the food energy consumed needs to approximate energy expenditure over time.

The three components of energy expenditure are **basal metabolism,** also called basal energy need, the thermic effect of food, and physical activity. For adults the basal energy need is estimated to be between 1300 and 1800 kilocalories per day (National Research Council, 1989), which, depending on activity levels, represents one-half to three-fourths of total energy expended. A small portion (6% to 10%) of the daily energy is expended in the thermic effect, or the process of converting food to energy. The remainder, physical activity, can be highly variable. The level of energy expended depends on the individual's body weight and the intensity and duration of the activity. In addition the various stages of growth increase children's need for additional food energy.

Macronutrients

The major components, functions, and sources of macronutrients and related compounds are listed in Table 1-1.

The primary function of dietary carbohydrates and lipids is to provide energy. Dietary protein also yields energy, but its primary role is to provide amino acids for synthesis of body protein and other essential compounds.

Protein

Dietary protein provides amino acids that are used to synthesize body proteins, which perform many important functions in the body. A major role is building and maintaining structural body tissues such as muscle, bone matrix, and connective tissue. Other nonstructural body proteins include serum proteins such as albumin, blood cell membranes, immune factors, enzymes, and some hormones. Proteins are found combined with other body compounds such as nucleic acids (DNA and RNA), carbohydrates (creating glycoproteins or mucoproteins), chromophores (creating chromoproteins such as rhodopsin for vision in dim light), lipids (creating lipoproteins), and metals (creating hemoglobin). Through this variety of structures, forms, and locations, proteins are essential to a multitude of functions in the body. In the typical American diet protein provides from 12% to 17% of the energy. In diets that provide sufficient energy to maintain body weight, this level exceeds recommended levels of intake.

Carbohydrate

Carbohydrate is of prime importance in the diets of people throughout the world. Carbohydrate, available in an abundance of foods, is the least expensive and quickest source of energy. Except for lactose or milk sugar, starches and sugars are obtained primarily from plant foods.

Over the last few decades consumption of sugar has increased. *Nutrition and Your Health,* a publication known as the Dietary Guidelines for Americans (Dietary Guidelines Advisory Committee, 2000; see pages 21-23), advises moderation of sugar intake because sugars may promote development of dental caries and because many foods high in sugar are low in nutrient density. From a practical standpoint, high consumption of sugary foods is incompatible with the goal of eating a nutritious diet at an energy intake level that maintains a healthful weight. As you will read later in this chapter, the U.S.

KEY TERMS

joule: the international unit of energy defined as work done by the force of 1 newton acting over a distance of 1 meter; kcal = 4184 joules

basal metabolism: the amount of energy expended by an individual at complete rest in a comfortable environment after fasting for 12 hours

Table 1-1 Macronutrients in Human Nutrition

Nutrient	Components	Functions	Sources
CARBOHYDRATE			
Disaccharides	Lactose, maltose, isomaltose	Provide energy (4 kcal/g)	Dietary sugars, milk, fruits
Oligosaccharides	3-10 sugar units		Dietary starches, grains, vegetables
Polysaccharides	Starch/glycogen		
Indigestible polysaccharides	Cellulose, hemicellulose, pectin, gum, mucilage, ligin	Maintain gastric motility, prevent constipation, and protect from some gastrointestinal disorders; may reduce serum cholesterol, blood glucose	Whole grains, cereal brans, some fruits and vegetables, dried beans
LIPIDS			
Triglycerides	Glycerol and 3 fatty acids	Provide energy (9 kcal/g)	Saturated fat: butter, margarine, whole-milk dairy products, meat, poultry, some fish
Fatty acids	Varied chain length		
Saturated	No double bonds		
Monounsaturated	1 double bond		Monounsaturated fat, olives, olive oil
Polyunsaturated	2 or more double bonds, omega-9, -6, -3 fatty acids		Polyunsaturated vegetable oils
Essential fatty acids	Omega-6 fatty acid-linoleic	Membrane formation: form 20- and 22-carbon fatty acids	Vegetable, safflower, sunflower, corn, soybean oils
	Omega-3 fatty acid-alpha linoleic	Elongation to DHA and EPA for a variety of body compounds	Flax seed, canola, and grapeseed oils; wheat germ; soya oil; fish (mackerel, tuna, salmon, sardines)
PROTEIN			
Complete proteins Partially complete proteins Incomplete proteins	Essential and nonessential amino acids	Synthesis of body proteins	Milk and milk products, meat, fish, poultry, eggs, nuts, legumes, soy beans, lentils

DHA = docosahexaenoic acid, is an omega-3 fatty acid with 22 carbons and 6 carbon-carbon double bonds. EPA = eicosapentaenoic acid, an omega-3 fatty acid with 20 carbons and 5 carbon-carbon double bonds. Both are present in fish oils and synthesized in the body from alpha-linolenic acid.

Department of Agriculture's (USDA) Continuing Survey of Food Intakes (CSFI) is a major tool for monitoring the nutrition intake of Americans. Data from the 1994 to 1996 survey revealed that Americans ages 2 years and older consumed the equivalent of 82 g of carbohydrate (328 kilocalories) per day from added sweeteners, which accounted for 16% of total energy intake (Guthrie and Morton, 2000). Male adolescents consumed the greatest amount of added sweeteners such as soft drinks, table sugar, syrups and sweets, sweetened grains, fruit drinks, and milk products. Using the same CSFI database, other researchers reported that 59% of high sugar consumers also overconsumed energy, but their intakes of other food groups (except fruit) was not consistently affected. In comparison to others consuming the same relative amount of energy, 41% of high sugar consumers compensated for the additional calories from sugar by reducing intake from fruit, vegetable, milk, and grain groups.

Dietary Fiber

Dietary fiber consists of nondigestible food plant and **lignin** in which the plant matrix is largely intact (Institute of Medicine [IOM], 2001b). There has been considerable interest in the potential health benefits of dietary fiber. **Epidemiologic** research on dietary fiber has suggested that dietary fiber may be important in the prevention of constipation, diverticulosis, and other gastrointestinal disturbances. It has been assumed that a diet high in fiber was a deterrent to the development of colon cancer. However, other studies found no association between a high-fiber intake and reduced risk of colon cancer. Recently several studies have shown that a diet containing high amounts of fiber from fruit, vegetables, and certain grains lowers blood glucose, insulin, and lipid levels in patients with non–insulin-dependent diabetes mellitus (Chandalia et al., 2000) and that dietary fiber supplements were associated with long-term reductions in total serum cholesterol and low-density lipoprotein-cholesterol (LDL-C) and increases in high-density lipoprotein (HDL)-cholesterol (Knopp et al., 1999).

Lipids and Fatty Acids

Lipids are an important source of energy and provide fatty acids for the synthesis of many body compounds. Most dietary lipids are in the form of **triglycerides.** The characteristics of individual dietary fats are determined by which fatty acids are present. Fatty acids have been classified, based on chain length and structure, as saturated (no double bonds between the carbon chains), monounsaturated (one double bond), and polyunsaturated (two or more double bonds). Polyunsaturated fatty acids (PUFAs) are further classified by the location of the double bonds in the carbon chain. Since the 1960s the type of dietary fat and its relationship to chronic disease has been an important and sometimes controversial issue. It was demonstrated that consumption of a diet high in saturated fatty acids raised total cholesterol (TC) and (LDL-C), which are established risk factors for coronary heart disease, and that monounsaturated fats (predominately from olive oil) have the potential of lowering levels of cardiovascular risk in some individuals (American Heart Association, 1999). The PUFAs are effective in reducing serum TC and LDL-C levels.

Fatty acids considered essential for humans are derived from linoleic acid (18 carbons, 2 double bonds) and alpha-linolenic acid (18 carbons, 3 double bonds). Linoleic acid is referred to as an omega-6 fatty acid and alpha-linolenic acid as an omega-3 fatty acid, indicating that the double bond occurs at the sixth and third carbons from the methyl (-CH_3) end of the fatty acid, respec-

KEY TERMS

dietary fiber: substances in plant foods that are not digested by the processes that take place in the gastrointestinal tract

lignin: a fibrous material found in the bran layer of grains and in stems and seeds of fruits and vegetables

epidemiologic: related to epidemiology, the study of behavior and disease across a population

triglycerides: a major form of lipid in the diet and body; it is composed of three fatty acids bonded to glycerol, an alcohol

clinical studies: studies in which an intervention is implemented and results are observed, usually in a blind and double-blind fashion

tively. Epidemiologic and **clinical studies** have documented an association between omega-3 fatty acids and the prevention and amelioration of many diseases (Connor, 2000); particularly heart disease (Brown and Hu, 2001; GISSI Investigators, 1999). These protective effects are attributed to their omega-3 PUFA content, particularly eicosapentaenoic acid (EPA) and docosahexaenoic acid (DHA). These PUFAs are incorporated into the cell membrane, where they influence membrane fluidity, receptor function, enzyme activity, cytokines, and eicosanoid production. Intakes of omega-3 PUFAs in the United States are estimated to range from 1.2 g/day to 2.2 g/day per person, and omega-6 PUFA intake is estimated at 11 g/day to 16 g/day per person (Simopoulos and Salem, 1999).

For more than three decades major treatment and education for health-promotion activities have encouraged reduced consumption of fat and saturated fat. As Americans attempted to reduce the saturated fat content of their diets, food producers promoted margarines and shortenings to replace food high in "saturated fatty acids," especially butter and lard. The promoted products were heralded as the healthy alternative to saturated fat products. However, the hydrogenation process that created semisolid fats from oils results in the formation of **trans fatty acids.** Although trans fatty acids cause only moderate increases in serum cholesterol, they have more negative effects on lipoprotein profiles, effects comparable to those of saturated fatty acids (Judd et al., 1994). In prevention and treatment of cardiovascular diseases, nutritionists recommend that consumers reduce intakes of *both* saturated fats and trans fatty acids.

Cholesterol. Cholesterol is a fat-like substance that is found in foods of animal origin. It is synthesized in the human body and is found in many tissues, such as brain and nervous system tissues. It is an important component of cell membranes and cholesterol, and its derivatives are also precursors of vitamin D and various hormones and bile acids. Elevated serum levels of cholesterol are associated positively with the risk of coronary heart disease (Klag et al., 1993).

> **KEY TERMS**
>
> **trans fatty acids:** fatty acids in which the double bond has one hydrogen on the opposite side of the double bond

Lipoproteins. Because lipids and cholesterol are not soluble in water, they move through the bloodstream as a component of lipoprotein molecules categorized as HDL, low-density lipoprotein (LDL), and very-low-density lipoprotein (VLDL). Cholesterol found in each of these lipoproteins is referred to as HDL-cholesterol (HDL-C), LDL-C, and VLDL-cholesterol (VLDL-C), respectively. The sum of cholesterol in the lipoproteins is the TC. Numerous studies have established that elevated TC and LDL-C levels are related to increased risk of coronary artery disease, but that increased HDL-C levels are inversely related to risk (Hausmann, 1996).

Water

Approximately 60% of the adult body is water. Although it is often overlooked, water is essential for almost all body functions. It serves as a solvent, a lubricant, and a medium for transporting nutrients to body cells and waste products for excretion. Water is essential in regulation of body temperature and facilitation of chemical processes. For most individuals thirst mechanisms automatically ensure adequate fluid intake, but under circumstances of rapid water loss from the body or impairment of the thirst sensation, fluid levels can become depleted, which may lead to dehydration.

Micronutrients

Minerals

Minerals are inorganic substances that are essential for diverse functions in the human body. Minerals are critical to hundreds of body reactions in cellular processes, water balance, and regulation of the nervous system. They are constituents of body compounds such as bone, hemoglobin, and enzymes and regulators of most body functions. Table 1-2 lists major functions and food sources of the minerals that are significant in human nutrition.

Table 1-2 MINERALS IN HUMAN NUTRITION

Mineral	Major Functions	Significant Food Sources
Calcium	Constituent of bones and teeth; muscle contraction, blood coagulation, transmission of nerve impulses, cell membrane permeability, enzyme activation	Milk, cheese, milk-based foods; tofu and soy milk; sardines, canned salmon and other fish with bones; legumes; dark green vegetables
Chloride	Major anion in extracellular fluid; fluid, acid-base balance, component of hydrochloric acid in the stomach	Table salt; fish; eggs; meats; milk; large amounts in processed foods
Chromium	Cofactor for insulin in glucose uptake by cells; glucose tolerance factor	Whole grains; legumes; brewer's yeast; animal protein
Copper	Formation of hemoglobin; part of cytochrome enzyme system for energy production; metalloprotein of enzymes	Whole grains; legumes; shellfish; meats; food content reflects soil content
Fluoride	Formation of bones and teeth; enhancement of resistance to tooth decay	Drinking water if naturally fluoride-containing; fluoridated water; marine fish; tea
Iodine	A component of thyroxine; regulation of basal metabolism, growth, development	Iodized salt; seafood; seaweed; dairy products; food content reflects soil content
Iron	Constituent of enzymes, hemoglobin, myoglobin; transport of oxygen and carbon dioxide; cellular oxidation (cytochrome compounds)	Meats, organ meats; shellfish; poultry; eggs; enriched and whole-grain cereals; dark green vegetables; dried fruits; legumes; nuts (may come from cast iron cookware)
Magnesium	Constituent of bones and teeth; catalyst in the conversion between ATP and ADP; protein synthesis; cation in intracellular fluid; function of nerves and muscles	Wheat bran, whole grains; meat; milk; nuts; leafy green vegetables; beans; seafood
Manganese	Component of enzymes in metabolic reactions involving protein, carbohydrate, and fat metabolism	Legumes; whole grains; nuts; fruits; vegetables; tea; cocoa powder; instant coffee
Molybdenum	Constituent of enzymes; xanthine oxidase, aldehyde oxidase, sulfite oxidase	Milk; whole grains; liver; legumes; leafy vegetables; food content reflects soil content
Phosphorus	Component of bones and teeth; organic compounds including proteins, lipids and nucleic acids; glucose absorption, buffer system, energy metabolism	Almost all foods, especially meat, fish, poultry; dairy products; eggs; legumes; whole grains; soft drinks; nuts
Potassium	Major cation in intracellular fluid; fluid, acid-base balance, muscle contraction; protein synthesis; glycogen formation	Most foods, especially vegetables; dried fruits; orange juice; bananas; whole grains; legumes; milk
Selenium	Component of enzymes: glutathione peroxidase; antioxidant with vitamin E	Seafood; whole grains; legumes; red meat; dairy products; food content reflects soil content
Sodium	Major cation in extracellular fluid; fluid, acid-base balance, cell membrane permeability, glucose absorption	Table salt, salt added to processed foods; baking soda, baking powder, seasonings; moderate amounts in meat, fish, poultry, vegetables, grains
Zinc	Component of over 70 metalloenzymes; protein digestion, acid-base balance, anaerobic carbohydrate metabolism, wound healing, taste and smell	Meat; seafood; poultry; eggs; cheese; milk; whole grains; beans

ADP = ammonium dihydrogenphosphate. ATP = adenosine triphosphate.

Vitamins

The term *vitamin* originated from the name used to designate the substance in whole grains that could prevent the deficiency disease beriberi. That substance was later identified as thiamin (vitamin B_1). Today *vitamin* designates the essential organic substances that the body is unable to manufacture and therefore must be consumed. These essential regulators of body metabolism occur in food and the body in exceedingly small quantities. Water-soluble and fat-soluble vitamins of significance in human nutrition are listed in Table 1-3. Vitamins have diverse chemical structures and may participate in one, several, or even hundreds of reactions in the body. The absence of any vitamin can lead to lowered tissue levels and eventually vitamin-specific deficiency signs and symptoms, and in extreme circumstances, it can lead to death.

Vitamins and Minerals in Today's Environment

As the science of nutrition expands and our knowledge of nutrients grows more refined, it becomes apparent that nutrients seldom act alone in the body. They are integrally related to one another. Macronutrients cannot be used without the assistance of micronutrients, and both categories interact to make body tissues, promote use of energy, and regulate body functions. Some dietary components, such as phytochemicals, carotenoids, carnitine, and glutamine, have relevance to human health in their potential to decrease risk of or prevent chronic diseases or developmental abnormalities. In the process of evaluating and reformulating its Recommended Dietary Allowances (RDAs), the Standing Committee on the Scientific Evaluation of Dietary Reference Intakes (DRI) of the Food and Nutrition Board (FNB) of the IOM (IOM, 2000a) addressed micronutrients (vitamins and minerals) by four nutrient groups: calcium and related nutrients; B vitamins and related nutrients; nutrients that function as antioxidants; and vitamin A, iron, and other nutrients. For simplicity the discussion of nutrient needs and recommendations throughout this text will follow the groupings established by the DRI Committee.

DIETARY STANDARDS

- *What are dietary standards?*
- *What are the DRIs?*
- *How are the DRIs used for individuals and groups?*

How many calories do I need to eat to maintain my weight? How much protein does a football player need while training? An analysis of my diet shows that I eat 10 grams of fiber a day. Is that good? How much formula should we feed babies each day to make sure they get all they need to grow? These queries about nutrient needs are representative of the myriad questions dietitians and nutritionists answer each day. In most instances they formulate responses using levels of energy and nutrients established in dietary standards. The Food and Agriculture Organization and the World Health Organization of the United Nations have established international dietary recommendations, and many countries have issued guidelines appropriate for their populations.

The science of nutrition attempts to answer the question: "what should we eat to be healthy?" That question can be addressed on two levels: the scientific level and the consumer level. At the scientific level, recommended amounts of essential nutrients and other dietary components have been established by expert groups such as the committees and subcommittees of the FNB of the IOM that developed the reports on micronutrient intakes used throughout this text. The dietary standards for consumers are represented by the recommendations for food consumption, particularly the 2000 Dietary Guidelines and the Food Guide Pyramid (FGP). They are discussed in the following section.

Dietary Reference Intakes

For more than half a century the RDAs have been the American "gold standard" for recommending food intake to meet energy and nutrient needs and against which dietary intakes are evaluated. The RDAs, established by the FNB and the IOM, part of the National Academy of Sciences (NAS), are levels of nutrient intake assumed to be sufficient to meet the needs of most

Table 1-3 VITAMINS IN HUMAN NUTRITION

Vitamin	Major Functions	Significant Food Sources
Vitamin A retinol	Maintenance of epithelial cells and mucous membranes; growth; reproduction; formation of other light-receptor pigments	*Vitamin A:* fortified margarine, butter fat, liver, egg yolk *Carotenoids:* dark green and yellow vegetables, yellow fruits
Vitamin D ergocholecalciferol (D_2), cholecalciferol (D_3)	Regulation of calcium and phosphorus absorption and metabolism	Fortified milk; fish oils; synthesis from dehydrocholesterol by exposure to sunlight
Vitamin E tocopherols	Antioxidant; protection of polyunsaturated fatty acids, vitamin A and ascorbic acid, and cell membranes; sharing of action with selenium	Plant oils; leafy green vegetables; wheat germ; whole grains; nuts
Vitamin K phylloquinone (K_1), menaquinone (K_2)	Activation (carboxylation) of proteins required for blood coagulation; protein in bone	Green leafy vegetables; liver; egg yolks; synthesis by intestinal bacteria
Thiamin	Coenzyme (TPP) to release energy from carbohydrates, fats and proteins; formation of ribose for DNA and RNA	Most foods (in moderate amounts); pork, liver; whole or enriched grains; legumes
Riboflavin	Coenzymes (FMN and FAD) in energy metabolism; conversion of tryptophan to niacin	Milk and milk products; liver; meat, fish, poultry, eggs; whole-grain and enriched breads and cereals
Niacin nicotinic acid nicotinamide	Coenzymes (NAD & NADP) in energy metabolism; fatty acid synthesis	Meats, poultry, fish; whole-grain and enriched breads and cereals (milk and eggs are sources of tryptophan, which is converted to niacin)
Vitamin B_6 pyridoxine pyridoxal pyridoxamine	Coenzyme (PLP) in amino acid and fatty acid metabolism; conversion of tryptophan to niacin; production of antibodies; hemoglobin synthesis; glucogen degradation	Meats, fish, poultry; legumes; green, leafy vegetables; whole-grain breads and cereals
Pantothenic acid	Component of coenzyme A; release of energy from carbohydrates, fats and proteins; synthesis of cholesterol, fatty acids, hemoglobin	Organ meats; whole-grain cereals; most foods
Biotin	Coenzyme in carboxylation; release of energy from carbohydrates, fats, amino acids; amino acid, fatty acid, purine synthesis	Egg yolks; milk; organ meats; legumes, synthesis by intestinal microorganisms
Folate	Formation of coenzymes for single carbon transfers in formation of nucleotides, heme	Dark green leafy vegetables; seeds; liver; kidney; fruits
Vitamin B_{12} cobalamin	Coenzyme in synthesis of amino acids, activation of folate coenzymes	Liver; meat; milk; eggs; cheese
Vitamin C ascorbic acid	Antioxidant; collagen synthesis; facilitation of iron absorption, incorporation into hemoglobin; amino acid metabolism; activation of folate	Fruits, especially citrus; tomatoes, cabbage, peppers, broccoli, spinach, potatoes

FAD = flavin adenine dinucleotide. FMN = flavin mononucleotide. NAD = nicotinamide adenine dinucleotide. NADP = nicotinamide adenine dinucleotide. PLP = pyridoxal phosphate. TPP = thiamine pyrophosphate.

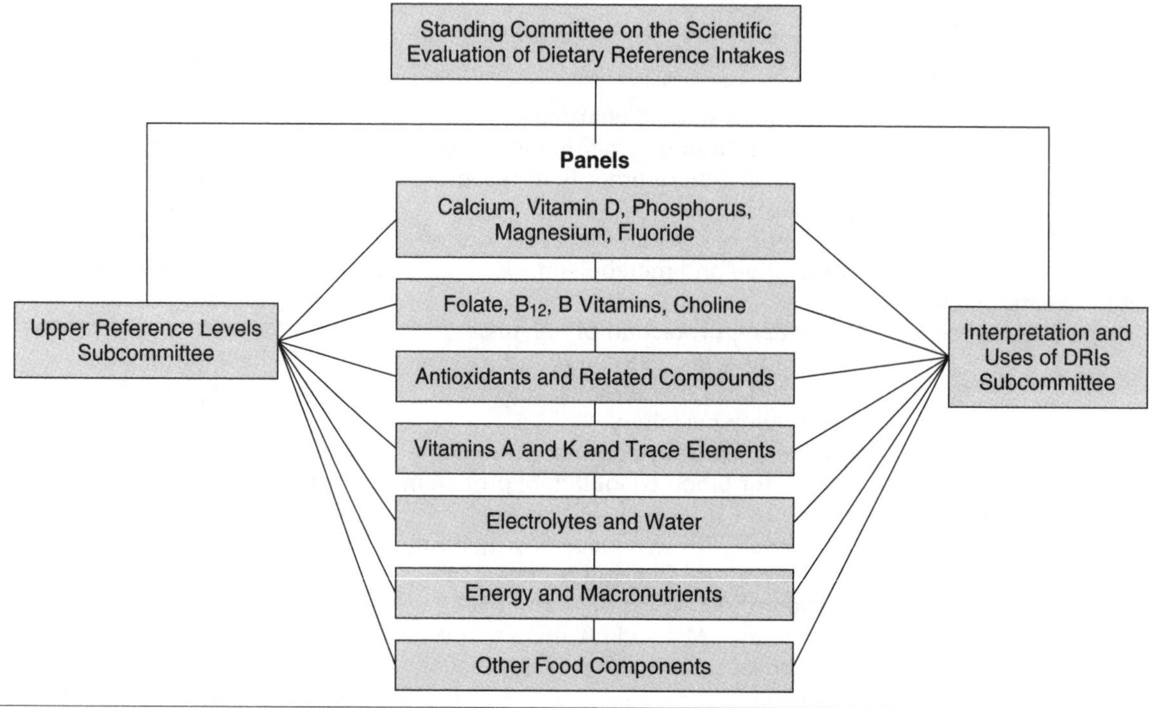

Figure 1-1 Structure of Dietary Reference Intake project. *(From Institute of Medicine: Dietary reference intakes for thiamin, riboflavin, niacin, vitamin B_6, folate, vitamin B_{12}, pantothenic acid, biotin and choline, Washington, DC, 1998, National Academy Press.)*

healthy individuals. In the last edition RDAs were established for energy and 26 nutrients (National Research Council, 1989).

Since publication of the 1989 edition of the RDAs, increases in knowledge of nutrition and the rapid accumulation of scientific data have dictated an expanded review of uses of the RDAs. Historically the RDAs have been determined on the basis of essentiality, the levels required to prevent deficiency symptoms plus a safety factor. But many nutritionists believed that the criterion of essentiality was too narrow for the current state of nutrition. In 1993 the FNB convened a symposium to consider the future of the RDA (FNB, 1994). After extensive interactions with the nutrition community, the FNB agreed to develop a radically new approach.

The result was a framework for the development of nutrient recommendations, the **DRIs.** Formulation of the DRIs has been a process of establishing a comprehensive set of reference values for dietary nutrient intakes for the healthy populations of the United States and Canada (FNB, 1994). As shown in Figure 1-1 the overall process is being coordinated by the Standing Committee on the Scientific Evaluation of Dietary Reference Intakes. Seven panels address specific nutrient categories and subcommittees handle upper reference levels and the interpretation and uses of DRIs. By late 2001 four panels have reported standards for vitamins and minerals. They are calcium and related nutrients (IOM, 1997); B complex vitamins (IOM, 1998); antioxidants and related compounds (IOM, 2000b); and vitamins A, K, iron, zinc, and other trace elements (IOM, 2001a). Be sure to check with your instructor about the levels of energy and macronutrients to be released in 2002.

The DRIs are designed to provide quantitative estimates of nutrient intakes for use in a variety of settings. They encompass current concepts about the roles of nutrients and food components in prevention of developmental abnormalities and reduction of the risk of chronic diseases (Mertz, 2000). For instance the current DRIs address intakes necessary to maintain adequate levels of the nutrients in the body and the relationships between calcium and osteoporosis, between folate and neural tube defects, and among vitamin B_6, folate, and cardiovascular disease. In addition information about nonessential but valuable components of food such as dietary fiber, carotenoids, and phytoestrogens are included.

To set realistic recommendations of any sort, an adequate database is critical. Because the objectives of the dietary recommendations depend on the extent of scientific data available at any time, the goals of the allowances become more ambitious and comprehensive with an increasing database.

The most ambitious objective, risk reduction for developmental abnormalities and major degenerative and **neoplastic diseases,** is the most difficult to handle in the scientific context of the DRIs. Such diseases have multiple causes, take decades to develop, and therefore demand studies and interventions over many years. Although the results of some long-term epidemiologic studies are emerging, they are difficult to interpret. At present risk reduction is the basis for the food-based dietary guidelines, but the results of present and future research can be expected to strengthen the database for addressing the disease risk reduction objective through the DRI as well. Rather than following a scheduled revision every 5 years as the RDA did until 1989, the recommendations for individual nutrients or nutrient groups of the DRI will occur when substantial new data demand changes (Mertz, 2000).

The DRIs differ from the RDAs in that nutrient recommendations are stated in four categories whenever possible instead of one. It is a generic term that encompasses four types of reference intake values for healthy individuals: **RDA, Estimated Average Requirement (EAR), Tolerable Upper Intake Level (UL),** and **Adequate Intake (AI).**

The RDA is to be used as a goal for the individual, and the UL is given to assist in advising individuals what levels of intake may result in adverse effects if habitually exceeded.

Of the four categories, the EAR and UL set lower and upper limits, respectively, of acceptable intakes (Figure 1-2). Neither is a recommendation in the strict sense. The EAR would cover the requirements of only one half of the population, and UL, "the maximal level of nutrient intake that is unlikely to pose risks of adverse health effects," falls just below the level of potentially dangerous excess (FNB, 1998, p. 6). It should not be inferred that nutrient intakes greater than the RDA are recommended as beneficial to an individual.

Using the Dietary Reference Intakes

Each report of DRIs for groupings of nutrients contains recommendations for interpretation and use. A separate DRI subcommittee, Interpretation and Uses of DRIs, (see Figure 1-1) will expand on the interpretation of new terms and concepts integral to the overall project and pro-

KEY TERMS

dietary reference intakes (DRIs): reference values that are quantitative estimates of nutrient intakes to be used for planning and assessing diets for healthy people

neoplastic diseases: diseases characterized by the growth of new and abnormal tissue, as in cancer

recommended dietary allowance (RDA): the dietary intake level of a nutrient needed to meet the requirement of *nearly all (97% to 98%) of the healthy population* of individuals in a particular life stage and sex

estimated average requirement (EAR): the average requirement of a nutrient intake value that is estimated to meet the requirement of *one-half of the healthy individuals* in a life stage and gender group

tolerable upper intake level (UL): the highest level of daily nutrient intake that is likely to pose *no risk of adverse health effects* to almost all individuals in the general population; as intake increases above the UL, the risk of adverse effects increases

adequate intake (AI): a recommended daily intake value based on observed or experimentally determined approximations or *estimates of nutrient intake by a group (or groups) of healthy people that are assumed to be adequate*—used when an RDA cannot be determined

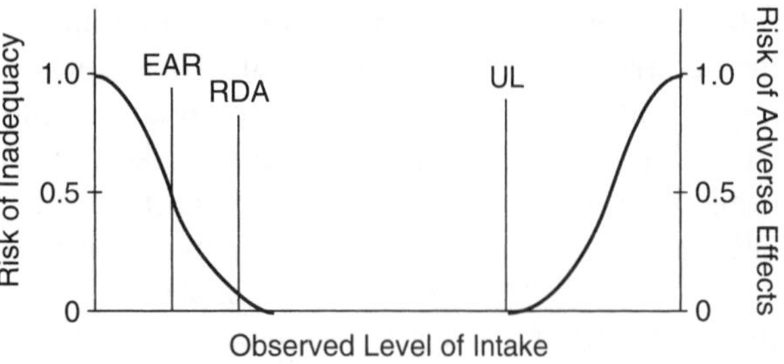

Figure 1-2 Dietary reference intakes. This figure shows that the Estimated Average Requirement (EAR) is the intake at which the risk of inadequacy is 50%. The Recommended Dietary Allowance (RDA) is the intake at which the risk of inadequacy is very small—only 2% to 3%. The Adequate Intake (AI) does not bear a consistent relationship to the EAR or the RDA because it is set without being able to estimate the average requirement. It is assumed that the AI is at or above the RDA. At intakes between the RDA and the Tolerable Upper Intake Level (UL), the risks of inadequacy and of excess are both close to zero. At intakes above the UL, the risk of adverse effects may increase. *(From Institute of Medicine: Dietary reference intakes for thiamin, riboflavin, niacin, vitamin B_6, folate, vitamin B_{12}, pantothenic acid, biotin and choline, Washington, DC, 1998, National Academy Press.)*

vide guidance for their uses in dietary assessment and planning of diets. These include dietary data assessment, food and nutrition assistance programs, standards and evaluations, nutrition education programs and food guides, food labeling, food fortification, and medical nutrition therapy. This method emphasizes the importance of balance among nutrients and highlights foods and food combinations appropriate to meet needs. It provides guidelines for design and evaluation of fortification policies, food analogues, and ready-to-eat meals.

When all the DRI reports have been issued, they will form a comprehensive set of reference values for nutrient intakes for healthy U.S. and Canadian populations. Table 1-4 outlines the uses of the DRI categories in planning or assessing dietary intake of individuals and groups. The table inside the front cover of this text provides summary data for Recommended Intakes for Individuals with RDA and AI for vitamins and elements. The DRIs are divided into 10 age categories, with divisions for sex after age 9 years. Recommendations for pregnancy and lactation recognize the unique role of age in reproduction with three age categories (14 to 18 years, 19 to 30 years, and 31 to 51 years). Based on increased research data related to older adults, the new DRI framework expands the age grouping of 51 years and above in the 1989 RDA to 50 to 70 years and 70 years of age and older. In using the values in this table, remember that although both RDA and AI are used, their definitions are different in that the AIs are estimates based on less scientific data than the RDAs.

Reference Weights and Heights

The requirement for many nutrients is based on body weight; therefore the RDAs and AIs are listed in terms of reference height and weight for each age group from 2 months to 6 months and by sex from age 9 years to 30 years. There is no evidence that body weight should change as adults age, if activity is maintained, so the reference weights for adults ages 19 years through 30 years are applied to all adult age groups. Reference weights and heights are based on anthropometric data collected from 1988 to 1994 as part of the Third National Health and Nutrition Examination Survey (NHANES III) in the United States.

Energy and Macronutrient Recommendations

The DRI panel on energy and macronutrients has not submittted its report at the time of this writing. The Recommended Energy Intakes for Median Heights and Weights from the 1989 RDA are shown in Table 1-5 (National Research Council, 1989). Recommended energy intake levels for the various age and gender groups are based on median heights and weights for the U.S. population from the Second National Health and Nutrition Examination Survey (NHANES II). The recommended energy levels represent average requirements for resting energy expenditure and an allowance for light to moderate activity. They must be adjusted for individual body size and activity level.

Table 1-4 USES OF DIETARY REFERENCE INTAKES FOR HEALTHY INDIVIDUALS AND GROUPS

Uses	For the Individual	For a Group
Planning	**RDA:** Aim for this intake.	**EAR:** Use in conjunction with a measure of variability of the group's intake to set goals for the mean intake of a specific population.
	AI: Aim for this intake.	
	UL: Use as a guide to limit intake: Chronic intake of higher amounts may increase risk of adverse effects.	
Assessment	**EAR:** Use to examine the possibility of inadequacy. Evaluation of true status requires clinical, biochemical, and/or anthropometric data.	**EAR:** Use in the assessment of the prevalence of inadequate intakes within a group.
	UL: Use to examine the possibility of overconsumption. Evaluation of true status requires clinical, biochemical, and/or anthropometric data.	

RDA = Recommended Dietary Allowance
EAR = Estimated Average Requirement
AI = Adequate Intake
UL = Tolerable Upper Intake Level

From Institute of Medicine: Dietary reference intakes for thiamin, riboflavin, niacin, vitamin B_6, folate, vitamin B_{12}, pantothenic acid, biotin, and choline, Washington, DC, 1998, National Academy Press.

NATIONAL HEALTH PROMOTION AND DISEASE PREVENTION

- *Describe the overall thrust of nutrition objectives of* Healthy People 2010.
- *How is progress toward these objectives measured?*

Healthy People 2010

More than 20 years ago the U.S. Department of Health and Human Services (HHS) released *Healthy People: The Surgeon General's Report on Health Promotion and Disease Prevention* and created the Healthy People Initiative (Moritsugu, 2000). It introduced the concept of forecasting national health goals with 10-year targets for improving various measures of the public's health status. The first *Healthy People* goals were issued in 1980 with 1990 targets. *Healthy People 2000,* issued in September 1990, drew on expanding scientific knowledge about disease prevention to identify three broad goals: increase years of healthy life, reduce health disparities among population groups, and increase access to preventive health services. The *Healthy People 2000* goals were supported by 319 objectives in 22 priority areas, including nutrition. In 1998 the Assistant Secretary for Health and the Surgeon General reported that 60% of the *Healthy People 2000* objectives had been met. Among the unmet goals was one to reduce the percentages of Americans who are overweight or obese. In fact the incidence of both obesity and overweight status increased dramatically across most segments of the population (see Chapter 14).

Table 1-5 MEDIAN HEIGHTS AND WEIGHTS AND RECOMMENDED ENERGY INTAKE

Category	Age (years) or Condition	Weight (kg)	Weight (lb)	Height (cm)	Height (in)	REE* (kcal/day)	Average Energy Allowance (kcal)† Multiples of REE	Per kg	Per Day††
Infants	0.0-0.5	6	13	60	24	320		108	650
	0.5-1.0	9	20	71	28	500		98	850
Children	1-3	13	29	90	35	740		102	1300
	4-6	20	44	112	44	950		90	1800
	7-10	28	62	132	52	1130		70	2000
Males	11-14	45	99	157	62	1440	1.70	55	2500
	15-18	66	145	176	69	1760	1.67	45	3000
	19-24	72	160	177	70	1780	1.67	40	2900
	25-50	79	174	176	70	1800	1.60	37	2900
	51+	77	170	173	68	1530	1.50	30	2300
Females	11-14	46	101	157	62	1310	1.67	47	2200
	15-18	55	120	163	64	1370	1.60	40	2200
	19-24	58	128	164	65	1350	1.60	38	2200
	25-50	63	138	163	64	1380	1.55	36	2200
	51+	65	143	160	63	1280	1.50	30	1900
Pregnant	1st Trimester								+0
	2nd Trimester								+300
	3rd Trimester								+300
Lactating	1st 6 months								+500
	2nd 6 months								+500

Reprinted with permission from Recommended Dietary Allowances, 10th ed. Copyright 1989 by the National Academy of Sciences. Courtesy of the National Academy Press, Washington, DC.
*Resting energy expenditure (REE); calculation based on FAO equations, then rounded.
†In the range of light to moderate activity, the coefficient of variation is ±20%.
††Figure is rounded.

Although the *Healthy People* goals are determined by the HHS, *Healthy People 2010* is a national health-promotion and disease-prevention initiative that brings together national, state, and local government agencies; nonprofit, voluntary, and professional organizations; business communities; and individuals. With a theme of "Healthy People in Healthy Communities," *Healthy People 2010* has two preeminent goals: increase quality and years of healthy life and eliminate health disparities (*Healthy People 2010,* 2001). These primary goals are supported by four enabling goals: promote healthy behaviors, promote health and safe communities, improve systems for personal and public health, and prevent and reduce diseases and disorders.

The four goals are organized into 28 focus areas and 467 objectives. Each of the 467 objectives has a target for improvements to be achieved by 2010. One focus area has a goal to promote health and reduce chronic disease associated with diet and weight (Box 1-1). More than one half of the other focus areas have implications for nutrition issues and policy. *Healthy People 2010* identifies a set of priorities that reflect 10 major public health concerns in the United States. These leading health indicators (Table 1-6) are intended to help everyone understand the importance of health promotion and disease prevention. These indicators were chosen based on their ability to motivate action, the availability of data to measure their progress, and their relevance as broad public health issues.

Box 1-1 *HEALTHY PEOPLE 2010* NUTRITION- AND OVERWEIGHT-RELATED OBJECTIVES

WEIGHT STATUS AND GROWTH

- Increase the proportion of adults who are at a healthy weight.
- Reduce the proportion of adults who are obese.
- Reduce the proportion of children and adolescents who are overweight or obese.
- Reduce growth retardation among low-income children under age 5 years.

FOOD AND NUTRIENT CONSUMPTION

- Increase the proportion of persons aged 2 years and older who consume at least three daily servings of vegetables with at least one third being dark green or orange vegetables.
- Increase the proportion of persons aged 2 years and older who consume at least six daily servings of grain products with at least three being whole grains.
- Increase the proportion of persons aged 2 years and older who consume less than 10 percent of kilocalories from saturated fat.
- Increase the proportion of persons aged 2 years and older who consume no more than 30 percent of kilocalories from total fat.
- Increase the proportion of persons aged 2 years and older who consume 2400 mg or less of sodium.
- Increase the proportion of persons aged 2 years and older who meet dietary recommendations for calcium.

IRON DEFICIENCY ANEMIA

- Reduce iron deficiency among young children, females of child-bearing age, and pregnant females.
- Reduce anemia among low-income pregnant females in their third trimester.

SCHOOLS, WORKSITES, AND NUTRITION COUNSELING

- Increase the proportion of children and adolescents aged 6 to 19 years whose intake of meals and snacks at school contributes to good overall dietary quality.
- Increase the proportion of worksites that offer nutrition or weight management classes or counseling.
- Increase the proportion of physician office visits made by patients with a diagnosis of cardiovascular disease, diabetes, or hyperlipidemia that include counseling or education related to diet and nutrition.

FOOD SECURITY

- Increase food security among U.S. households and in so doing reduce hunger.

From *Healthy People 2010*. www.healthypeople.gov. Accessed September 2, 2001.

NUTRITION MONITORING

- *How are data collected and used for nutrition monitoring?*

The National Nutrition Monitoring and Related Research Act of 1990 requires the federal government to develop a 10-year comprehensive plan for nutrition monitoring and related research. The plan, formulated by a joint USDA-HHS work group, serves as the basis for planning and coordinating the activities of federal and state agencies that provide information about the dietary and nutrition status of the U.S. population, including conditions that affect the dietary and nutrition status of individuals and the relationship between diet and health. The primary purpose of the 10-year plan is coordination to ensure that methods of collecting and reporting data are comparable for all participating agencies.

Table 1-6 *HEALTHY PEOPLE 2010:* LEADING HEALTH INDICATORS

Subject/Topic	Public Health Challenge
Physical activity	Promote regular physical activity
Overweight status and obesity	Promote healthier weight and good nutrition
Tobacco use	Prevent and reduce tobacco use
Substance abuse	Prevent and reduce substance abuse
Responsible sexual behavior	Promote responsible sexual behavior
Mental health	Promote mental health and well-being
Injury and violence	Promote safety and reduce violence
Environmental quality	Promote healthy environments
Immunization	Prevent infectious disease through immunization
Access to healthcare	Increase access to quality healthcare

Data from U.S. Department of Health and Human Services: Healthy People 2010: national health promotion and disease prevention objectives, Washington, DC, 2000, U.S. Dept of Health and Human Services.

Major measurement components of nutrition monitoring are nutrition and health-related measurements, food and nutrient composition, knowledge, attitude and behavior assessments, food composition and nutrient databases, and food supply determinations. The information accumulated for nutrition monitoring purposes goes into databases used for public policy decisions. It will be a basis for choices related to nutrition education; public health nutrition programs; food assistance programs; regulation of food enrichment and fortification; labeling of the food products; and food production, safety, and marketing. Such data were used in formulating *Healthy People 2010,* the 2000 Dietary Guidelines for Americans, Food Plans for Welfare and Food Stamp Programs, and regulations governing food programs. Nutrition monitoring is essential to provide data for future decision making regarding all aspects of public policy.

Most of the available information on the dietary intake or nutrition status of the American population has been accumulated from government surveys. Two of the most significant are the National Food Consumption Survey (NFCS) conducted by the USDA and the National Health and Nutrition Examination Surveys (NHANES) of the NCHS (NCHS, 2000).

The NFCS, conducted every 10 years, allows comparison of food intake of the American population across over time. The most recent, the 1987 to 1988 survey, collected demographic and 3-day food consumption data from approximately 8000 individuals. The information obtained from NFCS has been compared with various age- and sex-appropriate RDAs to assess adequacy of intake. The data have been used to explore relationships of nutrition to numerous socioeconomic factors including education, size of household, and geographic location. In 1985 the USDA initiated The Continuing Survey of Food Intake of Individuals (CSFI), a continuous annual survey of the food intake of women aged 23 through 50 and their children 1 through 5 years of age.

The NHANES is a series of national examination studies conducted approximately every 5 years on a random nationally representative sample of the American population. Information gathered includes diet, nutrition status, and health outcomes. Research techniques include interviews, standardized examinations, analyses of blood and urine samples, and anthropometric measurements (Chapter 2 discusses basic assessment techniques). These data allow an assessment of the status of the population and an investigation of possible relationships between dietary habits and specific heath problems.

The NHANES II survey was conducted between 1976 and 1980 on a representative population sample aged 6 months to 74 years. From 1982 to 1984 the NCHS also conducted a survey of food intake among the Spanish-speaking populations, now referred to as the Hispanic NHANES. NHANES III covered a 6-year period (1988 to 1994) and included dietary information and physiologic measurements on about 40,000 individuals 2 months of age and older from households in 81 counties across the United States. Also, NHANES III was designed to produce national data for African Americans, Mexican Americans, children, and older adults. Follow-up will be conducted on individuals who participated in the NHANES III to collect longitudinal information on health status. In 1999 a new NHANES survey began in which each year, approximately 5000 randomly selected residents in 12 to 15 counties across the country will participate.

The food intake data from the 1987 NFCS and the CSFI and the nutrition assessment data from the NHANES are coupled with data from vital statistics and epidemiologic studies conducted by the National Institutes of Health and various academic institutions to provide the basis for nutrition monitoring.

THE DIETARY GUIDELINES FOR AMERICANS AND THE FOOD GUIDE PYRAMID

- *What tools are available to assist consumers in selecting nutritious, healthy diets?*
- *Discuss the use of the Dietary Guidelines designed to promote long-term health for Americans.*
- *Explain the use of the FGP.*

To help Americans make healthy food choices, scientific concepts must be translated into simple dietary patterns to promote health and prevent or reduce the progression of chronic diseases with a nutrition-related source. Since 1980 the Dietary Guidelines for Americans from the USDA and HHS have provided advice for healthy Americans age 2 years and older.

The Dietary Guidelines for Americans is the cornerstone of federal food, nutrition, and health policy and programs in the United States (Dietary Guidelines Advisory Committee, 2000). Each federal department is mandated to use these guidelines in carrying out federal nutrition and health programs. The National Nutrition Monitoring and Related Research Act mandated that the Dietary Guidelines for Americans be reviewed at least every 5 years. The 2000 *Nutrition and Your Health: Dietary Guidelines for Americans* was formulated by an expert advisory committee appointed to review scientific evidence and make recommendations with input from experts in nutrition, the food industry, professional associations, consumer advocates, and the public (USDA and HHS, 2000).

Revisions of the guidelines sparked broad interest and some controversy. Most of the changes received support, but there were also disagreements. For example experts differed on the appropriate recommendations for salt. One group of scientists argued that scientific evidence does not warrant more restrictive advice for salt and supported retaining the moderation recommendation (McCarron, 2000), whereas another called for more stringent wording (Kaplan, 2000). Similar concerns arose on the sugar recommendations. But all agree that the new guidelines are designed to be consumer friendly and to contain specific scientific recommendations (Kennedy and Davis, 2000).

The new guidelines include a hierarchy of 10 individual guidelines grouped around three positive messages, the ABCs for health: "Aim for Fitness," "Build a Healthy Base," and "Choose Sensibly" (Figure 1-3).

The "Aim for Fitness" guidelines deal with healthy eating and regular physical activity to help people of all ages work productively, enjoy life, and feel good. They also help children to grow, develop, and do well in school. The first guideline within this message, "Aim for a Healthy Weight" (Figure 1-4), is supported by information that allows the consumer to calculate body weight and compare it to a body mass index chart in "Are You at a Healthy Weight?" (Figure 1-5). The second guideline emphasizes physical activity's importance for healthy living, more than just for weight maintenance. Benefits of physical activity are promoted and consumers are encouraged to sustain moderate physical activity for at least 30 minutes most days of the week. An important aspect of the physical activity guideline is the emphasis on its importance for children and adults.

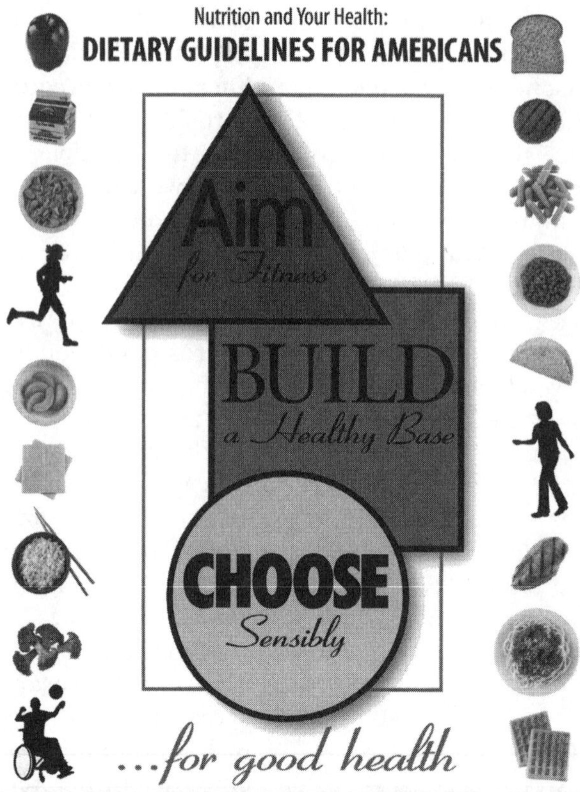

Figure 1-3 Nutrition and Your Health: Dietary Guidelines for Americans, 2000. Aim, Build, and Choose for Good Health. *(From USDA, USDHHS, Home and Garden Bulletin 232, 5th ed., 2000.)*

The "Build a Healthy Base" principles emphasize the use of the FGP (see Figure 1-4) for food choices. The new guidelines continue to emphasize balance, moderation, and variety in food choices, with a special emphasis on grain products, vegetables, and fruits. The guidelines include specific examples of foods that deliver given nutrients, including choices for vegetarians. The pyramid recommends grains, fruits, and vegetables as the foundation of meals and calls them the base for good nutrition and health, noting that they may reduce the risk of certain chronic diseases. For the first time the guidelines also emphasize taking steps to keep food safe to eat, particularly in the home. Recommendations include keeping preparation areas and utensils clean, separating raw and ready-to-eat foods, cooking food to a safe temperature, and chilling perishable foods promptly. The guidelines have long recognized and included the importance of a healthy diet. The new guidelines now highlight the integral relationships of physical activity and safe food handling to healthful eating patterns.

The FGP is a practical and flexible tool developed to help consumers make healthy food choices. Because it incorporates the 10 basic principles of the Dietary Guidelines for Americans, it is also an important tool in making food choices to reduce the risk of chronic disease (USDA, 2000). The pyramid is based on five food groups that form the foundation of a nutritionally adequate diet when the recommended number of servings from each group are consumed daily (Figure 1-6). Typical serving sizes for each group are outlined in Box 1-2. The number of servings appropriate for an individual depends on the caloric level he or she requires. Caloric needs and the number of servings vary with age, sex,

Aim for fitness

▲ Aim for a healthy weight—balance the calories you eat with physical activity.

▲ Get moving. Do 30 minutes or more of moderate physical activity most days or every day. Make physical activity part of your daily routine.

▲ Eat sensible portion sizes (see below) as one key to a healthy weight.

▲ Set a good example for children. Eat healthy meals and enjoy regular physical activities together. Children need at least 60 minutes of physical activity daily.

CHOOSE SENSIBLE PORTION SIZES

- If you're eating out, order small portions, share an entree with a friend, or take part of the food home (if you can chill it right away).
- Check product labels to see how much food is considered to be a serving. Many items sold as single portions actually provide 2 servings or more—such as a 20-ounce soft drink, a 12-ounce steak, a 3-ounce bag of chips, or a large bagel.
- Be especially careful to limit portion size of foods high in calories, such as cookies, cakes, other sweets, French fries, and fats, oils, and spreads.

Build a healthy base

Use the Food Guide Pyramid to help make healthy food choices that you can enjoy. For children 2 to 6 years old, see the Pyramid for Young Children. Figure 1-6 gives a quick guide to Pyramid food groups and servings.

■ Build your eating pattern on a variety of grains, fruits, and vegetables.

■ Include several servings of whole grain foods daily, such as whole wheat, brown rice, oats, and whole grain corn.

■ Enjoy five a day—eat at least 2 servings of fruit and at least 3 servings of vegetables each day. Choose dark green leafy vegetables, orange fruits and vegetables, and cooked dry peas and beans often.

■ Also choose foods from the milk and the meat and beans groups each day. Make low-fat choices most often.

■ It's fine to enjoy fats and sweets occasionally.

KEEP FOOD SAFE TO EAT

- Wash hands and surfaces often.
- Separate raw, cooked, and ready-to-eat foods while shopping, preparing, or storing.
- Cook foods to a safe temperature.
- Refrigerate perishable foods promptly.
- Check and follow the label.
- When in doubt, throw it out.

Choose sensibly

● Limit your use of solid fats, such as butter and hard margarines. Use vegetable oils as a substitute.

● Choose fat-free or low-fat types of milk products and lean meats and poultry. Eat cooked dry beans and peas and fish more often.

● Use the Nutrition Facts Label to help choose foods lower in total fat—especially saturated fat—as well as in cholesterol and sodium.

● Limit your intake of beverages and foods that are high in added sugars. Don't let soft drinks or sweets crowd out other foods you need, such as milk products or other calcium sources.

● To keep your sodium intake moderate, choose and prepare foods with less salt or salty flavorings.

● If you are an adult and choose to drink alcoholic beverages, do so sensibly—limit intake to one drink a day for women or two a day for men.

WHAT IS YOUR LIMIT ON FAT?

Total Calories per Day	Saturated Fat in Grams*	Total Fat in Grams*
1600	18 or less	53
2000**	20 or less	65
2200	24 or less	73
2500**	25 or less	80
2800	31 or less	93

*These limits are less than 10% of calories for saturated fat and 30% of calories for total fat.

**Percent Daily Values on Nutrition Facts Labels are based on a 2000-calorie diet. Values for 2000 and 2500 calories are rounded to the nearest 5 grams to be consistent with the Nutrition Facts Label.

Figure 1-4 Nutrition and Your Health: Dietary Guidelines for Americans, 2000. Aim, Build, and Choose for Good Health. *(From USDA, USDHHS, Home and Garden Bulletin 232, 5th ed., 2000.)*

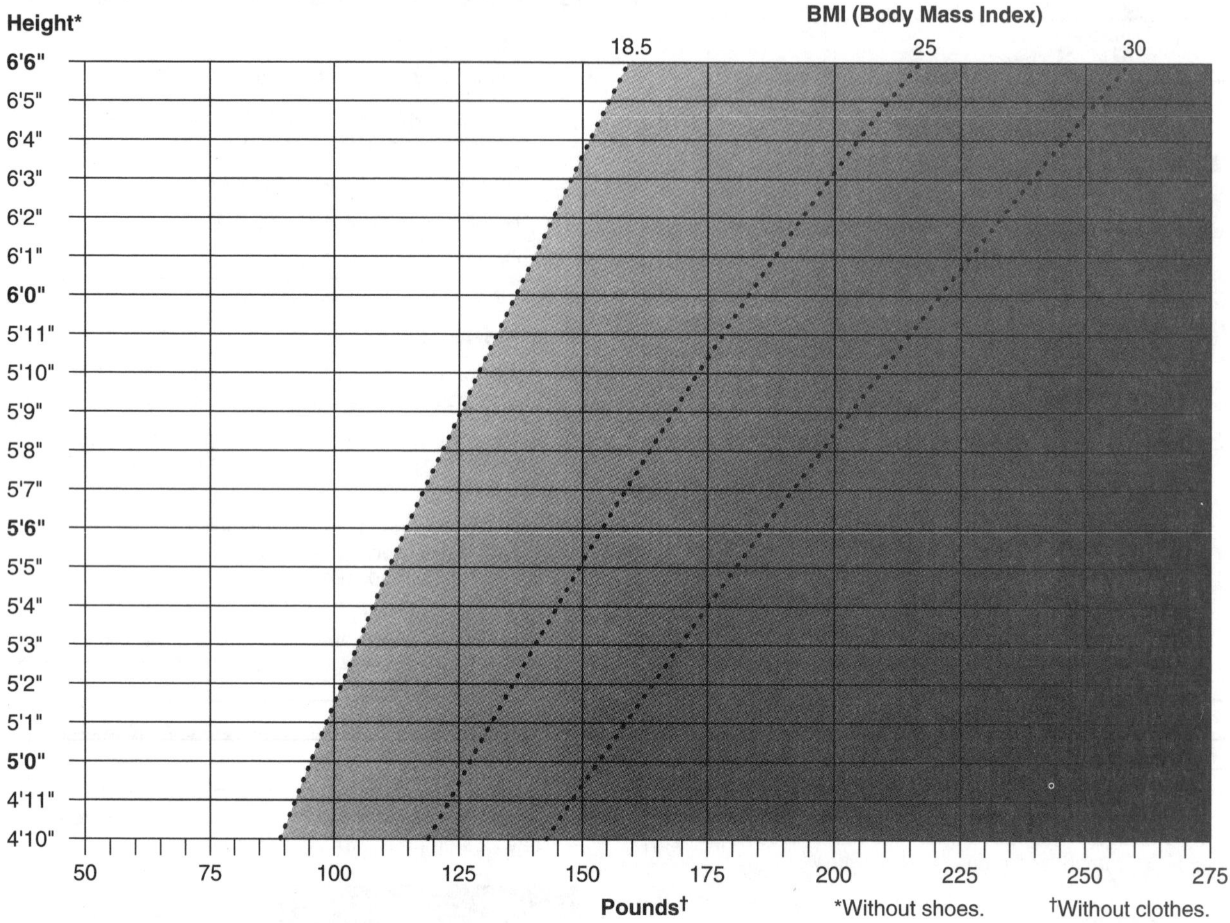

BMI measures weight in relation to height. The BMI ranges shown above are for adults. They are not exact ranges of healthy and unhealthy weights. However, they show that health risk increases at higher levels of overweight and obesity. Even within the healthy BMI range, weight gains can carry health risks for adults.

Directions: Find your weight on the bottom of the graph. Go straight up from that point until you come to the line that matches your height. Then look to find your weight group.

Healthy Weight BMI from 18.5 to 25 refers to healthy weight.

Overweight BMI from 25 to 30 refers to overweight.

Obese BMI 30 or higher refers to obesity. Obese persons are also overweight.

Figure 1-5 Nutrition and Your Health: Dietary Guidelines for Americans, 2000. Aim, Build, and Choose for Good Health. *(From USDA, USDHHS, Home and Garden Bulletin 232, 5th ed., 2000.)*

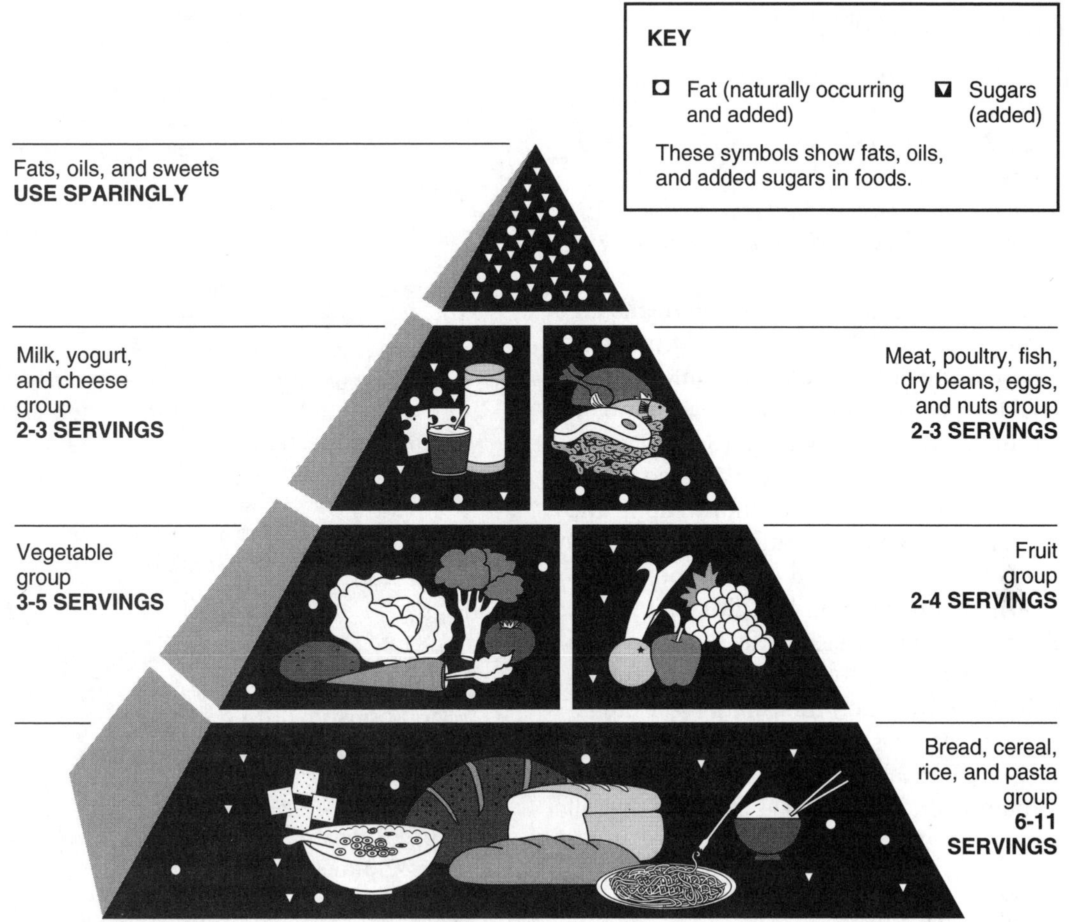

Figure 1-6 Nutrition and Your Health: Dietary Guidelines for Americans, 2000. Aim, Build, and Choose for Good Health. *(From USDA, USDHHS, Home and Garden Bulletin 232, 5th ed., 2000.)*

body size, and activity level. For most individuals, a diet that provides the recommended levels of nutrients will require at least the minimum number of servings recommended in Table 1-7.

The third group of guidelines, under the positive message "Choose Sensibly," uses four guidelines to incorporate recommendations to reduce consumption of fat, saturated fat, and cholesterol; to moderate consumption of sodium and sugar; and if an individual consumes alcoholic beverages, to drink in moderation (see Figure 1-4). The lower intakes of saturated fat and cholesterol are consistent with decreases in blood cholesterol and lower rates of coronary mortality over the past 30 years (Dixon and Ernst, 2001). Foods from the grain products group, with fruits and vegetables, are recommended to form the foundation of healthful diets. Such foods tend to be low in fat, saturated fat, cholesterol, added sugar, and sodium. These foods should be accompanied by lean and low-fat choices from the third tier. Foods at the tip of the FGP (i.e., fats, oils, and sweets) should be used sparingly because they are concentrated sources of fats and sugars that provide energy, but few nutrients.

Nutrition experts believe that implementation of the 10 principles will lead to improved health status and reduced risk of certain chronic diseases, such as coronary artery disease, stroke, diabetes mellitus, and some forms of cancer.

NUTRITION LABELING

- *Describe the information available to consumers from the nutrition label.*
- *What are the uses of Daily Reference Values (DRVs) and Recommended Dietary Intake (RDI)?*
- *What are the advantages of having regulations for nutrient claims and health claims on food products?*

In this era of health consciousness Americans are actively interested in what they eat. Unfortunately despite the vast quantity of nutrition information now available, it has not always been easy for consumers to make informed food choices. Nutrition labeling has helped. In response to the need for reliable, consistent, and useful information, the Nutrition Labeling and Education Act of 1990 mandated new food labels and established regulations governing nutrient and health claims for foods. Food labels are designed as a tool to help consumers select a healthy diet within the framework of the FGP. Nutrition information on the label of most foods uses serving sizes that reflect portions of food usually eaten. These labels provide information on how the food fits in an overall daily diet.

Nutrition Facts Panel

The nutrition label shown in Figure 1-7 illustrates the required format and content for nutrition labels. This "Nutrition Facts" panel contains information to help consumers fit the food into their overall daily diet. The nutrient content of the food is listed as a percentage of a standard amount referred to as the daily values (DV). The DVs give only one standard for all individuals over the age of 4 years, except pregnant and lactating women. They consist of two separate sets of reference values: DRV for macronutrients—carbohydrate, fat, protein, saturated fat, cholesterol, fiber, sodium, and potassium—and RDI for vitamins, other minerals, and protein for certain age groups (Table 1-8). Thus the DVs are a simpler set of standards than the DRI.

Percent Daily Value (%DV) shows how a food fits into the overall daily diet. Higher percentages reflect greater concentrations, and greater amounts, of nutrients. For most people the goal is to choose foods that add up to about 100% DV or more for total carbohydrate, dietary fiber, and vitamins and minerals, and 100% DV or less for total fat, saturated fat, cholesterol, and sodium. Defining nutrients as a %DV is intended to help consumers understand the role of individual foods in the context of the total daily diet.

The DVs for certain nutrients appear on package labels for both a 2000- and a 2500-calorie

Box 1-2 THE DAILY FOOD GUIDE: SAMPLE SERVING SIZES

A TYPICAL SERVING FOR FOODS IN EACH GROUP FORMS THE BASIS FOR RECOMMENDED NUMBER OF SERVINGS

Breads, Cereals, Rice, and Pasta

1 slice of bread
½ cup of cooked rice or pasta
½ cup of cooked cereal
1 ounce of ready-to-eat cereal

The amount of a food eaten may be more than one serving. For example, a dinner portion of spaghetti would count as two or three servings of pasta.

Vegetables

½ cup of chopped raw or cooked vegetables
1 cup of leafy raw vegetables

Fruits

1 piece of fruit or melon wedge
¾ cup of juice
½ cup of canned fruit
¼ cup of dried fruit

Milk, Yogurt, and Cheese

1 cup of milk or yogurt
1½ to 2 ounces of cheese

Meat, Poultry, Fish, Dry Beans, Eggs, and Nuts

2½ to 3 ounces of cooked lean meat, poultry, or fish

Count ½ cup of cooked beans, 1 egg, or 2 tablespoons of peanut butter as 1 ounce of lean meat (about ⅓ serving)

Fats, Oils, and Sweets

LIMIT CALORIES FROM THESE especially if you need to lose weight

From Food and Drug Administration, Rockville, Md, 1993.

Table 1-7 NUMBER OF SERVINGS FROM THE GROUPS IN THE FOOD GUIDE PYRAMID AT VARIOUS CALORIE LEVELS*

Food Group	About 1600	Calorie Level About 2200	About 2800
Bread	6	9	11
Vegetable	3	4	5
Fruit	2	3	4
Milk	2-3†	2-3†	2-3†
Meat	total of 5 oz	total of 6 oz	total of 7 oz

From Food and Drug Administration, Rockville, Md, 1993.
*The number of servings are appropriate for the calorie levels if low-fat, lean foods are chosen from the five major food groups and fats, oils, and sweets are used sparingly.
†Women who are pregnant or breast-feeding, teenagers, and young adults to age 24 need 3 servings.

Table 1-8 REFERENCES FOR DAILY VALUES ON NUTRITION LABELS

Reference Daily Intakes (RDI)*		Daily Reference Values (DRV)	
Nutrient	**Amount**	**Food Component**	**Basis for DRV**
Protein			
children 1-4 years	16 g	Total fat	30% of calories
infants <1 year	14 g	Saturated fatty acids	10% of calories
pregnant women	60 g	Cholesterol	300 mg
nursing mothers	65 g	Total carbohydrate	60% of calories
Vitamin A	5000 IU	Protein	10% of calories
Vitamin C	60 mg	Dietary fiber	11.5 g/1000 calories
Thiamin	1.5 mg		
Riboflavin	1.7 mg	Sodium	2400 mg
Niacin	20 mg	Potassium	3500 mg
Calcium	1.0 g		
Iron	18 mg		
Vitamin D	400 IU		
Vitamin E	30 IU		
Vitamin B_6	2.0 mg		
Folic acid	0.4 mg		
Vitamin B_{12}	6 μg		
Phosphorus	1.0 g		
Iodine	150 μg		
Magnesium	400 mg		
Zinc	15 mg		
Copper	2 mg		
Biotin	0.3 mg		
Pantothenic acid	10 mg		

Food Component	2000-Calorie Diet	2500-Calorie Diet
Total fat	65 g	80 g
Saturated fat	20 g	25 g
Cholesterol	300 mg	300 mg
Total carbohydrate	300 g	300 mg
Protein	50 g	65 g
Sodium	2400 mg	2400 mg
Potassium	3500 mg	3500 mg

From Food and Drug Administration, Rockville, Md, 1993.
*Based on the 1968 Recommended Dietary Allowances.

Check the food label before you buy

Food labels have several parts, including the front panel, Nutrition Facts, and ingredient list. The front panel often tells you if nutrients have been added—for example, "iodized salt" lets you know that iodine has been added, and "enriched pasta" (or "enriched" grain of any type) means that thiamin, riboflavin, niacin, iron, and folic acid have been added.

The ingredient list tells you what's in the food, including any nutrients, fats, or sugars that have been added. The ingredients are listed in descending order by weight.

Learn how to read the Nutrition Facts. Use the Nutrition Facts to see if a food is a good source of a nutrient or to compare similar foods—for example, to find which brand of frozen dinner is lower in saturated fat, or which kind of breakfast cereal contains more folic acid. Look at the % Daily Value (%DV) column to see whether a food is high or low in nutrients. If you want to limit a nutrient (such as fat, saturated fat, cholesterol, sodium), try to choose foods with a lower %DV. If you want to consume more of a nutrient (such as calcium, other vitamins and minerals, fiber), try to choose foods with a higher %DV. As a guide, foods with 5%DV or less contribute a small amount of that nutrient to your eating pattern, while those with 20% or more contribute a large amount. Remember, Nutrition Facts serving sizes may differ from those used in the Food Guide Pyramid (see Figure 1-6). For example, 2 ounces of dry macaroni yields about 1 cup cooked, or two (1/2 cup) Pyramid servings.

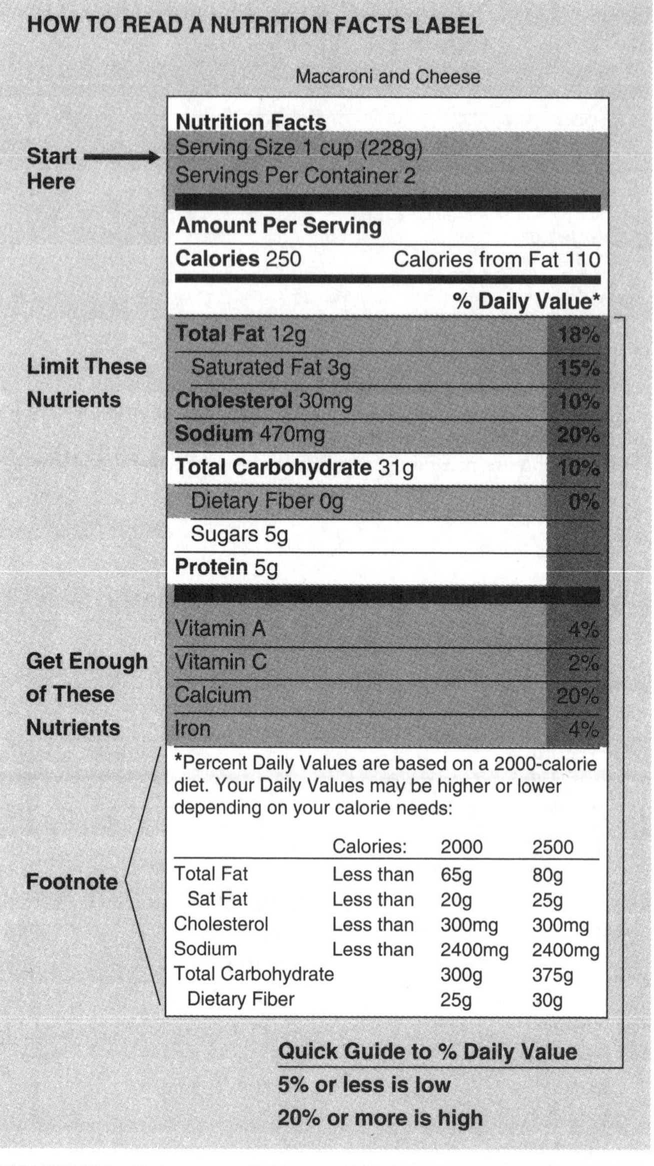

Figure 1-7 Nutrition and Your Health: Dietary Guidelines for Americans, 2000. Aim, Build, and Choose for Good Health. *(From USDA, USDHHS, Home and Garden Bulletin 232, 5th ed., 2000.)*

diet. Although the 2000-calorie diet is assumed to be appropriate for many women, teenage girls, and less active men and the 2500-calorie diet for many men, teenage boys, and very active women, the actual range of energy intakes is very wide and must be adjusted accordingly. For example the 65 g of fat listed for a 2000-calorie diet represents 30% of total kcal; however, a woman whose habitual intake is 1600 kilocalories who consumes 65 g of fat will be getting 36% of her energy from fat rather than the 30% or 53 g considered desirable.

Ingredient Labeling

Current labeling regulations require complete ingredient labeling on all processed, packaged foods, including standardized foods such as may-

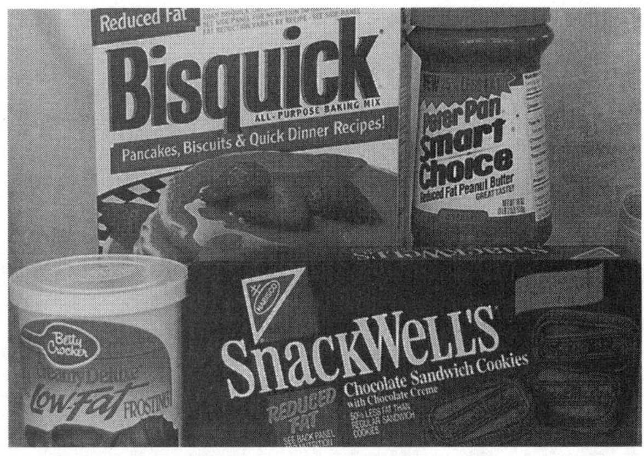

Figure 1-8 Examples of nutrient claims on food labels.

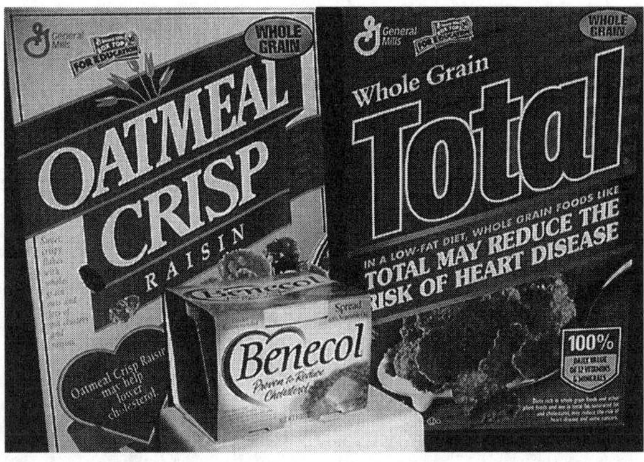

Figure 1-9 Examples of health claims on food labels.

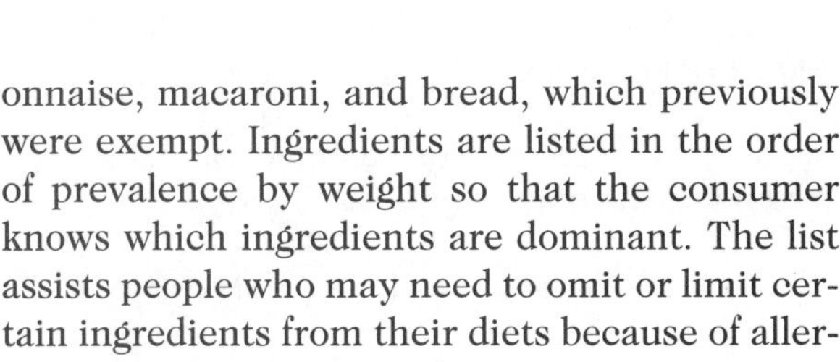

onnaise, macaroni, and bread, which previously were exempt. Ingredients are listed in the order of prevalence by weight so that the consumer knows which ingredients are dominant. The list assists people who may need to omit or limit certain ingredients from their diets because of allergies or intolerances.

Nutrient Content Claims

Certain terms defined by the FDA and the USDA can be used on the label to describe a food's nutrient content. Any term used to describe the nutrient content of a food means the same thing on every product on which it appears. Samples of such nutrient content claims are illustrated in Figure 1-8. The terms that can be used are *free, low, fewer, light* (or *lite*), *reduced, less, more,* and *high. Lean* and *extra lean* also have been defined and apply specifically to the fat content of meat, poultry, and fish. The definitions of these terms in regard to sugar, calories, fat, cholesterol, sodium, and fiber content appear in Box 1-3.

Health Claims

Under certain circumstances health claims linking a nutrient or a food to the risk of a disease or health-related condition are allowed on Food and Drug Administration (FDA)-regulated products. The FDA has strict requirements about when and how these claims can be used. Health claims may use only the terms *may* or *might* in discussing the relationship of a food to a disease, may not state the degree of risk, may state that other foods play a role in that disease, and must phrase the claim so that the consumer can understand the nutrient and the disease and the nutrient's importance in a daily diet. Currently the FDA allows statements about the relationships between a specific food or nutrient and the 12 health claims listed in Table 1-9. Samples of such health claims are shown in Figure 1-9.

Dietary Supplements

The Dietary Supplement Health and Education Act (DSHEA) of 1994 broadened the traditional definition of dietary supplements from essential dietary nutrients (such as vitamins or minerals) while distinguishing them from drugs or food additives. Dietary supplements are defined in the DSHEA as a product (other than tobacco) intended to supplement the diet that bears or contains one or more of the following ingredients: vitamin, mineral, an herb or other botanical, an amino acid, a supplement used by individuals to supplement the diet by increasing the total dietary intake, or a concentrate, metabolite, constituent, extract, or combination of any ingredient just described (Kurtzwell, 1998; Nesheim, 1998).

The DSHEA defines a dietary supplement as a product that is labeled as a dietary supplement and is not represented for use as a conventional food or as a sole item of a meal or the diet. These

Box 1-3 Approved Terms for Specific Nutrient Content Claims

NUTRIENT CONTENT CLAIMS

The regulations also spell out what terms may be used to describe the level of a nutrient in a food and how they can be used. These are the core terms:

- **Free.** This term means that a product contains no amount of, or only trivial or "physiologically inconsequential" amounts of, one or more of these components: fat, saturated fat, cholesterol, sodium, sugars, and calories. For example, "calorie-free" means fewer than 5 calories per serving, and "sugar-free" and "fat-free" both mean less than 0.5 g per serving. Synonyms for "free" include "without," "no" and "zero." A synonym for fat-free milk is "skim."
- **Low.** This term can be used on foods that can be eaten frequently without exceeding dietary guidelines for one or more of these components: fat, saturated fat, cholesterol, sodium, and calories. Thus, descriptors are defined as follows:
    - **low-fat:** 3 g or less per serving
    - **low-saturated fat:** 1 g or less per serving
    - **low-sodium:** 140 mg or less per serving
    - **very low sodium:** 35 mg or less per serving
    - **low-cholesterol:** 20 mg or less and 2 g or less of saturated fat per serving
    - **low-calorie:** 40 calories or less per serving.

  Synonyms for low include "little," "few," "low source of," and "contains a small amount of."
- **Lean and extra lean.** These terms can be used to describe the fat content of meat, poultry, seafood, and game meats.
    - **lean:** less than 10 g fat, 4.5 g or less saturated fat, and less than 95 mg cholesterol per serving and per 100 g.
    - **extra lean:** less than 5 g fat, less than 2 g saturated fat, and less than 95 mg cholesterol per serving and per 100 g.
- **High.** This term can be used if the food contains 20 percent or more of the Daily Value for a particular nutrient in a serving.
- **Good source.** This term means that one serving of a food contains 10 to 19 percent of the Daily Value for a particular nutrient.

From Food and Drug Administration, Rockville, Md, 2001.

products can be ingested as a capsule, powder, gelcap, tablet, liquid, or other form.

Under the Act, labels on supplements are permitted to carry statements that describe how the intended nutrient or dietary supplement may affect physiologic structure or function in human beings, such as "vitamin D is required for proper bone development," but the label must also carry the declaration, "this statement has not been evaluated by the FDA. This product is not intended to diagnose, treat, cure, or prevent any disease" (DSHEA, 1994).

According to the FDA, health claims such as the claim that a supplement reduces the risk of a specific disease must meet the standard of "significant scientific agreement" and are subject to FDA oversight. Companies have 30 days after they begin marketing a dietary supplement to file their health claims and substantiating evidence with the FDA.

Provisions to protect public health allow the FDA to prove a product is unsafe for human consumption by evaluating whether the product poses a "significant or unreasonable risk." The FDA can prohibit marketing of a product if it is deemed unsafe or if it has been adulterated. Supplement manufacturers are required to notify the FDA at least 75 days before marketing a non-food product for which history of use or evidence of safety does not exist. Manufacturers must establish that the dietary ingredients or products are reasonably safe when used under the conditions recommended or suggested on the product label.

Box1-3 Approved Terms for Specific Nutrient Content Claims—cont'd

- **Reduced.** This term means that a nutritionally altered product contains at least 25 percent less of a nutrient or of calories than the regular, or reference, product. However, a reduced claim can't be made on a product if its reference food already meets the requirement for a "low" claim.
- **Less.** This term means that a food, whether altered or not, contains 25 percent less of a nutrient or of calories than the reference food. For example, pretzels that have 25 percent less fat than potato chips could carry a "less" claim. "Fewer" is an acceptable synonym.
- **Light.** This descriptor can mean two things:
    - First, that a nutritionally altered product contains one-third fewer calories or half the fat of the reference food. If the food derives 50 percent or more of its calories from fat, the reduction must be 50 percent of the fat.
    - Second, that the sodium content of a low-calorie, low-fat food has been reduced by 50 percent. In addition, "light in sodium" may be used on food in which the sodium content has been reduced by at least 50 percent.

  The term "light" still can be used to describe such properties as texture and color, as long as the label explains the intent—for example, "light brown sugar" and "light and fluffy."
- **More.** This term means that a serving of food, whether altered or not, contains a nutrient that is at least 10 percent of the Daily Value more than the reference food. The 10 percent of Daily Value also applies to "fortified," "enriched," "added," and "extra and plus" claims, but in those cases, the food must be altered.

Alternative spelling of these descriptive terms and their synonyms is allowed—for example, "hi" and "lo"—as long as the alternatives are not misleading.

Healthy. A "healthy" food must be low in fat and saturated fat and contain limited amounts of cholesterol and sodium. In addition, if it's a single-item food, it must provide at least 10 percent of one or more of vitamins A or C, iron, calcium, protein, or fiber. Exempt from this "10-percent" rule are certain raw, canned, and frozen fruits and vegetables and certain cereal-grain products. These foods can be labeled "healthy" if they do not contain ingredients that change the nutritional profile, and, in the case of enriched grain products, conform to standards of identity, which call for certain required ingredients. If it's a meal-type product, such as frozen entrees and multicourse frozen dinners, it must provide 10 percent of two or three of these vitamins or minerals or of protein or fiber, in addition to meeting the other criteria. The sodium content cannot exceed 360 mg per serving for individual foods and 480 mg per serving for meal-type products.

Claims on Dietary Supplements

The FDA has published rules that define the types of statements that can be made concerning the effect of a dietary supplement on the structure or function of the body according to the DSHEA. Under the DSHEA, dietary supplements may bear "structure/function" claims—claims that the products affect the structure or function of the body—without prior FDA review. They may not, without prior FDA review, bear a claim that they can prevent, treat, cure, mitigate, or diagnose disease (a disease claim). The final rule precludes express disease claims (such as "prevent osteoporosis") and implied disease claims ("prevents bone fragility in post-menopausal women") without prior FDA review. The rule permits claims that do not relate to disease. These include health maintenance claims ("maintains a healthy circulatory system"), other nondisease claims ("for muscle enhancement," "helps you relax"), and claims for common, minor symptoms associated with life stages ("for common symptoms of PMS").

Under the DSHEA and existing regulations, dietary supplement manufacturers are already required to have, in their files, substantiation of any structure or function claims they make. They must also include a disclaimer on their labels that dietary supplements are not drugs and receive no FDA premarket approval. Finally they must notify FDA of the claims they are making within 30 days of marketing a dietary supplement.

Table 1-9 Approved Health Claims for Use on Food Labels

Nutrient/Food and Related Disease or Condition	Food Requirements	Model of Statement on Label
Calcium and osteoporosis	High in calcium; assimilable (bioavailable). Supplements must disintegrate and dissolve; phosphorus content cannot exceed calcium content.	Regular exercise and a healthy diet with enough calcium helps teens and young adult white and Asian women maintain good bone health and may reduce their high risk of osteoporosis later in life.
Sodium and hypertension	Low sodium.	Diets low in sodium may reduce the risk of high blood pressure, a disease associated with many factors.
Dietary fat and cancer	Low fat; fish and game meats must be *extra lean.*	Development of cancer depends on many factors. A diet low in total fat may reduce the risk of some cancers.
Dietary saturated fat and cholesterol/ coronary heart disease	Low saturated fat, low cholesterol, low fat. Fish and game meats must be *extra lean.*	While many factors affect heart disease, diets low in saturated fat and cholesterol may reduce the risk of this disease.
Fiber-containing grain products, fruits, and vegetables and cancer	Dietary fiber, low fat, good source of dietary fiber (without fortification).	Low-fat diets rich in fiber-containing grain products, fruits, and vegetables may reduce the risk of some types of cancer, a disease associated with many factors.
Fruits, vegetables, and grain products that contain fiber, particularly soluble fiber, and heart disease	Low saturated fat, low cholesterol, low fat. At least 0.6 g of soluble fiber per reference amount (without fortification).	Diets low in saturated fat and cholesterol and rich in fruits, vegetables, and grain products that contain some types of dietary fiber may reduce the risk of heart disease, a disease associated with many factors.
Fruits and vegetables and cancer	Low fat, good source (without fortification) of at least one of the following: vitamin A, vitamin C, or dietary fiber.	Low-fat diets rich in fruits and vegetables (foods that are low in fat and contain dietary fiber, vitamin A, or vitamin C) may reduce the risk of some types of cancer, a disease associated with many factors. Broccoli is high in vitamins A and C and is a good source of dietary fiber.

From U.S. Food and Drug Administration, Rockville, Md, 2001.

NUTRITION ACROSS THE LIFE SPAN

- *How do differentiation, growth, development, maturation, and aging progress across the life span?*
- *What are the nutrition-related characteristics of these stages?*

The continuum of life encompasses growth, development, maturation, and aging. With the exception of the brain and the nervous system, the cells of the body constantly form, function, age, and die only to be replaced by new cells. Throughout life, the body as a whole and its individual systems, organs, tissues, and cells grow, develop, function, and decline in this pattern. Across this sequence of life span events there are changes in body size, proportion, and composition.

In the first two decades of life, cell formation, **differentiation**, growth, and **development** predominate. Growth of an individual is a composite of the growth of many tissues and organs at

Table 1-9 Approved Health Claims for Use on Food Labels—cont'd

Nutrient/Food and Related Disease or Condition	Food Requirements	Model of Statement on Label
Folate and neural tube defects	Enriched cereal grains, some legumes, peas, leafy green vegetables.	Women who consume adequate amounts of folate throughout their childbearing years may reduce their risk of having a child with neural tube defects. Such birth defects, although uncommon, are serious. Fruits, dark green leafy vegetables, legumes, enriched grain products, fortified cereals, and supplements are good folate sources. Mothers of children with spinal cord birth defect should consult a physician before becoming pregnant again. Folate intake should be limited to 1000 μg/day.
Dietary sugar alcohol and dental caries	Sugarless candy and gum.	Frequent between-meal consumption of foods high in sugar and starches promotes tooth decay. The sugar alcohols do not promote tooth decay.
Dietary soluble fiber, such as that found in whole wheat and psyllium seed husk, and coronary heart disease	Oatmeal cookies, muffins, breads, and other foods made with rolled oats, oat bran, or whole oat flour; hot and cold breakfast cereals.	Diets low in saturated fat and cholesterol that include 3 g of soluble fiber from whole oats may reduce risk of heart disease.
Soy protein and coronary heart disease	Foods containing soy protein low in saturated fat and cholesterol.	Diets low in saturated fat and cholesterol that include 25 g of soy protein a day may reduce risk of heart disease. One serving of ___ provides ___ g of soy protein.
Plant sterol and plant stanol esters and coronary heart disease	Spreads and salad dressings, snack bars and dietary supplements in softgen form.	Foods containing at least 0.65 g/serving of sterol esters, eaten twice a day with meals for a daily total intake of at least 1.3 g as part of a diet low in saturated fat and cholesterol, may reduce the risk of heart disease. A serving of ___ supplies ___ g of sterol esters.

different rates. The early stages of the life span are characterized by rapid growth and development, which proceed in an orderly and predictable sequence. Growth is characterized by a period of **hyperplasia** and rapid cell differentiation. During this period, the tissue, organ, or individual is particularly susceptible to physical and environmental influences. For example an infant who has inadequate food intake during this critical period in brain growth may have fewer brain cells and compromised intellectual

KEY TERMS

differentiation: process of acquiring individual characteristics or functions; progressive diversification

development: the acquisition of function or progression to a more advanced stage of complexity for greater facility in function

hyperplasia: increase in the number of cells

development in the long run. As growth progresses hyperplasia is accompanied by **hypertrophy** and eventually hypertrophy predominates. A normal healthy infant, child, or adolescent grows and develops at a genetically predetermined rate that can be compromised or accelerated by environmental factors including undernutrition, imbalanced nutrient intake, or overnutrition.

Growth and development gradually decline as the individual moves into early adulthood. Some growth, such as that of bone, extends well into the third decade. After growth ceases and maturation is complete, the process of cell turnover becomes static, with formation and breakdown in a general state of equilibrium. Gradually with age, there is a net decrease in some body tissues and organs, resulting in a decline in functional cells. Aging is the regression of physiologic function accompanied by advancement of age. Although aging is a problem of the whole body, each organ independently loses its function, and as a result, the body becomes **senescent.** Individuals age at varying rates. The process is governed by genetics, race, and sex, but is influenced by early life events, social and behavioral factors, activity, substance use habits, and the accompanying pathologic conditions.

Although all humans have essentially the same nutritional needs, the concentration and balance may differ at various points in the life span. The stages of the life span and their nutrition-related characteristics are illustrated in Table 1-10. The rapid growth and development of the embryo and fetus depend on the maternal diet and reserves. Because of rapid growth and cell differentiation, embryos and fetuses are vulnerable to undernutrition and toxic substances such as alcohol and drugs.

The neonatal period (the first 30 days after birth) is a time of critical adjustments to the extrauterine environment. Energy and nutrient needs are high to maintain basal metabolism and support growth. Compared with *in-utero* growth, the changes of infancy are slow, but they are still demanding because body weight typically increases threefold in the first year of life. This is a period of high nutritional demand during which energy and nutrient requirements per unit of body weight are two to three times those of adults.

In terms of nutritional needs, infants and children are not simply small adults. Every stage of growth is thought to be influenced by nutrition. Although progress in growth is most often measured as physical growth (gains in stature and weight of individual infants, children, or adolescents), such measurements do not reflect changes in all of the components of growth. Although growth of skeletal muscle approximates that of the whole body, growth of many other tissues, such as reproductive organs, brain, and adipose tissue, follows very different patterns. After infancy a relatively slower but steady rate of growth and development prevails through childhood. The amounts of nutrients children require to sustain normal growth and development often exceed those required by adults. For example children need 50% more total calcium than adults do to promote adequate bone formation.

Adolescence is a period of very rapid growth. The total nutritional requirements of adolescents are greater than those of adults except during pregnancy and lactation, yet meeting nutritional needs of adolescents is complicated. Changes in physiologic, psychologic, and social development may compromise food habits. As a result this group is particularly vulnerable to poor nutrient intake and disordered eating.

Nutritional needs tend to stabilize in early adulthood. It is difficult to define stages of adulthood. It begins in the early twenties, but the transition to middle and old age has relatively few markers, and there is wide variability between individuals. Middle age traditionally was said to begin around age 40, but the generation of baby boomers who are now approaching 50 have stretched that definition. Similarly the definition of an older adult is arbitrary. The heterogeneous nature of the elderly population makes it difficult to define "old age" as a chronological milepost. In fact with increased longevity and population trends, the elderly are an ever-greater segment of the American population.

Across the period of adulthood, decreases in energy expenditure with no corresponding decrease in dietary intake contribute to acceler-

Table 1-10 PERIODS OF THE LIFE SPAN

Period	Approximate Ages or Time	Nutrition-Related Characteristics
Embryonic	8 weeks after conception	Rapid cell differentiation; development of specific tissues, organs, and systems
Fetal	Last 7 months of in-utero growth	Rapid growth; elaboration of tissues, organs; early functional activities of body systems
Neonatal	First month of postnatal life	Adjustments to postnatal environment; initiation of respiration; maintenance of body temperature and other functions; initial oral feeding
Infancy	Neonatal to 1 year	Rapid growth and development; maturation of functions
Late infancy	1-2 years	Decelerating growth rate; increased development, especially of motor skills; increased independence, including in eating
Childhood		
Preschool	2-6 years	Slow, steady growth; increased physical activity and coordination of motor functions; rapid cognitive development
School	Girls: 6-10 years Boys: 6-12 years	Steady growth; continued physical and cognitive development; increasing responsibility for own food habits
Adolescent		
Prepubertal	Girls: 10-12 years Boys: 12-14 years	Accelerated growth rate; rapid gains in weight and height; changes in hormone levels, reproductive organs
Pubertal	Girls: 12-14 years Boys: 14-16 years	Development of secondary sex characteristics; changes in body composition; increased need for independence
Postpubertal	Girls: 14-20 years Boys: 16-20 years	Maximum gains in height, continuing increases in bone mass; cognitive development; increased independence
Early adult	20-45 years	Growth and skeletal development completed; gradual decrease in energy expenditure
Middle age	45-65 years	Tendency to increased body weight; decreased physical activity; energy needs stabilize
Older adult	65+ years	Decreased physical activity and mobility over time; increased chronic disease, often multiple; increased use of medication

ated weight gain. During this time clinical signs of the slow, insidious processes of chronic disease begin to appear. For many adults these disorders may require substantial changes in diet or lifestyle. For some individuals the associated medical care and medication may diminish resources needed to obtain an adequate diet. Nutritional status may also be compromised by interactions between medications and diet.

TEXT OVERVIEW

This text explores each stage across the life span in the context of physiologic, social, psychologic, and cognitive development, which influence nutrition needs and food-related behaviors and practices. Unique characteristics and nutrition-related concerns are emphasized. This chapter addresses some of the basic information and skills needed to apply nutrition principles. The next two chapters discuss techniques for measuring and evaluating nutrition status and plan-

KEY TERMS

hypertrophy: enlargement from an increase in cell size

senescent: exhibiting signs of the process of growing old

ning and facilitating for changes in food-related behavior and improvement of nutrition status.

Chapters 4 through 6 address the special needs and concerns of the reproductive period, periconception, pregnancy, postpartum and lactation, and breast-feeding. Chapters 7 and 8 explore infancy and the special role of nutrition for the high-risk infant. Chapter 9 follows the chronological progression to puberty. Chapter 10 will address the significance of diet and nutrition of children with developmental delays and disabilities. Adolescence will be covered in Chapter 11. In each chapter interrelationships among physiologic, biochemic, and sociologic factors and their impact on nutrient recommendations and food behaviors are explored. Maintenance of nutrition status and promotion of health through maturity and aging are stressed in Chapters 12 and 13. Areas of nutrition that are common to many stages of the life span—eating dilemmas and physical activity and fitness—are discussed in the two final chapters. The student may wish to refer to segments of these chapters to enhance use of other parts of the book. Concerns such as dental health, smoking, and alcohol and other substance use are incorporated in individual chapters or sections. The Application sections following each chapter emphasize application of principles or expand on nutrition care, and illustrate how nutrition influences each stage of the life span.

Concepts to Remember

- Requirements for energy and nutrients are complex and vary over the life span.
- Food consumption patterns may be factors in developmental abnormalities and progression of some chronic diseases.
- Dietary standards (DRIs) define nutritional needs and serve as a basis for development of food guides, nutrition standards, food products and services, menu plans, nutritional counseling, and educational materials.
- *Healthy People 2010* identifies areas of health concerns and specifies of priority areas and public health objectives or targets to be met by the year 2010. Success in meeting the nutrition objectives is tracked by a National Nutrition Monitoring program that includes the NHANES and the Continuing Survey of Food Intake of Individuals.
- Food guides for promoting nutritional adequacy and long-term health include the Dietary Guidelines for Americans and the FGP.
- Current nutrition labeling regulations mandate a label format that provides consumers with a tool for selecting a healthy diet.
- Certain terms are defined by the FDA to describe a food's nutrient content.
- Under certain circumstances claims linking a food to the risk of disease or health-related conditions are allowed.
- The DSHEA of 1994 defines a dietary supplement, outlines specific statements that may appear on product labels, and shows the presentation of claims.
- All people have the same nutritional needs, but specific amounts vary at different stages of the life span.
- Across the life span, physiologic, psychologic, cognitive, and social development influence nutrition needs and food-related behaviors.

REFERENCES

American Heart Association: Scientific advisory on monounsaturated fatty acids and risk of coronary heart disease, Circulation 100:1253, 1999.

Bloomberg News Service: February 15, 2001. Radio report.

Brown AA and Hu FB: Dietary modulation of endothelial function: implications for cardiovascular disease, Am J Clin Nutr 73:673, 2001.

Chandalia M et al.: Beneficial effects of high dietary fiber intake in patients with type 2 diabetes mellitus, N Engl J Med 342:1392, 2000.

Connor W: Importance of n-3 fatty acids in health and disease, Am J Clin Nutr 71:171S, 2000.

Dietary Guidelines Advisory Committee: Report of the Dietary Guidelines Advisory Committee on the dietary guidelines for Americans, 2000. http//www.ars.usda.usda.gov.80/dgac/dgacguidexp.htm

Dietary Supplement Health and Education Act of 1994, Washington, DC, 1994, U.S. Food and Drug Administration.

Dixon LB and Ernst ND: Choose a diet that is low in saturated fat and cholesterol and moderate in total fat: subtle changes in a familiar message, J Nutr 131: 510S, 2001.

Food and Nutrition Board: How should the recommended dietary allowances be revised? Washington, DC, 1994, National Academy Press.

Food and Nutrition Board: Dietary reference intakes: a risk assessment model for establishing upper intake levels for nutrients, Washington, DC, 1998, National Academy Press.

GISSI Investigators: Dietary supplementation with omega-3-polyunsaturated fatty acids and vitamin E after myocardial infarction: results of the GISSI Prevention Trial, Lancet 354:447, 1999.

Guthrie JF and Morton JF: Food sources of added sweeteners in the diets of Americans, J Am Diet Assoc 100: 43-48,51, 2000.

Hausmann D: Angiographically silent atherosclerosis detected by intravascular ultrasound in patients with familial hypercholesterolemia and familial combined hyperlipidemia: correlation with high density lipoprotein, J Am Coll Cardiol 27:1562, 1996.

Healthy People 2010: www.healthypeople.gov, 2001.

Institute of Medicine: Dietary reference intakes for calcium, phosphorus, magnesium, vitamin D and fluoride, Washington, DC, 1997, National Academy Press.

Institute of Medicine: Dietary reference intakes for thiamin, riboflavin, niacin, vitamin B_6, folate, vitamin B_{12}, pantothenic acid, biotin and choline, Washington, DC, 1998, National Academy Press.

Institute of Medicine: Dietary reference intakes: applications in dietary assessment. A report of the Subcommittees on Interpretation and Uses of Dietary Reference Intakes and Upper Reference Levels of Nutrients and the Standing Committee on the Scientific Evaluation of Dietary Reference Intakes, Food and Nutrition Board, Washington, DC, 2000a, National Academy Press.

Institute of Medicine: Dietary reference intakes for vitamin C, vitamin E, selenium, and carotenoids, Washington, DC, 2000b, National Academy Press.

Institute of Medicine: Dietary reference intakes for vitamin A, vitamin K, arsenic, boron, chromium, copper, iodine, iron, manganese, molybdenum, nickel, silicon, vanadium and zinc, Washington, DC, 2001a, National Academy Press.

Institute of Medicine: Proposed definition of dietary fiber, Washington, DC, 2001b, National Academy of Sciences.

Judd JT et al.: Dietary trans fatty acids: effects on plasma lipids and lipoproteins of healthy men and women, Am J Clin Nutr 59:86, 1994.

Kaplan NM: The dietary guideline for sodium: should we shake it up? No! Am J Clin Nutr 71:1020, 2000.

Kennedy E and Davis CA: Dietary guidelines: the opportunity and challenges for reaching the consumer, J Am Diet Assoc 100:1462, 2000.

Klag MJ et al.: Serum cholesterol in young men and subsequent cardiovascular disease, N Engl J Med 328: 313, 1993.

Knopp RH et al.: Long-term blood cholesterol-lowering effects of dietary fiber supplement, Am J Prev Med 17:18, 1999.

Kurtzwell P: New FDA labeling rules for dietary supplements, FDA Consumer 32:2, 1998.

McCarron DA: The dietary guideline for sodium: should we shake it up? Yes! Am J Clin Nutr 71:1013, 2000.

Mertz W: Three decades of dietary recommendations, Nutr Rev 58:324, 2000.

Moritsugu KP: A report from the Office of the Surgeon General, J Am Diet Assoc 100:1013, 2000.

National Center for Health Statistics: Report of final mortality statistics, 1995. Monthly Vital Statistics Report 45(11): Suppl 2, 1997.

National Center for Health Statistics: Monthly Vital Statistics Report 48, 2000.

National Center for Health Statistics: Data 2010: the Healthy People 2010 database. http://www.cdc.gov/nchs/about/otheractupdate.2010/about.hp.htm, 1999.

National Research Council: Recommended dietary allowances, ed 10, Washington, DC, 1989, National Academy Press.

Nesheim MC: Regulation of dietary supplements, Nutrition Today 33:62, 1998.

Simopoulos AP and Salem LA: Essentiality of and recommended dietary intakes for omega-6 and omega-3 fatty acids in health and disease, Ann Nutr Metab 43: 127, 1999.

U.S. Department of Agriculture: Food guide pyramid, Washington, DC, 2000, U.S. Government Printing Office.

U.S. Departments of Agriculture and Health and Human Services: Nutrition and your health: dietary guidelines for Americans, ed 5, Home and Garden Bulletin No 232, Washington, DC, 2000, U.S. Government Printing Office.

INTERNET-BASED RESOURCES

Dietary Supplements: http://www.fda.gov

Health Claims: http://www.vm.cfsan.fda.gov~dms/fdcln.htnl

Healthy People in Communities: http://www.health.gov/healthypeople

Dietary Guidelines: http//www.ars.usda.usda.gov.80/dgac/dgacguidexp.htm

APPLICATION

Assessing and Interpreting Nutrition Research

Eating mayonnaise can protect women from strokes!
High-fiber diets don't prevent colon cancer!
Fruits and vegetables can prevent cancer!
Your grandmother can save her short-term memory with vitamin E!

Whether they're true or false, such headlines, lead-ins, or teasers for reports about nutrition research reach the public almost daily. They arrive through print, radio, television, and the Internet, all of which have a powerful role in disseminating information with implications for dietary intake and use of a variety of supplements.

A brief report of the newest published study is likely to be aired on the morning news, often before the journal containing the research article is in the hands of subscribers. (Editors of some professional and scientific journals publicize new findings through prepublication press releases to the media.) A follow-up of the news report might be a feature on the evening news or a more in-depth health report. Expanded coverage of the potential implications of the study for health and diet may be the topic for interviews or talk shows. In a few days there is another study to report and yesterday's news topic is shelved awaiting new information, which may confirm or refute its results.

In today's world the results of nutrition research studies are also important fodder for newspapers and the more than 10,000 periodicals that must have "new" or "fresh" and relevant information each day, week, or month of publication. News stories summarizing the latest published study appear as soon as possible after release. Within days there may be in-depth coverage in the feature section of a newspaper. Over the next few weeks **fillers,** prepared by news services, may appear in various sections of the newspaper. Periodicals often build feature articles or in-depth stories around nutrition research reports. These reports may include suggestions for improving health, such as specific food dietary programs and exercise regimens, menu and recipe ideas, and tips to implement change.

> **fillers:** news pieces of consumer interest that newspapers or news services prepare to be used as needed to fill empty spaces in page makeup

In addition thousands of websites provide a plethora of health and nutrition information. Some sites, particularly those maintained by professional organizations, universities, major medical centers, and government agencies (see the list of websites at the end of this Application), provide reliable and useful information. Numerous websites provide nutrition information offering a broad spectrum of products or services. It is important to recognize that much information gets published on the Internet without the vigorous scrutiny of **peer review** that journal articles receive (Kipp, 1996). In fact one of the nutrition-related priorities of *Healthy People 2010* focuses on the need to address the quality of information on websites (*Healthy People 2010,* 2001).

> **peer review:** a process in which a study's research design and results are reviewed by experienced researchers knowledgeable in the area of the research

> ***HEALTHY PEOPLE 2010* PRIORITY**
> Increase the proportion of health-related sites on the Internet that disclose information that can be used to assess the quality of the site.

Never have consumers had greater access to nutrition information. The benefit of broad dissemination of the results of nutrition research studies is heightened awareness of how diet influences health and the progression of disease. Consumers have an almost insatiable appetite for nutrition news. They get most of their nutrition information from media reports, but the proportion using the Internet is increasing significantly (American Dietetic Association, 2000). In fact Americans give more attention to news stories related to health and nutrition than to local events, sports, or business news (Center for Media and Public Affairs, 2000).

Most publications provide accurate and useful information. For individuals with a background in and concern about nutrition, media reports of research studies may be helpful or may be intriguing enough to prompt them to seek additional information. There is great variation in how complete the information is, how the research should be interpreted, and if, or how, the applications are presented. This variation may result in incomplete messages or mixed signals that confuse the public. Individuals who participated in the Center for Media and Public Affairs (2000) survey reported that they found stories about vitamin and mineral supplements and nutrition more confusing than stories about cancer, heart disease, and depression.

There may be even greater confusion associated with use of dietary supplements (as defined by the Dietary Supplement Health and Education Act [DSHEA] of 1994, see page 27). Currently these substances and products receive extensive media attention and coverage on their purported health-promoting or therapeutic qualities. However, there is only a limited amount of peer-reviewed research to support or negate the validity or reliability of such claims (Radimer et al., 2000).

Accurate and complete reporting of nutrition research is complicated by the fact that media staff typically have a limited understanding of nutrition research and short timelines. Pressure to write catchy headlines and sensational stories may twist inconclusive findings into meaningful discoveries. Sometimes scientific findings are presented prematurely without adequate interpretation or review. Providing nutrition information quickly is popular, but hurried reporting often fails to give the public an overall perspective of how the nutrition information fits with current nutrition knowledge and recommendations.

A study of the quantity and quality of the content of reports related to diet, nutrition, and food safety sponsored by the American Dietetic Association and International Food Information Council (1994) found that most stories tended to be general, lacking information about amounts of food or nutrient involved or data about causal relationships or statistical significance. Even interested consumers were handicapped when trying to judge the significance of the findings for themselves. Those in health professions and in the scientific community have begun to examine their roles and responsibilities related to the way that nutrition science is presented to the public (Wellman, 1999).

Print and electronic media coverage typically includes advertisements promoting foods, products, and services. These ads might promote or refute nutrition-health messages conveyed in the news. The manufacturers of mayonnaise products may be delighted to cite a study that suggests their product may protect the consumer from stroke. Manufacturers of food products are increasingly using research studies to promote their products through many advertising modes.

CHARACTERISTICS OF NUTRITION RESEARCH

The process of conducting and reporting research is universal. The researcher formulates a research question from which a **hypothesis** is generated. Study design and specific methods of

> **hypothesis:** a scientific prediction of what will happen; an educated guess

> **COMPONENTS OF THE RESEARCH ARTICLE**
>
> Introduction—statement of background and purpose
> Review of relevant literature
> Description of the study design and methods
> - What is the overall plan?
> - What techniques or procedures were used to collect data?
> - What safeguards were use to make sure that the data collected were valid and reliable?
>
> Results
> - Describe what was learned.
>
> Discussion, summary, conclusions
> - How do the results of the study relate to other research?
> - What are the implications or applications for that research?
>
> References cited

data collection are chosen to test the hypothesis. Data are collected in a systematic fashion and analyzed using appropriate statistical procedures. Data collection may take weeks, months, or even years. Upon completion of the project the researcher prepares and submits a manuscript of the research article to a scientific or professional journal. (Professional and scientific journals have an editorial staff and a large group of experienced researchers who review manuscripts and make recommendations.)

The article or research paper undergoes rigorous peer review. The manuscript may be returned to the authors for revision based on questions or comments from the reviewers. The following sections address some of the factors to be considered in interpreting reports of nutrition research.

Research Studies Are Seldom Equal

Research is undertaken to answer a specific question. However, most research issues are complex and a single research study is seldom definitive. Suppose the research question asks whether a diet high in dark green vegetables and dark yellow and orange fruits and vegetables reduce the risk of epithelial cell cancer. One researcher might conduct an epidemiologic, **retrospective study** of a large **nationally representative sample** from a population group. The researcher might find that, as a group, individuals who consumed ample amounts of fruits and vegetables had significantly lower rates of epithelial cancer than did those who consumed few fruits and vegetables. Such an observation may be a clue that dietary intake might be related to the incidence of cancer.

retrospective study: a study that collects information about something that has already occurred

nationally representative sample: selection of study subjects whose demographic characteristics reflect those of the American population

Another researcher might then conduct a **prospective study** of individuals who work in a specific industry where chemical exposure is known to increase the risk of epithelial cell cancer. At the beginning, or baseline, the individuals' fruit and vegetable consumption is determined and annual assessments are then conducted during a 5-year study. At the end of the study the progression of an existing cancer or development of new cases of cancer within the study group is determined. If there are no differences between the two groups in the number of cancers reported, the researcher may have to rethink the hypothesis and methodology of the study. If, conversely, the individuals who had low intakes of fruits and vegetables at baseline had a significantly higher occurrence of epithelial cell cancer, the study would support the research hypothesis.

prospective study: an ongoing study in which the data are collected at regular intervals

Meanwhile a third researcher in a laboratory may have isolated compounds from fruits and vegetables that appear to have protective effects related to cancer. This researcher's experimental design involves feeding high levels of the protective factor to mice who have epithelial cell cancer and feeding a similar compound that is actually a **placebo** to another group (the control group). If at the end of the study twice as many mice in the control group have died from cancer as compared with mice in the experimental group, the researcher might believe that the protective factors may be effective in reducing the mortality rate related to cancer.

placebo: a treatment that is an imitation (but without the protective factors, in this case) of that given as the treatment group

If the data accumulated from many animal and human studies begin to define a relationship between fruit and vegetable consumption and epithelial cancer, a **clinical trial** might be undertaken. There are numerous designs for clinical trials, but the overall concept is to compare clinical outcomes of individuals receiving a placebo with individuals receiving the **intervention** (treatment) compound believed to have protective effects. In most instances such a study would involve **random assignment** that is **blind** to the study subjects. The best research design for clinical trials uses random **double blind,** meaning that study subjects are randomly assigned to receive either the treatment or the placebo in such a way that the investigators do not know who is receiving which treatment.

clinical trial: a study in which the effectiveness of an intervention is studied with human subjects, using a control group and an experimental group

intervention: a treatment given to improve health or well-being

random assignment: a technique that ensures that each study subject has an equal chance of being selected for the intervention group or control group

blind: a setup in which the subjects are assigned to a group so they do not know if they are receiving a treatment or a placebo

double blind: random blinded assignments of subjects such that the investigators who judge outcomes do not know who is assigned to which group until the end of the study

Nutrition and Diet Recommendations Change over Time

Frequently a research study will answer only part of the question. To have broad application to dietary practices, even the most successful or landmark report requires the validation of additional studies. As understanding of nutrition and its relationship to health evolves, advice regarding food intake will also evolve. For nutrition researchers, practitioners, and policymakers, this is a reasonable and inevitable consequence of progress in nutrition research. The lay public, on the other hand, tends to view alterations in dietary recommendations as an indication of indecision on the part of the scientific community, which may become yet another source of confusion about what to eat to follow a healthful diet.

The Nutrition-Health Message Is Complex

Some dietary recommendations are relatively easy to understand and implement. For example Americans have been encouraged to limit their fat intake to no more than 30% of total calories. This recommendation has been incorporated into the Dietary Guidelines for Americans and many other health messages to the public. Its effectiveness is reflected in the decline in fat consumption in the United States over the last two decades.

On the other hand Americans are also being advised that the amount of dietary fat should be distributed in descending order of polyunsaturated fatty acids (at least 10%), monounsaturated fatty acids (at least 10%), and saturated fatty acids (less than 7%). Many individuals find this concept too complicated to implement. The message has become even more complicated in recent years, with research reports indicating that consumption of **omega-3 fatty acids** may reduce the risk of cardiovascular disease and that margarines and solid fats, produced by **hydrogenation** of vegetable oils, may be more atherogenic because of the formation of trans fatty acids. In frustration some consumers have decided to go back to eating butter.

omega-3 fatty acids: acids that are found in fish and marine oils, canola oil, and flax seed oils

hydrogenation: a process that converts vegetable oil to fats with higher melting points and greater stability (longer shelf life); it creates partially saturated fat by breaking the double bonds of polyunsaturated fatty acids. There is also rapid breaking and reforming of double bonds in monounsaturated fatty acids. The initial double bond is *cis,* and the new bond formed in this process is *trans,* which has a different relationship to the carbon chain.

H C=C H
R R
cis

H C=C R
R H
trans

Nutrition Research Is Subject to Interpretation

Participants in the promotion of nutrition information include government agencies; health professionals; advocacy groups; and producers of food, diet, and health products. Interpretation of nutrition research and its implications for diet and health may be influenced by the goals, agenda, and bias of the groups who attempt to influence eating behavior.

As discussed in this chapter, in the twenty-first century, government agencies are key players in nutrition. Their roles include research; food safety; food labeling; nutrition monitoring; administration of food, nutrition, and health programs; and dissemination of reliable information. The Food Guide Pyramid and the Dietary Guidelines for Americans are prominent among the educational initiatives from federal agencies. They are updated as a preponderance of scientific evidence dictates changes. However, critics say that their diet and health message, although accurate and useful, is often so general that consumers may not readily understand how to act on them.

Health professionals, especially registered dietitians (RDs), provide nutrition information through advice, education, and counseling (see Chapter 3). In these roles they may help consumers interpret and use nutrition information. Health-related volunteer organizations, whose overall goals often parallel those of government agencies, also have recommendations that may differ, if only slightly, from government agencies. Often, however, such differences may be a source of confusion to the consumer.

Some of the most distracting information comes from the food industry. A food producer emphasizes the nutritional attributes of the products it markets to further the goal of selling its product. When products to be sold are contrary to recommended nutrition practices, other features are promoted, in apparent lack of concern for nutrition.

Special interest groups may distort the nutrition message for their own purposes. Their agendas or perspectives frequently are dominated by the desire to sell products or materials or to support their points of view. These groups are very good at using scientific facts to build a case (sometimes fictional) for their cause. They add to the confusion and may actually mislead the consumer. The average consumer cannot be expected to understand the agendas and bias of these diverse groups.

To assist individuals in interpreting nutrition research information, a coalition of food and nutrition professionals (Food and Nutrition Science Alliance) encourages consumers to question the accuracy of nutrition statements marked by any combination of the following characteristics:

- Recommendations that promise a quick fix
- Dire warnings of danger from a single product or regimen
- Claims that sound too good to be true
- Simplistic conclusions drawn from a complex study
- Recommendations based on a single study
- Dramatic statements that are refuted by reputable scientific organizations
- Lists of “good” and “bad” foods
- Recommendations made to help sell a product
- Recommendations based on studies published without peer review
- Recommendations from studies that ignore differences among individuals or groups

The Time Between a Report of a Research Study and Dietary Recommendations Can Be Long

The current need for researchers to publish results as quickly as possible is motivated by technology that operates on instant access to information and the need of researchers to publish and gain recognition to secure or maintain funding or, in university settings, achieve promotion and tenure. For the media the perceived need to present the findings of major articles from scientific literature the day they are released reflects the race to be first with the facts. The payoff is increased circulation and more viewers and listeners, which translate into enhanced revenues from advertisers.

However, the results of a single research study rarely provide sufficient evidence to serve as a basis for recommending dietary changes. Too often it is the provocative nature of the findings rather than their scientific significance that determines which study will be headline news. It will be months, and more likely years, until other investigators **replicate** the research and conduct clinical trials.

replicate: to repeat the research to demonstrate that the results can be reproduced

Nutrition Research May Be Specific, But Diets Are Not

Understanding and using nutrition research information is compounded by the relatively specific nature of relationships between nutrition and health and the complexity of diets. In most instances evidence for these relationships is associated with long-term consumption patterns. Identification of nutrients related to specific diseases logically leads to the development of recommendations that focus on prevention of that disease. However, people do not eat one diet to reduce the risk for cardiovascular disease and another to prevent cancer. They eat meals and snacks. The challenge is to incorporate changes that may reduce the risk of disease into a diet that is nutritionally adequate and fits the lifestyle of the individual.

Ample evidence that the public responds to nutrition and health information reported by electronic and print media pushes those media to emphasize or highlight the potential of even modest research reports. One study does not refute an entire body of evidence, but the accumulation of many, sometimes hundreds, of studies may provide the basis for recommendations regarding dietary change.

In the conflicting agendas of media interests, many groups promote only their view of nutrition information, and persuasive advertising compete with personal concerns and reliable information about nutrition and health. Consumers are confused by conflicting views on nutrition issues that appear in the popular media. Increasing recognition of the effect of nutrition on lifetime health and well-being has led community health agencies, government agencies, the food industry, and a variety of health professions to give more attention to promotion of reliable nutrition information and nutrition education. Nutrition education and counseling are emerging as important professional focuses for the future.

In summary, always consider the source of nutrition news. Ask two questions: Is the person purveying the information qualified to speak on nutrition? Is the information based on valid scientific research? If not, find a better source.

NUTRITION INFORMATION WEBSITES

American Dietetic Association: http://www.eatright.org
Dietetians of Canada: http://www.dietitians.ca
Food and Drug Administration: http://www.vm.cfsan.fda.gov
National Council for Reliable Health Information: http://www.ncrhi.org
Tufts University Nutrition Navigator: http://www.navigator.tufts.edu
USDA Food and Consumer Services: http://www.usda.gov/fcs.htm
U.S. government health information site: www.healthfinder.gov

REFERENCES

American Dietetic Association: Position of the American Dietetic Association: food and nutrition misinformation (position statement), J Am Diet Assoc 95:705, 1995.

American Dietetic Association: 2000 Nutrition trends survey: executive survey, Chicago, 2000, American Dietetic Association.

The American Dietetic Association and International Food Information Council: How are Americans making food choices? 1994 update, prepared by the Gallup Organization, April 1994.

Capellano KL: Internet 101: a guide for food and nutrition professionals, Nutr Today 33:77, 1998.

Center for Media and Public Affairs: Food for thought III, a quantitative and qualitative content analysis of diet, nutrition and food safety reporting, Washington, DC, 2000, International Food Information Council Foundation.

Kipp DE et al.: The internet and the nutritional scientist, Am J Clin Nutr 64:659, 1996.

Radimer K et al.: Nonvitamin, nonmineral dietary supplements: issues and findings from NHANES III, J Am Diet Assoc 100:447, 2000.

Wellman NS et al.: Do we facilitate the scientific process and the development of dietary guidance when findings from single studies are publicized? An American Society for Nutritional Sciences controversy session report, Am J Clin Nutr 70:802, 1999.

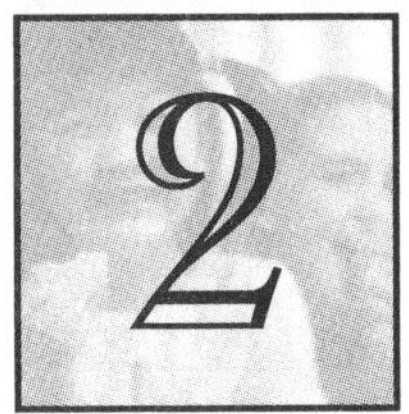

CHAPTER 2

Nutrition Screening and Assessment

Chapter Outline

The health and productivity of an individual or a population is related to nutrition well-being. Knowledge of nutrition status provides the basis for formulating individual nutrition care and community-based nutrition intervention and education programs.

Students of nutrition are familiar with large surveys such as the National Food Consumption Survey conducted by the U.S. Department of Agriculture (USDA) and the National Health and Nutrition Examination Surveys (NHANES) of the National Center for Health Statistics (NCHS), part of the continuing nutrition surveillance or monitoring system for the U.S. population. The same general techniques employed in such surveys are applicable to identify individuals at nutrition risk across all stages of the life span. Such assessment helps with the planning of nutrition intervention for improvement of nutritional status, or the health of the body as it relates to energy and nutrients.

THE NUTRITION CARE PROCESS

- *What is the role of nutrition assessment in the nutrition care process?*

Health status can be thought of on a continuous scale ranging from optimal health on one end to clinical disease or deficiency disease on the other. Nutritional factors can move individuals either way along this continuum (Hensrud, 1999). Historically nutrition screening has been an initial process of identifying patients at high risk so they can undergo further nutritional assessment to determine the need for prevention or treatment, often characterized as **medical nutrition therapy.** Although nutrition screening is standard practice in healthcare settings, the application of the concept has been extended to health-promotion activities to determine individuals who will benefit from educational intervention.

KEY TERMS

medical nutrition therapy: the use of specific nutrition interventions to prevent illness or treat an illness, injury, or condition

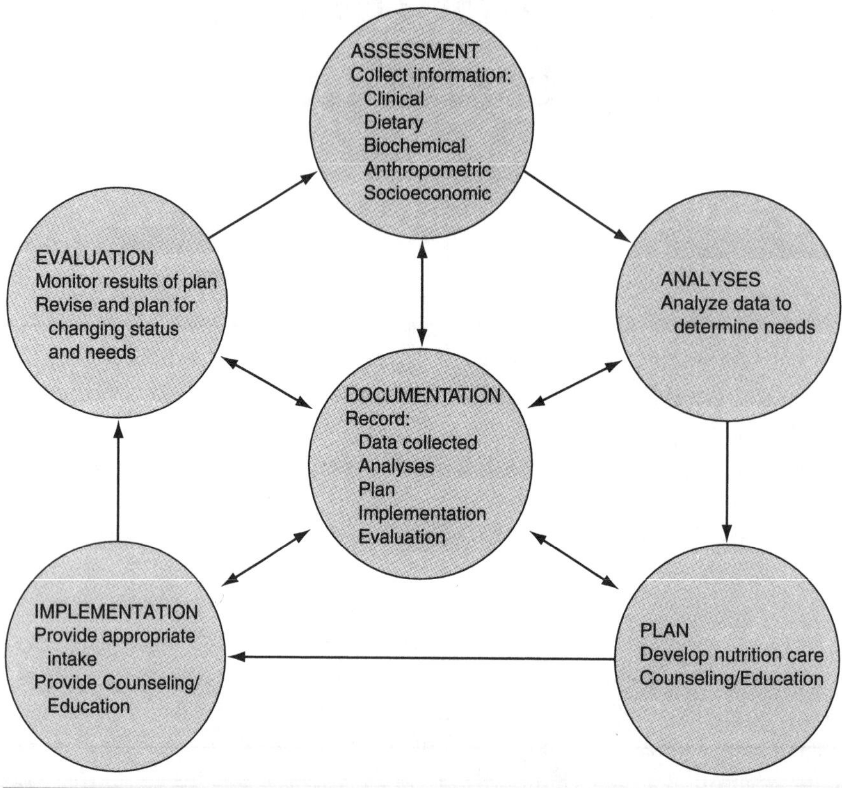

Figure 2-1 The nutrition care process.

Nutrition assessment initiates the nutrition care process (Figure 2-1), which is an organized series of activities that includes the following: identification of nutritional status, analysis of nutrition risk and associated problems or needs, planning to meet those needs, implementation of that plan, and evaluation of the effectiveness of the intervention (American Dietetic Association, 1994). Nutrition care for an ill or hospitalized person will be different from that designed to reduce the risk of nutrition problems in a healthy person, but the components of the nutrition care process are essentially the same.

OVERVIEW OF NUTRITION SCREENING AND ASSESSMENT

- *How does nutrition screening differ from nutrition assessment?*
- *Describe commonly used assessment techniques and the body compartments estimated.*
- *Which assessment techniques are useful in documenting nutrition deficiency?*

Nutrition Screening

Nutrition screening is the process of identifying individuals at high nutrition risk so more extensive nutrition assessment can be performed. To be cost effective nutrition screening must be a process that can be completed quickly with readily available information, but will be relevant to nutrition intervention. The Nutrition Screening Initiative (NSI) checklist shown in Figure 2-2 is a good example of a tool used to identify undernutrition in older adults in community settings. Other examples of community-based programs to identify individuals at potential nutrition risk include programs to screen individuals for diabetes at shopping malls, or simple questionnaires used in health clinics or physicians' offices. These programs identify individuals who may need further testing.

The Warning Signs of poor nutritional healthare often overlooked. Use this checklist to find out if you or someone you know is at nutritional risk.

DETERMINE YOUR NUTRITIONAL HEALTH

Read the statements below. Circle the number in the yes column for those that apply to you or someone you know. For each yes answer, score the number in the box. Total your nutritional score.

	YES
I have an illness or condition that made me change the kind and/or amount of food I eat.	2
I eat fewer than 2 meals per day.	3
I eat few fruits or vegetables or milk products.	2
I have 3 or more drinks of beer, liquor, or wine almost every day.	2
I have tooth or mouth problems that make it hard for me to eat.	2
I don't always have enough money to buy the food I need.	4
I eat alone most of the time.	1
I take 3 or more different prescribed or over-the-counter drugs a day.	1
Without wanting to, I have lost or gained 10 pounds in the last 6 months.	2
I am not always physically able to shop, cook, and/or feed myself.	2
TOTAL	

Total Your Nutritional Score. If it's —

0-2 **Good!** Recheck your nutritional score in 6 months.

3-5 **You are at moderate nutritional risk.** See what can be done to improve your eating habits and lifestyle. Your office on aging, senior nutrition program, senior citizens center or health department can help. Recheck your nutritional score in 3 months.

6 or more **You are at high nutritional risk.** Bring this checklist the next time you see your doctor, dietitian, or other qualified health or social service professional. Talk with them about any problems you may have. Ask for help to improve your nutritional health.

These materials developed and distributed by the Nutrition Screening Initiative, a project of:

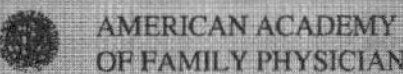

AMERICAN ACADEMY OF FAMILY PHYSICIANS

THE AMERICAN DIETETIC ASSOCIATION

NATIONAL COUNCIL ON THE AGING

Remember that warning signs suggest risk, but do not represent diagnosis of any condition. Turn the page to learn more about the Warning Signs of poor nutritional health.

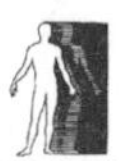

The Nutrition Screening Initiative
2626 Pennsylvania Avenue, NW, Suite 301
Washington, DC 20037

The Nutrition Screening Initiative is funded in part by a grant from Ross Laboratories, a division of Abbott Laboratories.

Figure 2-2 An example of a nutritional screening tool for community use. *(From Report of Nutrition Screening, I: Toward a common view, Washington, DC, 1991, The Nutrition Screening Initiative. Reprinted with permission by the Nutrition Screening Initiative, a project of the American Academy of Family Physicians, the American Dietetic Association, and the National Council on the Aging, Inc., and funded in part by a grant from Ross Products Division, Abbott Laboratories.)*

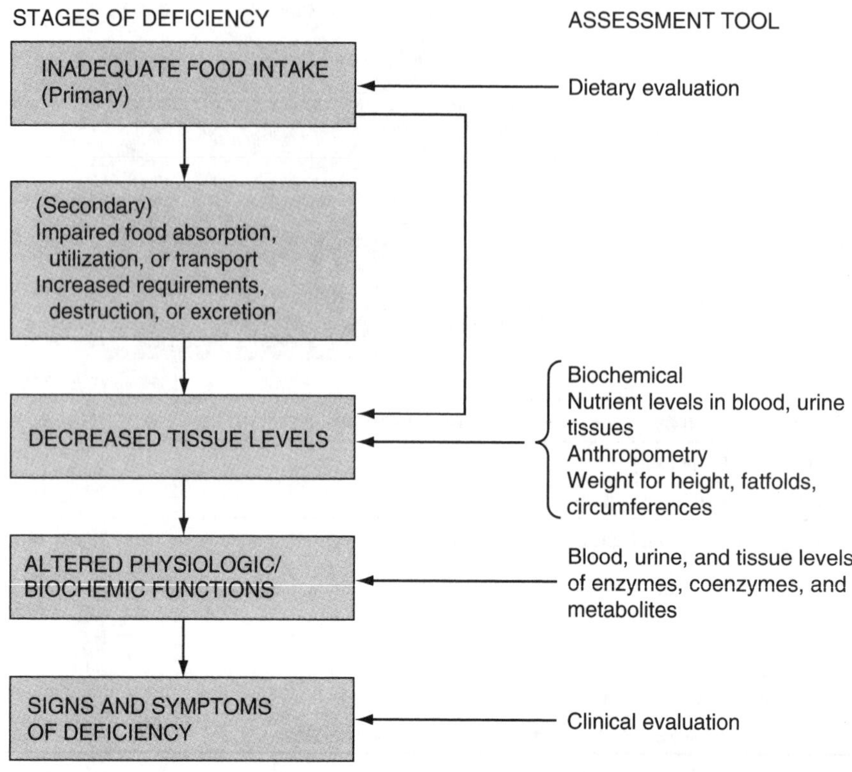

Figure 2-3 Sequence of events in prolonged nutrition inadequacy and appropriate assessment techniques.

Many health-promotion and health-education programs include simple screening tools. Nutrition screening has become routine in most hospitals because the Joint Commission on Accreditation of Healthcare Organizations (1998) requires that all hospital patients be screened within 24 hours of admission. A simple tool like the NSI questionnaire may be used after a patient is admitted and some facilities use a similar tool to call people at home for specific information before scheduled admission to the hospital (Schwartz and Gudzin, 2000).

Nutrition Assessment

Nutrition assessment is a more detailed evaluation and interpretation of multiple parameters that seeks to define the risk of developing nutrition-related medical complications. Nutrition intervention refers to any change or treatment that is designed to improve nutritional health. It could range from nutrition education (i.e., the "Five-a-Day" program that encourages people to consume at least five servings of fruits and vegetables each day to reduce the risk of cancer) (Anderson et al., 2001); to nutrition counseling to make general improvements in the diet; to counseling for implementation of specific dietary modifications to treat disease; to supplementation to improve energy and nutrient intake by providing complete nutrition in the form of liquid supplements, tube feedings, or **total parenteral nutrition.** The ultimate goal of nutrition screening and assessment activities is identification of risk factors in individuals that can be altered through nutritional intervention.

Nutrition screening uses some simple assessment techniques to identify characteristics known to be associated with nutrition problems and to recognize clients who may benefit from assessment and intervention. Nutrition assessment is the science of determining **nutrition status.** It is designed to identify individuals who, without change or intervention, will develop malnutrition. Malnutrition can refer to undernutrition (i.e., underweight status, poor protein status, or a vitamin deficiency) or overnutrition (i.e., obesity, hyperlipidemia, or vitamin toxicity). Tools of nutrition assessment are used in many settings by members of the healthcare team such as dietitians, dietetic technicians, nurses, physicians, or other healthcare professionals.

Development of a Nutrient Deficiency

Although deficiencies of single nutrients are rare, the sequence of occurrences in the development of a specific nutrient deficiency illustrates the progression to undernutrition (Figure 2-3). Assume that an individual's dietary intake of a certain nutrient is low. If the low intake continues over time, body tissue levels of that nutrient will decline. Continued inadequate intakes will cause impairment of certain body functions and, eventually, the lack of the nutrient will result in physical signs and symptoms of a deficiency. Nutrition assessment techniques are used to identify stages of this process.

For example a dietary interview with a client may reveal a low intake of thiamin, which could lead to a deficiency disease known as beriberi. An inadequate intake initially causes low tissue levels, which can be measured by blood or urine levels of the vitamin. Even lower tissue levels result in a decrease in the activity of thiamin-dependent enzymes such as transketolase. As the deficiency progresses, pyruvate (an intermediary product of glucose breakdown), which requires a thiamin-containing coenzyme for metabolism, increases in the blood. Eventually symptoms of beriberi, such as anorexia, depression, and changes in the function of the central nervous system, are observed.

Nutrient deficiencies that result because of an inadequate dietary intake, such as the one previously described, are primary deficiencies. Progression to a deficiency state may also occur when dietary intake appears to be adequate if requirements for the nutrient increase, if absorption or use of the nutrient is severely curtailed, or if nutrient losses increase. Such deficiencies are referred to as secondary deficiencies.

Nutrition Assessment Techniques

Nutrition assessment techniques may be used in a hospital, an extended care facility, a physician's office, an outpatient or community clinic, or they may be included as part of health-promotion activities. Nutrition assessment is based not on a single determination, but on a group or series of measurements and observations that provide an estimate of nutrition status. Techniques used for nutrition assessment must reflect nutrition status, be readily available in that particular healthcare or health-promotion setting, and be of reasonable cost. The assessment technique must also be repeatable so the impact of intervention can be monitored. Data collected for nutrition assessment, often categorized as anthropometric, laboratory or biochemical, clinical, and dietary data, are combined to provide an accurate picture of the individual's nutrition status.

Deficiencies of specific vitamins or minerals occur infrequently in people in developed countries. General malnutrition, which is associated with inadequate food intake or impaired use of food sources, is more common and involves status related to energy and several nutrients. Therefore nutrition assessment of individuals centers on their macronutrient status, particularly energy and protein status. Because iron deficiency is a concern for many age groups, iron status is often part of the nutrition assessment. But increasingly other micronutrients are attracting interest, such as folic acid, vitamin B_{12}, vitamin B_6, and zinc.

KEY TERMS

total parenteral nutrition: provides all the energy and nutrients an individual requires through infusion into the bloodstream

nutrition status: the degree to which physiologic needs for nutrients and energy are being met

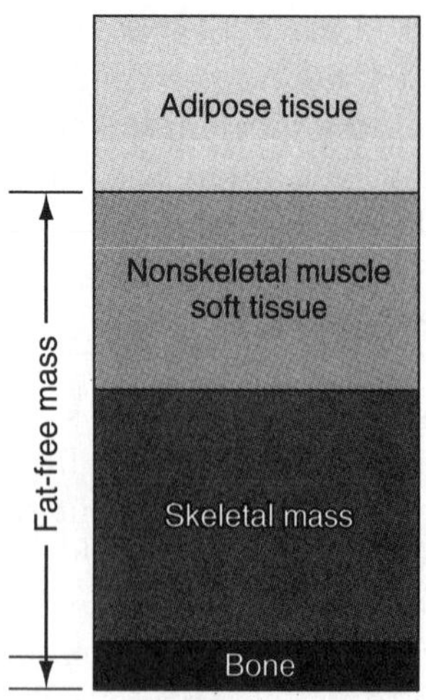

Figure 2-4 A tissue system model of body composition. *(From Wang Z-M, Pierson RN, and Heymsfield SB: The five-level model: a new approach to organizing body-composition research, Am J Clin Nutr 56:19, 1992. Copyright Am J Clin Nutr. American Society for Clinical Nutrition.)*

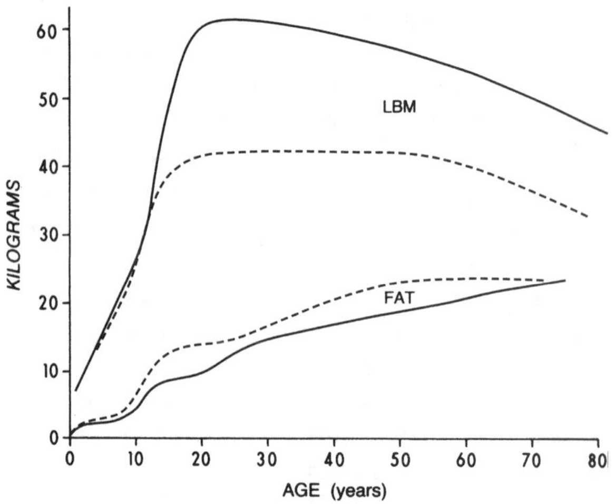

Figure 2-5 Average values for lean body mass (LBM) and fat across the life span. Solid lines represent males; broken lines represent females. *(Modified from Forbes GB: Body composition: influence of nutrition, disease, growth and aging. In Shils ME et al., editors: Modern nutrition in health and disease, Philadelphia, 1994, Lea & Febiger.)*

Body Macronutrient Components

The major body components are water, protein, fats, and minerals. For an assessment, macronutrients in the body can be divided into two compartments: body fat and fat-free mass. Fat, the major energy reserve, is the most variable component of the body. Body fat mass can be estimated from fatfold (skinfold) measurements at a variety of body sites, the most common of which is the triceps fatfold (TFF). Body fat is sensitive to acute malnutrition and can be used as an indirect estimate of energy balance.

The fat-free components of the body include bone, skeletal muscle mass, and nonskeletal soft tissue (Figure 2-4). **Somatic protein** and **visceral protein** are considered metabolically active because they can be drawn upon to meet body needs. The status of these proteins is assessed by different methods. Because the human body does not store protein as it does fat, decreases in body protein result in loss of structural units such as skeletal protein and visceral proteins such as plasma albumin. Nutritional assessment measurements must reflect these body compartments. Because the amount and proportion of lean body mass and body fat change across the life span (Figure 2-5), data related to these compartments are interpreted using gender- and age-specific standards.

Somatic protein (muscle mass) may be evaluated from anthropometric measurements and from the determination of the amount of creatinine, a metabolite of the use of energy in the creatine-phosphate bond for the work of muscle. Creatine is excreted in the urine. Visceral protein status is assessed by biochemical analyses of plasma proteins and immune proteins, most often the total lymphocyte count (TLC). Table 2-1 lists representative measurements of major body compartments used in nutrition assessment, which will be discussed in this chapter.

Application of Nutrition Assessment

The number of measurements and the level at which techniques are applied vary. A dietary interview in a health clinic or private-practice setting may be used to develop counseling plans to help a client adjust nutrient intake. A young child may be evaluated for eligibility for the

Table 2-1 PARAMETERS FOR EVALUATION OF NUTRITION STATUS

Body Compartment	Parameter

Adipose tissue	Weight for height
	Body Mass Index (BMI)
	Subcutaneous fatfolds
	  Triceps (TFF)
	  Subscapular (SSFF)

Somatic protein	Midarm muscle circumference (MAMC) Midarm muscle area (MAMA) Creatinine height index (CHI)

Visceral protein	Serum proteins
	  Albumin
	  Transferrin
	  Prealbumin (PA)
	  Retinol-binding protein (RBP)
	Immune proteins
	  Total lymphocyte count (TLC)

Iron	Hemoglobin (hgb), hematocrit (hct) Total iron binding capacity (TIBC) Serum ferritin Free erythrocyte protoporphyrin

Women, Infants, and Children (WIC) supplemental food program by using anthropometry (weight and height measurements), dietary intake, and a simple blood test. At another level, the hospitalized patient who is receiving total parenteral nutrition may be assessed using all the preceding measures plus a series of laboratory tests and the observation of physical signs and symptoms.

Nutrition assessment is the first step in the nutrition care process. It is a multifactorial approach in which several kinds of information are collected and used to evaluate an individual's nutrition status. In this introduction to nutrition assessment, anthropometric, biochemical, clinical, and dietary measurements are described and examples for use and interpretation are discussed.

ANTHROPOMETRY

- *What are the advantages and limitations of using anthropometric measurements for nutrition assessment?*
- *Which anthropometric measurements are commonly used, and how are they interpreted?*

Anthropometry is the measurement of physical dimensions of the human body. In the hands of an experienced practitioner, anthropometry is a useful technique for estimation of body composition. Several measures can be used to estimate body fat (energy) and somatic protein status. In undernutrition, skeletal muscle and fat stores are depleted earlier than proteins of organs; therefore low levels in these compartments can be an early indicator of nutritional depletion. The reliability of anthropometric measurements in estimating body fat and protein has been validated using densitometry (underwater weighing) (Durnin and Womersley, 1974; Gray et al., 1990; Jackson and Pollock, 1985).

Anthropometric techniques are rapid and repeatable. The required equipment (i.e., scales, tape measures, and calipers) is readily available,

KEY TERMS

somatic protein: protein within skeletal muscle
visceral protein: protein of the organs (viscera) and circulation

inexpensive, and portable. However, attaining accuracy and reliability in anthropometric measurements requires a skilled, careful measurer and quality equipment that is calibrated regularly. Standard techniques for anthropometry have been established. Those used most frequently are described briefly in this chapter. Errors of **accuracy** or imprecision are due largely to observer error. Measurers need to be trained in correct techniques. **Reliability** of measurements can be ensured by repeating measurements and recording them immediately to reduce the chance of error. If the two measurements are substantially different, a third reading should be made.

There are dozens of anthropometric measurements that can be used (Lohman et al., 1988). This introductory discussion includes only stature (height), weight, upper arm circumference, and TFF and subscapular fatfold (SSFF). The purpose of anthropometry in nutrition assessment is completing physical measurement of an individual and relating those data to standards that reflect population or reference data. Therefore anthropometric standards are likely to be sex and age-group specific.

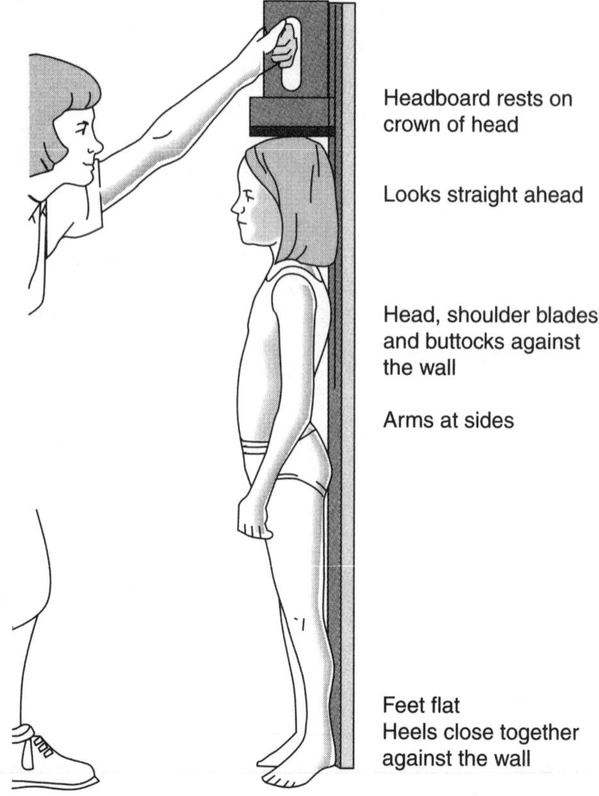

Figure 2-6 Accurate determination of height requires careful positioning of the subject.

Weight for Height

The most common anthropometric measurements, stature and weight, can be useful for preliminary assessment of energy and protein stores.

Height

Stature is a major component of body size and is important for evaluation of growth in children and weight status in adults. Measured heights are important in assessing body weight for height status. A recent study reported that self-reported heights are significantly different from measured heights, particularly in older adults (Kuczmarski et al., 2001). Accurate measurement of standing height requires a nonstretchable tape or measuring stick attached to a vertical surface and a moveable horizontal or right-angle headboard for reading. For measurement the subject stands erect, without shoes, with weight equally distributed on both feet and heels together and touching the vertical board (Figure 2-6). Arms hang freely at the sides of the trunk with palms facing the thighs. Looking straight ahead so that the line of vision is perpendicular to the body, the subject takes a deep breath and holds that position while the horizontal headboard is brought down firmly on the top of the head. Stature is recorded to the nearest 0.1 cm or ¼ inch.

Weight

Body weight is a composite measure of total body size and provides a rough evaluation of overall muscle mass and fat stores. It is important in screening for unusual growth, obesity, or undernutrition and is a component in equations that predict energy needs and body composition. Weight is measured on a leveled platform scale with a beam and moveable weights or an electronic scale. The subject, in minimal clothing and without shoes, stands with weight evenly distributed on both feet. Weight is recorded to the nearest 0.1 kg or ¼ lb.

Interpretation of Weight for Height

Measurements of stature and weight are interpreted by comparison to tables derived from a reference population or to the individual's former or usual weight. Gains in stature and weight in infants, children, and adolescents are important indicators of growth status and are discussed in Chapters 7, 9, and 11.

Usual body weight. In the healthcare setting recent changes in body weight can be an important indicator of nutrition status. Changes may be reported as percentage of body weight lost or of previous or usual body weight using the following calculations:

% weight change = [(usual weight − current weight)/usual weight] × 100

% usual weight = (current weight/usual weight) × 100

Body mass index. Body Mass Index (BMI) estimates total body mass. Because BMI is highly correlated with total body fat (Micozzi et al., 1986; Revicki and Israel, 1986), it is considered a general indicator of body fatness. BMI can be determined using this calculation:

$$\text{BMI} = \text{weight (kg)/height (m}^2\text{)}$$

For a 22-year-old male who is 183 cm tall and weighs 68 kg, the BMI is:

$$\text{BMI} = 68 \text{ kg}/1.83^2 = 20.2$$

Using the categories of BMI in Table 2-2, he would be considered of normal weight (BMI = 18.5-24.9), which is associated with the least risk of early death (National Institutes of Health, National Heart Lung and Blood Institute, 1998). Weights categorized as overweight and obese are associated with high blood lipid levels and increased risk of hypertension, diabetes mellitus, and cardiovascular disease (Kuczmarski et al., 2001). The BMI does not distinguish excess fat from muscularity as the source of excessive body weight (Frisancho and Flegel, 1983; Smalley et al., 1990). More direct indicators of obesity are body fatfolds (discussed in the following section), determination from body density measured by **hydrostatic weighing** or **bioelectric impedance (BIA)**, or **dual photon X-ray absorptiometry (DXA).**

Table 2-2 Body Mass Index Classification of Overweight Status and Obesity

Classification	BMI (kg/m²)
Underweight	<18.5
Normal	18.5–24.9
Overweight	25.0–29.9
Obesity, class I	30.0–34.9
Obesity, class II	35.0–39.9
Extreme obesity, class III	≥40

From National Institutes of Health, National Heart, Lung and Blood Institute: Clinical guidelines in the identification, evaluation, and treatment of overweight and obesity in adults—the evidence report, Obes Res 6(suppl 2):S51, 1998.

Height-weight tables. For adults the appropriateness of body weight for height can be assessed using reference height-weight tables. Height-weight tables have been generated from data from the insurance industry, the Metropolitan Life Insurance Tables, and data from the NHANES. Most tables reflect average or adjusted weights. The most frequently used height and weight reference tables, the 1983 Height and Weight Tables from the

KEY TERMS

accuracy: nearness of the measure to the true value
reliability: the extent to which the same measurement is obtained on repeated trials
hydrostatic weighing: weight in air is divided by loss of weight when submerged with corrections for density of water and air and for the volume of air in the lungs
bioelectric impedance (BIA): electrodes are attached to the wrist and ankle and a weak alternating current is applied; density is determined from resistance or the decrease in voltage detected by electrodes
dual photon X-ray absorptiometry (DXA): the body is scanned by two X-ray beams allowing calculation of estimates of bone mineral content, body fat, and soft lean tissue

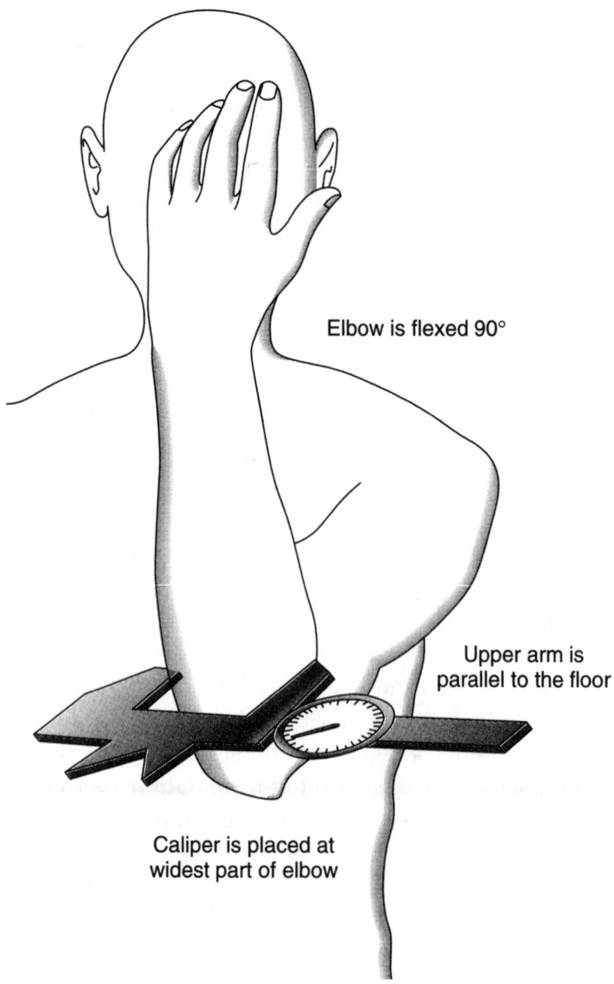

Figure 2-7 Elbow breadth is measured between the two prominent bones on the sides of the elbow.

Metropolitan Life Insurance Company (Metropolitan Life Insurance Company, 1983), are located in Appendix B. These tables provide weight ranges for height based on the 1979 Build Study, which included approximately 4 million policy holders of 25 insurance companies. Data from adults with significant disease were omitted. Weights for a given stature are those associated with the greatest longevity. The 1983 tables include weight ranges for small, medium, and large frame for each height. Interpretation of body weight for height can be enhanced by use of the appropriate frame size designation, especially in distinguishing between individuals who have large fat-free mass and those who have high body weights from excess fat.

Frame size is a concept based on skeletal dimensions, which reflect body build, but are not influenced by the degree of body fat. A variety of body breadth and diameter measurements, including ankle, elbow, wrist (breadth, not circumference), shoulder, and hip, have been suggested to represent body frame size (Himes and Bouchard, 1985; Mitchell, 1993). The frame measure for which reference data from a large population are available is elbow breadth. Elbow breadth is measured with a broad-faced sliding anthropometer while the right arm is extended and the forearm is bent upward at a 90-degree angle with the wrist toward the body (Figure 2-7). Measurement is made between the two prominent bones on either side of the elbow. Pressure is exerted to compress soft tissues and record the breadth to the nearest 1 mm. Elbow breadth correlates with fat-free body mass (Frisancho, 1990). Categories for frame size were determined from elbow breadth measurements of the subjects in NHANES I and II. The frame size designations that accompany the 1983 Height and Weight Tables were formulated by dividing the elbow breadth measurements into quartiles. Medium frame corresponds to elbow breadths between the twenty-fifth and seventy-fifth percentiles in each height category. Values above the seventy-fifth percentile and below the twenty-fifth percentile were designated as large and small frame, respectively (Frisancho and Flegel, 1983).

Reference Weight. Reference weight is the individual's actual weight expressed as a percentage of a reference weight. The Metropolitan Height and Weight Tables are used by selecting the appropriate frame size based on elbow breadth. Reference weight is a range for the individual's sex, height, and frame size. Usually the midpoint of this weight range is used to calculate the Metropolitan Relative Weight (MRW) as follows:

$$\text{MRW} = (\text{Current weight/reference weight}) \times 100$$

It should be noted that the Metropolitan Height and Weight Tables contain values for measure-

Box 2-1 Hamwi Formula for Quick Calculation of an Appropriate Body Weight

FORMULA FOR ESTIMATING AN APPROPRIATE BODY WEIGHT*

Females: 100 lbs for the first 5 feet of height and 5 lbs for every inch over 5 feet

Males: 106 lbs for the first 5 feet of height and 5 lbs for every inch over 5 feet

Example: A woman of medium frame with a height of 65 inches would be calculated as:

100 lbs for first 5 feet	= 100
5 lbs × 5 inches	= 25
Total	125 lbs

*If the individual is of large frame, add 10%. If the individual is of small frame, subtract 10%.

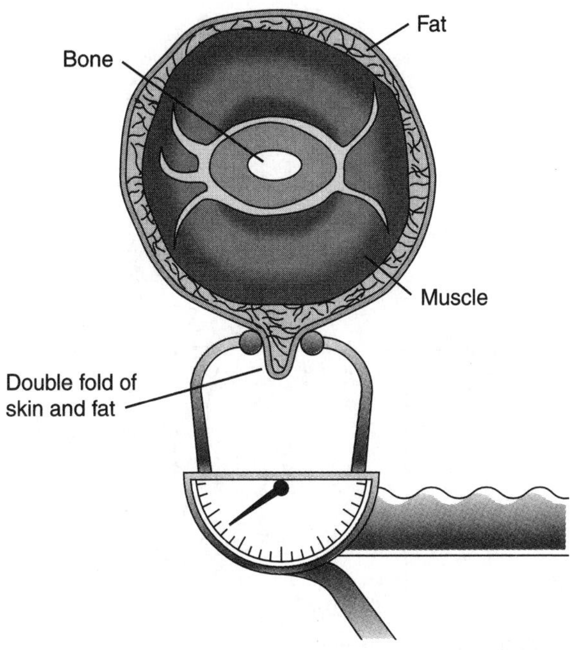

Figure 2-8 The fatfold measurement is a double thickness of fat and skin.

ments made with the subject wearing 1-inch heels and clothing weighing approximately 5 pounds for men and 3 pounds for women. These values are added when using the tables if barefoot height and nude weights are used.

For a 35-year-old man who is 72 in (183 cm) in stature with a medium frame and weighs 150 lb (68 kg), the reference weight range is 157 to 170 lb (71.3 to 77.2 kg). Using the midpoint of the range of weight for stature, his MRW is:

$$\text{MRW} = 68\ \text{kg}/74.3 \times 100 = 92 \text{ or } 92\%$$

Because overweight status and obesity are major health concerns in North America, it is important to acknowledge appropriate or healthy body weights. Such weights are those associated with the lowest mortality and morbidity. The Metropolitan Tables represent one such example.

There have been numerous efforts to devise a "quick" method to determine appropriate weight. One that commonly appears in textbooks and is often used by registered dietitians (RDs) is the Hamwi* formula (Box 2-1). Frequently the term *ideal weight* has been attached to the result of these calculations, which may be somewhat misleading. Alternatives might be *reference weight* or *appropriate weight.* With publication of the 2000 edition of the *Dietary Guidelines for Americans,* the term *healthy weight* has been used to designate weight for height associated with BMIs between 18.5 and 25. Deviations from that weight increase health risk (see Figure 1-5).

*Dr. George Hamwi was an endocrinologist at Ohio State University Medical Center in the 1960s.

Fatfolds

Body fatness is of interest for two reasons. Too little fat is associated with undernutrition and too much is associated with increased risk of chronic disease. Fatfold, sometimes called skinfold, measurements are indicators of body fat and energy reserves. Fatfolds can be measured on almost any site of the body where subcutaneous fat is present, but the most frequently measured fatfolds are those of the triceps, biceps, chest, subscapular area, suprailiac area, abdomen, and thigh. A fatfold is actually the thickness of a double fold of skin and subcutaneous adipose tissue (Figure 2-8). Calipers calibrated to exert standardized

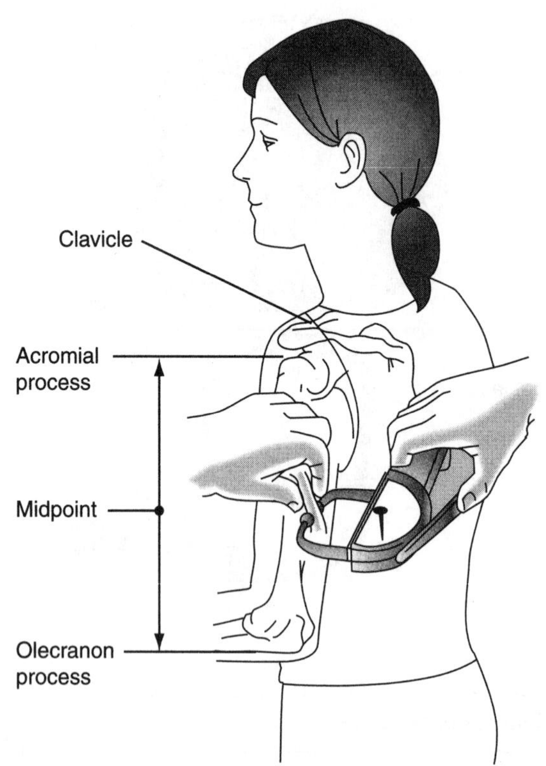

Figure 2-9 The triceps fatfold is measured at the midpoint between the acromial process and the olecranon process.

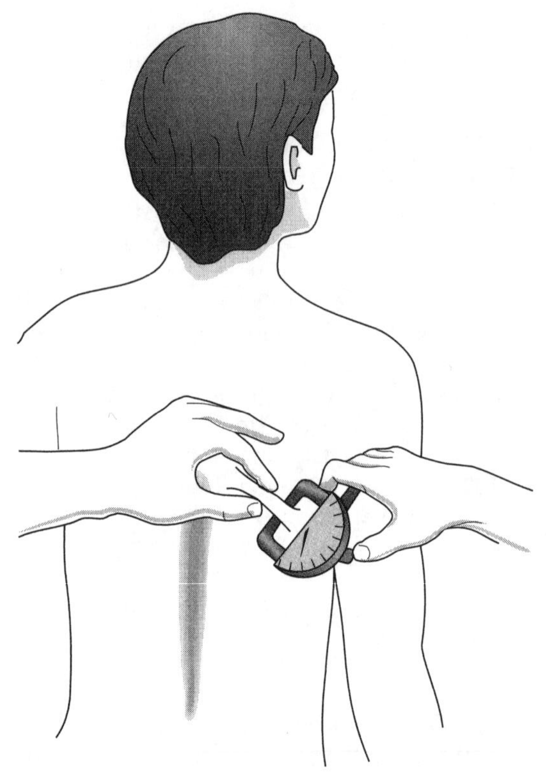

Figure 2-10 Measurement of the subscapular fatfold.

pressure per unit of jaw surface are used for the measurement. The fatfolds that are most readily measured and for which there are reference data from large population studies are the triceps and subscapular area.

Triceps Fatfold

The TFF is measured in the midline at the back of the arm, over the triceps muscle, at a point midway between the lateral projection (acromial process) of the shoulder and the tip of the elbow (Figure 2-9). The measurement is taken with the subject's right arm hanging loosely and comfortably at the side. The caliper is held in the measurer's right hand. Standing behind the subject, the measurer picks up the triceps skinfold approximately 1 cm above the marked midpoint. The tips of the calipers are applied to the fatfold at the marked level and the fold is measured to the nearest 0.1 mm.

Subscapular Fatfold

Figure 2-10 illustrates measurement of the SSFF. The subject stands with the arm relaxed to the side. The calipers are applied at the site along the axis of the inferior angle of the scapula and the fatfold is measured to the nearest 0.1 mm.

Interpretation of Fatfold Measurements

Fatfold measurements for a given individual are evaluated by comparison with age- and sex-specific percentile distribution of a reference population, in most instances using the data from the NHANES survey. Reference tables for TFF and SSFF are in Appendix B. If a 35-year-old man has a TFF of 9.0 mm and an SSFF of 16 mm, Appendix B reveals that 9.0 mm is equal to the twenty-fifth percentile for TFF and 16 mm is just below the fiftieth percentile for SSFF. This indicates that, compared with a reference population, this man's TFF is lower than 75% and higher than 24% of the reference population and his SSFF is almost at the midpoint for the reference population. Values below the tenth percentile or above the ninetieth percentile suggest very low or very high fat reserves and increased risk of malnutrition or obesity, respectively. Sometimes measurements fall between the percentiles shown on the tables and must be estimated from the data available. For a man of the same age a TFF of 7.9 mm falls between the fifteenth and twenty-fifth percentiles, or at approximately the twentieth percentile. Many clinicians believe that a more accurate representation of total body fat can be obtained by taking an average of two or more fatfolds, including peripheral and central fat reserves such as the TFF and the subscapular or suprailiac fatfolds. Durnin and Womersley (1974) have developed tables for predicting the percentage of total body fat from the sum of fatfolds (tricep, bicep, subscapular, and suprailiac fatfolds). These values were validated against percent of body fat obtained from hydrostatic weighing (see Appendix B).

Circumferences

Body circumferences can be measured easily with flexible, nonstretch tapes. Various body circumferences are used to calculate estimates of somatic protein and distribution of body fat.

Waist Hip Circumference

Excess body fat is a specific risk factor for many chronic diseases. Long-term research studies indicate that the site of fat storage, specifically abdominal as opposed to gluteal (hip) fat storage, is a major risk factor for mortality from cardiovascular diseases (Kannel et al., 1991) and endometrial cancer (Schapira et al., 1991). With the recognition that fat distribution is an indicator of risk, circumferential or girth measurements have new importance. Waist circumference is measured by using the smallest circumference between the nipples and the top of the thighs and hip circumference is defined as the largest circumference between the waist and the knees.

The waist-to-hip ratio (WHR), which differentiates between android and gynoid obesity, is calculated as follows:

$$\text{WHR} = \text{waist (cm)/hip (cm)}$$

A WHR of 1.0 or greater in men or 0.8 in women is indicative of android obesity and an increased risk of obesity-related diseases. Recent studies have suggested that waist circumference alone is as accurate a predictor of cardiovascular risk as the WHR.

Midarm Circumference

The TFF, an independent measure of body fat, is also used with the midarm circumference (MAC) to calculate two estimators of somatic protein status: midarm muscle circumference (MAMC) and midarm muscle area (MAMA) (Heymsfield et al., 1982). The MAC is measured at the same site as the TFF. The subject stands erect with the arm hanging freely at the side of the trunk, palm facing the thigh. A tape is placed around the arm so that it is touching the skin, but not compressing the soft tissues (Figure 2-11). The circumference is recorded to the nearest millimeter.

Midarm Muscle Circumference

The MAMC is calculated using the following formula:

$$\text{MAMC} = \text{MAC (mm)} - (\pi \times \text{TFF in mm})$$

with MAC and TFF given in millimeters. The MAMC for a 35-year-old man with a MAC of 304 mm (30.4 cm) and a TFF of 8.5 mm is calculated as follows:

$$\text{MAMC} = 304 - (3.14 \times 8.5)$$
$$\text{MAMC} = 277 \text{ mm or } 27.7 \text{ cm}$$

Midarm muscle area is calculated from the circumference of the upper arm and the TFF values using the following formulas:

$$\text{Females} \quad \text{MAMA(mm)}^2 = \frac{\text{MAMC(mm)}^2}{4\pi} - 6.5$$

$$\text{Males} \quad \text{MAMA(mm)}^2 = \frac{\text{MAMC(mm)}^2}{4\pi} - 10$$

In these equations π equals 3.14, MAC is in millimeters and TFF is in millimeters. The constants

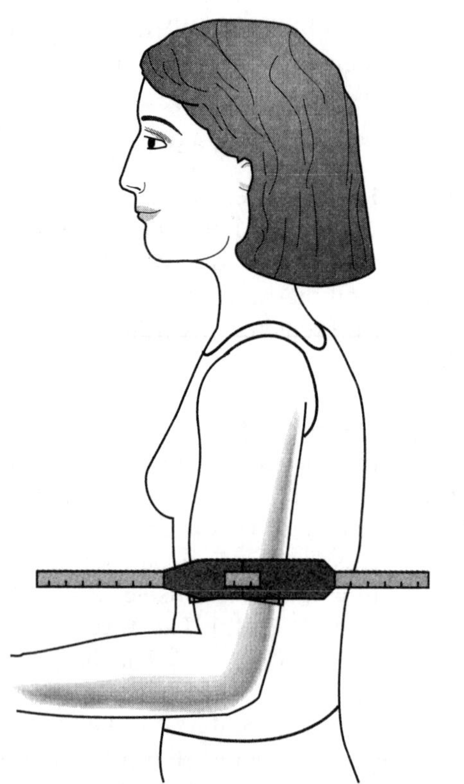

Figure 2-11 Midarm circumference is measured at the midpoint of the upper arm, which is the same site as the triceps fatfold.

(6.5 and 10) that are subtracted at the end of the calculation account for the presence of bone, nerves, and vascular tissue in the upper arm (Heymsfield et al., 1982).

The MAMA for the man in the previous example is calculated as follows:

$$\begin{aligned} \text{MAMA} &= [277^2/(4 \times 3.14)] - 10 \\ &= (7673/12.56) - 10 \\ &= 6109 - 10 \\ &= 6099 \text{ mm}^2 \text{ or } 60.9 \text{ cm}^2 \end{aligned}$$

The MAMC and MAMA are interpreted using the percentile distribution of the NHANES data in Appendix B. This Appendix B2 shows that a MAMC value of 27.7 is just above the twenty-fifth percentile and that a MAMA of 60.9 cm^2 is slightly below the tenth percentile.

LABORATORY MEASUREMENTS

- *What are the advantages and limitations of laboratory measurements for nutrition assessment?*
- *Describe three measures of visceral protein status and the significance of decreases in these measurements.*
- *What does a decreased level of serum ferritin, hemoglobin, or hematocrit tell about iron status?*

Laboratory tests for nutrition assessment must reflect body levels of the specific nutrient and be sensitive to a depletion of body stores. The measurements may be of nutrients or their metabolites (products of the metabolism of the nutrient), substances that contain the nutrient (i.e., hemoglobin for iron), enzymes that require the nutrient (i.e., transketolase for thiamin), or substances that result from abnormal metabolism from a deficiency of the nutrient (i.e., elevated pyruvate levels in thiamin deficiency). Laboratory tests are performed on available body tissues, usually blood or urine. Biochemical tests are the most objective and quantitative measures of nutrition status. They can detect nutrient deficits long before alterations in anthropometric measures or clinical signs or symptoms appear. Because biochemical tests may be influenced by non-nutrition factors such as diseases or medication use, they are used with other measures for assessment.

Measurements on Blood

Nutrients

Nutrients in blood may be measured in **plasma** or **serum** and in specific cellular components such as erythrocytes (red blood cells) or white blood cells (WBC). In most cases serum and plasma concentrations are similar. The potential effect of recent dietary intake on nutrient levels can be reduced by collecting fasting blood samples. Measurements of nutrients or products in blood are reported per unit of blood; that is, they are measured by gram, milligram, or microgram (μg) per deciliter (dL) or liter (L). Body hydration status may influence actual values reported. For example an individual who is dehydrated may appear to have high nutrient levels, but when body fluids are returned to normal, the values

Table 2-3 Laboratory Measurements for Assessment of Vitamin and Mineral Status

Nutrient	Laboratory Measurement
FAT-SOLUBLE VITAMINS	
Vitamin A	Serum carotene, retinol-binding protein, retinol, conjunctival impression cytology, dark adaptation
Vitamin D	Serum 25-OH vitamin D_3 Serum alkaline phosphatase
Vitamin E	Plasma alpha-tocopherol, erythrocyte hemolysis test
Vitamin K	Prothrombin time, plasma vitamin K, clotting factors
WATER-SOLUBLE VITAMINS	
Vitamin C	Serum vitamin C, neutrophil ascorbate
Thiamin	Transketolase activity in red blood cells with and without thiamin pyrophosphate (TPP) Urinary thiamin
Riboflavin	Erythrocyte glutathione reductase activity with and without flavin-adenine dinucleotide (FAD), plasma riboflavin, urinary riboflavin, and metabolites
Niacin	Urinary metabolites of niacin (N_1-methylnicotinamide and 2-pyridone)
Vitamin B_6	Plasma pyridoxal-5-phosphate, plasma pyridoxal, transaminase activity in red blood cells, plasma and urinary vitamin B_6 and 4-pyridoxic acid
Folate	Erythrocyte folate, plasma folate, plasma homocysteine
Vitamin B_{12}	Hematologic status, vitamin B_{12} in serum and red blood cells, urinary methylmalonic acid
Biotin	Serum biotin, urinary biotin
MINERALS	
Calcium	Bone mineral density or content
Copper	Serum copper
Iodine	Serum protein bound iodine (PBI), uptake of radioiodine $^{(131)}$
Iron	Serum ferritin, serum iron, total iron binding capacity (TIBC) or transferrin saturation, free protoporphyrin in red blood cells, hemoglobin, hematocrit, mean corpuscular volume, mean corpuscular hemoglobin
Magnesium	Serum magnesium, magnesium in red blood cells
Potassium	Serum potassium
Selenium	Plasma selenoprotein glutathione peroxidase
Zinc	Serum zinc, urinary zinc, hair zinc

may drop to normal or below normal levels. Laboratory tests have been developed for assessment of many nutrients (Table 2-3). For some nutrients blood tests may not be sensitive indicators of nutrition status because of large body stores (e.g., fat-soluble vitamins), or because blood levels are regulated by hormones (e.g., calcium).

Metabolites

Vitamins often function as coenzymes in the metabolism of carbohydrates, protein, or fat. The absence of a vitamin to synthesize a coenzyme may block a normal series of reactions, resulting in an increase of an intermediary product or

> **KEY TERMS**
>
> **plasma:** whole blood from which blood cells have been removed
>
> **serum:** whole blood that remains after cells and clotting factors have been removed

byproduct in the blood. For instance citing the example used earlier, an increase in pyruvate in the blood occurs when there is insufficient thiamin for carbohydrate metabolism to proceed normally. The presence of abnormal metabolic substances or abnormal amounts of certain products can be an indicator of an inadequacy.

Enzymes

Many nutrients are parts of enzyme systems and nutrient status may be assessed by measuring a coenzyme or the activity of an enzyme that requires the nutrient. To return to the initial example of a thiamin deficiency, the enzyme transketolase requires thiamin-containing coenzymes. If thiamin is deficient, enzyme activity is reduced. A reduced level of transketolase activity in red blood cells may indicate a deficiency of thiamin before metabolic changes or deficiency symptoms occur.

Functional Tests

Functional tests of nutrition status measure one or more physiologic processes that rely on a nutrient. Examples include determination of dark adaptation for vitamin A status or response to an injected antigen for protein status. Some functional tests are nonspecific, such as immune response; these tests may indicate general nutrition status, but do not allow identification of specific nutrient deficiencies.

Urine

The presence of nutrients or their metabolites in urine may be useful in assessing nutrition status. Urinary levels of many nutrients reflect dietary intakes. For example if an individual has adequate tissue levels of water-soluble vitamins, any intake in excess of the amount required for body turnover is excreted in the urine. If tissue levels are low, a larger portion of dietary intake is retained in the body and urinary excretion is proportionately less, suggesting a potential deficiency.

The presence of substances not normally excreted in the urine can be an indicator of decreasing levels of a nutrient in the body. For example folate- and vitamin B_{12}-containing coenzymes are required for the conversion of homocysteine to the amino acid methionine. If either vitamin is absent, metabolism is blocked, and homocysteine increases in the urine. An increase in its presence suggests a possible vitamin deficiency.

Somatic Protein

Illness, trauma, and stress result in a number of metabolic (catabolic) responses that result in breakdown of muscle protein. Coupled with malnutrition, such stresses can rapidly deplete protein reserves. Therefore protein status is a primary concern in nutrition assessment. Midarm muscle circumference and muscle area have been described as indicators of somatic protein status. Urinary products of protein metabolism or muscle metabolism have also been considered markers of protein status. These include urinary nitrogen, 3-methylhistidine in the urine, and urinary creatinine. Body protein is approximately 16% nitrogen. The amount of nitrogen excreted in the urine in a 24-hour period could be compared with dietary intake to estimate protein balance. The urinary excretion of the amino acid 3-methylhistidine is considered a marker of protein metabolism because the amino acid is found only in the proteins actin and myosin of muscle. During normal metabolism the amount of 3-methylhistidine excreted in the urine is related to protein mass. For each of these measures a 24-hour urine collection is required.

Urinary Creatinine

Creatinine is the urinary metabolite of the catabolism of creatine, a compound found almost exclusively in muscle that stores high-energy creatine phosphate for muscle contraction. The amount of creatinine excreted by a healthy adult in a 24-hour period is a relatively constant proportion of muscle mass (Keshaviah et al., 1994). Therefore muscle protein mass can be estimated by measuring the amount of creatinine excreted and comparing that amount to a population-based standard.

Table 2-4 gives creatinine excretion levels by height, frame size, and reference weight for men and women. Urinary creatinine excretion is expressed as the creatinine height index (CHI), which is a percentage of the standard.

Table 2-4 Standards for Creatinine Height Index

MEN

Height		Small Frame		Medium Frame		Large Frame	
in	cm	Reference Weight (kg)	Creatinine (mg/24 h)	Reference Weight (kg)	Creatinine (mg/24 h)	Reference Weight (kg)	Creatinine (mg/24 h)
61	154.9	52.7	1212	56.1	1290	60.7	1396
62	157.5	54.1	1244	57.7	1327	62.0	1426
63	160.0	55.4	1274	59.1	1359	63.6	1463
64	162.5	56.8	1306	60.4	1389	65.2	1500
65	165.1	58.4	1343	62.0	1426	66.8	1536
66	167.6	60.2	1385	63.9	1470	68.9	1585
67	170.2	62.0	1426	65.9	1516	71.1	1635
68	172.7	63.9	1470	67.7	1557	72.9	1677
69	175.3	65.9	1516	69.5	1598	74.8	1720
70	177.8	67.7	1557	71.6	1647	76.8	1766
71	180.3	69.5	1599	73.6	1693	79.1	1819
72	182.9	71.4	1642	75.7	1741	81.1	1865
73	185.4	73.4	1688	77.7	1787	83.4	1918
74	187.9	75.2	1730	80.0	1846	85.7	1971
75	190.5	77.0	1771	82.3	1893	87.7	2017

WOMEN

Height		Small Frame		Medium Frame		Large Frame	
in	cm	Reference Weight (kg)	Creatinine (mg/24 h)	Reference Weight (kg)	Creatinine (mg/24 h)	Reference Weight (kg)	Creatinine (mg/24 h)
56	142.2	43.2	778	46.1	830	50.7	913
57	144.8	44.3	797	47.3	851	51.8	932
58	147.3	45.4	817	48.6	875	53.2	958
59	149.8	46.8	842	50.0	900	54.5	981
60	152.4	48.2	868	51.4	925	55.9	1006
61	154.9	49.5	891	52.7	949	57.3	1031
62	157.5	50.9	916	54.3	977	58.9	1060
63	160.0	52.3	941	55.9	1006	60.6	1091
64	162.5	53.9	970	57.9	1042	62.5	1125
65	165.1	55.7	1003	59.8	1076	64.3	1157
66	167.6	57.5	1035	61.6	1109	66.1	1190
67	170.2	59.3	1067	63.4	1141	67.9	1222
68	172.7	61.4	1105	65.2	1174	70.0	1260
69	175.2	63.2	1138	67.0	1206	72.0	1296
70	177.8	65.0	1170	68.9	1240	74.1	1334

From Grant A, DeHoog S: Nutritional assessment and support, ed 4, Northgate Station, Seattle, WA, 1991. Reprinted with permission.

Table 2-5 Plasma Proteins for Nutrition Assessment

	Normal Value (range)	Half-Life (days)	Function	Nutritional Significance
Albumin	35-55 g/L	18-20	Maintains plasma oncotic pressure; carrier for small molecules.	Large body pool is 4-5 g/kg body weight. Indicator of long-term protein status and decreased protein intake.
Transferrin	2.0-4.0 g/L	8-10	Binds and transports iron in plasma; accepts iron from sites of hemoglobin destruction, storage sites, and iron absorbed from intestine.	Body pool is <0.1 g/kg body weight. Compared to albumin, smaller body pool and shorter half-life; better index of changes in protein status. Levels increase with iron deficiency, pregnancy, and estrogen therapy.
Prealbumin	2.0-4.0 g/L or 90-400 mg/L	2-3	Binds thyroxine, carrier for retinol-binding protein (also referred to as thyroxine-binding prealbumin).	Body pool is 0.01 g/kg body weight. Better indicator of recent dietary intake than overall nutrition status.
Retinol-binding protein (RBP)	21-64 mg/L	8-12 h	Liver protein; transports vitamin A in plasma; binds to prealbumin.	Body pool is 0.002 g/kg body weight. Responds quickly to protein energy deprivation and nutrition intervention; better indicator of recent dietary intake than overall nutrition status.
Total lymphocyte count (TLC)	1500-4000 cells/mm^3	4-6	20-40% of total white blood cells. Part of antigen-specific defenses of the immune system.	Good indicator of general malnutrition. Declines early in protein energy deficiency. Responds to nutrition intervention.

CHI is calculated as follows:

$$\% \text{ CHI} = \text{actual urinary creatinine} / \text{reference urinary creatinine} \times 100$$

A CHI of 60% to 80% is considered a moderate deficit; less than 60% is considered a severe deficit of body muscle mass (Blackburn, 1997). As with all tests, however, the results must be interpreted carefully, because urinary creatinine can be influenced by diet, exercise, drugs, stress, and kidney function.

Visceral Protein

Visceral proteins are those in the plasma, extracellular fluids, and body organs (i.e., liver, kidney, heart, pancreas, and other organs). They make up approximately 10% of body protein. Several measurements of proteins in the plasma are considered reliable indicators of visceral protein status. However, these proteins have many functions, including transport or storage of nutrients, fluid balance, acid-base balance, and immune responses. Therefore laboratory tests have some limitations and their interpretation must be considered in the context of an individual's overall health status. Several serum proteins and a measure of immunocompetence, the TLC, are discussed in this section.

Plasma Proteins

Plasma proteins that are used to monitor nutrition status are selected because they reflect protein status, have a rapid rate of synthesis and a constant catabolic rate (Spiekerman, 1993), and are responsive to protein and energy restriction and repletion (Young et al., 1990). The liver is the major site for synthesis of serum proteins and one of the first organs to be affected by protein undernutrition.

Approximately 50% to 60% of the plasma protein is albumin. Low concentrations of serum albumin are associated with increased risk of morbidity and mortality in hospitalized patients (Herrman et al., 1992). The level of serum albumin has been used as an indicator of visceral protein status. Because it has a **half-life** of about 20 days and has a large extravascular pool that can return to the blood when concentration drops, it is not considered as sensitive an indicator of changes in protein status as other protein measurements have become available (Carlson, 2000).

Several other circulating proteins synthesized by the liver have a shorter half-life and are useful for nutrition assessment, including serum transferrin, prealbumin, and retinol-binding protein. Table 2-5 shows the normal range of plasma protein levels for adults. Lower levels are associated with protein deficiency. Interpretation of serum protein values requires knowledge of the diagnosis and general condition of the client because serum protein levels can be influenced by many factors, including liver disease, medication, stress, exercise, and infection.

Immune Proteins

The relationship between nutrition and immune function is complex. Undernutrition can lead to impaired immunocompetence and infection. Because changes in immune response occur early in nutrition deficiency, tests of immune function can be indicators for assessment of nutrition status and an index of response to nutrition intervention. The most common laboratory test is a complete blood count (CBC). It counts erythrocytes (red cells), leukocytes (white cells), and platelets. A differential count gives the percentage of different types of WBC in the sample. The normal differential for WBC is 20% to 40% lymphocytes, 50% to 70% neutrophils, 1% to 4% eosinophils, 0% to 4% basophils, and 2% to 8% monocytes. Lymphocytes have a relatively short half-life and can therefore reflect short-term changes in protein status. The TLC can be calculated using the total WBC count and differential by applying the following equation:

$$\text{TLC} = \text{Total WBC} \times \%\ \text{lymphocytes}/100$$

Normal values for TLC are found in Table 2-5. Such data must be interpreted with caution because TLC can be influenced by radiotherapy, surgery, immunosuppressive medication, viral infections, and some medications.

Iron Status

Iron deficiency is the most frequent nutritional deficiency worldwide and the most common cause of anemia. Several laboratory tests can be used to identify iron deficiency anemia (Worwood, 1997). Early stages are characterized by progressive reduction in the amount of stored iron as measured by serum ferritin. With iron depletion, iron stores decline, resulting in a reduced iron supply to cells and a decreased concentration of iron carried in transferrin (decreased transferrin saturation). The **total iron binding capacity (TIBC)** increases. Concentrations of protoporphyrin, a precursor of heme, increase in erythrocytes when the iron supply is inadequate for normal hemoglobin synthesis. The final stage, iron deficiency anemia, occurs with depletion of iron stores and declining levels of circulating iron. It is characterized by reduced concentration of hemoglobin, which impairs the ability of erythrocytes to carry oxygen to body cells. Laboratory tests used to assess iron status are described in Table 2-6.

Hemoglobin is probably the most widely used screening test for iron deficiency anemia, but the hemoglobin level does not decline until iron reserves are exhausted. Hence hemoglobin is

KEY TERMS

half-life: the time in which one half the concentration of a substance in the plasma is turned over

total iron binding capacity (TIBC): the amount of iron that can be taken up by transferrin; a high TIBC indicates that amount of iron bound to the protein is low

Table 2-6 Laboratory Measurements for Assessment of Iron Status

Laboratory Measurement	Normal Value	Nutritional Significance
Plasma or serum iron	100 ± 60 μg/L	A measurement of iron stores. Found primarily in liver, spleen, and bone marrow. Declines as iron stores become depleted.
Transferrin saturation (Total iron binding capacity)	35% ± 10%	Transferrin saturation indicates iron available to tissues. Declines as iron deficiency progresses. Levels of <16% considered to be inadequate for erythropoesis.
Zinc protoporphyin (ZnPP)/erythrocyte protoprophyrin ratio	<80 μmol/mol	Protoporphyrin, a precursor of heme, becomes bound to zinc when iron is limited, as in iron deficiency.
Hemoglobin	Males 14-18 g/dL Females 12-16 g/dL	Index of the blood's oxygen-carrying capacity; does not decline until advanced stages of iron deficiency.
Hematocrit	Males 40%-54% Females 38%-46%	Percentage of cells that make up the total volume of blood; largely dependent on the number of RBCs.

diagnostic of deficiency, but not predictive of impending deficiency. Interpretation of hemoglobin levels is limited by variations in age, sex, race, and cigarette smoking. Decreased levels occur with deficiencies of vitamin B_{12} and folate and protein energy malnutrition. Levels also decline in response to chronic infection, inflammation, and hemorrhage. Changes in hematocrit levels in iron deficiency tend to parallel those of hemoglobin.

CLINICAL ASSESSMENT

- *At what stage are clinical signs appropriate for nutrition assessment?*
- *What are the limitations of using clinical observations in nutrition assessment?*
- *What is the nutrition-focused physical examination?*

Clinical evaluation for evidence of malnutrition consists of a medical history and a nutrition-focused physical examination. Clinical observation is useful only for the overt signs of the most advanced stages of malnutrition, after depletion of body stores. Consequently its usefulness is limited in identifying impending nutrition problems.

Clinical assessment is the most subjective of the nutrition-assessment measures. Accurate clinical assessment requires a trained, skilled observer to detect physical signs and interpret symptoms reported by the client that are indicative of malnutrition. Physical signs of malnutrition appear most quickly in tissues that turnover rapidly, such as skin and the tissues of the digestive tract. The most commonly observed tissues are superficial epithelial tissues, especially skin, eyes, hair, mucous membranes, teeth, and tongue. Critical physical signs and symptoms of nutritional deficiency are nonspecific and must be interpreted in conjunction with laboratory, anthropometric, and dietary data. Some of the physical signs of undernutrition are summarized in Table 2-7.

Awareness of the importance of nutrition in hospitalized patients has increased emphasis on a subjective global clinical assessment, emphasizing nutrition measures that can predict outcome in seriously ill patients (Jeejeebhoy, 1998). The more complete nutrition-focused physical examination uses a systems approach in performing an organized physical examination. Subjective global assessment classifications can aid in recognition of undernutrition based on the medical history and physical examination. More recently protocols for subjective global nutrition assessment have been developed for use in extended-care

Table 2-7 Clinical Signs Associated with Malnutrition

Body System/Normal Appearance	Clinical Finding	Possible Deficiency
HAIR		
Shiny; firm in the scalp	Lack of natural shine; dull and dry; sparse; loss of color; pluckable	PEM*
FACE		
Skin color uniform; smooth, healthy appearance	Pallor; dark skin over cheeks and under eyes; flakiness of skin of nose and mouth; swollen face; enlarged parotid glands; flaky dermatitis	PEM, vitamin A, vitamin B_{12}, iron folate
EYES		
Bright, clear, shiny; no sores at corners; membrane pink and moist	Membranes pale; night blindness; Bitot's spots (dull, dry lesions on conjunctiva); redness and fissuring of eyelid corners; dryness of eye membranes; cornea is dull and soft	Iron, vitamin A, riboflavin, vitamin B_6
LIPS		
Smooth, not chapped or swollen	Swelling of mouth or lips; lesions at corners of the mouth (cheilosis)	Niacin, riboflavin, protein, vitamin B_6, iron
TONGUE		
Deep reddish in appearance; surface papillae present	Swelling; scarlet and raw; purplish color; smooth; swollen sores	Vitamin B_6, niacin, iron, vitamin B_{12}, folate, riboflavin
TEETH		
No cavities; no pain	Missing teeth; gray or black spots (fluorosis); decay; unfilled cavities	Fluoride, poor dietary habits, poor oral hygiene (excess fluoride)
GUMS		
Healthy, red; do not bleed; not swollen	"Spongy," pale, bleed easily; receding	Vitamin C

Modified from Walker WW, Hendricks KM: Manual of pediatric nutrition, Philadelphia, 1985, WB Saunders.
*PEM 5 Protein-energy malnutrition.

Continued

environments (Gordon et al., 2000) and home-care services (Hammond, 1997). What is included in a subjective global assessment varies depending on the client, the setting, and the level of care. Figure 2-12 is an example of a nutrition-oriented subjective global assessment form used in a long-term care environment.

DIETARY INTAKE

- *Describe the techniques that can be used to estimate current or typical dietary intake.*
- *How is information regarding dietary intake interpreted and used?*
- *What are the limitations of using dietary information for assessment?*

Table 2-7 Clinical Signs Associated with Malnutrition—cont'd

Body System/Normal Appearance	Clinical Finding	Possible Deficiency
SKIN		
Smooth, firm; no rashes or spots	Dry, rough (xerosis); flakiness; sores; red swollen pigmentation of light-exposed areas; black and blue marks due to skin bleeding; scaling	Essential fatty acid, vitamin A, protein, vitamin C, vitamin K, niacin
NAILS		
Firm, pink	Nails are spoon-shaped (koilonychia); brittle, ridged	Iron
GLANDS		
Face and neck not swollen	Thyroid enlargement; parotid enlargement	Iodine, PEM, bulimia
MUSCLE		
Good muscle tone and posture	Muscle wasting; pain; weakness; twitching; cramps	Potassium, sodium PEM, vitamin B_6, magnesium, thiamin
BONES AND JOINTS		
Bone development appropriate for age	Epiphyseal thickening; deformities; bone pain	Calcium, vitamin D, vitamin C
CARDIOVASCULAR		
Normal heart rate and rhythms, normal blood pressure for age	Rapid heart rate, enlarged heart; abnormal rhythm	PEM, potassium, thiamin, magnesium
GASTROINTESTINAL		
No palpable organs; normal digestion	Liver enlarged; spleen enlarged; abnormal digestion; wasting	PEM, iron, niacin
NERVOUS		
Psychologically stable; normal reflexes	Mental irritability, disorientation; burning and tingling of hands and feet; loss of position and vibratory sense; weakness and tenderness of muscles; loss of ankle and knee reflexes	Thiamin, vitamin B_6, vitamin B_{12}, niacin

Modified from Walker WW, Hendricks KM: Manual of pediatric nutrition, Philadelphia, 1985, WB Saunders.
*PEM = Protein-energy malnutrition.

Reliable information about energy and nutrient intake is important in making an accurate nutritional assessment and planning intervention. As illustrated in the earlier description of the development of a thiamin deficiency, knowing how much of a nutrient an individual has eaten can contribute to identifying the potential for a deficiency. In advanced stages of deficiency, information about a person's dietary intake can suggest or confirm the cause of biochemical abnormalities or physical changes. Knowledge of food intake also helps plan nutrition care, counseling, and education.

Dietary intake data for large groups of people are important considerations in the development of dietary guidance in the Dietary

MEDICAL HISTORY	SGA Rating A	B	C
1. **Weight Change** Clothing Size _____ No Change _____ Change Overall loss in past month: _____ _____ 6 months _____ 1 year			
% Loss of usual weight _____ <5% _____ 5-10% _____ >10%			
Change in past 2 weeks _____ Increase (*gain*) _____ No change (*stabilization*) _____ Decrease (*continued loss*)			
2. **Dietary Intake** Reduction _____ Unintentional _____ Intentional Overall Change _____ No Change _____ Change Increase or Decrease			
Duration _____ Weeks _____ Months			
Diet change _____ Suboptimal solids (i.e., 75%, 50%, 25% intake) _____ Full liquid diet _____ Hypocaloric fluids _____ NPO (*starvation*)			
3. **Gastrointestinal Symptoms** (*persisting daily for >2 weeks*) _____ None _____ Diarrhea _____ Dysphagia/Odynaphagia _____ Nausea _____ Vomiting _____ Anorexia			
4. **Functional Impairment** Overall impairment _____ None _____ Mild _____ Severe			
Duration _____ Days _____ Weeks _____ Months			
Type _____ Ambulatory (Walking or Wheelchair) _____ Bedridden			

PHYSICAL EXAMINATION	SGA Rating Well (A)	Mild/Mod (B)	Severe (C)
5. **Muscle Wasting** _____ Bicep _____ Tricep _____ Quadricep _____ Deltoid _____ Temple			
6. **Subcutaneous Fat Loss** _____ Tricep _____ Chest _____ Eyes _____ Perioral _____ Interosseous _____ Palmar			
7. **Edema** _____ Hands _____ Sacral _____ Lower extremity			

(A) Well Nourished _____ **(B) Mild/Moderate Undernutrition** _____ **(C) Severe Undernutrition** _____

Figure **2-12** An example of an evaluation form for subjective global assessment. *(From Sacks GS et al: Use of subjective global assessment to identify nutrition-associated complications and death in geriatric long-term care facility residents, J Am Coll Nutr 19:570, 2000.)*

Reference Intakes (DRIs) and the Dietary Guidelines for Americans. Assessing the adequacy of energy and nutrient levels involves careful and complete collection of dietary intake data and an evaluation of the nutrient content using food group systems, tables of food composition, or computerized nutrient analysis programs.

Collecting Dietary Information

Information about food intake of groups or individuals can be obtained using one of several basic methods (Block et al., 1994; Briefel et al., 1997; Medlin and Skinner, 1988). Selection of an appropriate technique is guided by the purpose of the assessment and available resources, including time, personnel, and funds. Information may be confirmed or expanded using more than one tool or combination of tools. As with anthropometric measures, validity and reliability of dietary assessment tools are essential considerations (Kubena, 2000). Techniques for collecting dietary information involve having individuals record or remember their food intake (dietary history, 24-hour recall, and food frequency questionnaire).

Reliability of all these methods has been reviewed to determine if each method can provide the same estimate on different occasions (Johnson, 2000). Reviews of their reliability have included comparisons of repeated measures, comparisons of record or recall to observed intake, and comparisons of measures over time (Howat et al., 1994). These tests have discovered some limitations of tools for measurement of dietary intake from failure to get complete and accurate information. The errors are from inaccuracy caused by memory lapses of the individual, inability to judge portion sizes, failure to record foods faithfully, changes in food intake to simplify recording, decisions not to eat or record foods that might be considered unhealthy, or failure to record foods that were eaten in excessive amounts (Beaton et al., 1997).

Validity in the measurement of what people eat has been hampered by the lack of appropriate reference points reflecting intake. Because of the inherent limitations of self-reported dietary data, researchers have investigated biomarkers to confirm or validate dietary intake. For example total urinary nitrogen can be a marker for total protein intake. For several decades it has been recognized that risk of some cancers is inversely related to fruit and vegetable consumption. Consumption of green and yellow vegetables and dark yellow fruits can now be confirmed by measurement of increased levels of beta carotene in the blood as a biomarker of intake (Gerber et al., 2000).

Awareness of the underreporting of energy intake has resulted from studies comparing reported energy intake levels with maintenance of body weight across long-term studies and from comparisons of reported intake to prediction equations for energy expenditure (Johnson et al., 1998). The best documented finding of the information confirming underreporting of energy intake has come from studies using **doubly labeled water.** Measurements of doubly labeled water are expensive and may have limited practicality for routine assessment. Other biomarkers to confirm dietary reports of intake of specific nutrients are under investigation, but many may prove too expensive to be practical (Kubena, 2000).

Many techniques and tools can be used to estimate energy and nutrient intakes. Commonly used dietary evaluation techniques are described here.

Dietary History

Information about a person's food habits may be obtained from a comprehensive interview conducted by an RD. Information gathered in the diet or nutrition history includes not only the types and amounts of foods typically consumed, but also patterns of intake, use of supplements and alcohol, and relevant information about personal, psychosocial, and economic factors that influence food intake. Although the dietary interview is time-consuming and requires a skilled professional to obtain accurate information, it provides information about usual intake patterns that is essential in planning dietary changes. The process can be expedited by having the client complete a food frequency questionnaire or 24-hour dietary recall in advance of the personal interview.

Twenty-Four Hour Recall

The 24-hour dietary recall is more rapid and less expensive than the diet history. Clients are asked to recall the specific foods and amounts they have consumed during the previous 24-hour period. Forms or questions may be structured to obtain a complete description of intake. Photographs, food models, and measuring utensils can help the client judge the amounts of foods consumed. This method is not suitable for individuals who have difficulty remembering or estimating portion sizes.

Food Records

Carefully completed food records provide sufficiently detailed information for an analysis of energy and nutrient intake. The client is instructed in how to measure and record the food items he or she has eaten. Food records are usually kept for 2 to 7 days. The number of days needed to provide reliable information for nutrient analysis varies with the nutrient studied, but a minimum appears to be 3 days (Basiotis et al., 1987; Schlundt, 1988).

Food Frequency Questionnaire

The food frequency questionnaire can provide information about an individual's food intake over a specified time. It consists of a list of foods and a scale indicating the frequency of consumption of that food over a given period such as a week or month. An abbreviated food frequency checklist appears in Appendix B. A food frequency report is particularly useful when specific food items or groups that provide the nutrient of interest, such as fat, calcium, or vitamin A, can be identified (Briefel et al., 1992). The food frequency questionnaire has been used extensively in epidemiologic surveys to investigate potential relationships between specific nutrients and disease incidence or risk (Roidt et al., 1988).

Interpretation of Dietary Information

The limitations of self-reported dietary intake information have been recognized and crosschecks or a combination of methods are often used to obtain more representative data. Data obtained using the dietary methods previously described can be very useful in assessing nutrition status and planning nutrition care. The information they provide about food intake can be interpreted using several guides or standards, including food groups, the Dietary Guidelines, or DRIs. A quick, general evaluation of food intake data can be made by comparing the foods and number of servings with a food group plan. The simplest and most frequently used system is the five groups of the Food Guide Pyramid (Figure 2-13). A comparison of dietary intake to recommended amounts in food groups can identify potential inadequacies of protein, iron, calcium, riboflavin, and vitamins A and C, but is limited in estimating energy and other nutrients.

If the information provided on dietary intake is complete and accurate, a more precise evaluation can be made by determining the quantities of nutrients in the food consumed. Energy and nutrient levels can be determined using one of several computerized nutrient analysis programs available. (A sample printout of a nutrient analysis appears in Table 2-11 at the end of this chapter.)

Standards for Evaluation of Nutrient Intake

The Healthy Eating Index (HEI) is a summary measure of an individual's overall diet quality on a scale from 0 to 100 based on 10 components (Bowman et al., 1998) (Table 2-8). Measurements of five components determine the degree to which a person's diet conforms to the Food Guide Pyramid recommendations for the major food groups: grains, vegetables, fruits, milk, and meat and beans. Four components measure compliance with recommendations for total fat, saturated fat, cholesterol, and sodium consumption.

KEY TERMS

doubly labeled water: a method of measuring total energy expenditure in free-living individuals that uses two stable isotopes of water, oxygen-18 and deuterium; based on the difference in the turnover rates in urinary elimination of these isotope measures, CO_2 production is measured, from which energy production can be calculated

Food Consumed (Mixed foods will count in more than 1 group)	Food Group				
	Milk	Meat	Vegetables	Fruit	Grains
Total Servings					
Minimum Recommended Servings	2	2	3	2	6

Assessment:

Figure 2-13 Food group evaluation chart using the Food Guide Pyramid.

The final component measures the extent of variety in the diet, measured by the number of different foods eaten in a quantity that contributes at least one-half serving. The HEI was used to assess the dietary status of Americans using food consumption data from the USDA's Continuing Survey of Food Intake of Individuals in 1994 (Bowman et al., 1998). The overall score was 63.8. An HEI score greater than 80 implies a "good" diet, an HEI score between 51 and 80 implies a diet that "needs improvement," and a score less than 51 implies a "poor" diet.

Table 2-8 COMPONENTS OF THE HEALTHY EATING INDEX

Component	Score Ranges	Criteria for Minimum Score of 10
1. Grain consumption	0-10 points	9 servings*
2. Vegetable consumption	0-10 points	4 servings
3. Fruit consumption	0-10 points	3 servings
4. Milk consumption	0-10 points	2 servings
5. Meat consumption	0-10 points	2.4 servings
6. Total fat intake	0-10 points	<30% of energy from fat
7. Saturated fat intake	0-10 points	<10% of energy from saturated fat
8. Cholesterol intake	0-10 points	<300 mg
9. Sodium intake	0-10 points	<2400 mg
10. Food variety	010 points	8 different items in a day

From The Healthy Eating Index, 1994-1996. Center for Nutrition Policy and Promotion, USDA, 2000.
*Number of servings will depend on the Recommended Energy Allowance. The table assumes 2200 kcal/day as recommended for women 25 to 50 years of age.

One of the stated purposes for the DRIs is planning and assessing diets for healthy people (Institute of Medicine, 1998) (see Chapter 1, page 19 to 24). The Recommended Dietary Allowance (RDA), or average daily intake level that is sufficient to meet nutrient requirements for nearly all healthy people, and the Adequate Intake (AI), a recommended daily intake value based on an observed or experimentally determined approximation of nutrient intake by a group of healthy people, are recommendations for individual intake. The RDAs are based on the Estimated Average Requirement (the level of intake below which a deficiency would occur) plus a coefficient of variation. Therefore diets below the RDA are not necessarily deficient, but do fall below an accepted standard for health. Such a comparison must be interpreted with discretion. In addition the RDAs and AIs are formulated for most healthy individuals and may not be appropriate for individuals with stress, disease, or illness.

The RDAs for energy and protein are based on body size. In assessment of dietary intakes, energy and protein adequacy should be evaluated on the basis of actual body weight, if it is within acceptable limits, or reference weight. This is particularly important for both overweight and underweight adults and for children, who, at any particular age, may vary widely in size and in energy and protein needs.

A number of tools can be used to screen and assess individuals for malnutrition. It is important that the measurement reflect nutrition status, be accurate and reliable, and be completed in a timely fashion. Most assessments use more than one tool to identify individuals at risk. This chapter has emphasized this process in assessing undernutrition. The identification of risk for overnutrition will be discussed in subsequent chapters.

NUTRITION ASSESSMENT ACROSS THE LIFE SPAN

Throughout this chapter nutrition screening and assessment have been discussed in relation to adult needs. Standards for comparison are based on adult populations and the same techniques and principles are applied across the life span. Their application in growth and development, reproduction, and aging are discussed in individual chapters, with age- and sex-specific standards for evaluation.

Nutrition screening and assessment are important in formulating and providing nutrition guidance and care to all age groups, from infancy to old age. Each stage presents unique physiologic demands, social and psychologic factors, and health concerns that affect nutrition status. Some general characteristics of various stages of the life span and the measurements recommended for nutrition screening appear in Table 2-9.

Table 2-9 APPROPRIATE MEASUREMENTS FOR NUTRITION SCREENING ACROSS THE LIFE SPAN

		Measurements			
Stage	Characteristics	Anthropometry	Biochemical	Clinical	Dietary
Infancy	Birth weight, rapid growth and development	Weight/length, head circumference	Hemoglobin, hematocrit	Color; response to stimuli; overall growth rate	Bottle or breast-feeding, supplemental feedings; sources of iron, fluoride, vitamin D
Childhood	Slow, steady growth; increased physical activity; development of food habits; increased social interaction; skill development	Weight/height, arm circumference fatfolds	Hemoglobin, hematocrit	Skin color, texture, musculature; subcutaneous fat; oral cavity; overall growth rate	Food intake, appetite, feeding/snacking patterns, food jags, pica; food/nutrient supplements
Adolescence	Rapid growth and development, sexual maturation; increasing independence	Weight/height, changes in body composition, fatfolds	Hemoglobin, hematocrit	General appearance: hair, skin, eyes, musculature, body fat/patterns; oral cavity; secondary sex characteristics	Food intake, where and with whom; fad diets; snacking; nutrient supplements; substance use/abuse
Pregnancy	Weight gain/fetal growth and development; maternal physiologic changes	Prepregnancy weight, gestational weight gain	Hemoglobin, hematocrit, glucose tolerance test, protein in urine	General appearance; blood pressure; pattern of weight gain; edema	Appetite, food intake, pica, iron/folate intake; nausea, vomiting, heartburn, constipation; smoking, alcohol intake
Lactation	Milk production; maternal—infant bonding; weight loss; changes in body composition	Gestational weight gain, postpartum weight loss, current weight status	Hemoglobin, hematocrit	Appearance, hair, skin, eyes, muscle tone; weight changes	Energy and nutrient intake; breast-feeding/supplemental feedings; feeding difficulties
Adult	Stable weight or weight gain; decreased physical activity; increased risk for chronic disease; tendency to increase body fat	Weight for height; recent weight changes; fatfolds, abdominal/gluteal circumference ratio	Hemoglobin, hematocrit, blood glucose, blood lipid levels	General appearance, hair, skin, and eyes; blood pressure; dental health; weight history	Food intake, especially fat, saturated fat, sugar, fiber, calcium; snacking habits; nutrient supplements; alcohol intake; dieting patterns
Older Adult	Tendency to lose muscle mass, increase body fat; age-related physical changes; concerns about income/healthcare costs; increased incidence of chronic diseases and medication use	Weight for height, recent weight change, fatfolds	Hemoglobin, hematocrit, blood glucose, blood lipid levels	Skin color, pallor; dentition; blood pressure; physical changes	Food intake and patterns; nutrient supplements; ability to purchase/prepare food; changes in food habits; dietary restrictions

Modified from Davis J, Sherer K: Applied nutrition and diet therapy for nurses, ed 2, Philadelphia, 1994, WB Saunders.

Concepts to Remember

- The goal of nutrition screening is to identify individuals who may benefit from assessment and intervention.
- Nutrition assessment is a process or series of measurements used to identify individuals at nutritional risk.
- Nutrition assessment, the first step in the nutrition care process, forms the basis for planning and implementing nutrition care, providing counseling and education, and evaluating the effectiveness of intervention.
- Measurements selected for nutrition assessment must reflect body status and must be readily available at a cost that allows them to be repeated for monitoring the impact of intervention.
- Data used for nutrition assessment are based on anthropometric and biochemical measurements, clinical evaluation, and assessment of dietary intake and food patterns.
- Most individuals who are at nutrition risk have compromised energy and protein status. Nutrition assessment focuses on determination of the adequacy of energy and somatic and visceral protein status, but can be expanded to include other vitamins and minerals, especially iron.

REFERENCES

American Dietetic Association: ADA's definitions for nutrition screening and nutrition assessment, J Am Diet Assoc 94:838, 1994.

Anderson JV et al.: Five a day fruit and vegetable intervention improves consumption in a low income population, J Am Diet Assoc 101:195, 2001.

Basiotis PP et al.: Number of days of food intake records required to estimate individual and group nutient intakes with defined confidence, J Nutr 117:1138, 1987.

Beaton GH et al.: Errors in the interpretation of dietary assessments, Am J Clin Nutr 65:1100S, 1997.

Blackburn GL et al.: Nutritional and metabolic assessment of the hospitalized patient, JEPN 1:11, 1997.

Block GL et al.: Validation study of two food frequency questionnaires with WIC women and children, Am J Public Health 84:53, 1994.

Bowman SA et al.: The healthy eating index, 1994-1996, Fam Econ Nutr Rev 11:2-14, 1998.

Briefel RR et al.: Assessing the nation's diet: limitations of the food frequency questionnaire, J Am Diet Assoc 92:959, 1992.

Briefel RR et al.: Dietary methods research in the Third National Health and Examination Survey: underreporting intakes, Am J Clin Nutr 65:1203S, 1997.

Carlson T: Laboratory data in nutrition assessment. In Mahan LK and Escott-Stump S, editors: Krause's food, nutrition & diet therapy, Philadelphia, 2000, WB Saunders.

Durnin JVGA and Womersley J: Body fat assessed from total body density and its estimation from skinfold thickness: measurements on 481 men and women aged from 16 to 72 years, Br J Nutr 32:77, 1974.

Frisancho AR: Anthropometric standards for the assessment of growth and nutritional status, Ann Arbor, MI, 1990, University of Michigan Press.

Frisancho AR and Flegel PN: Elbow breadth as a measure of frame size for U.S. males and females, Am J Clin Nutr 37:311, 1983.

Gerber M et al.: Profiles of a healthful diet and its relationship to biomarkers in a population from Mediterranean Southern France, J Am Diet Assoc 100:164, 2000.

Gordon SS et al.: Use of subjective global assessment to identify nutrition-associated complications and death in geriatric long-term care facility residents, J Am Coll Nutr 19:570, 2000.

Gray DS et al.: Skinfold thickness measurements in obese subjects, Am J Clin Nutr 51:571, 1990.

Hammond KA: Physical assessment: a nutritional perspective, Nurs Clin North Am 32:779, 1997.

Hensrud DD: Nutrition screening and assessment, Med Clin North Am 83:1525, 1999.

Herrman FR et al.: Serum albumin level on admission as a predictor of death, length of stay and readmission, Arch Intern Med 152:125, 1992.

Heymsfield SB et al.: Anthropometric measurement of muscle mass: revised equations for calculating bone-free arm muscle area, Am J Clin Nutr 36:680, 1982.

Himes JH and Bouchard C: Do the new Metropolitan Life Insurance weight-height tables correctly assess body form and body fat relationships?, Am J Public Health 75:1067, 1985.

Howat PM et al.: Validity and reliability of reported dietary intake data, J Am Diet Assoc 94:2, 1994.

Institute of Medicine: Dietary reference intakes for thiamin, riboflavin, niacin, vitamin B_6, folate, vitamin B_{12}, pantothenic acid, biotin, and choline, Washington, DC, 1998, National Academy Press.

Jackson AS and Pollock ML: Practical body composition, Phy Sport Med 13:76, 1985.

Jeejeebhoy KN: Nutritional assessment, Gastroenterol Clin North Am 27:361, 1998.

Johnson RK: What are people really eating and why does it matter?, Nutr Today 35:4, 2000.

Johnson RK et al.: Literacy and body fatness are associated with underreporting of energy intake in U.S. low-income women using the multiple-pass, 24-hour recall: a doubly labeled water study, J Am Diet Assoc 98:1136, 1998.

Joint Commission on Accreditation of Healthcare Organizations: Comprehensive accreditation manual for hospitals: the official handbook, Oakbrook Terrace, IL, 1998, Joint Commission on Accreditation of Healthcare Organizations.

Kannel WB et al.: Regional obesity and risk of cardiovascular disease: the Framingham study, J Clin Epidemiol 44:183, 1991.

Keshaviah PR et al.: Lean body mass estimation by creatinine kinetics, J Am Soc Nephrol 4:1475, 1994.

Kubena KS: Accuracy in dietary assessment: on the road to good science, J Am Diet Assoc 00:775, 2000.

Kuczmarski MF et al.: Effects of age on validity of self-reported height, weight and body mass index: findings from the third National Health and Nutrition Examination Survey, 1988-1994, J Am Diet Assoc 101:28, 2001.

Lohman TG et al.: Anthropometric standardization reference manual, Champaign, IL, 1988, Human Kinetics Books.

Medlin C and Skinner JD: Individual dietary intake methodology: a 50-year review of progress, J Am Diet Assoc 88:1250, 1988.

Metropolitan Life Insurance Company: Metropolitan height and weight tables, Statistical bulletin of the Metropolitan Life Insurance Company, 64(Jan-Jun):3, 1983.

Micozzi MS et al.: Correlations of body mass indices with weight, stature, and body composition in men and women in NHANES I and II, Am J Clin Nutr 44:725, 1986.

Mitchell MC: Frame size in older adults: a comparison of four measurements, J Am Diet Assoc 93:53, 1993.

National Institutes of Health, National Heart Lung and Blood Institute: Clinical guidelines on the identification, and treatment of overweight and obesity in adults—the evidence report, NIH Publication NO 98-4082, Bethesda, MD, 1998, National Institutes of Diabetes and Digestive and Kidney Diseases, 6:515, 1998.

Revicki DA and Israel RG: Relationship between body mass indices and measures of body adiposity, Am J Clin Nutr 76:992, 1986.

Roidt L et al.: Association of food frequency questionnaire estimates of vitamin A intake with serum vitamin A levels, Am J Epidemiol 128:645, 1988.

Schapira DV et al.: Upper-body fat distribution and endometrial cancer risk, JAMA 266:1808, 1991.

Schlundt DG: Accuracy and reliability of nutrient intake estimates, J Nutr 118:1432, 1988.

Schwartz DB and Gudzin D: Preadmission nutrition screening: expanding hospital-based nutrition services by implementing earlier nutrition intervention, J Am Diet Assoc 100:81, 2000.

Smalley KJ et al.: Reassessment of body mass indices, Am J Clin Nutr 52:405, 1990.

Spiekerman AM: Proteins used in nutritional assessment, Clin Lab Med 13:353, 1993.

Worwood M: Laboratory assessment of iron status—an update, Clin Chim Actat 259:3, 1997.

Young VR et al.: Assessment of protein nutritional status, J Nutr 120:1469, 1990.

ADDITIONAL RESOURCES

Gibson RS: Principles of nutritional assessment, New York, 1990, Oxford University Press.

Lee RD and Nieman DC: Nutritional assessment, St. Louis, 1996, Mosby.

Simko MD et al.: Nutrition assessment: a comprehensive guide for planning intervention, ed 2, Gaithersburg, MD, 1995, Aspen.

APPLICATION

A Case for Nutrition Assessment

Information from anthropometric, biochemical, clinical, and dietary measurements or observations described in this chapter can be used to develop a profile of the nutrition status of an individual. This application is designed to demonstrate the following:

- The use of anthropometric, biochemical, clinical, and dietary information to evaluate the nutritional status of an individual
- The use of the nutritional assessment as a basis for recommendations to improve nutritional status

THE CASE

Katherine is a 22-year-old graduate student who was admitted to the hospital following a skiing accident. She was alert and in some pain, but her only obvious injury was a broken ankle. Her ankle was placed in a cast and she was given some medication for pain before discharge. Because of her general appearance and low body weight, an appointment was made for a nutritional evaluation in the outpatient clinic the following week. She was told not to eat before coming to the appointment and was instructed to bring a 24-hour urine sample.

When Katherine arrived in the clinic a blood sample was drawn and sent to the laboratory for analyses, she was weighed and measured, a physician completed a physical examination, and the RD conducted a dietary interview.

ANTHROPOMETRY

Height: 168 cm (5′6″)
Weight: 47.7 kg (105 lbs)
(weight 6 months ago was 59.1 kg)
MAC: 21.2 cm
TFF: 10.5 mm (1.05 cm)
SSFF: 7.4 mm (0.74 cm)
Elbow breadth: 69.9 mm (2¾ in)

BIOCHEMICAL (LABORATORY) FINDINGS

Hemoglobin: 100 g/L
Hematocrit: 0.32 or 32%
Prealbumin: 155 mg/L
WBC: 4000 mm^3
Differential: lymphocytes 25%

CLINICAL EVALUATION

Katherine's medical history revealed that she had a broken arm at age 10 and an appendectomy at age 15. Her mother has diabetes mellitus. A summary of Katherine's physical examination follows: patient appears to be pale and underweight with limited musculature and fat. Her hair is dull and skin is dry, scaling, and rough. All other parameters appear to be normal.

Dietary Intake

The dietary history completed by the dietitian revealed the following facts. Katherine lives with a roommate in a small apartment off campus. Her basic income is a monthly stipend as a graduate teaching associate, but she earns a small amount tutoring part time. She maintains that she doesn't have enough money to buy adequate amounts of food and that she is too busy to eat. She does not like to cook and is not particularly interested in food. Her typical weekday intake is usually obtained from a cafeteria on campus or a nearby fast-food restaurant.

TYPICAL WEEKLY INTAKE

7 AM: black coffee
10 AM: black coffee plus a donut or muffin
Noon: sandwich (hamburger or ham); French fries or potato chips; diet cola or iced tea with lemon
Afternoon: coffee or diet cola
6 PM: 2 cups mixed green salad of lettuce, spinach, and endive; l oz cheese; one hard-cooked egg; fat-free dressing; 6 to 8 saltines or a roll (no butter or margarine)
8 to 11 PM: several diet colas

Weekends are different in that Katherine sleeps in and does not eat until noon. Lunch is often a sandwich, as indicated, or a very late breakfast with sausage, eggs, and toast or bacon and waffles. She denies consuming alcoholic beverages and takes no medication except an occasional aspirin. She denies taking any vitamin or mineral supplements or dietary supplements. Her food preferences are for sandwiches with mustard only—no lettuce or tomato. She will eat green salads, but does not drink milk and maintains that she cannot afford fruit or fruit juices.

Assessment

Because the results from laboratory data are not usually available immediately, assessment, planning, and intervention counseling are likely to involve two or more sessions. In a counseling session the dietitian uses dietary information and other assessment data as the basis for planning and implementing intervention. The process of implementing dietary change is discussed in Chapter 3. In this application the anthropometric, biochemical, clinical, and dietary information obtained from Katherine are used to evaluate energy, visceral and somatic protein status, and to consider vitamin and mineral status.

A Reminder: *The following information is available related to the compartments to be studied:*

- *Energy reserves: indirect estimate from weight for height or fatfolds*
- *Visceral protein: serum albumin, serum, transferrin, and TLC*
- *Somatic protein: MAC with TFF to estimate midarm muscle circumference and midarm muscle area*
- *Iron status: serum transferrin, hemoglobin, and hematocrit*
- *Confirming and supporting information provided by dietary intake data and clinical signs*

Body Energy Reserves

Body energy reserves can be assessed indirectly using body weight or weight for height; in this case it can be calculated from percent of usual body weight, MRW, or BMI. To use the Metropolitan Height and Weight Table (Appendix B), frame size must be determined. An elbow breadth of 69.6 mm (2¾ in) indicates a "large" frame size. For a woman of large frame size who is 168 cm (5'6" or 5'7" with the 1-inch heels assumed in the chart), a reference weight range is 133 to 147 lb. Using 140, the midpoint of that range, the dietitian can calculate the MRW.

% Usual Body Weight = current weight/previous weight
= 105/130 lb
= 81% of usual weight (6 months ago)

MRW = 105/140 = 75%

BMI = $47.7/1.68^2$ = 16.9

Calculation of the BMI reveals that Katherine would be categorized as underweight.

Fatfolds. Body fat reserves can be assessed by comparing Katherine's fatfold values to those from a reference population. Consulting Appendix B reveals that Katherine's TFF of 10.5 mm is equal to the fifth percentile value. Her SSFF is 7.4, which is below the tenth percentile value of 6.5 mm.

Energy Intake. A typical daily intake determined from Katherine's dietary history can be used to estimate caloric intake. The dietitian's quick estimation was that Katherine's energy intake ranged from 1000 to 1400 kcal. For their next session she will have a printout of the computerized diet analysis to share with Katherine. The computer printout reveals that for a typical day, Katherine consumed 1008 kcal, a level well below the recommended for her age and body size (Table 2-10).

Somatic Protein

Katherine's MAC (21.2) and TFF (1.05 cm) are used to determine midarm muscle circumference. A comparison of 18.2 cm to reference values from NHANES data given in Appendix B reveals that her value is equal to the fifth percentile for her age and sex.

MAMC = MAC − π × TFF

Table 2-10 COMPUTERIZED SUMMARY OF CALORIES AND NUTRIENTS IN A TYPICAL DIET FOR KATHERINE

Analysis: Untitled % RDA: Katherine Cost:			Wgt: 3146 g (111 oz.) Water: 93%		
Calories	1008	56%	Folate	196 μg	109%
Protein	37.2 g	98%	Pantothenic	2.14 mg	31%
Carbohydrates	113 g	43%	Vitamin C	20.8 mg	35%
Fat—Total	46.3 g	77%	Vitamin D	.927 μg	9%
Saturated Fat	16.1 g	80%	Vit E-Alpha E	3.91 mg	49%
Mono Fat	14 g	70%	Calcium	488 mg	41%
Poly Fat	12.3 g	61%	Copper	.536 mg	21%
Omega 3 FA	.969 g	—	Iron	8.06 mg	54%
Omega 6 FA	11.3 g	—	Magnesium	154 mg	55%
Cholesterol	306 mg	102%	Manganese	2.09 mg	60%
Dietary Fiber	5.54 g	31%	Phosphorus	723 mg	60%
Total Vit A	453 RE*	57%	Potassium	1971 mg	99%
A—Retinol	184 RE	—	Selenium	55.9 μg	102%
A—Carotenoid	269 RE	—	Sodium	2201 mg	92%
Thiamin-B_1	.725 mg	80%	Zinc	4.98 mg	42%
Riboflavin-B_2	1.04 mg	95%	Complex Carbs	79 g	—
Niacin-B_3	11.5 mg	96%	Sugars	28.7 g	—
Niacin Equiv.	11.5 mg	96%	Alcohol	0 g	—
Vitamin B_6	.463 mg	29%	Caffeine	604 mg	—
Vitamin B_{12}	1.69 μg	84%	Water	2936 g	—

*RE = retinol equivalents.

Midarm muscle area is calculated from the MAMC. Comparison of this value with Appendix B reveals that Katherine's MAMA is well below the fifth percentile level, suggesting low somatic protein status.

MAMC = MAC − π × TFF
MAMC = 18.2

$$\text{MAMA} = \frac{\text{MAMC}^2}{4\pi} - 6.5$$

$$\text{MAMA} = \frac{18.2^2}{12.56} = 26.3\text{ cm}$$

263 mm − 6.5
= 256.5

Visceral Protein

Comparison of Katherine's level of 155 mg/L for prealbumin to values shown in Table 2-5 indicates levels below the normal range, suggesting moderate depletion of visceral protein. Another indicator, the TLC, can be determined from the total white cell count and the percentage of lymphocytes. According to Table 2-5, such a level is below normal values, suggesting malnutrition. Katherine's typical daily intake of protein is near or only slightly below the recommendation.

TLC = WBC × % lymphocytes/100
4000 × 25/100 = 1000

Vitamin and Mineral Status

Katherine's levels of hemoglobin (100 g/L) and hematocrit (32%) are in the deficient range. Although she does consume beef or pork and an egg on a regular basis and some dark green leafy vegetables, the actual amount of iron consumed in the absence of other dietary sources is low. Evaluation of the dietary intake in comparison to the Food Guide Pyramid (see Figure 2-13) reveals other potential low intakes of nutrients such as calcium, riboflavin, and zinc, which may not be apparent in the other assessment parameters. The printout from a computerized diet program shows a summary of Katherine's intake that can be compared with dietary standards (RDA or AI) (Table 2-11).

Clinical Evaluation

The clinical signs observed for Katherine must be interpreted with caution because they are subjective and can indicate a number of situations or conditions other than malnutrition. In this case pallor is consistent with iron deficiency anemia and the general condition of the hair and skin indicates a possibility of inadequate protein intake and deficiencies of other nutrients.

SUMMARY OF NUTRITION ASSESSMENT

The following might represent a summary of the calculation and data that can be used for nutritional assessment in this case. It should be pointed out that to explore many kinds of data, several tests or measurements have been reported for each body compartment in this case. In an actual situation it is unlikely that all of this information would be available for one individual.

Katherine appears to be at nutrition risk. Her energy reserves are compromised, as evidenced by a loss of body weight of almost 20% in the last 6 months and an MRW of 75. The TFF and SSFF values are below the tenth percentile. The dietary history confirms a low energy intake. A persistent intake at this level would be a major contributor to continued weight loss.

Measures of somatic protein status suggest low reserves. The MAC (18.2 cm) is below the fifth percentile and MAMA (256.5 mm^2) falls below the fifteenth percentile. Visceral protein levels of serum transferrin (1.55 mg/L or 155 mg/dL) and TLC (1000) are below normal values and suggest moderate deficit. The dietary history suggests that daily protein intake is near or only slightly below the standard. However, that level would not be sufficient to meet the needs of an individual who is in negative energy balance and who continues to lose weight. Therefore it would be reasonable to assume that protein intake is inadequate relative to her current need. Hemoglobin and hematocrit levels (100 g/L or 10 g/dL and 32%, respectively) indicate iron deficiency. This finding is supported by dietary intakes below the level recommended. Intake levels of several other nutrients, including calcium, riboflavin, and zinc, are below the standard.

NUTRITION CARE PLAN

Katherine needs to improve her dietary intake to avoid progressive malnutrition. There is no question that nutrition intervention is appropriate. She needs to increase her total food consumption to provide sufficient kilocalories to prevent continued weight loss and nutrient deficiencies. Her increased intake should include 2 servings of dairy products, 3 to 4 servings of whole grain breads and cereals, 3 to 4 servings of fruits and vegetables, and 1 serving of lean meat, fish, poultry, or meat alternative per day.

If other causes of iron deficiency are ruled out, Katherine needs a supplement of ferrous iron until her hemoglobin and hematocrit levels return to normal values.

Implementation

If Katherine were admitted to the hospital, part of the nutrition care plan would be to provide a balanced diet and encourage its consumption. Because the assessment occurred in an outpatient setting, the nutrition care plan will concentrate on recommendations for dietary improvement using nutrition education and counseling.

Evaluation

The effectiveness of the nutrition care and counseling of Katherine will be evaluated in two ways.

Table 2-11 GRAPHIC COMPARISON OF KATHERINE'S DIETARY INTAKE TO DIETARY STANDARD

Analysis: Untitled
% RDA: Katherine
Cost:

Wgt: 3146 g (111 oz.)
Water: 93%

Nutrient	Values	Goal %
Calories	1008	56%
Protein	37.2 g	98%
Carbohydrates	113 g	43%
Fat—Total	46.3 g	77%
Saturated Fat	16.1 g	80%
Mono Fat	14 g	70%
Poly Fat	12.3 g	61%
Omega 3 FA	.969 g	—
Omega 6 FA	11.3 g	—
Cholesterol	306 mg	102%
Dietary Fiber	5.54 g	31%
Total Vit A	453 RE*	57%
A—Retinol	184 RE	—
A—Carotenoid	269 RE	—
Thiamin-B_1	.725 mg	80%
Riboflavin-B_2	1.04 mg	95%
Niacin-B_3	11.5 mg	96%
Niacin Equiv.	11.5 mg	96%
Vitamin B_6	.463 mg	29%
Vitamin B_{12}	1.69 μg	84%
Folate	196 μg	109%
Pantothenic	2.14 mg	31%
Vitamin C	20.8 mg	35%
Vitamin D	.927 μg	9%
Vit E-Alpha E	3.91 mg	49%
Calcium	488 mg	41%
Copper	.536 mg	21%
Iron	8.06 mg	54%
Magnesium	154 mg	55%
Manganese	2.09 mg	60%
Phosphorus	723 mg	60%
Potassium	1971 mg	99%
Selenium	55.9 μg	102%
Sodium	2201 mg	92%
Zinc	4.98 mg	42%
Complex Carbs	79 g	—
Sugars	28.7 g	—
Alcohol	0 g	—
Caffeine	604 mg	—
Water	2936 g	—

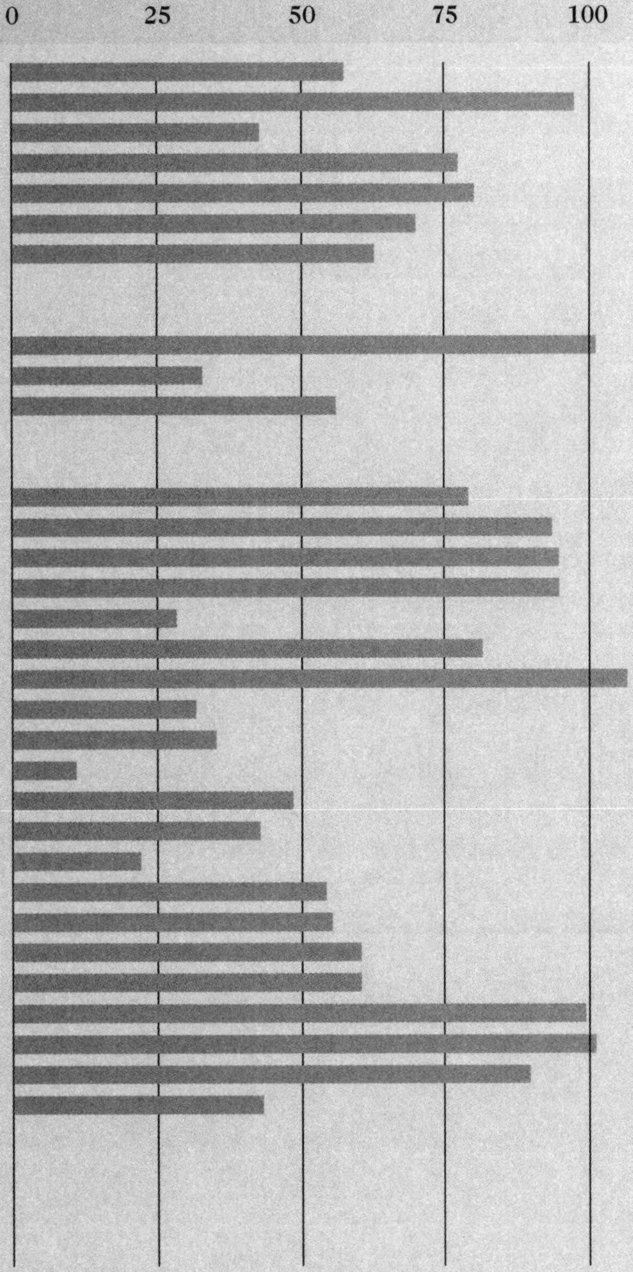

*RE = retinol equivalents.

First the effectiveness of the counseling will be judged on the changes she makes in her dietary intake. These, in turn, should be reflected in improvement in the nutritional assessment parameters measured in the initial assessment (anthropometry and biochemical indices).

Documentation

A summary of the assessment of Katherine's nutritional status and the nutrition care plan will be recorded in her chart in the clinic. When she returns for follow-up visits her progress will be evaluated and documented in the medical record.

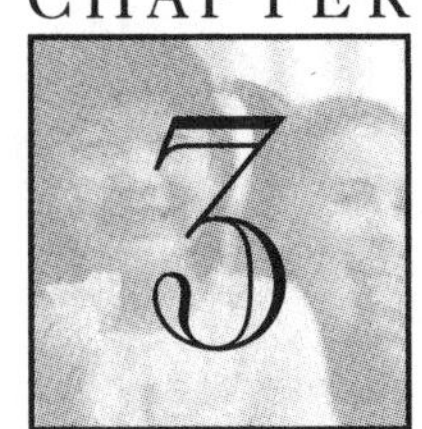

CHAPTER 3

Promoting Dietary Change

Gail Kaye

Chapter Outline

Clarice is a 46-year-old Hispanic female who is severely obese. Two years ago, she was treated for breast cancer. Clarice has gained a significant amount of weight in the past year, which has exacerbated her diabetes and caused hypertension. She takes medication for both medical conditions. As explained by her physician, the dose for both medications was increased because of her weight gain. Clarice has a family history of obesity, diabetes, hypertension, breast cancer, and colon cancer. She is frightened about her health.

Clarice lives with her husband and her four children, who range in age from 10 to 21 years of age. She does all the food shopping, meal planning, and food preparation. She has worked full time as an accountant for the past 20 years for the same company in the same office building. At this facility vending machines provide soda, candy, and other high-calorie, high-fat items. The only eating establishments accessible to workers at lunchtime are fast-food establishments. Clarice typically selects foods from the vending machines for breakfast and goes to a fast-food establishment for lunch. There is not an exercise facility at her place of employment. The nearest exercise facility is approximately 20 minutes from her work and her home.

Clarice has been involved with numerous weight-loss programs. Although she has successfully lost weight with each program, at the completion of each program she regained the weight she had lost and gained additional pounds. Despite attempts to change, her dietary intake is high in total kilocalories and total and saturated fat. She does not consume the recommended amounts of fruits and vegetables. Clarice has attempted numerous exercise programs; however, consistent participation has been difficult.

How should you converse with this client? In a formal or informal manner? Should you evaluate if she believes her current lifestyle (including dietary practices) is threatening her health? Is it important to talk about previous attempts to change dietary behaviors, noting what worked and what didn't and how change was evaluated? What about her perception of those dietary behaviors she believes would be beneficial to change currently and her ability to execute these changes? Should these concerns be considered and discussed? Should you or Clarice decide the treatment goals, or should goal setting be a collaborative, ongoing process? What are Clarice's expectations about results? What about assessing her readiness to change? How would you assess it and how would you use this information? Is there one best way to discuss the rationale for treatment and what type of information is best used to do so? How do you help cultivate hope in Clarice? Is it important to discuss her social environment including her social network, work environment, home environment, and her current life circumstances? Should you help her evaluate whether her community and place of employment support healthy lifestyles and discuss what to do if they don't?

To answer these questions and important others, this chapter reviews the psychotherapy-outcomes literature. Key variables or factors noted to facilitate change in client behavior will be noted and discussed. A review of important public health and health-promotion strategies for initiating behavior change will be presented next, followed by a summary of results from a systematic review of the current literature on interventions aimed at modifying dietary behavior related to cancer risk. Intervention components noted to facilitate changes in dietary behaviors will be highlighted and compared with the factors and variables noted in the previous two sections. Directions for future research will also be noted.

FACTORS THAT FACILITATE CHANGES IN CLIENT BEHAVIOR

- *Do information or psychologically based interventions really work?*
- *What are the variables associated with treatment success?*
- *Are there practical **helper**-initiated practices that can foster desired behavior change for clients?*

Data from more than 40 years of outcomes research in the field of psychotherapy clearly indicate that psychologically based or informed interventions do work (Bergin and Garfield, 1994; Hubble et al., 1999; Seligman, 1995). Using the extensive review and analysis of outcomes data by Lambert (1992), Hubble et al. (1999) identified four empirically based common factors associated with treatment success: client variables and extratherapeutic events such as environment; relationship factors; expectancy and placebo effects; and techniques. Data indicate that as much as 40% of improvement in clients can be attributed to client variables and extratherapeutic factors and that relationship factors, expectancy and placebo effects, and techniques account for 30%, 15%, and 15% of client improvements, respectively (Asay and Lambert, 1999). For each of the four factors key findings and practical implications for helpers follow.

Box 3-1 CLIENT CHARACTERISTICS THAT CAN AFFECT THERAPEUTIC OUTCOMES

Age
Sex
Psychosocial Development
Ego Strength
Interpersonal Skill
Intellectual Capacity
Personality
Client Expectations
Education
Health Status
Risk for Disease
Ethnicity
Religious Background

Client Variables and Extratherapeutic Events

Psychotherapy outcomes data (Asay and Lambert, 1999; Lambert, 1992) indicate that client variables and extratherapeutic events contribute as much as 40% of the effect on client improvement. Box 3-1 provides a partial list of client variables that can affect therapeutic interventions. Comprehensive reviews of client variables associated with treatment outcomes can be found in Bergin and Garfield (1994). The literature indicates that clients who do the best with therapeutic interventions and who maintain treatment gains believe that *the changes made in treatment were the results of their own efforts.* Within this framework the helper is best seen as someone who helps the client mobilize, channel, and focus naturally occurring powers of healing and personal agency. In other words, counseling, therapy, or therapeutic helping is best described as "professionally coached self-change" (Prochaska et al., 1994).

Practical Implications for Helpers: Client Variables

Given these findings it is important that helpers listen carefully to their clients, respect their frame of reference, and genuinely collaborate with them. As noted by Tallman and Bohart (1999, p. 117):

> Collaboration means more than client participation and compliance. It means that therapy (therapeutic interventions) must be thought of as the meeting of two minds, each possessing its own expertise and competence, with goals and solutions cocreated through mutual dialogue, instead of being chosen and applied to the client by the helper.

Box 3-2 lists practical suggestions for helpers to use to enhance key client variables associated with positive changes.

Extratherapeutic Events

The environments in which clients live (extratherapeutic factors) can be sources of support and sabotage. The data clearly indicate that many clients improve and change without formal intervention (Hubble et al., 1999; Prochaska et al., 1992). Significant numbers of clients have been successfully helped by family, friends, teachers, and clergy who provide a variety of hope-instilling and supportive techniques (Asay and Lambert, 1999).

Practical Implications for Helpers: Extratherapeutic Events

Helpers are best advised to view a goal of intervention as helping clients mobilize components of their environment to assist them with desired changes. For example Schlossberg (1984, 1989) describes different types (intimate relationships, family units, networks of friends, institutions, and communities) and functions (affect, affirmation, aid, and honest feedback) of social support that can be mobilized to facilitate desired behavior change (Box 3-3). Box 3-4 lists other practical suggestions that helpers can use to help clients use components of their environment to achieve desired changes.

Box 3-2 Practical Ways for Helpers to Enhance the Client Variables Associated with Positive Change

Acknowledge and maximize client competencies.
- Treat clients as though they are capable and have strengths and resources necessary to solve their problems (Watzlawick, 1986). Responsibility for the cure is the client's business (cited in Ansbacher and Ansbacher, 1956, p. 336).
- Actively listen and identify the client's strengths and resources.

Help clients to develop a change focus.
- Listen to and validate client change for the better (Hubble et al., 1998) (pretreatment, between sessions, and at end sessions). For example ask what is different and what is better.
- Welcome and explore new and different client perspectives, behaviors, and experiences.
- Acknowledge and validate changes and the client's participation in that change.

Data from Hubble M et al.: Directing attention to what works. In Hubble M, Duncan B, and Miller S, editors: The heart and soul of change, what works in therapy, Washington, DC, 1999, American Psychological Association.

Relationship Factors

Empiric findings suggest that the relationship between the helper and the client accounts for nearly 30% of client improvements. Data indicate that a positive therapeutic relationship is a necessary component of successful psychologic or information-based interventions, but typically not a sufficient component. Simply stated, *if the client's view of the relationship is positive, change is more likely to occur* (Duncan et al., 1997).

Practical Implications for Helpers: Relationship Factors

Because the client's perception of the relationship (as opposed to the helper's) is most relevant to the outcome of intervention, it is important that the helper listens attentively and

KEY TERMS

helper: counselor or therapist

Box 3-3 Different Types of Social Support

AFFECT

An expression that someone respects, likes, or loves you.

AFFIRMATION

An expression that someone agrees that what you are doing is understandable, appropriate, or both.

AID

An expression that someone will actually supply you with information, time, or some other intangible aid.

HONEST FEEDBACK

An expression that someone will offer guidance and support.

- Confirmatory feedback lets an individual know he or she is on course (Egan, 1982).
- Corrective feedback provides an individual with information to get back on course (Egan, 1982).
- Motivating feedback points out consequences of adequate or inadequate program implementation (Egan, 1982).

From Schlossberg N: Counseling adults in transition, New York, 1984, Springer; Egan G: The skilled helper: model, skills, and methods for effective helping, Monterey, Ca, 1982, Brooks/Cole.

communicates understanding, liking, and respect for the client *as defined by the client.* In other words helpers need to communicate with clients in ways that the client (not the helper) believes are helpful, supportive, and positive. As noted by Hubble et al, (1999, p. 418), achieving this requires notable skill and flexibility on the part of the helper:

> [It] demands a higher measure of flexibility on the part of the therapist and a willingness to change one's relational stance to fit with the client's perceptions of what is most helpful. Some clients...will prefer a formal or professional manner over a casual or warmer one. Others might prefer more self-disclosure...greater directiveness, a focus on their symptoms, or a focus on the possible meanings beneath them...a faster or perhaps a more laid-back pace for therapeutic work.

Box 3-4 Questions Helpers Can Use to Help Clients Evaluate their Social Network (Environment)

- What are some helpful aspects of your current social support network?
- Are you getting the affect, affirmation, and aid you need?
- Will your existing supportive network be disrupted by changes you plan to make? If so, what is the effect of the disruption and how will you manage these effects?

From Schlossberg N: Overwhelmed: coping with life's ups and downs, New York, 1989, Lexington Books.

Providers of service must attend to the clients' perceptions and feelings, including dissatisfaction about the therapeutic intervention and the provider of care *throughout* the therapeutic intervention. This includes discussing and clarifying different perceptions and establishing agreement on what is needed and helpful (Hubble et al., 1999).

To help ensure a positive view of the therapeutic relationship, Hubble et al. (1999) also recommend that providers of care accommodate a client's stage and theory of change. Prochaska and DiClemente (1982) offer a stage-of-change model that helpers can use. Empirical data support their belief that the process of change unfolds over time and involves progression through six stages: precontemplation, contemplation, preparation, action, maintenance, and termination (Box 3-5). In this context readiness for change or motivational readiness is a dynamic process that can be influenced by others, including helpers. By understanding a client's stage of change, helpers can tailor their interventions to match the client's motivational readiness. Unlike stages of human development, there is no innate drive that causes persons to progress from one stage to another. Instead principles of change need to be applied (Prochaska, 1999) (Box 3-6). Most relevant to a helper is Principle 6, which calls for matching particular processes of change with specific stages of change.

Consciousness raising, dramatic relief, and environmental reevaluation are change processes

Box 3-5 Stages of Change

STAGE: PRECONTEMPLATION
Description: Client does not intend to change or take action in the near future (next 6 months); may be uninformed or underinformed about the consequences of behavior; may have tried to change without success and become demoralized.

STAGE: CONTEMPLATION
Description: Client intends to change or take action within the next six months; is aware of pros and cons of change; may be ambivalent (chronic contemplation with behavioral procrastination).

STAGE: PREPARATION
Description: Client intends to take action in the immediate future, such as within the next month; typically has taken some action within the past year to develop a plan of action (e.g., go to support group, seek out counselor, or buy self-help book).

STAGE: ACTION
Description: Client has made specific, overt modifications in lifestyle within the past 6 months.

STAGE: MAINTENANCE
Description: Client is working to prevent relapse, but does not apply change processes as frequently as does a person in the action stage.

STAGE: TERMINATION
Description: Client experiences zero temptation and 100% self-efficacy (confidence that one is competent in performing a task or behavior that leads to a desired outcome).

From Prochaska J, Redding C, Evers K: The transtheoretical model and stages of change. In K Glanz, F Lewis, B Rimer, editors: Health behavior and health education: theory, research, and practice, San Francisco, CA, 1997, Jossey-Bass.

Box 3-6 Principles of Change

PRINCIPLE 1
The advantages of changing must increase for people to progress from precontemplation to contemplation.

PRINCIPLE 2
The disadvantages of changing must decrease for people to progress from contemplation to action.

PRINCIPLE 3
The pros and cons must cross over for people to be prepared to take action.

PRINCIPLE 4
The "strong principle" of progress holds that to progress from precontemplation to effective action, the advantages of changing must increase one standard deviation (Prochaska, 1994).

PRINCIPLE 5
The "weak principle" of progress holds that to progress from contemplation to effective action, the disadvantages of changing must decrease one-half standard deviation.

PRINCIPLE 6
Particular processes of change need to be matched to specific stages of change.

From Prochaska J: How do people change and how can we change to help many more people. In Hubble M et al.: The heart and soul of change, what works in therapy, Washington, DC, 1999, American Psychological Association. Adapted with permission.

best used with clients in the precontemplation and contemplation stages. Self-reevaluation is recommended for use with clients in the contemplation and preparation stages. Self-liberation is best employed to assist clients in the preparation and action stages. Finally contingency management, helping relationships, counterconditioning, and stimulus control are change processes recommended for clients in the action and maintenance stages (Box 3-7).

Although a client's theory of change tends to emerge over time, it can be accessed by asking clients what their goals are, how to best to accomplish these goals, and what role the therapeutic relationship can play in helping them achieve these goals. With this perspective, treatment is best viewed as a working partnership between the helper and the client. Both work together to construct interventions that help

Box 3-7 Processes of Change

PRECONTEMPLATION AND CONTEMPLATION STAGES

Consciousness Raising: Increase awareness and information about the causes, consequences, and cures for a particular problem.

Dramatic Relief: Induce emotional arousal (fear, inspiration, guilt, and hope) about current behavior and relief that can come from changing.

Environmental Reevaluation: Combine emotional and cognitive assessments of how behavior affects social environment and how changing would affect that environment.

CONTEMPLATION AND PREPARATION STAGES

Self-Reevaluation: Combine affective and cognitive assessments of self-image, free from a particular problem.

PREPARATION AND ACTION STAGES

Self-Liberation: Believe that one can change and commit or recommit to act on that belief.

ACTION AND MAINTENANCE STAGES

Counterconditioning: Learn healthier behaviors to replace problem behaviors.

Contingency Management: Systematically use reinforcements or punishments (less common) for taking steps in a particular direction.

Stimulus Control: Modify environment to increase cues that prompt healthier responses and decrease cues that are tempting.

Helping Relationships: Combine caring, openness, trust, acceptance, and support for changing.

Modified from Prochaska J: How do people change and how can we change to help many more people. In Hubble M et al.: The heart and soul of change, what works in therapy, Washington, DC, 1999, American Psychological Association.

the client reach his or her goals. Box 3-8 provides practical questions helpers can ask clients to clarify goals, gain ideas about helpful interventions, and learn how the therapeutic relationship can facilitate achieving noted goals and interventions.

Box 3-8 Practical Helper-Initiated Questions to Clarify Client's Theory of Change (Goals, Interventions, and Role of the Therapeutic Relationship)

- What is your goal in coming here?
- What do you (hope, wish, or think) will be different because of our meeting together?
- What do you want to change about your (life or problem)?
- What would have to be minimally different in your life to consider our work together a success?
- What will be the first sign to you that you have taken a solid step on the road to improvement even though you might not yet be out of the woods?
- What ideas do you have about what needs to happen for improvement to occur?
- Many times people have a pretty good hunch about what is causing a problem and what will resolve it. Do you have a theory of how change is going to happen here?
- In what ways do you see me and this process being helpful to attaining your goals?
- How does change usually happen in your life?
- What do you usually do to initiate change?
- What have you tried to help the problem or situation so far? Did it help? How did it help? Why didn't it help?

From Hubble M et al.: Directing attention to what works. In Hubble M, Duncan B, and Miller S, editors: The heart and soul of change, what works in therapy, Washington, DC, 1999, American Psychological Association.

Expectancy and Placebo Factors: The Dynamics of Hope

Lambert (1992) suggests that expectancy and placebo factors account for 15% of the improvements for clients who engage in psychologically based or information-based interventions. Lambert et al. (1993) reviewed studies to compare the effect size of psychotherapy and placebo interventions in relation to nontreatment controls. They found that the average placebo effect size was 0.42 for placebo (minimal) interventions and 0.82 for psychotherapy.

In percentage improvement rates, the average client who undergoes placebo treatment is better off than 66% of nontreatment controls, whereas the average client who undergoes treatment is better off than 79% of nontreatment controls. The question remains: how and why does placebo intervention work?

Snyder et al. (1999) cite clinical evidence that hope is the factor that fosters positive expectancy and placebo effects. They define hope as a way that people think about goals. First are the thoughts that individuals have about their ability to generate one or more workable solutions to their goals. This is called *pathways thinking*. Second are the thoughts that people have about their ability to initiate and continue executing solutions they have selected to help them reach their goals. This is called *agency thinking*. With this model stress, negative emotions, and difficulties in coping are the result of being unable to generate solutions or work toward achieving the desired goals. Therapeutic interventions work by fostering agency thinking (e.g., "I can do it") and pathways thinking (e.g., "Here is how I will do it"). The therapeutic relationship (emotional and confiding relationship) and the setting (perception of the helper as effective in facilitating change) foster agency thinking. The therapeutic rationale (a convincing myth that explains why the client is experiencing symptoms and how therapeutic procedures will ameliorate symptoms) and therapeutic ritual (procedures used by the helper) foster pathways thinking (Snyder et al., 1999).

Practical Implications for Helpers: Relationship Factors

To enhance placebo-based expectancy and hope, Hubble et al. (1999) offer the following suggestions. Helpers are advised to use "healing rituals" that they believe are effective and should show interest in the outcomes or results of selected practices. Treatments should be oriented to the future and should enhance a client's sense of personal control. It has long been known that people who believe they can influence or modify the course of life events are better able to adapt and cope with adversity, regardless of the accuracy of these beliefs. Box 3-9 provides sample questions that helpers can use to assist clients with envisioning a better future.

Box 3-9 Practical Helper-Initiated Questions to Assist Clients with Envisioning a Better Future

- What will be different when eating excessive amounts of concentrated sweets and overeating are behind you?
- What will be the smallest sign that eating excessive amounts of concentrated sweets and overeating are getting better?
- What will be the first sign that eating excessive amounts of concentrated sweets and overeating are getting better?
- When you are no longer eating excessive amounts of concentrated sweets and when you are not overeating, what will you be doing more of instead?
- Who will be the first person to notice that you have achieved a victory over this problem?
- What will that person notice about you that will tell him or her that the victory is achieved?
- Where do you suppose you will be when you first notice the changes? What will have taken place just before the changes that will have helped them to happen? What will happen later that will help maintain them?

Modified from Hubble M et al.: Directing attention to what works. In Hubble M, Duncan B, and Miller S, editors: The heart and soul of change, what works in therapy, Washington, DC, 1999, American Psychological Association.

Techniques and Models

Long thought to be the pivotal contributors to effective psychologic- or information-based interventions, specific techniques and models actually account for only about 15% of the improvements seen in clients, according to recent evidence. In fact in the psychotherapy outcomes literature, there is little evidence that one psychotherapeutic approach is better than another for assisting clients with needed behavior change (Bergin and

Garfield, 1994; Seligman, 1995). However, techniques and models can and do affect the outcomes of the helping process. They can provide needed structure and focus, which are essential elements of the therapeutic endeavor. One of the best predictors of negative outcomes is a lack of structure and focus during the helping process (Hubble et al., 1999).

Practical Implications for Helpers: Models and Techniques

Helpers have a wide array of choices when considering therapeutic techniques and models. A concern is what technique or model to select. The data indicate that the particular technique or model used is less important than the degree to which the technique or model is consistent with the client's theory of change and expectations for treatment.

Summary of Factors that Facilitate Change

Based on the psychotherapy outcomes literature, four empirically based common factors are associated with treatment success: client variables and extratherapeutic events (environment), relationship factors, expectancy and placebo effects, and techniques (Hubble et al., 1999). As much as 40% of improvement in clients may be attributed to client variables and extratherapeutic events, whereas relationship factors, expectancy and placebo effects, and techniques are thought to account for 30%, 15%, and 15% of client improvements, respectively (Asay and Lambert, 1999). Helper-initiated practices can help to cultivate these common factors.

Could any other body of information lend helpful perspectives on facilitating dietary changes? The fields of public health and health promotion offer such perspectives.

PUBLIC HEALTH, HEALTH PROMOTION, AND DIETARY CHANGES

- *How do public health and health-promotion programs promote behavior change, including changes in dietary behaviors?*
- *What is the ecologic approach for promoting behavior change?*
- *What are the targets of intervention for strategies designed to facilitate change in individuals, their social networks, and the organizations in which they work and play? Are the targets the same or different?*
- *How might the ecologic approach be used to develop a behavior change program for obese adolescents?*

Public health and health-promotion programs can help individuals, families, organizations, and communities to improve their health, reduce their risk of disease, manage their chronic diseases, and improve their quality of life and self-reliance (National Institute of Health and National Cancer Institute, 1997). Public health and health-promotion programs are viable intervention strategies for promoting dietary changes, given the connection between diet and disease and diet and disease prevention.

Health Promotion and the Ecologic Perspective

Not all health-promotion programs and initiatives are successful at achieving desired outcomes, including dietary changes. Programs most likely to succeed are based on a clear understanding of the identified health concern (e.g., obesity or diabetes) and the environmental context in which it occurs. In other words, understanding the individual and the environment in which the individual operates is critical when designing intervention programs (National Institute of Health and National Cancer Institute, 1997).

It is also important to approach public health problems using multiple levels of intervention (e.g., individual and community) and to ensure appropriate integration of interventions both within and across various levels. Contemporary health-promotion efforts often include educational activities and advocacy, organizational change efforts, policy development, economic supports, or environmental change. This multiple-perspective approach has been referred to as an ecologic perspective (McLeroy et al., 1988).

The ecologic perspective of health promotion holds that behavior can be affected by and can affect multiple levels of influence. In other words

Table 3-1 AN ECOLOGIC PERSPECTIVE: LEVELS OF INFLUENCE

Concept	Definition
INTRAPERSONAL FACTORS	Individual characteristics that influence behavior, such as knowledge, attitudes, beliefs, and personality traits
INTERPERSONAL FACTORS	Interpersonal processes, and primary groups including family, friends, peers, that provide social identity, support, and role definition
INSTITUTIONAL FACTORS	Rules, regulations, policies, and informal structures, which may constrain or promote recommended behaviors
COMMUNITY FACTORS	Social networks and norms, or standards, which exist as formal or informal among individuals, groups, and organizations
PUBLIC POLICY	Local, state, federal policies and laws that regulate or support healthy actions and practices for disease prevention, early detection, control, and management

National Institute of Health and National Cancer Institute: Theory at a glance: a guide for health and promotion practice, 1997. http://oc.nci.nih.gov/services/Theory_at_glance/HOME.html

behavior both influences and is influenced by the social environment (National Institute of Health and National Cancer Institute, 1997). McLeroy et al. (1988) identified five levels of influence for health-related behaviors and conditions: intrapersonal, or individual, factors; interpersonal factors; institutional factors; community factors; and public policy (Table 3-1). This approach highlights the importance of thinking about health problems and interventions at multiple levels and clarifies three different targets, or levels of intervention: the individual, the interpersonal, and the community.

Interventions that Promote Individual Change

In addition to the previously discussed stage-of-change model (Prochaska, 1999; Prochaska and DiClemente, 1982; Prochaska et al., 1992; Prochaska et al., 1994), the Health Belief Model (HBM) (Becker and Maiman, 1975; Rosenstock, 1966) and Consumer Information Processing (CIP) theory (Bettman, 1979) focus on aspects of the individual in an attempt to effect individual change.

The focus of the HBM (Becker and Maiman, 1975; Rosenstock, 1966) is an individual's perceived threat of a health problem and the individual's evaluation of recommended behaviors for preventing or managing the problem (Table 3-2). The HBM has been used effectively to design messages (e.g., print, electronic, and mass media messages) to persuade individuals to make healthy decisions.

Bettman (1979) developed one of the well-known models of CIP. The focus of the CIP is the processes that individuals use to acquire and use information for decision making (Table 3-3). The CIP uses two key assumptions: the amount of information individuals can process is limited; and to make faster and easier decisions or to improve usability of information, individuals combine bits of information into chunks and create a series of decision rules accordingly. The CIP models can be used to examine why people use or do not use health information and to design better health information pieces (National Institute of Health and National Cancer Institute, 1997).

Interventions that Promote Change at the Interpersonal Level

Interventions designed to promote change in the relationships between people are founded on the assumption that individuals live in environments in

Table 3-2 KEY CONCEPTS: HEALTH BELIEF MODEL

Concept	Definition	Application
PERCEIVED SUSCEPTIBILITY	One's opinion of chances of getting a condition	Define population(s) at risk, risk levels; personalize risk based on a person's features or behavior; heighten perceived susceptibility if too low
PERCEIVED SEVERITY	One's opinion of how serious a condition and its sequelae are	Specify consequences of the risk and the condition
PERCEIVED BENEFITS	One's opinion of the efficacy of the advised action to reduce risk or seriousness of impact	Define action to take; how, where, when; clarify the positive effects to be expected
PERCEIVED BARRIERS	One's opinion of the tangible and psychologic costs of the advised action	Identify and reduce barriers through reassurance, incentives, assistance
CUES TO ACTION	Strategies to activate "readiness"	Provide how-to information, promote awareness, reminders
SELF-EFFICACY	Confidence in one's ability to take action	Provide training, guidance in performing action

National Institute of Health and National Cancer Institute: Theory at a glance: a guide for health and promotion practice, 1997. http://oc.nci.nih.gov/services/Theory_at_glance/HOME.html

Table 3-3 KEY CONCEPTS: CONSUMER INFORMATION PROCESSING MODEL

Concept	Definition	Application
INFORMATION-PROCESSING CAPACITY	Individuals' limitations in the amount of information they can acquire, use, and remember	Choose the most important and useful points to communicate, whether orally or in print materials
INFORMATION SEARCH	Processing of acquiring and evaluating information; affected by motivation, attention, and perception	Provide information so it takes little effort to obtain, draws consumer's attention, and is clear
DECISION RULES/HEURISTICS	Rules of thumb, developed and used to help consumers select among alternatives	Learn key ways to synthesize information in ways that have meaning and appeal for your audience
CONSUMPTION AND LEARNING	Internal feedback based on outcome of choices, and use in future decisions	Keep in mind that people have probably made related choices in the past, and are not "empty vessels"
INFORMATION ENVIRONMENT	Amount, location, format, readability, and processability of relevant information	Design information tailored to the audience; place it conveniently for use

National Institute of Health and National Cancer Institute: Theory at a glance: a guide for health and promotion practice, 1997. http://oc.nci.nih.gov/services/Theory_at_glance/HOME.html

Table 3-4 KEY CONCEPTS: SOCIAL COGNITIVE THEORY

Concept	Definition	Application
RECIPROCAL DETERMINISM	Behavior changes result from interaction between person and environment; change is bidirectional	Involve the individual and relevant others; work to change the environment, if warranted
BEHAVIORAL CAPABILITY	Knowledge and skills to influence behavior	Provide information and training about action
EXPECTATIONS	Beliefs about likely results of action	Incorporate information about likely results of action in advice
SELF-EFFICACY	Confidence in ability to take action and persist in action	Point out strengths; use persuasion and encouragement; approach behavior change in small steps
OBSERVATIONAL LEARNING	Beliefs based on observing others like self and/or visible physical results	Point out others' experience, physical changes; identify role models to emulate
REINFORCEMENT	Responses to a person's behavior that increase or decrease the chances of recurrence	Provide incentives, rewards, praise; encourage self-reward; decrease possibility of negative responses that deter positive changes

National Institute of Health and National Cancer Institute: Theory at a glance: a guide for health and promotion practice, 1997. http://oc.nci.nih.gov/services/Theory_at_glance/HOME.html

which the thoughts, feelings, and behaviors of others can affect their own thoughts, feelings, and behaviors. A commonly used theory for interpersonal intervention is Social Cognitive Theory (SCT), or Social Learning Theory (SLT) (Bandura, 1977). A fundamental assumption of SCT and SLT is the supposition that people and their environment are in constant interaction. Behavior is explained as a three-way, dynamic, reciprocal process in which personal factors, environmental influences, and behavior continuously interact. People learn from their own experiences and from observation of others' actions (Bandura, 1977). Key concepts of SCT and SLT are noted in Table 3-4.

Interventions that Promote Change at the Community Level

Interventions that promote community-wide changes in health behavior include community organization, diffusion of innovations, and organizational change.

Community organization is a process that helps community groups identify common problems and goals and interventions. This process also helps community groups mobilize resources and develop and implement strategies so identified goals can be reached. Specific strategies used to achieve these ends include locality development, social planning, and social action. With locality (community) development, a broad cross-section of people in the community identify and solve their own problems. Social planning involves using experts to help with problem solving. Social action aims to help disadvantaged or oppressed groups identify common problems, attract attention to these problems, and obtain power to meet their identified needs (National Institute of Health and National Cancer Institute, 1997). Key concepts of community organization are noted in Table 3-5.

Table 3-5 KEY CONCEPTS: COMMUNITY ORGANIZATION

Concept	Definition	Application
EMPOWERMENT	Process of gaining mastery and power over oneself/one's community, to produce change	Give individuals and communities tools and responsibility for making decisions that affect them
COMMUNITY COMPETENCE	Community's ability to engage in effective problem solving	Work with community to identify problems; create consensus, and reach goals
PARTICIPATION AND RELEVANCE	Learners should be active participants, work should "start where the people are"	Help community set goals within the context of preexisting goals, and encourage active participation
ISSUE SELECTION	Identifying winnable, simple, specific concerns as focus of action	Assist community in examining how they can communicate the concerns, and whether success is likely
CRITICAL CONSCIOUSNESS	Developing understanding of root causes of problems	Guide consideration of health concerns in broad perspective of social problems

National Institute of Health and National Cancer Institute: Theory at a glance: a guide for health and promotion practice., 1997 http://oc.nci.nih.gov/services/Theory_at_glance/HOME.html

Table 3-6 KEY CONCEPTS: DIFFUSION OF INNOVATIONS

Concept	Definition	Application
RELATIVE ADVANTAGE	The degree to which an innovation is seen as better than the idea, practice, program, or product it replaces	Point out unique benefits: monetary value, convenience, time saving, prestige, etc.
COMPATIBILITY	How consistent the innovation is with values, habits, experience, and needs of potential adopters	Tailor innovation for the intended audience's values, norms, or situation
COMPLEXITY	How difficult the innovation is to understand and/or use	Create program/idea/product to be uncomplicated, easy to use and understand
TRIALABILITY	Extent to which the innovation can be experimented with before a commitment to adopt is required	Provide opportunities to try on a limited basis, e.g., free samples, introductory sessions, money-back guarantee
OBSERVABILITY	Extent to which the innovation provides tangible or visible results	Assure visibility of results: feedback or publicity

National Institute of Health and National Cancer Institute: Theory at a glance: a guide for health and promotion practice, 1997. http://oc.nci.nih.gov/services/Theory_at_glance/HOME.html

Table 3-7 Organizational Change: Stage Theory

Concept	Definition	Application
PROBLEM DEFINITION (AWARENESS STAGE)	Problems recognized and analyzed; solutions sought and evaluated	Involve management and other personnel in awareness-raising activities
INITIATION OF ACTION (ADOPTION STAGE)	Policy or directive formulated; resources for beginning change allocated	Provide process consultation to inform decision makers and implementers of what adoption involves
IMPLEMENTATION OF CHANGE	Innovation is implemented, reactions occur, and role changes occur	Provide training, technical assistance, and problem-solving aid
INSTITUTIONALIZATION OF CHANGE	Policy or program becomes entrenched in the organization; new goals and values are internalized	Identify high-level champion, work to overcome obstacles to institutionalization, and create structures for integration

National Institute of Health and National Cancer Institute: Theory at a glance: a guide for health and promotion practice, 1997. http://oc.nci.nih.gov/services/Theory_at_glance/HOME.html

The main focus of the diffusion-of-innovations theory is to identify how new ideas, products, and social practices spread within a society or from one society to another. This goal involves examining the innovation (new idea, technology, product, and practice) and the communications channels and social systems used to diffuse it (National Institute of Health and National Cancer Institute, 1997). Important characteristics of innovations are noted in Table 3-6. Communication channels are important aspects of the diffusion-of-innovations theory. Often opinion leaders (e.g., physicians or community leaders) mediate the impact of mass-media messages. For example when opinion leaders support and reiterate information presented in the mass media, consumers are more likely to act on this information than if no opinion leader supported the mass media presentation (National Institute of Health and National Cancer Institute, 1997).

Within the context of health promotion, organizational change and development strategies focus on identifying the processes and strategies that increase the chance that health-promoting policies and programs will be adopted and maintained within an organization (National Institute of Health and National Cancer Institute, 1997). Many approaches focus on changing social norms and values to mediate desired changes (Hornstein et al., 1971). Organizations go through various stages as they change. Similar in concept to Prochaska's stage-of-change model, stage-appropriate interventions can help facilitate the process of change within an organization. Key concepts of the stage theory of organizational change are listed in Table 3-7.

Designing Comprehensive Intervention Programs: Practical Application Summary

The most powerful approaches for promoting health behaviors (including dietary changes) borrow from the ecologic perspective of health promotion in their attempts to help individuals and communities make needed changes and to recognize the reciprocal causation between individuals and their environment. However, no specific set of interventions or theories will be practical and useful for all behavior change and health-promotion programs. Instead different variables (e.g., the type of behavior being addressed or the target audience) will influence which interventions and theories may work best. For example consider the development of a program to reduce adolescent obesity. Although the stage-of-change model might be a very useful component for program development, the HBM would likely be less promising because adolescents do not typically think of weight concerns in terms of their long-term health impact. Similarly the CIP model would likely be less useful for this problem because the information that obesity can cause health problems is widely available and does not appear to be causally related to eating practices. However, using social learning theory (SLT) for program planning would likely be beneficial because of its focus on the interchange among personal, environment, and behavioral factors, an especially important perspective when working with adolescents. Similarly community organization and organizational change strategies could affect the availability of healthy food choices and policies related to the provision of nutritious low-calorie, low-fat snacks and meals within school and community settings (Box 3-10).

Box 3-10 Practical Applications of Models for Program Development

STAGES OF CHANGE

By evaluating the stage of change for overweight adolescents, appropriate types of strategies (e.g., consciousness raising versus self-liberation) could be planned to foster behavior change among at-risk youth.

SOCIAL LEARNING THEORY

It would be helpful to examine how the social environment, including peer attitudes, influences eating and exercise behavior (i.e., overeating of empty kilocalorie or high-calorie, high-fat food items; choosing to not engage in interscholastic or intramural sports). The expectations (beliefs about the results of action) associated with unhealthy eating behaviors or lack of physical activity would be useful to understand. Observational learning and reinforcement could be important intervention strategies to help obese adolescents engage in healthy eating and exercise behaviors.

COMMUNITY ORGANIZATION

A coalition of concerned parents, community leaders, and teens (including those who are obese) could be organized to help explore the problems of obesity in the community. Among other things, this group might review the structures (e.g., restaurants, grocery stores, parks, athletic facilities, and bike paths) available that promote healthy eating and exercise behaviors.

ORGANIZATIONAL CHANGE

A team of concerned teachers, community leaders, dietitians, and obese adolescents could review school-based nutrition and exercise policies.

Adapted from National Institutes of Health and National Cancer Institute: Theory at a glance: a guide for health promotion practice. http://oc.nci.nih.gov/services/Theory_at_glance/HOME.html.

Summary of Public Health Strategies

Public health and health-promotion programs are useful intervention strategies for promoting dietary changes. The ecologic perspective emphasizes the importance of using multiple levels of influence (individual, interpersonal, and community) to develop successful intervention programs. Intervention models that promote behavior change at the individual level include the stages-of-change model (Prochaska, 1999; Prochaska and DiClemente, 1982; Prochaska et al., 1992; Prochaska et al., 1994), HBM (Becker and Maiman, 1975; Rosenstock, 1966), and CIP theory (Bettman, 1979). Interventions that promote change at the interpersonal level include SLT (Bandura, 1977) and those that promote change at the community level include community organization, diffusion of innovations, and organizational change (National Institute of Health and National Cancer Institute, 1997).

Are there any applied examples of interventions directed toward changing dietary behaviors? If so what are the variables associated with successful interventions? Are they similar to the four factors noted to facilitate individual behavior change? Do successful programs reflect important public health and health-promotion principles, including the ecologic perspective?

INTERVENTIONS TO MODIFY DIETARY BEHAVIOR RELATED TO CANCER RISK: EXAMPLES FROM THE FIELD

- *What types of interventions help individuals reduce their dietary fat intake and increase their consumption of fruits and vegetables?*
- *Are these findings consistent with what we know helps facilitate behavior change in individuals?*
- *Are these findings consistent with the fundamental principles of major public health and health-promotion strategies?*

The Agency for Healthcare Research and Quality (AHRQ) sponsors an "Evidence-Based Practice Program." Using 12 evidence-based practice centers, this program develops scientific information that other organizations can use to develop clinical guidelines, performance measures, and other quality improvement tools (AHRQ, 2000b).

In 1999 AHRQ contracted with the Research Triangle Institute and University of North Carolina at Chapel Hill Evidence-Based Practice Center to review relevant scientific literature on the efficacy of interventions to modify dietary behavior related to cancer risk and to produce an evidence report and technology assessment (ER/TA) on this topic. The objective of the review was to answer the following three questions:

- Is there evidence that one type of intervention or combination of interventions is more effective than another in helping individuals or groups modify their diets to consume more fruits and vegetables and less fat?
- What is the evidence for the efficacy of dietary interventions by population subgroup, particularly groups defined by ethnicity and sex?
- What conclusions (if any) can be reached about the cost effectiveness of these types of interventions (AHRQ, 2000a)?

To address the research questions, investigators from Research Triangle Institute synthesized and summarized results from 92 studies that reported the impact of interventions designed to decrease dietary fat intake or increase the consumption of fruits and vegetables. Interventions of all types (e.g., individual dietary counseling, group nutrition classes, and social support groups) and in all settings (e.g., school, workplace, healthcare, and community) were included. Adults, adolescents, and children who were generally healthy and those who were at elevated risk of cancer or chronic disease were included as well. The following two sections summarize key findings (AHRQ, 2000a).

Modifying Fruit and Vegetable Intake

Approximately one third of the studies (i.e., 39 of 92 studies) reported results of interventions designed to modify fruit and vegetable intake. The results of evaluation indicated the following:

- Dietary interventions were positively associated with changes in fruit and vegetable intake.
- When fruit and vegetable intake were measured individually, changes in fruit intake were larger.
- The median difference between intervention and control groups in the change in daily servings of fruits and vegetables was an average increase in fruit and vegetable intake of 0.6 servings per day.

Investigators also found that interventions were more successful at increasing fruit intake for children and vegetable intake among adults. Studies conducted with higher disease risk populations were more likely to report more statistically significant increases in fruit and vegetable intake than studies conducted with the general population.

Several intervention characteristics were associated with a greater likelihood for significant findings in modifying fruit and vegetable intake:

- Theory-based interventions
- Study quality
- Social support component
- Goal-setting activities
- Interactive activities involving food

Modifying Dietary Fat Intake

Approximately 77% of the articles reviewed (i.e., 80 of 104 articles) reported results for dietary fat. Using three different analytic techniques, investigators found that dietary interventions were positively associated with changes in intake of fat. For median differences in total fat intake between treatment and control groups, researchers noted a 7.3% reduction in the percentage of calories from fat. A subset of articles that used biochemical indicators (e.g., plasma cholesterol) showed that the decrease in total fat intake was significantly correlated with decreases in total blood cholesterol. However, changes in saturated fat intake were not associated with statistically significant decreases in total blood cholesterol. Studies conducted with high disease risk populations were not more likely to yield statistically significant results with regard to overall fat intake, although the magnitude of change for saturated fat intake was higher among high disease risk populations.

Unlike the results reported for fruit and vegetable outcomes, theory-based interventions and study quality were not associated with an increased likelihood of significant effects. However, intervention characteristics associated with a greater likelihood for significant findings for modifying dietary fat intake included the following:

- Social support component
- Goal-setting activities
- Interactive activities involving food
- Culturally or ethnically specific interventions

Concepts to Remember

- Four factors: Client variables and extra therapeutic events, relationship factors, expectancy and placebo effects, and techniques are associated with treatment success.
- Clients who respond to therapeutic interventions and who maintain treatment gains below the changes made in treatment were the results of their own efforts.
- If the clients' view of the relationship is positive, change is more likely to occur.
- Public health and health-promotion programs can help individuals, families, organizations, and communities to improve health, reduce risk of disease, manage chronic disease, and improve quality of life and self-reliance.
- Community organization is a process that helps community groups identify common goals and interventions.
- The most powerful approaches for promoting health behaviors recognize the reciprocal causation between individuals and their environment.

REFERENCES

Agency for Healthcare Research and Quality: Efficacy of interventions to modify dietary behavior related to cancer risk. Summary, evidence report/technology assessment: number 25. AHRQ Publication No. 01-E028, Rockville, MD, 2000a, Agency for Healthcare Research and Quality. http://www.ahrq.gov/clinic/dietsumm.htm

Agency for Healthcare Research and Quality: Evidence-based practice centers: overview. AHRQ Publication No. 00-P013, Rockville, MD, 2000b, Agency for Healthcare Research and Quality. http://www.ahrq.gov/clinic/epc/

Ansbacher H and Ansbacher R: The individual psychology of Alfred Adler, New York, 1956, Basic Books.

Asay T and Lambert M: The empirical case for the common factors in therapy: quantitative findings. In Hubble M, Duncan B, and Miller S, editors: The heart and soul of change, what works in therapy, Washington, DC, 1999, American Psychological Association.

Bandura A: Social learning theory, Englewood Cliffs, NJ, 1977, Prentice-Hall.

Becker M and Maiman L: Sociobehavioral determinants of compliance with health and medical care recommendations, Med Care 13:10-24, 1975.

Bergin A and Garfield S: Handbook of psychotherapy and behavior change, New York, 1994, Wiley.

Bettman J: An information processing theory of consumer choice, Reading, MA, 1979, Addison-Wesley.

Duncan B, Hubble M, and Miller S: Psychotherapy with impossible cases: the efficient treatment of therapy veterans, New York, 1997, Norton.

Egan G: The skilled helper: model, skills, and methods for effective helping, Monterey, CA, 1982, Brooks/Cole.

Hornstein H et al.: Organizational development: cultural change as a strategy of social intervention. In Hornstein H et al., editors: Social intervention: a behavioral science approach, New York, 1971, The Free Press.

Hubble M et al.: Directing attention to what works. In Hubble M, Duncan B, and Miller S, editors: The heart and soul of change, what works in therapy, Washington, DC, 1999, American Psychological Association.*

Hubble MA et al.: S.W.A.T.: "Special" words and tactics for critical situations, Crisis Intervention and Time-Limited Treatment 4:179-195, 1998.

Lambert M: Implications of outcome research for psychotherapy integration. In Norcross J and Goldstein M, editors: Handbook of psychotherapy integration, New York, 1992, Basic Books.

Lambert M et al.: Psychotherapy versus placebo. Poster presented at the annual meetings of the Western Psychological Association, Phoenix, AZ, April 1993.

McLeroy K et al.: An ecological perspective on health promotion programs, Health Educ Q 15:351-377, 1988.

National Institute of Health and National Cancer Institute: Theory at a glance: a guide for health promotion practice, 1997. http://oc.nci.nih.gov/services/Theory_at_glance/HOME.html

Prochaska J and DiClemente C: Transtheoretical therapy: toward a more integrative model of change, Psychother Theory Res Pract 19:276-288, 1982.

Prochaska J et al.: In search of how people change: applications to addictive behaviors, Am Psychol 47:1102-1114, 1992.

Prochaska J et al.: Changing for good, New York, 1994, William Morrow.

Prochaska J: How do people change and how can we change to help many more people. In Hubble M et al.: The heart and soul of change, what works in therapy, Washington, DC, 1999, American Psychological Association.

Rosenstock I: Why people use health services, Milbank Memorial Fund Q 44:94, 1966.

Schlossberg N: Counseling adults in transition, New York, 1984, Springer.

Schlossberg N: Overwhelmed: coping with life's ups and downs, New York, 1989, Lexington Books.

Seligman M: Effectiveness of psychotherapy: the Consumer Reports study, Am Psychol 50:965, 1995.

Snyder C et al.: Hope as a psychotherapeutic foundation of common factors, placebos, and expectancies. In Hubble M, Duncan B, and Miller S, editors: The heart and soul of change, what works in therapy, Washington, DC, 1999, American Psychological Association.

Tallman K and Bohart A: The client as a common factor: clients as self-healers. In Hubble M, Duncan B, and Miller S, editors: The heart and soul of change, what works in therapy, Washington, DC, 1999, American Psychological Association. Quotes copyright © 1999 by the American Psychological Association.

Watzlawick P: If you desire to see it, learn how to act. In Zeig J, editor: The evolution of psychotherapy, New York, 1986, Brunner/Mazel.

APPLICATION

Evidence Report and Technology Assessment

This evidence review supports the belief that a wide variety of dietary interventions—administered in different settings to persons of different sex, age, and ethnicity—can help people modify selected dietary behaviors for cancer risk reduction to increase consumption of fruits and vegetables and to decrease dietary fat intake. Collectively, the following intervention components appear helpful in facilitating these changes:

- Theory-based interventions
- Study quality
- Social support
- Goal-setting activities
- Interactive activities involving food
- Culturally or ethnically specific interventions

COMPARISON OF EVIDENCE REPORT/TECHNOLOGY ASSESSMENT RESULTS, CHANGE-PROMOTING INDIVIDUAL FACTORS, AND PUBLIC HEALTH AND HEALTH-PROMOTION PRINCIPLES

The results noted in the AHRQ ER/TA (AHRQ, 2000a) appear to show that both the individual factors and key public health and health-promotion principles were associated with intervention success (Table 3-8).

Regarding intake of fruits and vegetables, individual factors associated with successful outcomes in the ER/TA data included age and psychosocial development and disease risk (AHRQ, 2000a). The ecologic perspective (theory-based intervention), HBM (perceived health risk), and SCT (social support, goal-setting, and interactive activities with food) were public health and health-promotion principles associated with successful outcomes.

For intake of dietary fat, individual factors noted in the ER/TA report that were associated with successful outcomes included disease risk and culture and ethnicity (client variables) (AHRQ, 2000a). The HBM (perceived health risk) and SCT (social support, goal setting, and culture and ethnic-specific interventions) were public health and health-promotion principles associated with successful outcomes.

Although certain variables that can be considered individual factors or key public health and health-promotion principles were associated with intervention success, several other variables that could fit into these categories were not reported. Tables 3-9 and 3-10 list examples of some factors that the ER/TA did not include. Investigators who compiled the ER/TA reviewed numerous studies. Understandably the ER/TA could not include detailed information about each study and every possible factor.

It is legitimate to wonder whether these other unreported factors and principles were considered as intervention variables. Were they considered when interventions were being planned? If they were included in program interventions, were they measured and evaluated? Had they been measured and evaluated, would they have been found to be significant contributors to successful outcomes? For example did helpers assist study participants in developing a change focus (client variable)? Was their stage of change evaluated, and if so, were interventions delivered that matched the individuals' noted stage of change (client variables and relationship variables)? Were study participants assisted with evaluation of their social networks to determine if they had sufficient affirmation, aid, assistance, and honest feedback (extratherapeutic variables)? Were pathways and agency thinking evaluated in study participants, given that these processes are known to foster hope (expectancy and placebo variables)? Was the educational information used in the interventions formally evaluated? For example how many important points were presented? Were materials presented in ways that were meaningful to the target group (CIP)? Were study participants engaged in the development and evaluation of programs designed to affect their health problems (community organization)? Did any interventions include organizational efforts? Did they facilitate change in community and organizational structure and policies to better support healthy eating (organizational development)?

Understandably it is neither feasible nor pertinent to evaluate all these potential variables. However, with regard to promoting dietary changes, by evaluating some of these important variables, such as stage of change, pathway and agency thinking, types of social support, and organizational development efforts, we will likely improve our ability to identify what type of intervention program works best for whom and when.

Table 3-8 COMPARISON OF RESULTS FROM EVIDENCE REPORT/TECHNOLOGY ASSESSMENT REPORT WITH CHANGE PROMOTING INDIVIDUAL FACTORS AND PUBLIC HEALTH AND HEALTH-PROMOTION PRINCIPLES

Target of Interventions, ER/TA	Factors and Principles Associated with Behavior Change	Study Variables Associated with Successful Outcomes, ER/TA
Intake of Fruits and Vegetables	Individual Factors	
	Client Variables	Age/psychosocial development Disease risk
	Public Health/Health-Promotion Principles	
	Ecologic perspective: program planning, multiple levels of influence, and coordinated interventions	Theory-based interventions
	Health Belief Model	Perceived health risk?
	Social Cognitive Theory	Social support Goal setting Interactive activities with food
Intake of Dietary Fat	Individual Factors	
	Client Variables	Disease risk Culture/ethnicity
	Public Health/Health-Promotion Principles	
	Health Belief Model	Perceived health risk?
	Social Cognitive Theory	Social support Goal-setting Culture/ethnicity-specific interventions

Data from Agency for Healthcare Research and Quality: Efficacy of interventions to modify dietary behavior related to cancer risk. Summary, evidence report/technology assessment: number 25. AHRQ Publication No. 01-E028, Rockville, Md, 2000, Agency for Healthcare Research and Quality. http://www.ahrq.gov/clinic/dietsumm.htm

Table 3-9 CHANGE-PROMOTING INDIVIDUAL FACTORS AND PUBLIC HEALTH AND HEALTH-PROMOTION PRINCIPLES NOT REPORTED IN THE EVIDENCE REPORT/TECHNOLOGY ASSESSMENT REPORT FOR INTAKE OF FRUITS AND VEGETABLES

Factors and Principles Associated with Behavior Change	Study Variables Associated with Successful Outcomes, ER/TA
INDIVIDUAL FACTORS	
Client Variables	Age/psychosocial development
	Disease risk
Extratherapeutic Events	Not reported
Relationship Factors	Not reported
Expectancy and Placebo Factors	Not reported
Techniques and Models	Not reported
PUBLIC HEALTH/HEALTH-PROMOTION PRINCIPLES	
Ecologic Perspective	Theory-based interventions
Stages of Change	Not reported
Consumer Information Processing	Not reported
Health Belief Model	Perceived health risk?
Social Cognitive Theory	Social support
	Goal-setting
	Interactive activities with food
Community Organization	Not reported
Diffusion of Innovation	Not reported
Organizational Change	Not reported

Data from Agency for Healthcare Research and Quality: Efficacy of interventions to modify dietary behavior related to cancer risk. Summary, evidence report/technology assessment: number 25. AHRQ Publication No. 01-E028, Rockville, Md, 2000, Agency for Healthcare Research and Quality. http://www.ahrq.gov/clinic/dietsumm.htm

Table 3-10 CHANGE-PROMOTING INDIVIDUAL FACTORS AND PUBLIC HEALTH AND HEALTH-PROMOTION PRINCIPLES NOT REPORTED IN EVIDENCE REPORT/TECHNOLOGY ASSESSMENT REPORT FOR INTAKE OF DIETARY FAT

Factors and Principles Associated with Behavior Change	Study Variables Associated with Successful Outcomes, ER/TA
INDIVIDUAL FACTORS	
Client Variables	Disease risk
	Culture/ethnicity
Extratherapeutic Events	Not reported
Relationship Factors	Not reported
Expectancy and Placebo Factors	Not reported
Techniques and Models	Not reported
PUBLIC HEALTH/HEALTH-PROMOTION PRINCIPLES	
Ecologic Perspective	Not reported
Stages of Change	Not reported
Consumer Information Processing	Not reported
Health Belief Model	Perceived health risk?
Social Cognitive Theory	Social support
	Goal setting
	Culture/ethnicity-specific interventions
Community Organization	Not reported
Diffusion of Innovation	Not reported
Organizational Change	Not reported

Data from Agency for Healthcare Research and Quality: Efficacy of interventions to modify dietary behavior related to cancer risk. Summary, evidence report/technology assessment: number 25. AHRQ Publication No. 01-E028, Rockville, Md, 2000, Agency for Healthcare Research and Quality. http://www.ahrq.gov/clinic/dietsumm.htm

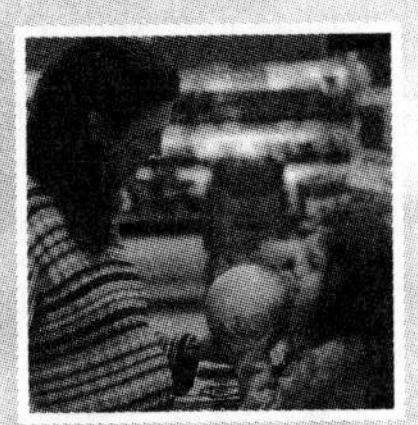

PART **TWO**

REPRODUCTION

CHAPTER

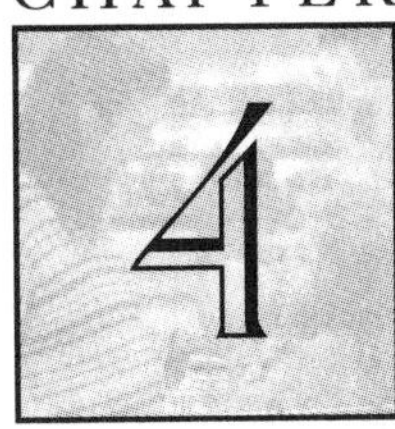

Pregnancy

Chapter Outline

Melissa is a 24-year-old accountant. She is 165 cm (65 in) tall, physically active, and concerned about being healthy. When her home pregnancy test was positive, Melissa immediately made an appointment at the obstetric clinic in her healthcare program.

Two weeks later, after a physical examination, the obstetrician pronounced her in excellent health, but at 52 kg (114 lb), a little underweight. When Melissa told her that she was having some difficulty with nausea and vomiting, the obstetrician reassured her that was normal and had the nurse give her a list of suggestions for controlling nausea. She gave Melissa a prescription for prenatal vitamins with iron and sent her to have some blood work done at a laboratory down the hall.

At her appointment the next month, Melissa's weight had dropped to 51 kg (112 lb). She said the nausea had subsided, but that she didn't want to gain too much weight. Concerned, the physician made an appointment for her to see the dietitian, Amy Smith, the following week. Melissa liked Amy right away. Amy measured her height, weight, and fatfolds, and they chatted about how Melissa felt and what she ate. Amy asked Melissa if she was taking the prenatal vitamin with the iron supplement. Melissa assured her she did because she wants to do everything right for her baby. Amy then pointed out that Melissa should also pay attention to her weight gain to help the fetus grow normally. She suggested that because Melissa was underweight when she became pregnant, she should gain a total of 28 to 40 pounds. Amy gave Melissa a chart to monitor her weight gain and, using a Food Guide for pregnancy, they discussed foods she needed to eat to achieve that weight. Melissa met with Amy again the following month.

By the fifth month, Melissa had gained 5.5 kg (13 lb) and said she felt great. The blood tests were repeated. Melissa felt good and she was gaining weight at the rate Amy had suggested. At about 7 months, Melissa weighed 61.5 kg (135 lb). She and her husband attended prenatal classes, which helped prepare them for the labor and delivery. The classes included information about diet and exercise. They had a tour of the hospital labor and delivery areas.

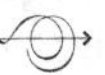

Soon Melissa was going for office visits every 2 weeks and then weekly. She called Amy about problems she was having with constipation and indigestion. Amy assured her that they were common during late pregnancy and made some suggestions about increasing the fiber and fluid content of her diet to relieve constipation and making some changes in her evening meal pattern to reduce heartburn. By the end of her pregnancy, Melissa had gained 17 kg (37 lb) and her new baby daughter weighed 3.4 kg (7.5 lb).

The greatest assurance of a baby's healthy start in life is a mother who has been well nourished throughout her life and during pregnancy. Pregnancy is a critical period of rapid growth and development for the fetus and high physiologic and metabolic demands are made on the mother. Nutrition deserves special consideration to make sure that it is not a limiting factor in maternal or infant health.

THE FEMALE REPRODUCTIVE CYCLE

- *Describe the sequence of changes in the menstrual cycle and the role they play in preparation for pregnancy.*
- *What hormones regulate the follicular and luteal phases in the ovary and the proliferative and secretory stages in the uterus?*
- *What is the premenstrual dysphoric disorder (PDD)?*
- *Can diet play a role in the treatment of PDD?*

The onset of menarche, usually between 11 and 14 years of age in girls living in developed countries, begins the female reproductive cycle, which continues until **menopause.** The female reproductive years are characterized by monthly cyclic changes in the secretion of the female hormones and corresponding changes in the ovaries and uterus. This pattern, called the menstrual cycle, usually lasts about 28 days. It is characterized by formation of a mature ovum that is released from one of the ovaries each month and a uterine **endometrium,** which is prepared for implantation of a fertilized ovum. If the ovum is released and fertilization does not occur, these preparations are discarded (menstruation) and the cycle repeats itself.

KEY TERMS

menopause: the span of time during which the menstrual cycle wanes and gradually stops, around age 50

endometrium: mucous membrane lining the uterus

gonadotropic hormones: hormones that has a stimulating effect on ovary and testes

progesterone: steroid hormone that causes changes in the endometrium preparatory to implantation

Hormones

The menstrual cycle is synchronized by the **gonadotropic hormones** from the anterior pituitary gland. The follicle-stimulating hormone (FSH) stimulates growth and maturation of follicles in the ovary and luteinizing hormone (LH) stimulates development of the ruptured follicle into the corpus luteum and signals ovulation. Two other significant hormones, estrogen and **progesterone,** are produced by the ovary under the stimulation of FSH and LH.

Follicular/Proliferative Phase

Figure 4-1 depicts the various stages of the menstrual cycle in the ovaries and uterus. At the beginning of each cycle, the onset of menstruation, the concentrations of FSH and LH from the anterior pituitary increase. These increases initiate accelerated growth of the cells in the ovarian follicles, ovum, and surrounding layers of cells (follicular phase). The ovum enlarges and develops into a mature follicle. Additional layers of cells

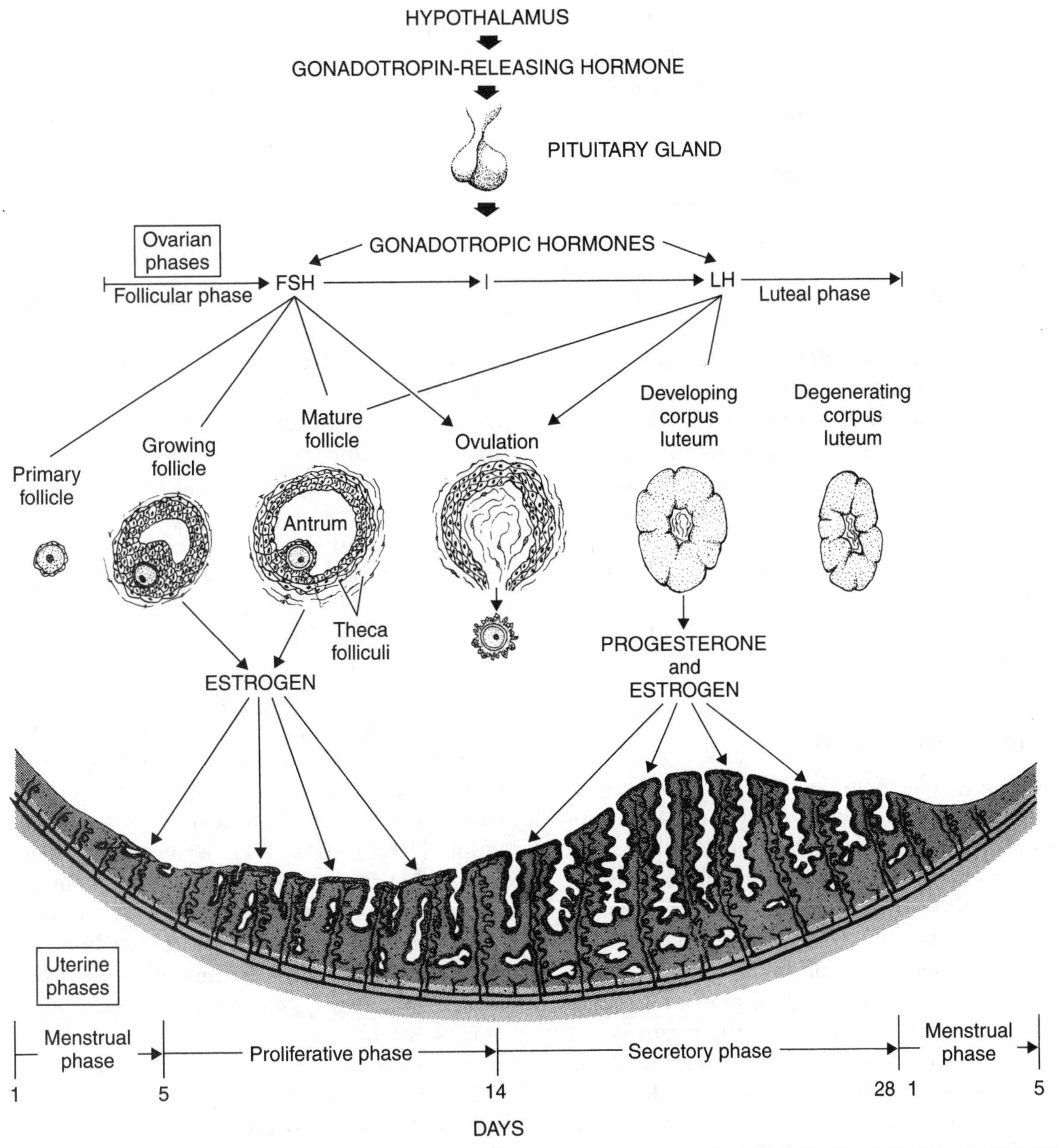

Figure 4-1 Hormones and phases of the menstrual cycle. The ovarian cycles are controlled by the pituitary gland, which in turn is controlled by gonadotropin-releasing hormone produced by neurosecretory cells in the hypothalamus of the brain. This schematic drawing illustrates the interrelations among the hypothalamus of the brain, the pituitary gland, the ovaries, and the endometrium of the uterus. One complete menstrual cycle is shown. Follicle-stimulating hormone (FSH) and luteinizing hormone (LH), which are released by the pituitary gland, stimulate the ovaries. Hormones from the ovaries (estrogen and progesterone) then promote changes in the structure and function of the endometrium. This process is called the menstrual cycle. Thus, the cyclical activity of the ovary is intimately linked with changes in the uterus. *(Modified from Moore KL and Persaud TVN: The developing human, ed 5, Philadelphia, 1993, WB Saunders.)*

develop around the ovum and secrete a fluid that contains a high concentration of estrogen. After approximately 12 days, the secretion of LH and FSH increases. The LH causes some cells in the follicle to **luteinize** and increase secretion of progesterone. In this environment—rapid growth of the follicle during a prolonged phase of excessive estrogen, followed by diminishing estrogen secretion and increasing secretion of progesterone—**ovulation** occurs about 14 days after the onset of menstruation.

The cycle begins simultaneously in the uterus, with most of the uterine endometrium being shed during menstruation. Estrogen released from the ovarian follicle initiates the proliferative phase, which lasts for approximately 2 weeks and ceases with ovulation. This phase stimulates rapid cell proliferation of the uterine lining and endometrium. The endometrium thickens and develops an extensive vascular system in preparation for implantation of the ovum should fertilization occur.

Luteal/Secretory Phase

In the ovary, cells of the follicle that remained after expulsion of the ovum from the follicle undergo rapid physical and chemical change and become a **corpus luteum.** In this luteal phase of the cycle, the corpus luteum secretes progesterone and estrogen, which causes a feedback decrease in secretion of both FSH and LH. Therefore during this period no new follicles begin to grow in the ovary. When the ovum is not fertilized, the corpus luteum **involutes** and the lack of estrogen feedback suppression allows the anterior pituitary gland to secrete greater quantities of FSH and LH. The FSH and LH initiate growth of new follicles and the next ovarian cycle begins.

The progesterone and estrogen secreted in large quantities by the corpus luteum during the luteal phase initiate the secretory phase in the uterus. This phase involves cellular proliferation, which results in swelling and increased secretion of the endometrium. These changes produce an endometrium containing large nutrient reserves that can provide favorable conditions for implantation of a fertilized ovum. If fertilization does not occur, approximately 2 days before the end of the monthly cycle, the ovarian hormones estrogen and progesterone decrease sharply. Menstruation follows and the cycle begins again.

Premenstrual Dysphoric Disorder

Premenstrual **dysphoria** affects as many as 40% of American women in their reproductive years (Daugherty, 1998). Every month millions of women experience symptoms such as headaches, mood swings, breast swelling, acne, depression, irritability, and food cravings just before their menstrual periods. Often referred to as premenstrual syndrome (PMS), the cluster of varied symptoms—mood, physical, cognitive, or a combination thereof—that appears during the luteal phase has been designated as PDD by the American Psychiatric Association (1994).

Overall approximately 80% of women complain of some premenstrual symptoms, but only 3% to 5% of cycling women can be categorized with true PDD (American College of Obstetricians and Gynecologists, 1995) according to the 11 criteria established by the American Psychiatric Association (1994) (Box 4-1). Diagnosis of PDD requires that 5 of the 11 symptoms must be severe premenstrually with postmenstrual remission and the 5 must include at least one dysphoric symptom (irritability, mood swings, anxiety, or depression). Multiple physical symptoms are considered one symptom.

The cause of the disorder is unknown and, over the last four decades, more than 50 treatment options have been suggested to be effective. Nutrient metabolism and status may play a role in regulating normal menstrual cycles. Variations in energy intake, protein, fat, and carbohydrate have been correlated with the cycle phase. Interest currently centers on differences in tryptophan metabolism between follicular and luteal phases.

Many women who suffer from PDD have cravings for sweets and increased consumption of carbohydrate-rich foods. A double-blind crossover study tested the effect of a high-carbohydrate bev-

Box 4-1 Criteria for Premenstrual Dysphoric Disorder

1. Markedly depressed mood, feelings of hopelessness, or self-deprecating thoughts
2. Marked anxiety, tension, feeling of being "keyed up" or "on edge"
3. Marked affective liability (e.g., feeling suddenly sad or tearful or feeling increased sensitivity to rejection)
4. Persistent and marked anger or irritability or increase in interpersonal conflicts
5. Decreased interest in usual activities (e.g., work, school, friends, hobbies)
6. Subjective sense of difficulty in concentrating
7. Lethargy, easy fatigability, or marked lack of energy
8. Marked change in appetite, overeating, or specific food cravings.
9. Hypersomnia or insomnia
10. A subjective sense of being overwhelmed or out of control
11. Other physical symptoms, such as breast tenderness or swelling, headaches, joint or muscle pain, a sensation of bloating, weight gain

The disturbances *must* markedly interfere with work or school or with usual social activities and relationships with others (e.g., avoidance of social activities, decreased productivity and efficiency at work or school).

The disturbances *must not* be an exacerbation of the symptoms of another disorder (e.g., major depressive disorder, panic disorder, dysthymic disorder, or a personality disorder).

erage and a placebo on PDD symptoms across three menstrual cycles (Sayegh et al., 1995). Compared with the placebo, the carbohydrate beverage decreased self-reported depression, anger, confusion, and carbohydrate craving and improved memory word recognition 90 to 180 minutes after ingestion. Results suggest that the psychologic and affective symptoms of PMS can be relieved by consuming a carbohydrate-rich beverage known to increase serum tryptophan levels.

Because no specific cause has been identified for PMS, treatment has been difficult and controversial. More than 30% of affected women have shown improvement of symptoms when given a placebo. Premenstrual dysphoria shares many of the features of depression and anxiety states that have been linked to serotoninergic dysregulation. Deficiencies in **serotonin**-mediated brain neurotransmitters may be responsible, in part, for symptoms of dysphoria. In fact treatment of premenstrual dysphoria with serotonin reuptake inhibitors (antidepressants) reduces symptoms of tension, irritability, and dysphoria (Johnson, 1998). These drugs are easily tolerated and free of major side effects. Other antidepressants are sometimes used. Treatment is often designed to improve or eliminate the symptoms. Tranquilizers may be useful to relieve anxiety, analgesics may relieve headaches, and diuretics may help with fluid retention.

For many women with mild symptoms, supportive counseling and general self-care measures such as exercise and adoption of improved nutrition can be successful strategies (Bendich, 2000). These changes include exercise, avoidance of tobacco and excess alcohol, relaxation training, psychotherapy, and consumption of a balanced diet. They are associated with an improvement in general health, which could make PDD more tolerable.

Key Terms

luteinize: the process after ovulation by which an ovarian follicle transforms into a corpus luteum

ovulation: process in which an ovum is discharged from an ovary

corpus luteum: mass formed in the ovary by a follicle after it has matured and lost the ovum; the corpus luteum secretes progesterone

involutes: regresses

dysphoria: excessive disquiet, agitation, and restlessness

serotonin: a neurotransmitter synthesized from tryptophan that is important in appetite control, sleep regulation, and sensory perception

NUTRITION AND REPRODUCTION

- *How can prepregnancy nutrition intervention improve pregnancy outcome?*
- *What is* ***periconceptional*** *nutrition?*
- *What disorders can be treated before conception to improve pregnancy outcomes?*

Periconceptional Nutrition

The birth, growth, and development of a healthy infant depends on a woman's health and well-being before conception and the amount and quality of care received during pregnancy and recovery from labor and delivery. Preconceptual care is an organized, comprehensive program that identifies and reduces women's medical, psychologic, social, and life-style reproductive risks before conception (Institute of Medicine [IOM], 1985; U.S. Public Health Service Expert Panel on the Content of Prenatal Care, 1989).

Components of preconceptual care are essentially the same as those of the nutrition care process discussed in Chapter 2. The purpose of nutrition risk assessment is to identify women at risk for an unfavorable pregnancy outcome. Health promotion, counseling, and medical modalities are used for intervention to reduce risk. High-risk behaviors such as smoking and alcohol or substance abuse can be identified and counseling or treatment initiated (Walker and Wilging, 2000). For some women, dietary changes before conception can reduce risk and have a positive influence on pregnancy outcome. Women with medical conditions such as diabetes mellitus (see page 158) or phenylketonuria (see page 154) have improved pregnancy outcomes with strict preconceptional metabolic control. Preconceptional modification of exposure to medications or other substances known to be **teratogens** reduces the risk of anomalies in the newborn. In recent years the dramatic increase in the use of nutrient supplements and dietary supplements may result in excess consumption of some nutrients, such as vitamin A, that increase risk of birth defects (Voyles et al., 2000). An important function of preconceptional nutrition risk assessment is to determine dietary intake, including use of such products.

Preconceptional assessment of nutrition status also identifies conditions or practices such as bulimia, anorexia, pica, hypervitaminosis, vegetarianism, and extremes of body weight that may compromise nutrition status. Once identified, nutrition counseling and, in some cases, treatment of underlying conditions can be initiated. Nutrient supplements may be recommended. For example multivitamins containing folate taken during the preconceptional period have been associated with a reduced recurrence of birth defects of the **neural tube** and are recommended for all women who may become pregnant (Botto et al., 1999; Centers for Disease Control, 1991).

EFFECT OF NUTRITION ON REPRODUCTION

- *How is pregnancy outcome defined for mother and infant?*
- *How can nutrition or diet influence pregnancy outcome?*

Multiple Risk Factors

Although most experts agree that nutrition is a factor in successful reproduction, the accumulation of direct evidence of a correlation between nutrition and reproductive performance is complicated by variations in age, parity, socioeconomic and education status of the mother, and her health and use of healthcare resources. Women most likely to be poorly nourished also have other risk factors for poor pregnancy outcome because of cultural, socioeconomic, or lifestyle factors. Although human studies on the effect of undernutrition on reproduction are limited, evidence has accumulated from observations of civilian populations subjected to semistarvation during World War II and populations that have experienced famine. In the last two decades additional information has been contributed from studies of women at nutrition risk who received supplemental food, nutrition counseling, or both. These findings include observations from several developing countries and the United States and Canada.

Undernutrition

Severe and acute undernutrition in previously well-nourished women is associated with a reversible decline in fertility rates (Stein et al., 1975). Severe undernutrition superimposed on previous marginal nutrition is associated with low fertility rates and, when conception occurs, an increase in **preterm births** and neonatal deaths (Winkvist et al., 1992).

Severe undernutrition at the time of conception and during early pregnancy can be manifested in birth defects. Although undernutrition that occurs later in **gestation** is less likely to result in birth defects, infants are likely to experience **fetal growth restriction** and be of **low birth weight.** Mild to moderate undernutrition has less impact on fertility, but may have far-reaching, and as yet undefined, effects on maternal and child health.

Intervention Studies

In developing countries intervention studies of pregnant women who improved their diets or who received nutrient or caloric supplements have shown moderate improvements in birth weight, infant survival, and childhood growth and development. In developed countries the results of intervention programs have been mixed. The beneficial effect of food supplements on maternal weight gain and fetal growth appears to depend on the prior energy deficiency of the mother and the extent to which the supplement compensates for that deficit. In a program in Montreal, nutrition supplementation and counseling were shown to improve pregnancy outcome (Rush, 1981). Similarly the Special Supplemental Food Program for Women, Infants, and Children (WIC) has documented changes in pregnancy outcome in poor women at nutritional risk (Rush et al., 1988) (see the Application at the end of Chapter 5). Although gains in infant birth weight have been lower than predicted from levels of supplementation, even modest changes in birth weight can have significant impact for reducing **perinatal** mortality and impairment (Susser, 1991).

Information regarding the effect of undernutrition on the male's reproductive role is limited. Malnutrition is associated with decreased libido and a reduction in the number, motility, and lifespan of sperm (Stein et al., 1975). Malnutrition during puberty can delay growth and development. For example Prasad has demonstrated dwarfism, hypogonadism, and iron deficiency anemia in zinc-deficient men in Egypt and Iran (Prasad, 1988).

Factors Related to Pregnancy Outcome

A successful pregnancy can be defined in terms of many outcome measures, the most significant of which are perinatal mortality, infant birth weight, and gestational age. A number of nutritional factors are related to reproductive performance. The nutrition status of a woman reflects her own birth status and her early nutrition and development. For example there is a correlation between a mother's birth weight and the weight of her infant (Klebanoff and Yip, 1987). Maternal height also has been related to infant birth weight and some researchers suggest that this correlation reflects maternal growth and, indirectly, long-term nutritional adequacy (Parsons et al., 1991).

KEY TERMS

periconceptional: the period from 1 month to 3 months before pregnancy through the first 6 weeks after delivery

teratogens: any agents that cause malformation in the fetus and birth defects

neural tube: tube formed in embryonic period from which the brain and spinal cord develop

preterm birth: birth occurring after a gestation of less than 37 weeks

gestation: period from conception to birth

fetal growth restriction: failure to grow at usual rate for time in the uterus; also called intrauterine growth retardation

low birth weight: a birth weight of less than 2500 g

perinatal: ranging from the twenty-eighth week of gestation to 28 days after birth

Maternal weight at the time of conception and gestational weight gain are the strongest predictors of infant birth weight (Abrams and Selvin, 1995; Mitchell and Lerner, 1989b). Underweight women are more likely to have low-birth-weight infants (Mitchell and Lerner, 1989a), higher fetal and neonatal mortality rates, more complications (Naeye, 1979), and perhaps higher risk of preterm delivery. Obese women have a greater risk of hypertension, diabetes, complications during labor and delivery, **postterm** births, and late fetal death (Cnattingius et al., 1998). During pregnancy many social, economic, education, and lifestyle factors can cause inadequate dietary intakes and poor gestational weight gain, increasing the risk of an unfavorable outcome (Hickey, 2000). In addition diets that are low in energy are likely to be below recommended intake levels for other nutrients. Inadequate prenatal care is associated with increased risk of preterm delivery (Krueger and Scholl, 2000).

PREGNANCY

- *Define ovulation, fertilization, and implantation.*
- *Describe the sequence and timing of critical phases of embryonic and fetal development.*
- *How is the developing embryo or fetus nourished?*
- *What are the functions of the placenta?*
- *Outline the physiologic changes of pregnancy.*
- *How might maternal undernutrition influence these changes?*

KEY TERMS

postterm: birth occurring after a gestation of 42 weeks
peritoneal cavity: space between the membranes lining the walls of the abdomen and pelvic cavities
zygote: fertilized ovum
morula: solid mass of cells formed by cleavage of a fertilized ovum
blastocyst: a stage in the developing embryo in which the cells are organized in a single layer to form a hollow sphere
trophoblastic: *tropho,* meaning food, nourishment; *blastic,* meaning immature stage in cellular development

During pregnancy a single fertilized cell grows into millions of cells of complex tissues, organs, and systems in just 40 weeks. Such rapid growth makes the developing fetus vulnerable to nutritional inadequacies. Diet deserves special consideration during pregnancy to ensure that it does not limit the growth and development of the fetus or the health of the mother.

Conception and Implantation

When ovulation occurs, the ovum, with its attached cells, is expelled directly into the **peritoneal cavity** and enters one of the fallopian tubes (Figure 4-2). Fertilization of the ovum normally takes place soon after the ovum enters the fallopian tube. After fertilization approximately 3 days are required for transport of the **zygote** through the tube into the uterus. Several stages of division occur before the zygote reaches the uterus. The first divisions produce a solid sphere of cells, the **morula,** but during subsequent divisions the cells pull away from the center and form a hollow cavity (Figure 4-3). This is referred to as a **blastocyst.** The developing ovum remains in the uterine cavity 4 to 5 days before it implants in the endometrium. Therefore implantation occurs 7 or 8 days after ovulation. During this time the nutrition needs of the ovum are met from the endometrial secretions.

Implantation is initiated by **trophoblastic** cells that develop over the surface of the blastocyst (Figure 4-4). These cells secrete proteolytic enzymes that digest and liquefy the cells of the endometrium. Fluid and nutrients released from these cells are absorbed into the blastocyst via phagocytosis by the trophoblastic cells. These substances provide the sustenance for further growth. At the same time, additional trophoblastic cells form cords of cells that extend into deeper layers of the endometrium and attach. This is implantation. Once implantation has taken place the trophoblastic and other cells proliferate rapidly and, with cells from the mother's endometrium, form the placenta and the various membranes of pregnancy.

As trophoblastic cells invade the endometrium, the stored nutrients are used by the

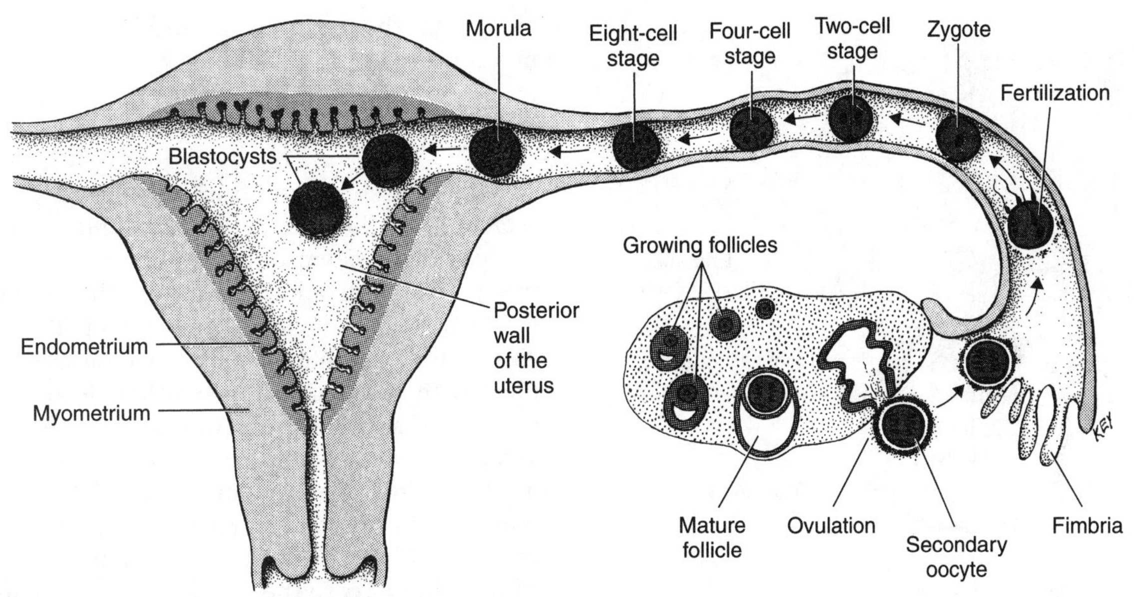

Figure 4-2 The beginning of human development, ovulation, conception, and blastocyst formation. Diagrammatic representation of ovulation, fertilization, and human development during the first week. Stage 1 of development begins with fertilization and ends when the zygote forms. Stage 2 (days 2 to 3) comprises the early stages of division, from two to about six cells of the morula. Stage 3 (days 4 to 5) consists of the free, unattached blastocyst. Stage 4 (days 5 to 6) is represented by the blastocyst attaching to the posterior wall of the uterus, a common site of implantation. The blastocysts have been sectioned to show their structure. *(From Moore KL and Persaud TVN: The developing human, ed 5, Philadelphia, 1993, WB Saunders.)*

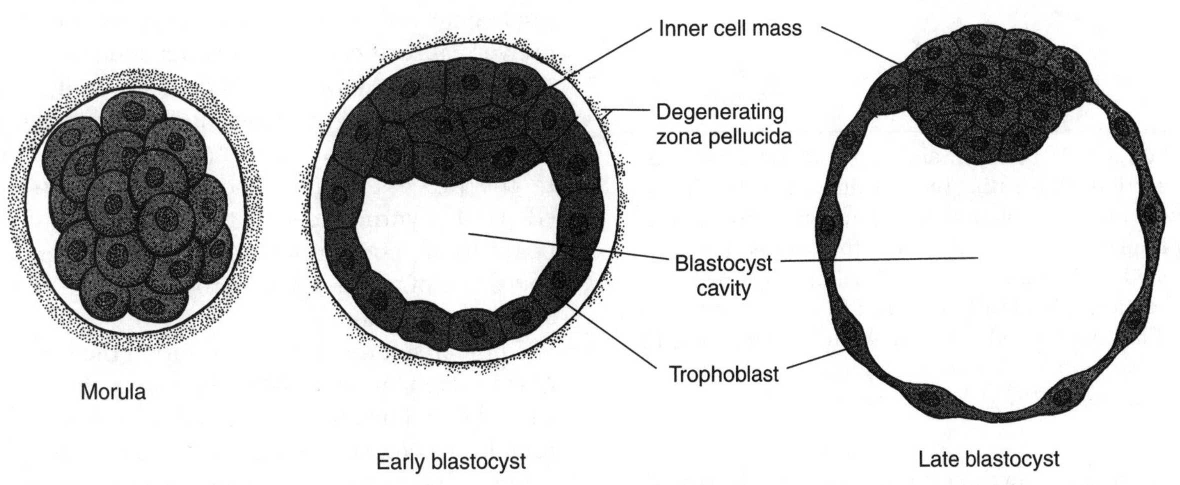

Figure 4-3 Formation of the embryoblast. The morula enters the uterus. The cells separate into two parts—an outer cell layer called the trophoblast and a centrally located cell mass on embryoblast. *(From Moore KL and Persaud TVN: The developing human, ed 5, Philadelphia, 1993, WB Saunders.)*

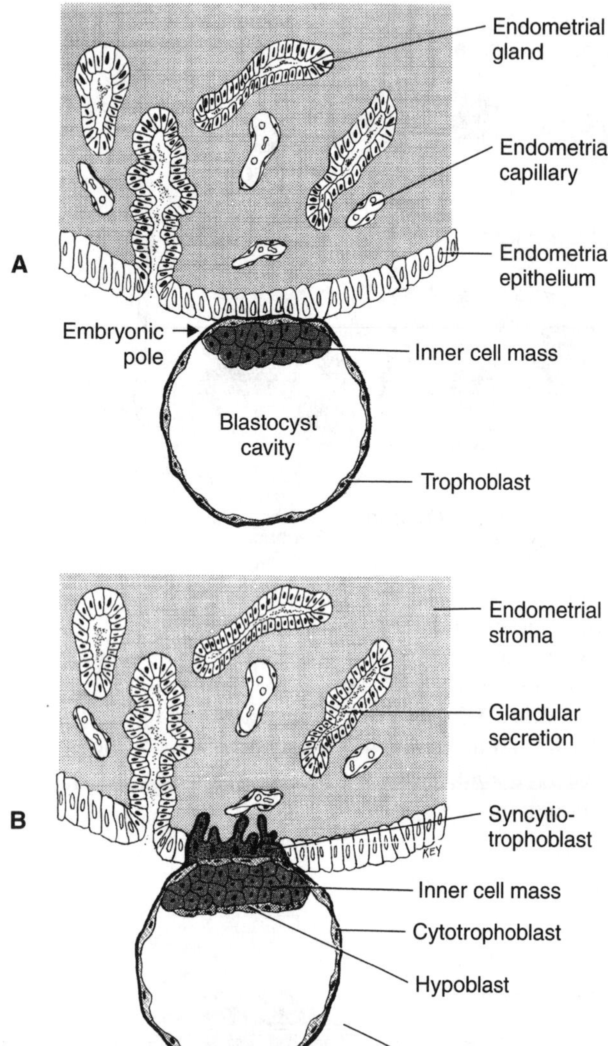

Figure 4-4 Attachment and implantation. Drawings of sections illustrating the attachment of the blastocyst to the endometrial epithelium and early stages of implantation. **A**, 6 days: the trophoblast is attached to the endometrial epithelium. **B**, 7 days: the syncytiotrophoblast has formed from the trophoblast and has penetrated the epithelium. *(From Moore KL and Persaud TVN: The developing human, ed 5, Philadelphia, 1993, WB Saunders.)*

embryo for growth and development. During the first week after implantation, the endometrium is the only source of nutrients to the embryo and it continues to contribute a large measure of its nutrition for 8 to 12 weeks. During this time the placenta gradually begins to increase its efficiency in the transfer of nutrients from the mother.

The Placenta

As trophoblastic cords from the blastocyst are attaching to the uterus, blood capillaries from the vascular system of the embryo are growing into cords that will become part of the placenta. By the sixteenth day after fertilization, blood begins to flow. Simultaneously blood **sinuses** supplied with blood from the mother develop between the surface of the uterine endometrium and the trophoblastic cords. Thus the villi carrying fetal blood are surrounded by sinuses containing maternal blood (Figure 4-5). Over time the fetal villi subdivide and form many branches, which will increase the exchange by providing a larger surface area. The fetus is surrounded by a fluid-filled sac called the amniotic sac. Within the sac the **umbilical cord** extends through the abdomen of the fetus to the placenta.

The major function of the placenta is to allow diffusion of oxygen and nutrients from the maternal blood across the placental membrane to the blood of the growing fetus and to allow diffusion of carbon dioxide and metabolic excretory products such as urea, uric acid, and creatinine from the fetus back to the mother. The trophoblastic cells in the placental membrane can actively absorb certain nutrients such as amino acids, calcium, inorganic phosphate, and ascorbic acid, resulting in higher quantities in the fetal blood than in the maternal circulation. Early in the process human chorionic gonadotropin (HCG) is synthesized by the placenta and appears to support implantation. The placenta is also a site of synthesis of estrogen, progesterone, and other hormones.

In the first few months of gestation the placenta grows much more rapidly than does the fetus. During this time quantities of substrates including protein, calcium, and iron are stored in the placenta to be used later for fetal growth. This function of the placenta in early pregnancy has been compared with that of the liver in adults. Later in gestation these metabolic functions of the placenta become less important as the fetal liver progressively assumes this important role on its own.

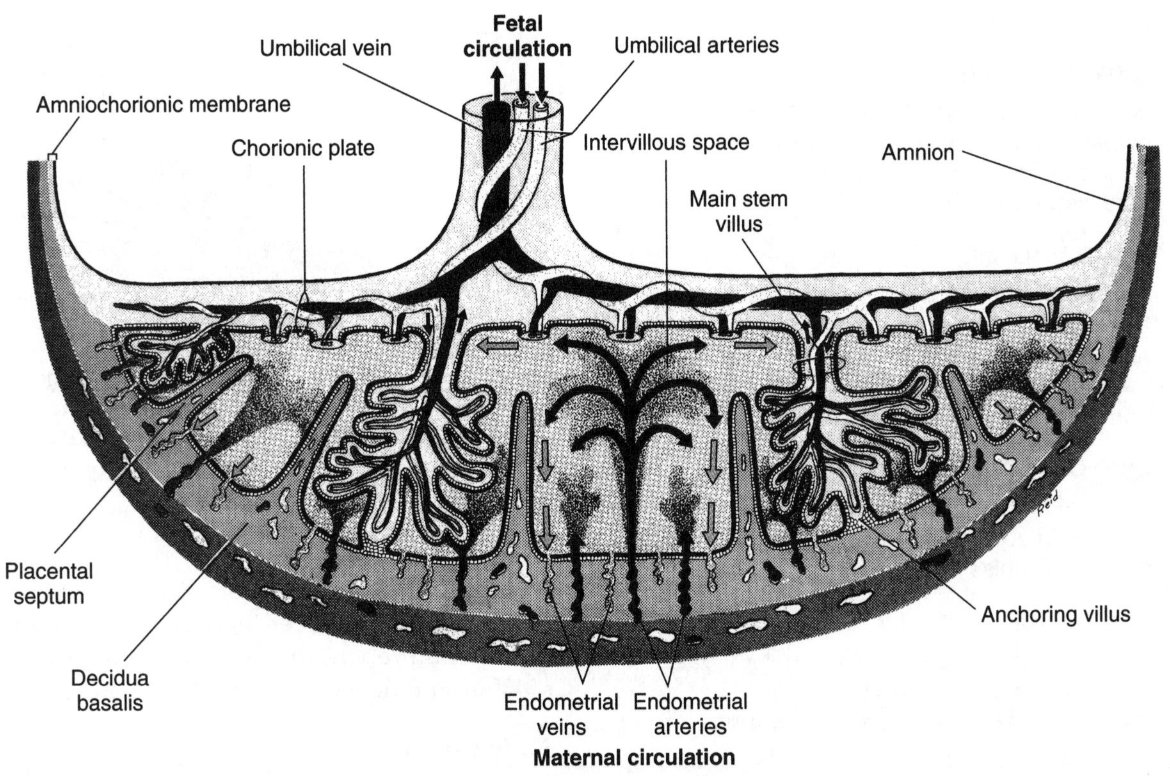

Figure 4-5 Schematic drawing of a section through a full-term placenta shows: (1) the relation of the villous chorion (fetal part of the placenta) to the decidua basalis (maternal part of placenta); (2) the fetal placental circulation; and (3) the maternal–placental circulation. Maternal blood flows into the intervillous space in funnel-shaped spurts, and exchanges occur with the fetal blood as the maternal blood flows around the branch villi (branches of stem villi). The main exchange of material between the mother and embryo/fetus occurs through the branch villi. The inflowing arterial blood pushes venous blood out into the endometrial veins, which are scattered over the entire surface of the decidua basalis. Note that the umbilical arteries carry poorly oxygenated fetal blood to the placenta and that the umbilical vein carries oxygenated blood to the fetus. *(From Moore KL and Persaud TVN: The developing human, ed 5, Philadelphia, 1993, WB Saunders.)*

Physiologic Changes of Pregnancy

Many visible changes occur in a woman's body during pregnancy. Most women gain between 11 and 16 kg (25 to 35 lb). The dimensions of the uterus expand 150 fold, changing the woman's center of equilibrium, and the breasts enlarge in preparation for lactation. In late pregnancy water is retained, causing feet and ankles to swell. These changes are accompanied by a diversity of adaptations in the anatomic, metabolic, and physiologic functions of the mother, to provide for the growing demands of the **conceptus.** Some of these changes are outlined in Box 4-2. In most instances physiologic activity is increased, but smooth muscle (urinary and gastrointestinal tracts) demonstrate decreased activity. Many of these changes occur during the first half of gestation to meet the metabolic demands of the placenta and fetus and to prepare for future needs. Changes during the latter half

KEY TERMS

embyro: the developing organism from 1 week after conception to the eighth week of gestation
sinuses: cavities or hollow spaces
umbilical cord: structure through which fetal veins and arteries reach the placenta
conceptus: product of conception (embryo or fetus)

Box 4-2 Physiologic Changes of Pregnancy

BODY COMPOSITION

Increase in body weight—15 to 40 pounds
Increase in maternal and fetal protein
Increase in maternal fat stores
Increase in body fluid

BLOOD VOLUME

Increase of about 50% in plasma volume
Increase of 18%-30% in red cell volume
Decrease in concentration of blood components, especially albumin, hemoglobin, hematocrit

CARDIOVASCULAR

Increase of 30% to 50% in cardiac output
Increase in stroke volume
Increase in pulse rate

RESPIRATION

Increase in tidal volume—amount of gases exchanged with each breath
Slight increase in respiratory rate; more efficient exchange of gases in alveoli

METABOLISM

Increase of about 15% in basal metabolic rate
Increase in oxygen-carrying capacity of the blood

KIDNEY

Increase in blood flow through the kidneys
Increase in glomerular filtration rate
Increase in excretion of glucose, amino acids, and water-soluble vitamins
Decrease in ability to excrete water, leading to edema of legs and ankles

GASTROINTESTINAL

Increase in appetite
Nausea and vomiting
Altered taste
Increase in absorption of nutrients
Decrease in emptying of the stomach; esophageal regurgitation and heartburn
Decrease in muscle tone, leading to increased water absorption from the colon, contributing to constipation

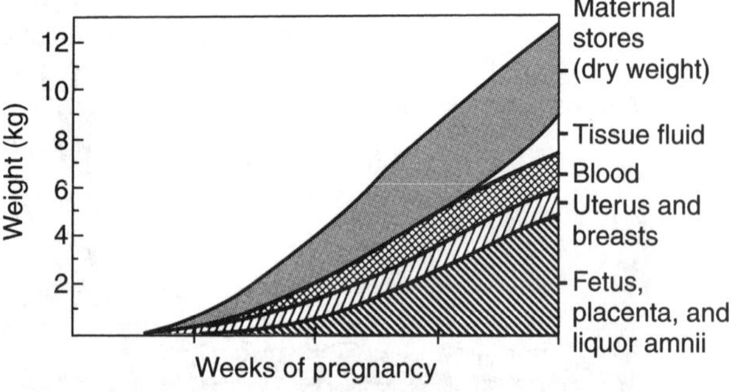

Figure 4-6 Components of gestational weight gain. *(Reprinted with permission from Maternal nutrition and the course of pregnancy, copyright 1970 by the National Academy of Sciences. Courtesy of the National Academy Press, Washington, DC.)*

of pregnancy help meet increasing fetal requirements and prepare the mother for the demands of labor and delivery and for lactation.

Body Composition

Many changes in body composition take place during pregnancy. An average weight gain of 12.5 kg, associated with a typical 40-week pregnancy, amounts to an approximate 20% increase in body weight. Most weight gain occurs during the last 20 weeks of gestation. About 40% of this weight gain is represented by the fetus, placenta, and amniotic fluid (Figure 4-6), and 60% is the maternal weight change (Forbes, 1962). The 6 kg to 8 kg (13 to 18 lb) of maternal weight that accumulate, particularly in the last 20 weeks, include increased fluid volume, protein deposition, and fat stores. These changes are from increased mammary, uterine, kidney, and heart tissue volume, and an increase in total fluid volume and body fat (Forbes, 1987). Changes in fat stores are somewhat more difficult to quantify. It has been estimated that approximately one third of the total gestational weight gain, or 3 kg to 6 kg (6 to 13 lb) is fat. Measurement of body fat using densitometry indicates that the increase in the percentage of body fat during gestation ranges from 2.6% to 8%. Women who gained more than 8.5 kg (19 lb) during pregnancy had greater fat accumulation than those who gained less weight.

Blood Volume

Perhaps the most striking maternal physiologic alteration of pregnancy is the 45% to 50% increase in blood volume. Hypervolemia begins in the first trimester, increases rapidly in the second trimester, and plateaus at about the thirtieth week. The increase is needed to provide for extra blood flow to the uterus, extra metabolic needs of the fetus, and increased perfusion of other organs, especially the kidneys. The increase in blood volume is accompanied by a smaller increase in red cell volume and concentration of various blood proteins, lipids, and enzymes. Therefore hemoglobin concentration falls during pregnancy until about the thirtieth week. This fall results because plasma volume increases more than does red cell volume, in a phenomenon often referred to as hemodilution. Iron supplementation during pregnancy modifies, but does not obliterate, the usual fall in hemoglobin and hematocrit levels during pregnancy (Figure 4-7).

If the increases in blood volume are inadequate, there will be smaller increases in cardiac output, resulting in decreased blood flow to the placenta and reduced transfer of nutrients to the fetus. Such a series of events that compromise fetal growth can be from a number of factors, including maternal undernutrition. In this case high levels of hemoglobin or hematocrit may indicate a reduction in volume expansion and be associated with increased fetal risk.

Cardiovascular Changes

During pregnancy, cardiac output increases approximately 40%, reaching its maximum at 20 to 24 weeks and continuing at this level until term. There is little change in systolic blood pressure, but diastolic pressure declines somewhat. Peripheral resistance declines markedly and blood flow increases to the uterus, placenta, and kidney.

Metabolism

As a consequence of the increased secretion of many different hormones during pregnancy, the basal metabolic rate of the mother increases about 15% during the latter half of pregnancy. Hormone changes also result in alterations in carbohydrates, protein, and fat use. Fat becomes

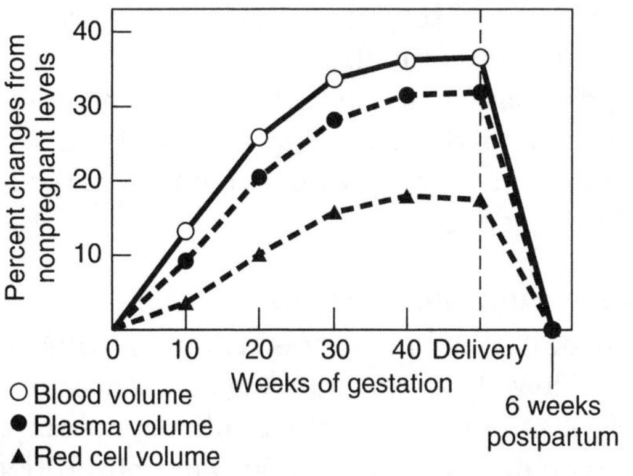

Figure 4-7 Changes in blood volume, plasma volume, and red cell volume during pregnancy. *(From Peek TM and Arias F: Hematologic changes associated with pregnancy, Clin Obstet Gynecol 22(4):785, 1979.)*

the major source of fuel for maternal tissue, whereas the main source of fetal energy is glucose, which is transported across the placenta by facilitated diffusion. Late in the third trimester the fetus metabolizes about 7 g of protein, 35 g of glucose, and 1.7 g of fat each day (Rosso, 1983). If maternal blood glucose is low, the fetus will use more fatty acids to meet energy needs.

Respiration

Because of the increase in basal metabolic rate and increased body size, the total amount of oxygen used by the mother increases, reaching approximately 20% above nonpregnant levels. The growing uterus presses upward against the diaphragm so the total expansion of the diaphragm is decreased. Consequently the respiratory rate is increased to maintain adequate ventilation.

Kidney Function

The rate of filtration of blood by the kidneys increases about 50% in early pregnancy and the level remains high until term. Therefore renal blood flow and clearance of waste products are increased, which tends to increase the loss of glucose, amino acids, and some water-soluble vitamins in the urine. Although the rate of urine formation is slightly increased, water is not excreted as well during pregnancy. This is a consequence of increased production of steroid hormones by the placenta and adrenal cortex, which enhances reabsorption of sodium, chlorine, and water by renal tubules. Hormones secreted during pregnancy have a direct effect on relaxing ureters and the enlarging uterus displaces the urinary bladder upward, leading to increased urinary frequency.

Gastrointestinal Systems

Gastrointestinal motility is reduced during gestation. Slowed gastric emptying and transit of food through the intestinal tract enhances absorption of some nutrients. Increased water absorption in the colon may lead to constipation. Esophageal peristalsis is decreased and gastric **reflux** is more prevalent because of slower gastric emptying time and relaxation of muscle between the esophagus and the stomach. Later in pregnancy this phenomenon is compounded by elevation of the stomach from the enlarged uterus, possibly resulting in heartburn.

Embryonic Development

The development of the placenta, fetal membranes, and amniotic sac allows the uterus to expand and support the growing embryo and fetus (Figure 4-8). The embryonic period encompasses development from implantation of the fertilized ovum to the eighth week of gestation. Growth during this period results from an increase in cell number, called hyperplasia. During this **critical period** of **organogenesis** fetal tissue differentiates into three primitive cell layers—the endoderm, mesoderm, and ectoderm—that eventually become organs and tissues. The endoderm, the innermost layer of embryonic cells, develops into the gastrointestinal tract, lungs, and glandular organs. The middle layer, the mesoderm, forms into voluntary muscles, the skeleton, and the cardiovascular and renal systems. The ectoderm, the outside layer, evolves into the brain, nervous system, hair, and skin. There is a specific timetable for development of each body organ or system (Figure 4-9). Thus specific tissues or organs have critical needs for specific nutrients at different periods. During critical periods the organism is vulnerable to inadequate development or **congenital anomalies** if required nutrients are not available or if it is exposed to teratogenic substances such as drugs, alcohol, radiation, or excess vitamin A.

Embryosis is a period when a woman may not even be aware that she is pregnant. It is also a time when food intake may be reduced by the nausea common to early pregnancy. A mother who has adequate nutrient reserves at the time of conception will be at lesser risk during this period than one with poor or marginal status.

At the end of 4 weeks the embryo weighs about 1 ounce and is less than 1 inch long. Many of the major organs have begun to develop and the heart has begun to beat. During this time nourishment is obtained from the degenerating cells of the wall of the uterus and, to some extent, from blood exchanges via the developing placenta. By week 8 placental exchange provides most nutritional needs and all of the major organs and systems have been differentiated and organized. Cellular development of these structures will be completed in the following months.

KEY TERMS

reflux: movement of some of the stomach contents back into the esophagus
critical period: a period during which specific development takes place; if developmental changes fail to occur during this period "catch-up" will not be complete
organogenesis: development of specific tissues, such as kidney, brain, heart, lungs
congenital anomalies: birth defects

Fetal Growth and Development

The remaining 7 months of gestation are known as the fetal growth period. The hyperplastic growth that characterized the embryonic period continues. In fact the cells of most organs continue to divide after birth, but the rate varies. Fetal growth is also characterized by hypertrophy. At this time needs are high for both quantity and quality of nutrients. A severe nutrient deficiency is less likely to result in a congenital defect than in the embryonic stage, but inadequate dietary intake can contribute to preterm birth or fetal growth restriction. During the third

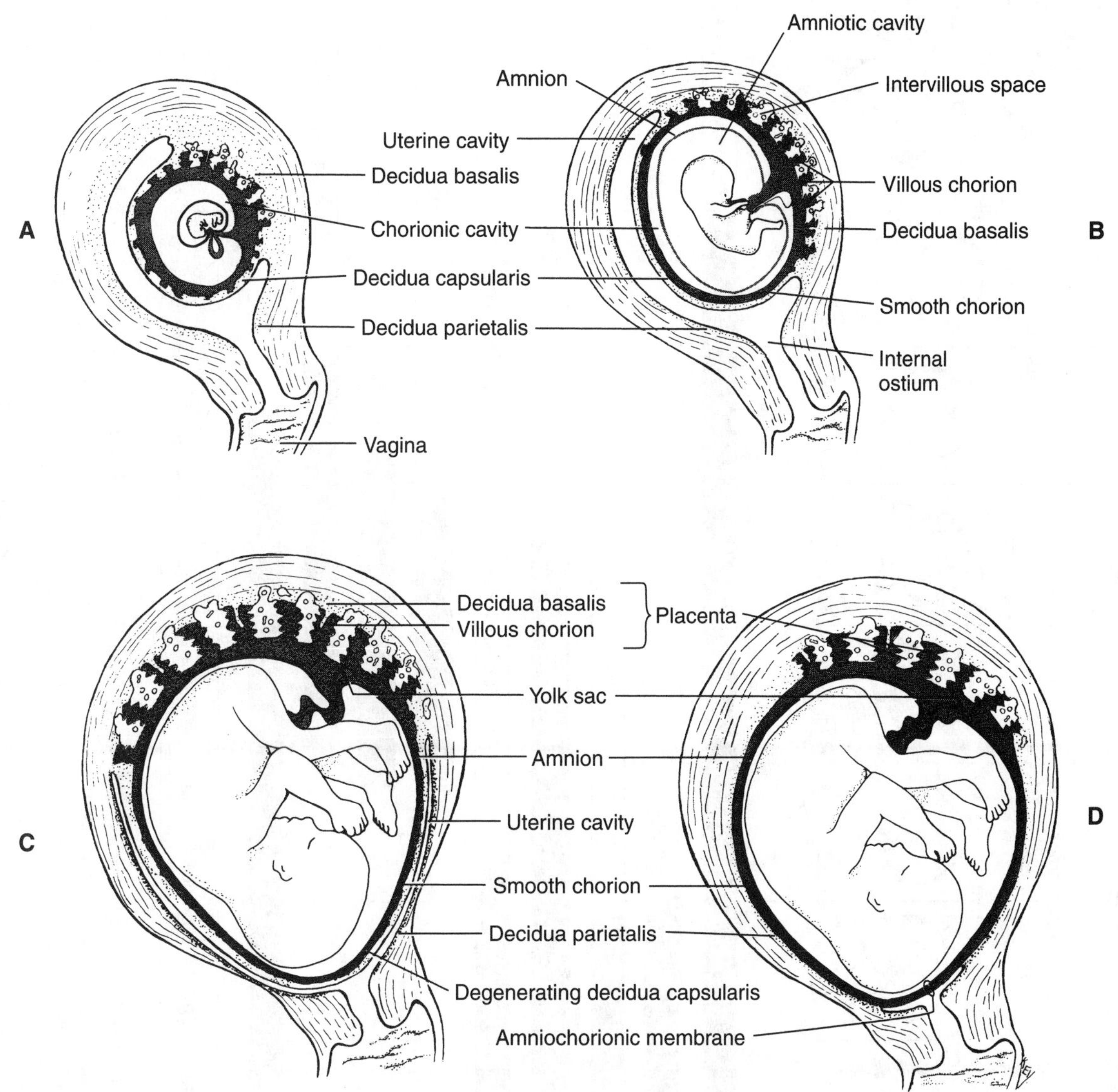

Figure 4-8 The fetus in amniotic sac showing the placenta and umbilical cord. Drawing illustrates development of the human placenta and fetal membranes. Sagittal sections of the gravid uterus from the 5th to the 22nd weeks show the changing relations of the fetal membranes to the deciduas. In **D** the amnion and chorion are fused with each other and the deciduas parietalis, thereby obliterating the uterine cavity. Note in **B** to **D** that chorionic villi persist only where the chorion is associated with the deciduas basalis—that is, where the placenta forms. *(From Moore KL and Persaud TVN: The developing human, ed 5, Philadelphia, 1993, WB Saunders.)*

trimester the fetus gains more than two thirds of its full-term birth weight. As much as 23 g to 25 g accumulate daily in the final days of gestation. On average the healthy full-term infant is about 51 cm (20 in) in length and weighs 3.4 kg (7.5 lb). Stages of development in fetal growth are shown in Figure 4-9.

ENERGY AND NUTRIENT REQUIREMENTS

- *How do energy needs increase during pregnancy?*
- *For which nutrients do requirements increase during pregnancy?*
- *What are appropriate pregnancy weight gains for underweight, normal weight, and overweight women?*

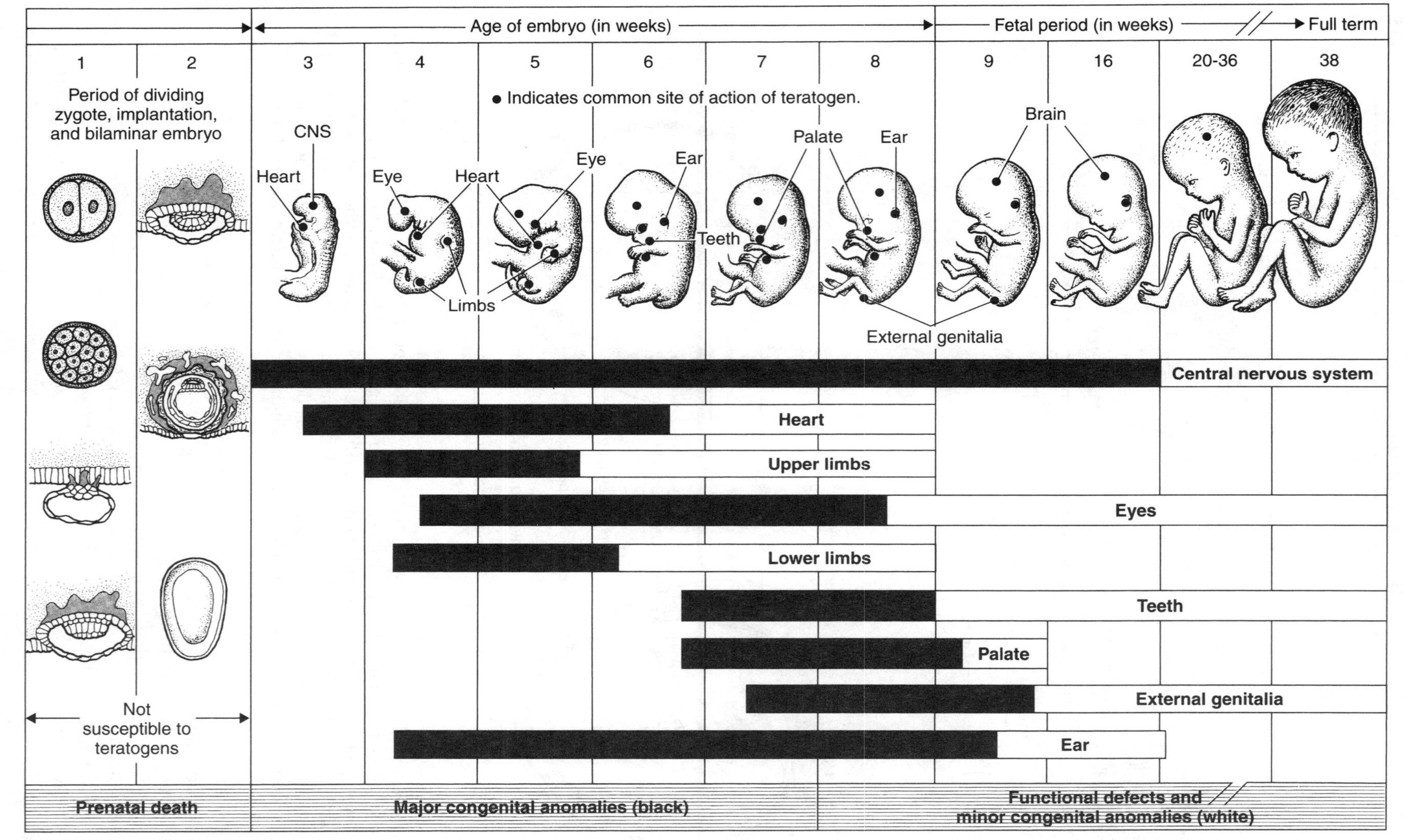

Figure 4-9 Schematic illustration of the critical periods in human development. During the first 2 weeks of development, the embryo is usually not susceptible to teratogens. During these preembryonic stages, a teratogen damages either all or most of the cells, resulting in the embryo's death, or damages only a few cells, thereby allowing the conceptus to recover and the embryo to develop without birth defects. The black areas denote highly sensitive periods when major defects may be produced (e.g., absence of limbs). White areas indicate stages that are less sensitive to teratogens when minor defects may be induced (e.g., hypoplastic thumbs). *(From Moore KL and Persaud TVN: The developing human, ed 5, Philadelphia, 1993, WB Saunders.)*

- *Plan a menu that would be appropriate to meet the nutrient and energy needs of a normal-weight pregnant woman.*
- *What nutrient supplements are recommended during pregnancy?*

Pregnancy is sometimes referred to as a hypermetabolic state because of the increased need for energy and nutrients to support growth of the fetus, placenta, and maternal tissue. Profound physiologic changes that cause hemodilution result in changes in nutrient turnover and homeostasis affects requirements during pregnancy (Allen, 2001). Fetal demand for nutrients occurs primarily during the last half of pregnancy when more than 90% of growth occurs. Nutrient requirements vary substantially among individuals within a population.

For most nutrients recommended intake during pregnancy is the sum of the recommendation for nonpregnant women and the amount of the nutrient deposited in maternal and fetal tissues plus an additional percentage because the efficiency of utilization for tissue growth is less than 100% (Allen, 2001).

Energy

The increased energy cost of gestation includes a 25% increase in basal energy requirements—energy for growth of the fetus, accessory tissues, and maternal supporting tissue and the energy needed for the additional work of the mother required by her increased body weight. Estimates of total energy need for pregnancy range from 60,000 kcal to 170,000 kcal (King, 2000). Energy recommendations are based on the assumption that pregnancy costs 85,000 kcal for a mother who gains 12.5 kg (27.5 lb) and gives birth to an infant weighing 3.3 kg (7.5 lb) (Durnin, 1987). Daily caloric recommendations of an additional 300 kcal are determined by dividing the energy cost of gestation by the approximate duration of pregnancy (280 days) (IOM, 1985). In 1996 an international working group revised the estimated energy cost of gestation to 71,702 kcal or 239 kcal/day (Allen et al., 1996). Decrements in physical activity in late pregnancy probably make 200 kcal/day a realistic intake. For the normal-weight woman added energy intake is probably not required for the first trimester; 200 to 300 kcal per day is an appropriate increase for the second and third trimesters.

Maternal Weight Gain

The components of gestational weight gain are shown in Figure 4-6. The amount of weight gained is inversely related to maternal fatness—body mass index (BMI)—of the woman at conception. Less than one half of the weight gain is accounted for by the fetus, placenta, and amniotic fluid (Forbes, 1962). The remainder is found in maternal reproductive tissues, fluid, blood, and stores. The maternal stores are largely composed of body fat, although there is some increase in the lean body mass other than reproductive tissues. Maternal fat stores are gained primarily between the tenth and thirtieth week of gestation—before fetal energy demands peak. Approximately 3.3 kg of fat is deposited as maternal stores, providing an energy reserve of approximately 30,000 kcal (King, 2000).

Gestational weight gain is often monitored as an indicator of the adequacy of the maternal diet. Over the last several decades an appropriate weight gain during pregnancy has been the subject of much discussion. In 1970 the Food and Nutrition Board (National Research Council, 1970) recommended a gestational weight gain of 10 kg to 12 kg (22 to 27 lb). Since that time experts have recognized that optimal pregnancy outcome reflects an interaction between gestational weight gain and the **pregravid** weight status of the mother. A report from the Collaborative Perinatal Project of more than 50,000 pregnancies found that the relationship between gestational weight gain and perinatal mortality was strongly influenced by pregravid weight (Naeye, 1979). As shown in Figure 4-10, mothers who were underweight before pregnancy had the lowest perinatal mortality when they gained at least

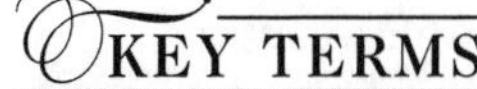

KEY TERMS

pregravid: before pregnancy

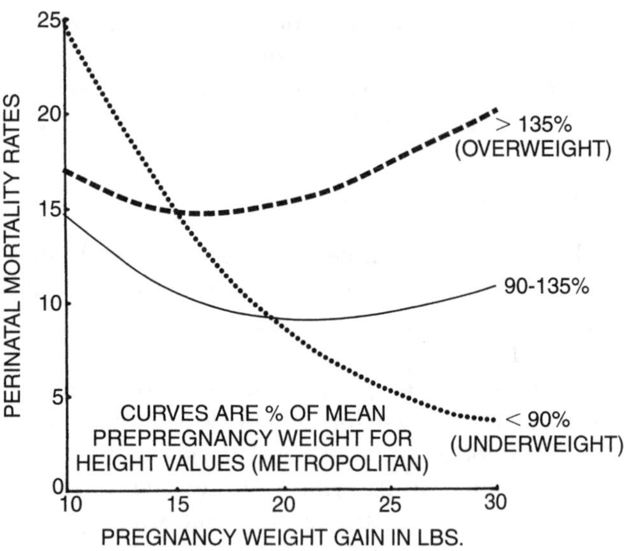

Figure 4-10 Perinatal mortality rates of overweight, normal weight, and underweight mothers as related to weight gain during pregnancy. *(From Naeye RL: Weight gain and the outcome of pregnancy, Am J Obstet Gynecol, 135:3, 1979.)*

Table 4-1 RECOMMENDED TOTAL WEIGHT GAIN RANGES FOR PREGNANT WOMEN, BY PREPREGNANCY BODY MASS INDEX (BMI)

Weight-for-Height Category	Recommended Total Gain* kg	lb
Low (BMI[†] <19.8)	12.5-18	28-40
Normal (BMI 19.8-26.0)	11.5-16	25-35
High (BMI 26.0-29.0)	7.0-11.5	15-25
Obese (BMI >29.0)	≥6.0	15

Adapted from Institute of Medicine: Nutrition during lactation, Washington, DC, 1991, National Academy Press.
*Young adolescents and African American women should strive for gains at the upper end of the recommended range. Short women (<157 cm [62 in]) should strive for gains at the lower end of the range.
[†]BMI is calculated in metric units.

16 kg (30 lb), whereas obese women had the lowest perinatal mortality when they gained only 7 kg (15 to 16 lb) (Naeye, 1979). Similar relationships between pregravid weight and **antenatal** weight gain have been observed for infant birthweight (Abrams et al., 1986; Mitchell and Lerner, 1989b). Low weight gains, especially in underweight women, are associated with increased risk of perinatal mortality and fetal growth restriction. High weight gains, particularly in obese women, are associated with increased birth weight and a greater likelihood of prolonged labor, complicated delivery, birth trauma, and **asphyxia.**

KEY TERMS

antenatal: before birth
asphyxia: lack of oxygen in the body caused by interruption in breathing, which causes unconsciousness

The pregnant woman who restricts weight gain to avoid accumulating body fat impairs, to some extent, normal fetal growth and development. Recommended weight gains are associated with infant birth weights between 3.5 kg and 4.0 kg, the birth weights with the lowest rates of infant mortality.

Healthy women who deliver full-term infants weighing between 3 kg and 4 kg (6.5 to 8.8 lb) have normal weight gains that range from 11 kg to 15 kg (25 to 35 lb). Guidelines from the IOM (1990) of the National Academy of Sciences (NAS) specify appropriate ranges for gestational weight gain based on maternal prepregnancy weight-for-height and age. Prepregnancy weight-for-height is categorized by BMI into underweight, normal weight, and overweight as a guide for suggested weight gain (Table 4-1). A chart incorporating these recommendations for underweight, normal weight, and overweight women is provided in Figure 4-11. It is characterized by a gradual steady increase over the second and third trimesters.

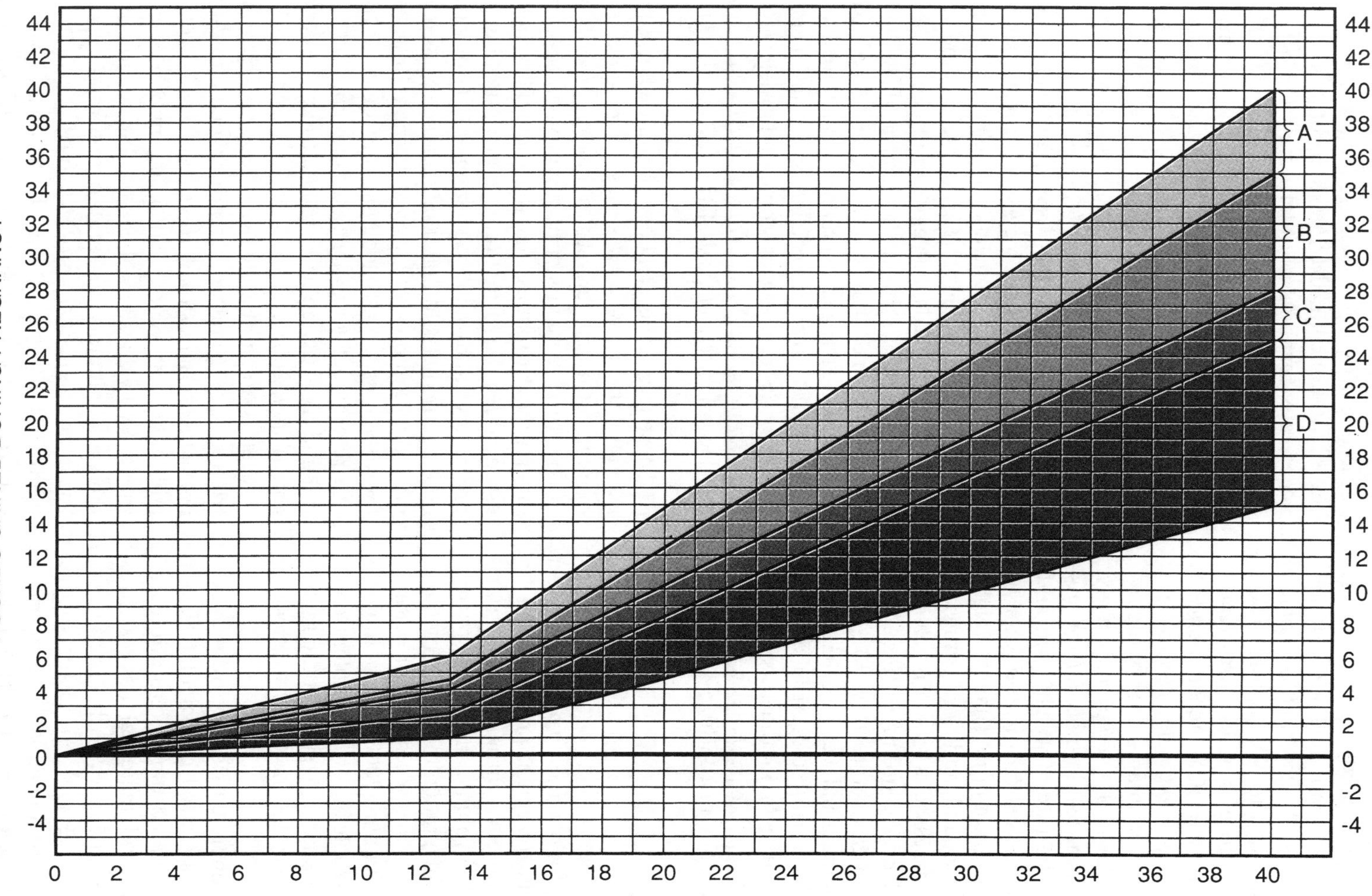

Figure 4-11 Recommended weight gain during pregnancy based on maternal BMI. For a woman with a BMI between 19.8 and 26, weight gain should be in the B-C range (26-35 lb). For the underweight woman (BMI < 19.8) weight gain should be in the A-B range (28-40 lb). The overweight woman (BMI > 26) should gain in the D range (15-25 lb). *(From the National Dairy Council: Great beginnings: the weighting game graph, Rosemont, Il, 1991, National Dairy Council. Courtesy of NATIONAL DAIRY COUNCIL®. Adapted from the National Academy of Sciences: Nutrition during pregnancy, Washington, DC, 1990, National Academy Press.)*

In the decade since the NAS weight gain recommendations, the impact of maternal weight gain has remained under study. Abrams et al. (2000) conducted a systematic review of studies that examined fetal and maternal outcomes since the publication of the NAS report. They confirmed that in those studies, pregnancy weight gains within the IOM recommended ranges (see page 118) were associated with best outcomes for mothers and infants. One of the reports reviewed was a study of approximately 3000 white women from San Francisco (Abrams and Selvin, 1995). The rate of weight gain and birth weight were regressed on the trimester of weight gain. Each kilogram of pregnancy weight gain during the first, second, and third trimester of weight gain was assessed with statistical increases in birth weight. According to these calculations, fetal weight gains were 18 g, 33 g, and 17 g per kilogram of maternal weight gain in the first, second, and third trimesters, respectively. Thus maternal weight gain in the second trimester was more strongly correlated with fetal growth than weight gain in the first and third trimesters.

Protein

The protein needs of a pregnant woman include synthesis of fetal and placental protein and increased maternal protein synthesis to support the expansion of blood volume and growth of the uterus and breasts. Adaptation in protein metabolism appears to occur in anticipation of maternal and fetal needs (Kalhan, 2000). Shifts in maternal protein metabolism are complex and change throughout gestation to support the rapid fetal protein synthesis in the third trimester (King, 2000).

The 1989 Recommended Dietary Allowance (RDA) for protein was based on calculation of total protein accumulated during gestation in the fetus, placenta, and maternal tissues, including blood. For a pregnancy with a maternal weight gain of 12.5 kg and an infant birth weight of 3.3 kg, the total need is 925 g of protein, or an RDA of an additional 10 g (total recommendation 60 g). Needs for synthesis of fetal proteins are small during the first trimester, but the maternal requirements for expanded blood volume and tissue growth are substantial. Over the second and third trimesters fetal demands accelerate, reaching as much as 10 g of protein per day in late pregnancy (Rosso, 1983). Most pregnant women in industrialized countries consume at least the recommended intake of protein (Allen, 2001).

Lipids

Essential long-chain polyunsaturated fatty acids play important roles as precursors of prostaglandins and as structural elements of cell membranes. These fatty acids must be consumed in the diet as parent fatty acids, linoleic acid (18:2n-6) found in vegetable oils, and alpha-linolenic acid (18:3n-3), which is found mostly in fish and seed oils. Throughout gestation accretion of maternal, placental, and fetal tissue occurs and, consequently, requirements of pregnant women and their developing fetuses are high. This is particularly true for docosahexaenoic acid (DHA [22:6n-3]) (Otto et al., 2000).

These fatty acids can be desaturated and elongated in the body to a series of longer-chain, more unsaturated derivatives that are precursors of structural elements of highly proliferating and differentiating tissues, making these fatty acids essential for the formation of new tissues during pregnancy and fetal development (Hornstra, 2000). The diet and maternal stores are likely to meet the requirement for most women. However, for women with multiple fetuses or women at risk of preterm delivery, increased amounts of the n-3 and n-6 fatty acids in the diet may be desirable (Allen, 2001).

Dietary Reference Intake values for micronutrients for pregnant women are divided into three age categories: less than 18 years, 19 to 30 years, and 31 to 50 years. The RDA and Adequate Intake (AI) values have been established for vitamins and minerals in a series of four reports published between 1997 and 2001 (IOM, 1997, 1998, 2000, 2001). Table 4-2 lists the RDAs and AIs for nonpregnant women and for three age groups of pregnant women.

Table 4-2 Dietary Reference Intakes: Recommended Intakes for Pregnant Women*

	Age Group			
	Pregnant			Not Pregnant
Nutrient	<18 years	19-30 years	31-50 years	19-30 years
Calcium (mg)	1300	1000	1000	1000
Phosphorus (mg)	**1250**	**700**	**700**	**700**
Magnesium (mg)	**400**	**350**	**360**	**310**
Vitamin D (μg)	5	5	5	5
Fluoride (mg)	3	3	3	3
Thiamin (mg)	**1.4**	**1.4**	**1.4**	**1.1**
Riboflavin (mg)	**1.4**	**1.4**	**1.4**	**1.1**
Niacin (mg)	**18**	**18**	**18**	**14**
Vitamin B_6 (mg)	**1.9**	**1.9**	**1.9**	**1.3**
Folate (μg)	**600**	**600**	**600**	**400**
Vitamin B_{12} (μg)	**2.6**	**2.6**	**2.6**	**2.4**
Pantothenic Acid (mg)	6	6	6	5
Biotin (μg)	30	30	30	30
Choline (mg)	450	450	450	425
Vitamin C (mg)	**80**	**85**	**85**	**75**
Vitamin E (mg)	**15**	**15**	**15**	**15**
Selenium (μg)	**60**	**60**	**60**	**55**
Vitamin A (μg)	**750**	**770**	**770**	**700**
Vitamin K (μg)	75	90	90	90
Chromium (μg)	29	30	30	25
Copper (μg)	**1000**	**1000**	**1000**	**900**
Iodine (μg)	220	220	220	150
Iron (mg)	**27**	**27**	**27**	**18**
Manganese (mg)	2	2	2	1.8
Molybdenum (mg)	**50**	**50**	**50**	**45**
Zinc (mg)	**13**	**11**	**11**	**8**

Adapted with permission from the following Institute of Medicine publications: Dietary reference intakes for calcium, phosphorus, magnesium, vitamin D, and fluoride (1997); Dietary reference intakes for thiamin, riboflavin, niacin, vitamin B_6, folate, vitamin B_{12}, pantothenic acid, biotin, and choline (1998); Dietary reference intakes for vitamin C, vitamin E, selenium, and carotenoids (2000); and Dietary reference intakes for vitamin A, vitamin K, arsenic, boron, chromium, copper, iodine, iron, manganese, molybdenum, nickel, silicon, vanadium, and zinc (2001). Washington, DC, National Academy Press.

Calcium and Related Nutrients

Calcium, phosphorus, and magnesium are accumulated by the fetus in substantial quantities, mainly during the last trimester. A total of approximately 25 g to 30 g of calcium are deposited in fetal tissue. Daily accumulation increases across gestation and may reach 250 mg to 300 mg late in the third trimester. Human pregnancy is associated with major changes in calcium, bone metabolism, and bone mineral status before and after gestation. Calcium balance studies of pregnant women indicate that substantial increases in absorption and a positive calcium balance begin in the first trimester. This positive balance continues throughout gestation, but does not increase substantially. Therefore in late pregnancy the needs of the fetus must be met by increased calcium retained from early pregnancy or by mobilization of calcium from the skeleton of the mother (Prentice, 2000).

The current AI for calcium during pregnancy is 1300 mg per day for mothers 18 years and younger and 1000 mg for mothers over 18 years (see Table 4-2). There is particular concern regarding calcium intake of women under 25 years of age because mineralization of their bones is probably still being completed. If calcium intakes of young women are low, dietary calcium should be increased. If that is not practical, a supplement of 600 mg of calcium should be given (IOM, 1990). Individuals who cannot drink milk need to consume alternate sources of calcium or calcium supplements.

The RDA for phosphorus during pregnancy has been set at 1300 mg for young mothers and 1000 mg for pregnant women over 19 years of age.

Approximately 1 g of magnesium is accumulated by the fetus during gestation. In the last trimester magnesium is deposited at the rate of 6 mg per day. Assuming an absorption rate of 50%, the RDA is 400 for women less than 18 years, 350 for women 19 to 30 years, and 360 mg for women between 31 and 50 years—an increase of 40 mg to 90 mg over the recommended value for nonpregnant women. There have been numerous anecdotal reports that magnesium supplements can provide relief from leg cramps often experienced by pregnant women. One controlled study reported that magnesium supplements did provide relief of leg cramps in pregnant women, but did not increase serum magnesium levels (Dahle et al., 1995). Excess magnesium appeared to be excreted in the urine.

Vitamin D

No increased need for vitamin D during pregnancy has been established (Salle et al., 2000). However, it is important that sufficient vitamin D is available to promote calcium deposition in the growing fetus. The fetus is dependent on the mother for its supply of 25-hydroxy vitamin D, which crosses the placenta and is converted to 1,25-dihydroxy vitamin D by the fetus. The placenta synthesizes 1,25 dihydroxy vitamin D and maternal serum levels are more than double in late pregnancy. Calcium absorption is increased. The AI for vitamin D for pregnant women of all ages is 5 micrograms, the same level recommended for nonpregnant women. Fortified milk (400 IU or 10 micrograms of cholecalciferol per quart) is one of the few dietary sources of vitamin D, so women who avoid milk and have little exposure to sunlight may have low intakes. Supplements of 10 μg of vitamin D are recommended for women who follow a vegan diet and 5 μg per day are recommended for pregnant women who consume little vitamin D-fortified milk. Supplements greater than the AI should be avoided because of potential toxicity.

Fluoride

Fluoride accumulates in the external tooth enamel and provides protection against dental caries. Its effect appears to be greatest during the first 2 years after tooth eruption. Although fluoride in the mother's bloodstream can cross the placenta, maternal fluoride supplementation during pregnancy has not been recommended because of insufficient evidence of prenatal benefit (IOM, 1990).

B Complex Vitamins and Choline

Thiamin, Niacin, and Riboflavin

Thiamin, niacin, and riboflavin function primarily in the release of energy from carbohydrate, lipid, and protein and are needed in increased amounts during pregnancy. The increase in the RDA for these vitamins is proportional to the 300 kcal increase recommended for pregnancy.

Vitamin B_6

Blood levels of both vitamin B_6 and the active coenzyme pyridoxal phosphate (PLP) are lower than those of nonpregnant women throughout pregnancy, especially in the third trimester. These levels of vitamin B_6 may reflect either inadequate intake or normal hormonal changes of pregnancy. The RDA is 1.9 mg, an increase of 0.6 mg over that recommended for nonpregnant women. Pyridoxal is actively transported from maternal circulation to the placenta, where it is converted to PLP. Fetal PLP concentrations are higher than those in the mother because significant sequestering of vitamin B_6 occurs.

Folate

Folate requirements increase substantially during pregnancy to support reactions requiring single carbon transfer and rapid cell division in maternal and fetal tissue. Prolonged inadequate intakes of folate can lead to megaloblastic bone marrow and eventually megaloblastic anemia.

The RDA for folate for pregnant women of all ages is 600 μg or 600 dietary folate equivalents on the basis of maintenance of normal red cell folate concentrations (Bailey, 2000). Folate can be obtained in a diet that includes fruits and vegetables and fortified or whole-grain cereals (Box 4-3). For women at greatest risk of inadequate intake from lack of knowledge or financial resources or because of abuse of alcohol, cigarettes, or drugs, supplementation may be appropriate. As discussed on page 106, 400 μg of folate are recommended for all women who might become pregnant. Such levels are associated with a decline in the incidence of neural tube defects (NTDs). However, NTDs occur before closure of the neural tube—between postconceptional days 15 and 28—long before most women know they are pregnant.

Vitamin B_{12}

Concentrations of vitamin B_{12} in the blood begin to decline early in the first trimester, at levels greater than can be accounted for by hemodilution. The placenta accumulates B_{12}, which is transferred to the fetus. Serum B_{12} concentration of the newborn is twice that of the mother, decreasing to adult concentrations in the second half of infancy. It is estimated that the fetal demands for vitamin B_{12} are approximately 50 μg, or 0.2 mcg per day. Body stores of the adequately nourished mother are approximately 3000 μg, so the drain of meeting the additional requirement for fetal needs is small. The RDA is 2.6 μg per day. A woman who has followed a vegan diet without vitamin B_{12} supplementation or fortified foods will have inadequate stores of vitamin B_{12} and will require a supplement to protect her fetus (IOM, 1990).

Antioxidant Nutrients

Vitamin E

Actual requirements for vitamin E during pregnancy have not been determined. Blood levels of tocopherol increase during pregnancy. The RDAs for vitamin E for all age groups of pregnant women are the same as that for nonpregnant women.

Box 4-3 Dietary Folate Equivalents (DFEs)

1 DFE = 1.0 μg of food folate
0.6 μg of folic acid from fortified food
0.5 μg of supplemental folate taken on an empty stomach

Vitamin C

Vitamin C is believed to be transported across the placenta. Fetal and infant blood levels of vitamin C are 50% higher than maternal levels. A daily increase to 80 mg or 85 mg of vitamin C is recommended to meet the increased demands on the mother's body pool.

Iron

Increased iron is needed throughout pregnancy for the synthesis of an expanded red cell mass, growth of placenta and fetus, and replacement of blood lost during delivery. Some iron is saved by the absence of losses through menstruation and enhanced absorption (Barrett et al., 1994). On the average, an additional 6 mg/day of iron needs to be absorbed during pregnancy. Iron is retained by the fetus (300 mg), deposited in the placenta (60 mg), and used for synthesis of additional maternal erythrocytes. The total iron requirement of pregnancy is estimated to be 1000 mg, or 3 mg per day over the 280 days of gestation. Iron transfer to the fetus is regulated by the placenta and most occurs after week 30 of gestation. That figure corresponds to the time of peak efficiency of maternal absorption. During pregnancy hemodilution and increased requirements cause a drop in hemoglobin levels in the first and second trimester and then a gradual increase during the third trimester. Iron supplementation is associated with a smaller decline in hemoglobin and hematocrit levels in early pregnancy and higher levels in the last trimester. The indications for and benefits of supplemented iron for mother and infant have come under recent scrutiny.

Large doses of supplemental iron are associated with some negative side effects and with increased oxidative damage. Although daily iron supplements provide protection against a decline in the iron pool in pregnant women, they

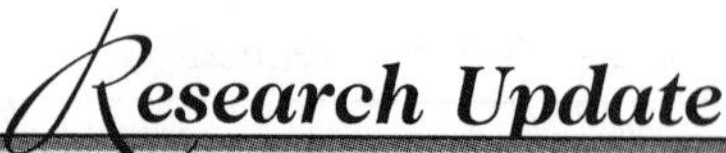

Is Homocysteine a Biomarker for Adverse Pregnancy Outcomes?

Homocysteine is a sulfur-containing amino acid that is the demethylated derivative of the essential amino acid methionine. Homocysteine is metabolized through two main pathways: remethylation to methionine or transsulfuration to cysteine. A defect in either of these pathways leads to an accumulation of homocysteine. An inborn error from a deficiency of the enzyme cystathionine β-synthase, which is required for metabolism of homocysteine, results in marked elevations of homocysteine in both plasma and urine, mental retardation, and premature death from atherosclerosis.

Women with untreated cystathionine β-synthase deficiency experience fetal loss in approximately 50% of pregnancies. Mild forms of hyperhomocysteinemia may be from one of two conditions: reduced enzyme activity of methylenetetrahydrofolate reductase (MTHFR) or deficiencies of folate, vitamin B_{12}, or vitamin B_6 that cause homocysteine to accumulate because remethylation to methionine requires folate and vitamin B_{12} and transsulfuration to cysteine requires vitamin B_6.

The most common and debilitating birth defects in the world are NTDs. In the last decade research has established that periconceptual folic acid reduces the first occurrence and the reoccurrence of NTDs (Scholl and Johnson, 2000). It appears that NTDs are caused by an interaction of multiple genes superimposed on a high-risk environment. Folate deficiency can occur because of poor folate intake or because the metabolic requirement for folate is increased or dietary absorption is decreased. A metabolic effect of folate deficiency is an elevation of plasma homocysteine. High concentrations of homocysteine have been associated with increased spontaneous abortion and pregnancy complications—namely, preterm delivery (Mills et al., 1996).

Genetic and geographic factors seem to play a role in the etiology of NTDs (Fleming, 2001). Because most women are not folate deficient, it has been hypothesized that supplementation with folic acid is overcoming a metabolic defect in folate metabolism. Numerous studies have reported that mothers of children with NTDs had significantly higher homocysteine levels than mothers in the research control groups, suggesting that there are probably multiple mutations in the MTHFR gene or other factors that contribute to NTDs (Caudill, 2000). Folic acid supplements alone have been shown to effectively lower homocysteine levels, even in the absence of a folate deficiency.

Preliminary data suggest that a mutation of the gene may be a maternal risk factor for Down syndrome (see Chapter 10). James et al. (1999) found that mothers with this mutation had significantly higher homocysteine concentrations and a 2.6-fold higher risk of having a child with Down syndrome than did mothers without the mutation. These researchers detected higher homocysteine levels in mothers of children with Down syndrome, even with normal genotype. This finding suggests that elevated homocysteine alone may be a biological marker of increased risk (Fleming, 2001).

The results of a recent prospective study suggest that elevated homocysteine may also be a marker for and possibly a cause of or contributor to additional adverse pregnancy outcomes, including premature delivery and very low birth weight (Vollset et al., 2000). If these data are confirmed by future investigations, folate fortification of the U.S. food supply may reduce the incidence of several adverse pregnancy outcomes (Caudill, 2000). Studies of dietary intakes and circulating folate levels for mothers who had preterm delivery found that low intakes of folate were associated with maternal characteristics reflecting poor nutrition status, including poor energy intake, low gestational weight gain, and iron deficiency (Scholl et al., 1996). These researchers found that poor dietary folate intake and low serum folate levels at 28 weeks of pregnancy were significantly associated with a more than threefold increase in risk of low birth weight and preterm delivery. These observations persisted after controlling for maternal age, parity, ethnicity, smoking, gestational weight gain, and intake of energy and other nutrients.

Observational studies of folate during pregnancy suggest a potential benefit of positive folate status—namely, improved birth weight and gestational age. However, randomized trials of folic acid supplementation have shown less uniform benefit (Scholl and Johnson, 2000). It appears that routine supplementation may benefit women who are potentially at risk, either from common genetic polymorphisms that alter folate metabolism or from environmental factors associated with poor intake.

are associated with more side effects and with poor compliance because of gastrointestinal distress. Supplementation alternatives may be use of delayed-release preparations or intermittent oral iron supplementation. Another option is a lower-dose iron supplement that would cause fewer symptoms (Beard, 2000).

In a review of several studies on maternal anemia and iron deficiency, Allen (2000) found evidence that maternal iron deficiency anemia increases risk of preterm delivery, low-birth-weight infants, and possibly poor iron status in infants. Minimal incidence of these unfavorable outcomes is associated with hemoglobin concentrations of 95 g/L to 105 g/L (Steer, 2000). However, such associations could be influenced by confounding factors such as socioeconomic status, health status, life-style, and difficulty in separating anemia from hemodilution. Other researchers have reported no statistical differences in pregnancy outcome between women who received routine iron supplementation and those who received it only for anemia (Hemminki and Merilainen, 1995).

Assuming an iron absorption level of 10%, the IOM (1990) recommended routine iron supplementation of 30 mg of elemental iron during the second and third trimesters for all pregnant women. Some experts have suggested that iron supplements are appropriate only for women with low iron status. Iron status can be determined by measuring plasma **ferritin** levels in addition to hemoglobin (Milman et al., 1995). Supplemental iron (120 to 180 mg/day) has been recommended for women with low plasma ferritin until hemoglobin levels become normal. There is substantial evidence that iron supplementation during pregnancy increases iron stores of the infant through approximately 6 months of age (Allen, 2000).

Vitamin A and Other Nutrients

Zinc

Severe zinc deficiency can have a devastating effect on pregnancy outcome including growth retardation, teratogenic effects, and fetal death (King, 2000). The role of zinc in protein synthesis, cell division, hormone metabolism, and immunocompetence makes it essential for fetal growth. The fetal need for zinc is approximately 100 mg, with the daily accumulation increasing from about 0.1 mg per day during the first trimester to 0.7 g during the third trimester. Increased intestinal absorption is the major mechanism by which fetal needs are met. Transfer of zinc to the fetus depends on maintenance of maternal levels. The RDA for zinc has been set at 11 mg to 13 mg. Usual intakes among American women appear to be 8.8 mg to 14.4 mg per day, but vegetarians may consume much less from low intake and poor absorption from a cereal-based diet. Zinc supplementation may be appropriate for women with poor zinc status, women under acute stress, those who smoke or abuse alcohol, or women with poor gastrointestinal function (IOM, 1990). Studies of the relationship of maternal zinc status to pregnancy outcome have been inconsistent. In a study of 3500 women who had plasma zinc levels determined at 16 weeks gestation found no association between plasma zinc and pregnancy outcome (Tsunenobu et al., 2000). Although the benefits of zinc supplementation needs further investigation, it is important that zinc intakes meet recommendations (Allen, 2000).

Iodine

An increase of 70 μg per day in the allowance for iodine is recommended to cover the additional requirements. Iodized salt can provide sufficient iodine for pregnant women.

Vitamin A

Vitamin A is required for growth, embryogenesis, and differentiation of epithelial tissue. The concentration of retinol in the fetal liver is low and vitamin A supplements do not increase it appreciably. Fetal needs for vitamin A could easily be met by mobilization of less than 10% of usual maternal stores (IOM, 1990).

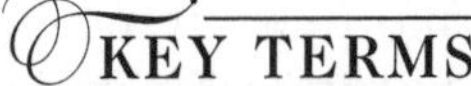

KEY TERMS

ferritin: a storage protein for iron, primarily in the liver and other iron-storage cells

An excess intake of retinal or isoteretinoin (13-cis-retinoic acid [accutane]), which is used to treat severe acne, has been shown to be associated with birth defects including abnormalities of the central nervous system and craniofacial and cardiovascular defects (Azais-Braesco and Pascal, 2000). Supplements greater than the RDA for vitamin A should be avoided. However, there is no evidence that high dietary intakes of carotenoids are toxic to mother or fetus.

Vitamin K

The transfer of vitamin K from mother to fetus appears to be minimal. The newborn has low blood levels of vitamin K, prothrombin, and other vitamin K-dependent clotting factors regardless of maternal intake. Because prenatal supplementation with vitamin K does not appear to effectively increase fetal levels, no increase in the AI is recommended for pregnancy.

ASSESSMENT OF NUTRITION STATUS

- *How do parameters of nutrition assessment differ for pregnant women?*
- *What measurements or standards are unique to pregnancy?*

Prentice and Goldberg have suggested that pregnancy is the most nutritionally sensitive period of the life span and that the time at which nutritional interventions can reap the greatest benefits need to be identified (Prentice and Goldberg, 2000). Basic principles and techniques for nutrition assessment were presented in Chapter 2. This section addresses their application in pregnancy. Women who enter prenatal care early provide clinicians a unique opportunity to assess and monitor nutrition status and to provide nutrition education throughout the reproductive cycle. Nutrition education during this time may have long-term consequences for the mother, her infant, and her family. Unfortunately many women who are at greatest nutritional risk do not enter prenatal care until late in pregnancy, if at all. Some receive healthcare for the first time when they are ready to deliver. Therefore the effectiveness of nutrition assessment and intervention is contingent on successful outreach programs to involve women in healthcare early in pregnancy.

Anthropometry

The only anthropometric measurements consistently available for pregnant women are height, prepregnancy weight, and a series of weight measurements during gestation. Prepregnant weight and antenatal weight gain are interrelated predictors of infant birth weight and the pattern of gestational weight gain can have clinical value. Monitoring of weight changes during gestation is especially important for underweight and obese women because their pregnancy outcome can be improved by achieving recommended weight gains (see Table 4-1). Charts or grids for gestational weight gain, as shown in Figure 4-11, can be helpful in tracking the pattern of weight gain.

It is difficult to obtain reproducible measurements of fatfold thickness in the prenatal care setting. Even reliable measurements have limited usefulness because there are no reference standards for skinfold thickness measurements for pregnancy.

Biochemical Assessment

As blood volume expands during pregnancy, the fluid volume increases more than do the cellular components. This hemodilution means that normal values for red blood cells, hemoglobin, and hematocrit are lower for pregnant women than for nonpregnant women (Table 4-3). It may be necessary to interpret levels of other nutrients and metabolites in this context as well.

Clinical Assessment

The initial prenatal visit provides the opportunity to identify factors that may increase the risk of an unfavorable outcome of pregnancy. Nutrition-related factors to be considered include anthropometric measures, age, signs of anemia, and chronic disease. During routine prenatal visits, urine is screened for sugar and pro-

Table 4-3 LABORATORY VALUES FOR SCREENING FOR ANEMIA IN WOMEN

	Nonsmokers		Smokers 0.5-1 pack/day		Smokers >1 pack/day	
Pregnancy Status	Hemoglobin (g/dL)	Hematocrit (%)	Hemoglobin (g/dL)	Hematocrit (%)	Hemoglobin (g/dL)	Hematocrit (%)
Nonpregnant	12.0	36	12.3	37	12.5	37.5
Pregnant						
First trimester	11.0	33	11.3	34	11.5	34.5
Second trimester	10.5	32	10.8	33	11.0	33.5
Third trimester	11.0	33	11.3	34	11.5	34.5

From Centers for Disease Control: CDC criteria for anemia in children and childbearing-age women, MMWR Morb Mortal Wkly Rep 38:400, 1989.

tein. Blood pressure is measured and clinical signs of edema are sought. These are useful in identifying women at risk for gestational diabetes or pregnancy-induced hypertension (see Chapter 5).

Dietary Assessment

Routine assessment of dietary practices is recommended for all pregnant women (IOM, 1990). The typical pattern of intake can be determined effectively using a food frequency questionnaire, dietary record, or dietary history questionnaire (see Chapter 2). Low intake of specific groups of foods, such as those rich in iron or calcium, can be identified quickly. Specific characteristics that indicate risk of an inadequate diet and therefore low weight gain (Hickey, 2000) include the following:

- Low income with inadequate access to food
- Young maternal age in **primiparas**
- Avoidance of a specific food group or groups because of intolerance, fad diets, or cultural practices
- Adherence to a diet that includes no animal tissue or products
- Consumption of substantial amounts of alcohol or use of tobacco or illicit drugs
- A life-style that is unlikely to support adequate acquisition, preparation, or consumption of food
- Diet restriction in an attempt to control weight
- Pica (consumption of nonfood substances such as clay or laundry starch)
- Low educational attainment and unmarried
- Unhappiness with being pregnant

Identification of poor dietary practices should result in initiation of appropriate intervention via counseling, supplementation, or referral to food assistance programs as appropriate. The *Healthy People 2010* Nutrition Related Objectives include reduction of anemia in low-income pregnant women and iron deficiency in pregnant females (U.S. Department of Health and Human Services, 2000).

A DIET PLAN FOR PREGNANCY

- *Outline diet intake for one day to meet the nutrition recommendations for a pregnant woman.*
- *What is the role of nutrient supplements during pregnancy?*

The requirements for energy and most nutrients increase during pregnancy. However, for the normal-weight woman, the increase in energy needs is less than 15% and the increased need for nutrients may range from none for vitamin A to 50% for iron to more than 200% for folate.

KEY TERMS

primiparas: women who are pregnant for the first time

Food Guide

A diet plan based on the food pyramid that is appropriate for pregnant and lactating women appears in Figure 4-12. As in any food group plan, it is important to select the recommended number of servings from a variety of foods within each food group. Choices should emphasize foods low in fat and rich in complex carbohydrates to spare protein needed for growth. Inadequate energy intake restricts weight gain, but may also compromise fetal growth and development as amino acids are mobilized to meet energy needs. Emphasis must be placed on sources of calcium, a mineral that even nonpregnant women have difficulty getting in sufficient amounts.

Nutrient Supplements

Except for iron, the nutrient requirements of the pregnant woman can be met by a balanced, varied diet. A multivitamin and mineral supplement is *not* a substitute for a balanced diet. Supplements should be recommended only when a deficiency is indicated or when it appears, after nutritional consultation, that dietary changes will not be made (Box 4-4). In addition, supplements may be recommended for complete vegetarians, women carrying more than one fetus, smokers, drinkers of alcoholic beverages, and drug abusers (IOM, 1990).

DIET-RELATED CONCERNS DURING PREGNANCY

- *How do the gastrointestinal symptoms of pregnancy influence overall food intake?*
- *What dietary changes can be made to alleviate the nausea, vomiting, constipation, and heartburn of pregnancy?*
- *How can cravings and aversions influence food intake?*
- *What are the advantages of monitoring physical activity during pregnancy?*

KEY TERMS

palliative: reducing the severity of symptoms

Nausea and Vomiting

The nausea and vomiting that frequently occur in the early months of pregnancy are referred to as *morning sickness,* but they are not confined to the morning. Morning sickness usually begins about 6 weeks after the start of the last menstrual period and commonly disappears 6 weeks to 8 weeks later. The cause of the nausea and vomiting of early pregnancy is unknown. Hormones that increase in early pregnancy have been implicated. Some studies have reported that women who experienced this discomfort during early pregnancy had higher blood levels of estrogen. Also levels of HCG, produced by the corpus luteum, rise in the first trimester of pregnancy and then fall about the fourteenth or fifteenth week—just about the time the nausea and vomiting diminish for most women. Time seems to be the only cure and treatment is **palliative.**

Approximately two thirds of pregnant women experience some nausea during pregnancy and about one half of those with nausea also vomit. These unpleasant conditions may be a positive prognostic indicator for a favorable pregnancy outcome. In a study of 9098 pregnancies researchers at the National Institutes of Health found that mothers who vomited had a 17% lower risk of a preterm delivery and a 30% lower risk of having a miscarriage or stillbirth than women who did not (Klebanoff and Yip, 1987).

The nausea of pregnancy is the only kind of nausea that improves with food on the stomach. Part of prevention is to keep the stomach filled, but not overfilled. Other suggestions to reduce nausea include eating small, frequent meals, separating consumption of fluids and solid foods, consuming easily digested carbohydrates, and avoiding highly seasoned or strong-flavored foods.

Although the nausea and vomiting of early pregnancy are usually mild and do not substantially reduce total food intake, excessive vomiting can cause an acute loss of fluid and electrolytes resulting in dehydration. If vomiting is prolonged there is the potential for significant losses of protein and other nutrients and medical intervention may be required.

Grain Products

6 to 11 servings a day

- Grain products provide energy, vitamins, and minerals.
- Whole grain products, like whole wheat breads, are good sources of **folic acid**.
- Limit pastries, doughnuts, and cookies because they are high in fat.

Choose these Grain Products

1 slice **whole grain bread**

3/4 cup ready-to-eat **enriched cereal**

1/2 cup oatmeal, grits, or cooked wheat

1 pancake or waffle

1/2 cup spaghetti or noodles

1/2 cup rice, enriched or brown

2 tortillas

1 pita

1 muffin or biscuit

4 soda-type crackers

2 rice cakes

Vegetables

3 to 5 servings a day

- Vegetables provide vitamins and minerals.
- Leafy green vegetables and beans are good sources of **folic acid**.
- Fresh vegetables are best, but frozen or canned vegetables are okay.
- Avoid fried vegetables like french fries.

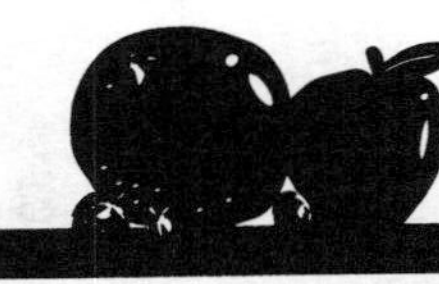

Choose these Vegetables

1 cup brussels sprouts

1 cup **broccoli**

1/2 cup **spinach**

1/2 cup chopped green pepper

1 cup **collard greens, kale**, or **cabbage**

1/2 cup carrots

1/2 cup squash

1/2 cup eggplant

1/2 cup **green beans**

1/2 cup **sweet peas**

1/2 baked potato

1 small sweet potato

1 medium tomato

4-6 medium spears **asparagus**

Fruits

2 to 4 servings a day

- Fruits provide vitamins and minerals.
- Limit fruit drinks with added sugar. Real fruit juice has more of the vitamins you need.

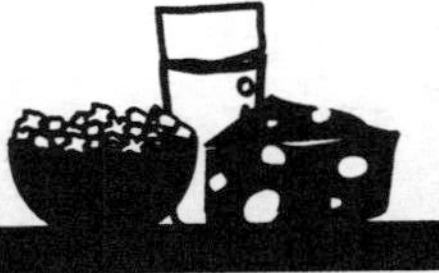

Choose these Fruits

1 **orange**

1/2 cup orange or grapefruit juice

1-1/4 cups cubed watermelon

3/4 cup **strawberries**

1 small **banana**

1 apple

1 guava

1 mango

2 tablespoons dried fruit

Milk and Milk Products

2 to 3 servings a day*

- Calcium builds bones and teeth.
- Limit nondairy milk substitutes. Coffee creamers and condensed milk have low nutritional value.
- If you can't digest the sugar in milk, or are lactose-intolerant, there are special products in the dairy section you can buy.

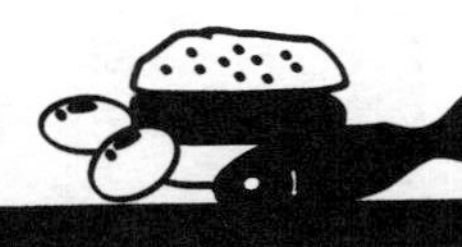

Choose these Milk and Milk Products

1 cup milk: whole, lowfat, skim, powdered, or buttermilk

1 cup **yogurt**

1 cup cottage cheese

2 1" cubes cheese

1 cup pudding or custard

1-1/2 cups soup made with milk

1 cup ice milk or ice cream

* Women who are pregnant or breast-feeding, teenagers, and young adults need 3 servings of milk and milk products daily.

Meat and Protein Foods

2 to 3 servings a day

- Protein builds strong muscles and blood.
- Liver is an excellent source of **folic acid**.
- Limit high fat and processed meats such as hot dogs, bologna, sausage, spare ribs, corned-beef hash, turkey wings, and bacon.

Choose these Meat and Protein Foods

Beef

Lamb

Pork

Liver

Chicken

Turkey

Fish

Shellfish

2 eggs

1 cup canned baked beans

1 cup dried **peas/beans**

1 cup tofu

1/4 cup peanut butter

1/2 cup nuts

Sample Menus

Breakfast

Orange juice

Bran flakes with peaches

Muffin or biscuit

Milk

Lunch

Glass of vegetable juice

Egg salad on lettuce

Two slices of pumpernickel bread

Tomato slices

Dinner

Baked chicken

Mixed green salad

Baked sweet or white potato

Milk

Whole wheat roll

Apple

Figure 4-12 Good food guide. (Bold type indicates foods that are sources of folic acid.) *(From The March of Dimes: Eating for two: nutrition during pregnancy, White Plains, NY, 1992, The March of Dimes. Adapted from the Food Guide Pyramid, U.S. Department of Agriculture.)*

Box 4-4 Recommendations for Nutrient Supplements During Pregnancy

GENERAL POPULATION

30 mg ferrous iron daily during the second and third trimesters

This is equal to 150 mg of ferrous sulfate
300 mg of ferrous gluconate
100 mg of ferrous fumarate

Take between meals or at bedtime on an empty stomach to facilitate iron absorption.

Potential side effects: heartburn, nausea, upper abdominal discomfort, constipation, and diarrhea. The risk of side effects is proportional to the amount of elemental iron in various soluble ferrous iron compounds. Side effects are much less likely with 30 mg.

OTHER SUPPLEMENTS

Recommended only when assessment of dietary practices indicates inadequacies and when dietary intervention seems to be ineffective.

300 μg per day of folate when there are doubts about the adequacy of dietary folate, as in women who consume little fruit, juices, whole-grain or fortified cereals, or green vegetables.

Recommended for pregnant women who do not ordinarily consume an adequate diet and those in high-risk categories such as women carrying more than one fetus, heavy cigarette smokers, and alcohol and drug abusers. A multivitamin supplement should contain the following during the second and third trimester:

Iron	30 mg	Vitamin B_6	2 mg
Zinc	15 mg	Folate	300 μg
Copper	2 mg	Vitamin C	50 mg
Calcium	250 mg	Vitamin D	5 μg

Take between meals or at bedtime to promote absorption.

IRON DEFICIENCY

If results of routine determination of hemoglobin and hematocrit at first prenatal visit indicate a deficiency:

60-120 mg of ferrous iron/day

When hemoglobin returns to normal: 30 mg/day

NUTRIENT SUPPLEMENTATION IN SPECIAL CIRCUMSTANCES

Vitamin D: 10 μg (400 IU) daily for complete vegetarians and others with a low intake of vitamin D-fortified milk. This is especially important for women who live at northern latitudes in winter and for others with minimal exposure to sunlight and, thus, reduced synthesis of vitamin D in the skin.

Calcium: 600 mg daily for women under age 25 whose daily dietary calcium is less than 600 mg. It should be taken at mealtime.

Vitamin B_{12}: 2.0 μg daily for complete vegetarians.

Zinc and copper: When therapeutic levels of iron (>30 mg/day) are given to treat anemia, supplementation with 15 mg of zinc and 2 mg of copper is recommended because iron may interfere with the absorption and utilization of those trace minerals.

Adapted from Subcommittee on Dietary Intake and Nutrient Supplements During Pregnancy. Committee on Nutritional Status During Pregnancy and Lactation, Food and Nutrition Board, Institute of Medicine, National Academy of Sciences: Nutrition during pregnancy, Washington, DC, 1990, National Academy Press.

Heartburn

The term *heartburn* is a misnomer because it has nothing to do with the heart. However, the burning pain in the lower esophagus caused by the reflux of food and acid from the stomach can indeed feel like heart pain. Two factors contribute to heartburn during gestation. The hormone-mediated changes of pregnancy result in relaxation of the **lower esophageal sphincter** and the growing fetus puts increasing pressure on the stomach. Heartburn can be averted by eating small, frequent meals, avoiding highly seasoned foods, and avoiding lying down soon after meals. Occasionally discomfort can be relieved by antacids, if prescribed by the physician.

Constipation

Constipation is a common complaint of pregnancy, especially during the last trimester. This problem results from reduced intestinal motility, which slows passage of unabsorbed food residue through the large bowel, resulting in increased absorption of water. The feces become dry, hard, and difficult to expel. In addition, the enlarging uterus exerts pressure on the bowel. Decreased physical activity and a diet low in fiber also contribute to the problem. Measures to reduce constipation include adequate fluid intake and increased dietary fiber. For some women the problem is persistent and the physician may recommend bulking agents or stool softeners to facilitate laxation.

Cravings and Aversions of Pregnancy

A variety of dietary and life-style changes occur during pregnancy. Although many women make positive changes that will improve the nutritional quality of their diets, many dietary changes are based on alterations in taste or appetite, cultural patterns, or the mother's perceived value of specific dietary components.

Many women experience changes in food preferences during pregnancy. A mother's conscious choice not to consume certain foods or beverages during pregnancy is referred to as food *avoidance.* Food *aversions* are distaste for foods or beverages that are normally consumed, but not tolerated during pregnancy. Approximately one half of pregnant women report an aversion to one or more foods or beverages, most frequently coffee, alcoholic beverages, highly seasoned foods, and fried foods.

Food cravings, which occur more frequently than food aversions, are not limited to any particular foods or food groups. They may range from the proverbial pickles to ice cream—although not necessarily together. The foods most frequently craved are sweets, chocolate, ice cream, cake, and candy. Other common cravings include spicy foods such as pizza or Mexican food and fruits and vegetables. There are few explanations for why cravings occur during pregnancy, but they are not from nutrient deficiencies. Suggested causes are changes in senses of taste and smell, metabolic changes, and responses to increased physical needs. Food cravings and aversions may disappear in late pregnancy and are seldom experienced after delivery. They often reappear in a later pregnancy or may be replaced by a craving for or aversion to different foods or beverages.

Exercise during and After Pregnancy*

In the last 30 years women have made tremendous achievements in the world of sports and athletics. One effect of such achievements is that more women choose to remain athletically competitive or at least athletically active for a longer period, encompassing the reproductive years. Many women remain physically active throughout pregnancy and the postpartum period.

Various physiologic and anatomic changes occur during pregnancy and lactation, which may influence or be influenced by physical activity (Clapp, 2000; Pivarnik, 1998). Although studies have been done on the effects of pregnancy and lactation on exercise, less is known about the effects of exercise on pregnancy and lactation (Rosenbloom, 2000). Even less is known about the impact of nutrition on exercising pregnant or lactating women (Clapp, 1998). Most health professionals derive recommendations for these women from the general knowledge base of the two disciplines of sports nutrition and obstetrics.

*This section contributed by Dr. Diane L. Habash.

KEY TERMS

lower esophageal sphincter: group of muscles located between the esophagus and stomach

Research Update

Pica during Pregnancy

Pica is the ingestion of nonfood substances such as clay (geophagia) or laundry starch (amylophagia) (IOM, 1990). A familiar example is the consumption of dirt or paint chips by young children. Pica is not limited to any one geographic area, race, sex, culture, or social status, but it does appear to have a predilection for underdeveloped areas and populations of low socioeconomic status.

The etiology of pica is poorly understood. Theories range from a learned pattern of behavior for relieving the nausea and vomiting of pregnancy to the body's instinctive search for a source of nutrients it is lacking. Pica is probably shaded by both cultural and physiologic bases and it is associated with poor nutrition status, particularly deficiencies of iron and zinc, and culturally ingrained food preferences.

Although pica has been associated with reduced maternal hemoglobin levels at birth (Rainville, 1998), the substances the victims crave are rarely rich in iron. For example people who eat tremendous quantities of ice (pagophagia) are often deficient in iron, but ice adds only water to their diets. In some cases pica itself contributes to the deficiency. Some clays contain substances that bind with iron and decrease its absorption. A cause-and-effect relationship has not been established. Not everyone with iron or zinc deficiency has pica, nor does everyone with pica have iron or zinc deficiency.

The most commonly reported pica in pregnant women in the United States involves the eating of dirt, clay, starch, or ice. Clay eating is especially common among Southern African-American women and may be a holdover from African culture. However, poverty and poor nutrition clearly aggravate the problem. The custom has followed the migration of the African-American population from the South, so that clays from a favorite "clay hole" may be mailed to relatives who have moved away. Clay consumption varies from a few lumps a day to a quart or more. Because the preferred clay is not often available in big cities, the craving is often transferred to laundry starch (cornstarch). Starch eating, like clay eating, interferes with iron absorption, but can also add a great many calories to the diet. Consumption of a pound of starch each day, which contains about 1600 kilocalories, is not unusual.

There is no question that pica has the potential of having adverse effects on the mother and fetus. Pica may be associated with the following:

- Displacement of essential nutrients or kilocalories from food
- Reduced absorption of required nutrients
- Ingestion of toxins or parasites
- Intestinal obstruction or bowel perforation
- Weight gain from excess calories from starch

The best defense against the negative effects of pica is to encourage a balanced, nutritious diet and to make pregnant women aware of the dangers of consuming large quantities of nonfood substances.

Changes of pregnancy that affect exercise often are slow and subtle. For example the greatest effect of pregnancy is the increasing body weight. This change can alter the center of gravity and thus balance, making certain types of exercise more difficult and more stressful for weight-bearing joints (i.e., ankle, knee, and hip). Women are cautioned to participate in activities to which they have been accustomed to before pregnancy. Activities that require excessive twists and turns or directional changes or those that risk abdominal trauma should not be initiated during pregnancy (Rosenbloom, 2000).

The increased blood volume of pregnancy usually makes aerobic activity easier because of the increased amount of blood and oxygen pumped by the heart to working muscles. Potentially an increased blood volume can affect blood pressure and heat distribution, both important for the viability of the fetus (Clapp et al., 1987). Uterine blood flow does appear to be reduced during exercise. However, this fact does not seem to have a detrimental effect on the fetus because the natural improvement in oxygen uptake, elevated maternal cardiac output, and increased total blood volume are sufficient compensation for exercising muscles and the fetus (Clapp, 2000; Sady and Carpenter, 1989).

As in nonpregnant women, working muscles of pregnant women use glucose as a source of fuel. After 20 minutes to 30 minutes of aerobic exercise, maternal blood glucose decreases, reducing placental blood levels and risking the glucose supply to the fetus. If the mother continues to exercise the fetus may be forced to use predominantly fatty acids for fuel. As a precaution dietitians who work with exercising pregnant women suggest that a carbohydrate snack be consumed before exercise to sustain blood glucose levels (Clapp, 1998; Rosenbloom, 2000; Soultanakis et al., 1996). Further research on nutrition effects and the effects of type, intensity, and duration of exercise will help healthcare professionals provide counseling for active pregnant women.

Benefits of exercise during pregnancy include a positive self-image (Jarski and Trippett, 1990), maintenance of aerobic fitness (Wolfe et al., 1989), shorter labor and quicker, easier delivery (Jarski and Trippett, 1990), and more vaginal deliveries with fewer surgical interventions (Wolfe et al., 1989). There are also several potential benefits from exercise during pregnancy that have not been unequivocally proved by research. There is some suggestion that exercise during pregnancy may improve Apgar scores of infants and enhance motor skills and performance on standardized tests of intelligence in offspring.

There are few formal guidelines for pregnant women who choose to exercise during pregnancy. Box 4-5 outlines some considerations for women who choose to exercise during pregnancy and postpartum. After pregnancy, regardless of lactation status, many women begin to exercise to enhance return to prepregnancy weight. Whether or not exercise places the lactating infant at risk by limiting the quality and quantity of milk has been the subject of continuing research. Health professionals have suggested that women who are lactating should restrict weight loss to less than 2 kg per month (McCrory, 2000) to ensure adequate milk quality and quantity for their infant. Research completed to date indicates that women who do not diet (or restrict energy intake), but who increase energy expenditure by exercising 3 to 5 days per week, may lose up to 0.5 kg per week over a 12- to 14-week period without compromising milk volume or composition (Dewey et al., 1994; Habash and Mitchell, 1994) and without having a negative effect on infant growth (Lovelady et al., 2000; McCrory, 2001). When the diet was restricted to 1800 kcal per day in a group of sedentary lactating women, mean weight loss was about 0.5 kg per week over 10 weeks and lactation was again not affected (Dusdieker et al., 1994).

Box 4-5 Nutrition Considerations for Women Who Choose to Exercise during Pregnancy and Postpartum

- Sufficient energy to sustain growth of the fetus as well as the physical activity of the mother
- 2 to 3 servings of meat or protein alternate daily (equivalent of 6 to 7 ounces)
- 3 to 4 servings of calcium-rich foods daily
- Limit on dietary fat to approximately 30% of total calories
- Liberal amounts of fluid before, during, and after exercise
- Multivitamin/mineral supplement recommended by physician to obtain adequate iron and folic acid

POSTPARTUM: REPLENISHING NUTRIENT STORES

- *What are the nutrition concerns unique to the postpartum woman?*
- *What are appropriate dietary recommendations?*
- *What is an appropriate weight loss in postpartum women?*

Basic nutrition concerns during the postpartum period are related to support for lactation, replenishment of nutrient stores, and return to pregravid weight status. Nutrition services for pregnant women should be extended into this period. Breast-feeding is discussed in Chapter 6.

Nutrient stores, especially calcium, vitamin B_6, and folate, may be diminished during the gestational period. Continuation of prenatal multivitamin supplements for several weeks can assist in establishing nutrient reserves. Women who had multiple infants, are of low body weight, had poor gestational weight gain, smoke cigarettes, or use or abuse substances that may compromise nutrition status may benefit from continued nutrition counseling and use of supplements. Mothers whose diets are inadequate despite nutrition counseling should be encouraged to continue to take the multivitamin-mineral supplement that was prescribed during pregnancy.

Requirements for dietary iron decrease to nonpregnant levels after delivery unless the mother had excessive blood loss during delivery. As blood volume returns to pregravid levels, hemoglobin and hematocrit values rise. Iron salvaged from the breakdown of red blood cells can, in part, be recycled for synthesis of hemoglobin.

Postpartum Body Weight

Current gestational weight gain recommendations (7 to 18 kg) are associated with infants with birth weights between 3 kg and 4 kg and the lowest incidence of infant mortality. Average gestational weight gain is approximately 12.5 kg and, for most women, all but 1 kg or 2 kg of this weight is lost by 6 months to 12 months postpartum (IOM, 1990). However, approximately 12% of the more than 50,000 women studied in the National Collaborative Perinatal Project were 6.8 kg or more above their prepregnancy weights 2 years after delivery (Greene et al., 1988). Some women have increased body weight following pregnancy and one study of WIC participants found an association between antenatal weight gain, particularly during the first pregnancy, and retained weight in the postpartum period (Parker and Abrams, 1993). This finding was especially true for African-American women.

Approximately one third (3.5 kg) of the average gestational weight gain is fat (Sadurskis et al., 1988). This increase in maternal body fat is not associated with increased birth weight, however, and may present a risk of retained excess body fat for the mother (Villar et al., 1992). Studies that have followed lactating postpartum women for up to 6 months have found that only 1 kg to 2 kg of body fat are mobilized during the period of breast-feeding. It has been observed that 12 months after delivery as much as 2 kg of body fat deposited during pregnancy remained. Retention of gestational gains in weight and fat have the potential to contribute to long-term obesity in some women.

Interventions for weight reduction in the postpartum period may be important in prevention of long-term obesity in women. Evidence shows that nutrition counseling to reduce caloric intake can be effective in accomplishing weight loss in postpartum women without interfering with milk production (Dusdieker et al., 1994). Aerobic exercise or weight training has the potential to decrease body fat and protect lean body mass. Boardley and others (1995), in studying WIC participants 7 to 12 months postpartum, found that energy intakes and activity levels were significant predictors of weight loss. During pregnancy many women have marked changes in health norms and behaviors, including eating behaviors. Continuation of nutrition, exercise, and health programs after birth has the potential to improve the nutrition status of the mother and her infant. Additional efforts are needed, particularly culturally specific intervention strategies, in the postpartum period to have an effect on the prevalence of overweight status in at-risk mothers.

Concepts to Remember

- Periconceptional nutrition care is important in providing the mother with the best possible foundation for a favorable pregnancy outcome and successful lactation.
- Pregnancy outcome is influenced by the mother's growth patterns and nutrition status at conception and dietary intake during pregnancy.
- During the first 2 weeks after fertilization, a blastocyst develops and is implanted in the uterine wall and the placenta begins to develop.
- The embryonic period, from 2 weeks to 8 weeks after conception, is critical for cell differentiation and organogenesis.
- The placenta synthesizes many important substances and provides an area for exchange of nutrients from mother to fetus and waste product from fetus to mother.

- Reproductive success is influenced by many factors.
- The rapid growth and development of the embryo and fetus create substantial physiologic and metabolic demands on the mother.
- Nutrition deserves special consideration during the reproductive interval to make sure that it is not a limiting factor in maternal or infant health.
- Early prenatal care, a varied, balanced diet, and appropriate weight gain during pregnancy are important determinants of a favorable outcome.
- The physiologic changes of pregnancy involve almost every body system and support growth of maternal tissues and fetal growth and development.
- Prepregnancy weight and gestational weight gain, indirect indicators of nutrition status, are strong predictors of birth weight and therefore of infant mortality and morbidity.
- Current recommendations for weight gain during pregnancy, based on maternal pregravid weight, range from 6 kg for overweight women to 18 kg for underweight women.
- Caloric needs are estimated to be approximately 300 kcal per day over prepregnancy intake for the second and third trimesters.
- For pregnant women the RDA and AI levels increase for protein and most vitamins and minerals.
- Except for iron, nutritional needs can be met from dietary sources. An iron supplement of 30 mg ferrous iron is recommended for all pregnant women.
- Other supplements are indicated only when careful assessment of dietary intake indicates a major lack of one or more key nutrients.
- Moderate exercise across the reproductive interval can be beneficial during gestation and the postpartum period.
- It is important to maintain maternal nutrition status, especially blood glucose levels, during exercise.
- The nutrition needs of the mother after delivery require special attention to support replenishing of nutrient reserves and return to pregravid weight.

REFERENCES

Abrams B and Selvin S: Maternal weight gain pattern and birth weight, Obstet Gynecol 86:163, 1995.

Abrams B et al.: Pregnancy weight gain: still controversial, Am J Clin Nutr 71:1233S, 2000.

Allen LH: Anemia and iron deficiency: effects on pregnancy outcome, Am J Clin Nutr 71:1280S, 2000.

Allen LH: Pregnancy and lactation. In Present knowledge of nutrition, ed 8, Washington, DC, 2001, ILSI Press.

Allen LH et al.: Report of the Working Group on Energy Requirements of Pregnancy and Lactation, Eur J Clin Nutr 50:S190, 1996.

American College of Obstetricians and Gynecologists: Premenstrual syndrome (ACOG committee opinion), Int J Gynecol Obstet 50:80, 1995.

American Psychiatric Association: Diagnostic and statistical manual of mental disorders, ed 4, Washington, DC, 2000, American Psychiatric Association.

Azais-Braesco V and Pascal G: Vitamin A in pregnancy: requirements and safety limits, Am J Clin Nutr 71: 1325S, 2000.

Bailey LB: New standards for dietary folate for pregnant women, Am J Clin Nutr 71:1304S, 2000.

Barrett JF et al.: Absorption of non-haem iron from food during normal pregnancy, BMJ 309:79, 1994.

Beard JL: Effectiveness and strategies of iron supplementation during pregnancy, Am J Clin Nutr 71:1288S, 2000.

Bendich A: The potential for dietary supplements to reduce premenstrual syndrome (PMS) symptoms, J Am Coll Nutr 19:3, 2000.

Boardley DJ et al.: The relationship between diet, activity, and other factors and post partum weight change by race, Obstet Gynecol 86:834, 1995.

Botto LD et al.: Neural-tube defects, N Engl J Med 341:1509, 1999.

Caudill MA: Current and emerging issues in folate nutriture, Nutr Today 35:206, 2000.

Centers for Disease Control: Recommendations for the use of folic acid to reduce the number of cases of spina bifida and other neural tube defects, MMWR Morb Mortal Wkly Rep 41:1, 1991.

Clapp JF: The effect of dietary carbohydrate on the glucose and insulin response to mixed caloric intake and exercise in both nonpregnant and pregnant women, Diabetes Care 21:B107-B112, 1998.

Clapp JF: Exercise during pregnancy: a clinical update, Clin Sports Med 19:273-286, 2000.

Clapp JF et al.: Thermoregulatory and metabolic responses to jogging prior to and during pregnancy, Med Sci Sports Exerc 19:124, 1987.

Cnattingius S et al.: Prepregnancy weight and the risk of adverse outcomes, N Eng J Med 338:147, 1998.

Dahle LO et al.: The effect of oral magnesium substitution on pregnancy-induced leg cramps, Am J Obstet Gynecol 173:175, 1995.

Daugherty JE: Treatment strategies for premenstrual syndrome, Am Fam Physician 58:183, 1998.

Dewey KG et al.: A randomized study of the effect of aerobic exercise by lactating women on breast-milk volume and composition, N Engl J Med 330:449, 1994.

Durnin JVGA: Energy requirements of pregnancy: an integration of the longitudinal data from the five-country study, Lancet 2:1131, 1987.

Dusdieker LB et al.: Is milk production impaired by dieting during lactation? Am J Clin Nutr 59:833, 1994.

Fleming A: The role of folate in prevention of neural tube defects: human and animal studies, Nutr Rev 59:S13, 2001.

Forbes GB: Methods for determining body composition of the human body, Pediatrics 29:477, 1962.

Forbes GB: Human body composition: growth, aging, nutrition and activity, New York, 1987, Springer-Verlag.

Greene GW et al.: Postpartum weight change: how much of the weight gained in pregnancy will be lost after delivery? Obstet Gynecol 71:701, 1988.

Habash DL and Mitchell MC: Exercise training in postpartum women: changes in body mass index, percent body fat, and fat distribution [abstract], Annual Meeting of the American College of Nutrition, Atlanta, GA, 1994.

Hemminki E and Merilainen J: Long-term follow-up of mothers and their infants in a randomized trial on iron prophylaxis during pregnancy, Am J Obstet Gynecol 173:205, 1995.

Hickey CA: Sociocultural and behavioral influences on weight gain during pregnancy, Am J Clin Nutr 71: 1364S, 2000.

Hornstra G: Essential fatty acids in mothers and their neonates, Am J Clin Nutr 71:1262S, 2000.

Institute of Medicine: Preventing low birth weight, Washington, DC, 1985, National Academy Press.

Institute of Medicine: Nutrition during pregnancy: weight gain and nutrient supplements. Report of the Subcommittee on Nutritional Status and Weight Gain During Pregnancy, Subcommittee on Dietary Intake and Nutrient Supplements During Pregnancy, Committee on Nutritional Status During Pregnancy and Lactation. Food and Nutrition Board, Washington, DC, 1990, National Academy Press.

Institute of Medicine: Dietary reference intakes for calcium, phosphorus, magnesium, vitamin D and fluoride, Washington, DC, 1997, Institute of Medicine.

Institute of Medicine: Dietary reference intakes for thiamin, riboflavin, niacin, vitamin B_6, folate, vitamin B_{12}, pantothenic acid, biotin, and choline, Washington, DC, 1998, National Academy Press.

Institute of Medicine: Dietary reference intakes for vitamin C, vitamin E, selenium and carotenoids, Washington, DC, 2000, National Academy Press.

Institute of Medicine: Dietary reference intakes for vitamin A, vitamin K, arsenic, boron, chromium, copper, iodine, manganese, molybdenum, nickel, silicon, vanadium and zinc, Washington, DC, 2001, National Academy Press.

James SJ et al.: Abnormal folate metabolism and mutation in the methylenetetrahydrofolate reductase gene may be maternal risk factors for Down syndrome, Am J Clin Nutr 70:495, 1999.

Jarski RW and Trippett DL: The risks and benefits of exercise during pregnancy, J Fam Pract 30:185, 1990.

Johnson SR: Premenstrual syndrome therapy, Clin Obstet Gynecol 41:405, 1998.

Kalhan SC: Protein metabolism in pregnancy, Am J Clin Nutr 71:1249S, 2000.

King JC: Physiology of pregnancy and nutrient metabolism, Am J Clin Nutr 71:1218S, 2000.

King JC: Determinants of maternal zinc status during pregnancy, Am J Clin Nutr 71:1334S, 2001.

Klebanoff MA and Yip R: Influence of maternal birth weight on rate of fetal growth and duration of gestation, J Pediatr 11:287, 1987.

Krueger PM and Scholl TO: Adequacy of prenatal care and pregnancy outcome, J Am Osteopath Assoc 100: 485, 2000.

Lovelady CA et al.: The effect of weight loss in overweight, lactating women on the growth of their infants, New Engl J Med 342:449-453, 2000.

McCrory MA: Aerobic exercise during lactation: safe, healthful, and compatible, J Hum Lact 16:95-98, 2000.

McCrory MA: Does dieting during lactation put infant growth at risk? Nutr Rev 59:18-27, 2001.

Mills JL et al.: Homocysteine and neural tube defects, J Nutr 126:756S, 1996.

Milman N et al.: Iron status markers and serum erythropoietin in 120 mothers and newborn infants, Acta Obstet Gynecol Scand 73:200, 1995.

Mitchell MC and Lerner E: A comparison of pregnancy outcome in overweight and normal weight women, J Am Coll Nutr 8:617, 1989a.

Mitchell MC and Lerner E: Weight gain and pregnancy outcome in underweight and normal weight women, J Am Diet Assoc 89:634, 1989b.

Naeye RL: Weight gain and the outcome of pregnancy, Am J Obstet Gynecol 135:3, 1979.

National Research Council: Recommended dietary allowances, ed 10. Report of the Subcommittee, Food and Nutrition Board, Commission on Life Sciences, Washington, DC, 1989, National Academy Press.

National Research Council, Food and Nutrition Board: Maternal nutrition and the course of pregnancy, Washington, DC, 1970, National Academy of Sciences.

Otto SJ et al.: Changes in maternal essential fatty acid profile during early pregnancy and the relation of the profile to diet, Am J Clin Nutr 73:302, 2000.

Parker JD and Abrams B: Difference in postpartum weight retention between black and white mothers, Obstet Gynecol 81:768, 1993.

Parsons MT et al.: Pregnancy outcomes in short women, J Reprod Med 34:357, 1991.

Pivarnik JM: Potential effects of maternal physical activity on birth weight: brief review, Med Sci Sports Exerc 30:400-406, 1998.

Prasad AS: Zinc and growth development and the spectrum of human zinc deficiency, J Am Coll Nutr 7:377, 1988.

Prentice A: Maternal calcium metabolism and bone mineral status, Am J Clin Nutr 71:1312S, 2000.

Prentice AM and Goldberg GR: Energy adaptations in human pregnancy: limits and long-term consequences, Am J Clin Nutr 71:1226S, 2000.

Rainville A: Pica practices of pregnant women are associated with lower maternal hemoglobin level at delivery, J Am Diet Assoc 98:293, 1998.

Rosenbloom CA, Ed.: Sports nutrition. A guide for the professional working with active people, SCAN, 463-476, 2000.

Rosso P: Nutritional needs of the human fetus, Clin Nutr 2:4, 1983.

Rush D: Nutritional services during pregnancy and birthweight: a retrospective matched pair analysis, Canadian Med Assoc J 125:567, 1981.

Rush D et al.: The national WIC evaluation: evaluation of the Special Supplemental Food Program for Women, Infants, and Children. V. Longitudinal study of pregnant women, Am J Clin Nutr 48:439, 1988.

Sadurskis A et al.: Energy metabolism, body composition, and milk production in healthy Swedish women during lactation, Am J Clin Nutr 48:44, 1988.

Sady SP and Carpenter MW: Aerobic exercise during pregnancy, Sports Med 7:357, 1989.

Salle BL et al.: Perinatal metabolism of vitamin D, Am J Clin Nutr 71:1317S, 2000.

Sayegh R et al.: The effect of a carbohydrate-rich beverage on mood, appetite, and cognitive function in women with premenstrual syndrome, Obstet Gynecol 86:520, 1995.

Scholl TO et al.: Dietary and serum folate: their influence on the outcome of pregnancy, Am J Clin Nutr 63:520, 1996.

Scholl TO and Johnson WG: Folic acid: influence on the outcome of pregnancy, Am J Clin Nutr 71:1295S, 2000.

Soultanakis HN et al.: Prolonged exercise in pregnancy: glucose homeostasis, ventilatory and cardiovascular responses, Semin Perinatol 20:315-327, 1996.

Steer PJ: Maternal hemoglobin concentration and birth weight, Am J Clin Nutr 71:1285S, 2000.

Stein Z et al.: Famine and human development: the Dutch hunger winter of 1944/1945, New York, 1975, Oxford University Press.

Susser M: Maternal weight gain, infant birth weight and diet: causal sequences, Am J Clin Nutr 53:1384, 1991.

Tsunenobu T et al.: Maternal plasma zinc concentrations and pregnancy outcome, Am J Clin Nutr 71:104, 2000.

U.S. Department of Health and Human Services: Healthy People 2010: national health promotion and disease prevention objectives, Washington, DC, 2000, U.S. Department of Health and Human Services.

U.S. Public Health Service Expert Panel on the Content of Prenatal Care: Caring for our future: the content of prenatal care, Washington, DC, 1989, U.S. Department of Health and Human Services.

Villar J et al.: Effects of fat and fat-free mass deposition during pregnancy on body weight, Am J Obstet Gynecol 167:1344, 1992.

Vollset SE et al.: Plasma total homocysteine, pregnancy complications, and adverse pregnancy outcomes: the Hordaland Homocysteine Study, Am J Clin Nutr 71:962, 2000.

Voyles LM et al.: High levels of retinol intake during pregnancy during the first trimester of pregnancy results from use of over-the-counter vitamin/mineral supplements, J Am Diet Assoc 100:1068, 2000.

Walker LO and Wilging S: Rediscovering the "M" in "MCH": maternal health promotion after childbirth, J Obstet Gynecol Neonatal Nurs 29:229, 2000.

Winkvist A et al.: A new definition of maternal depletion syndrome, Am J Public Health 82:691, 1992.

Wolfe LA et al.: Prescription of aerobic exercise during pregnancy, Sports Med 8:273, 1989.

APPLICATION

Nutrition Care for Pregnant Women

Improved pregnancy outcome is a national priority in the United States that is reflected in the *Healthy People 2010* goals. Nutrition is an essential component of any effort to improve delivery of healthcare. The *Healthy People 2010* nutrition-related objectives include the following (U.S. Department of Health and Human Services, 2000):

- Reduce the proportion of low-birth-weight and very-low-birth-weight infants
- Increase the proportion of pregnant women who receive early and adequate prenatal care
- Increase the proportion of mothers who achieve recommended weight during their pregnancy
- Increase the proportion of mothers who breast-feed their babies
- Increase abstinence from alcohol among pregnant women
- Reduce the incidence of fetal alcohol syndrome (FAS)
- Reduce iron deficiency anemia among pregnant females and anemia among low-income pregnant females in the third trimester

The introduction to this chapter describes nutrition care for a healthy woman experiencing an uncomplicated pregnancy. Nutrition services (e.g., assessment, counseling, education, and referral to programs and resources) are an integral part of healthcare across the reproductive interval (IOM, 1992b). Basic client-centered, individualized nutrition care should be an integral part of the primary care provided to every woman (IOM, 1992a). This care is the responsibility of primary care providers such as physicians, midwives, and nurse practitioners, who may provide the nutrition care or delegate it to another member of the healthcare team. A registered dietitian (RD) can provide nutrition counseling and education to clients and serve as a resource person for training and consultation for healthcare professionals and others who provide basic nutrition services or work directly with women.

All pregnant women, especially those in high-risk categories (see Chapter 5), need prenatal care including dietary counseling to eat well-balanced meals, gain sufficient weight to support fetal growth, take prenatal supplements as prescribed, and abstain from using cigarettes and alcohol.

The benefits of nutrition intervention are documented (Krueger and Scholl, 2000; Rush, 1988). For example the National Maternal and Infant Health Survey found that mothers who reported receiving nutrition advice, including information about weight gain, supplement use, avoidance of alcohol, and breast-feeding, had a significantly lower incidence of low-birth-weight infants than did other mothers (Kogan et al., 1994). Mothers who received nutrition education, food supplements, and prenatal care through Medicaid and WIC had reduced neonatal and infant deaths (Carver and Moss, 1999). The cost of providing effective nutrition services to women can be offset by savings in infant and maternal medical care costs produced by these and other interventions.

CHARACTERISTICS OF CARE

The characteristics of healthcare for women are as follows (IOM, 1992b):

- Healthcare is structured for easy access
- Community providers are familiar with the cultural backgrounds and social circumstances of the clients
- Providers are aware of the influences of their own culture on their attitudes toward women and delivery of service
- Healthcare is centered on the woman's needs, preferences, culture, and resources
- Providers convey respect and concern for the woman
- The woman and the provider or team set goals jointly

Quality nutrition care, by definition, centers on the needs and concerns of the individual woman. Information from and about the woman is essential for making decisions concerning nutritional care. Successful client-centered prenatal care depends on supportive networks of people within the healthcare system and in the community. Family members and friends are a significant source of support and may have a strong impact on the dietary habits and the nutritional well-being of the woman.

Continuity in nutritional care enhances its quality (IOM, 1992a). The progression of care should build on previous learning as the woman moves from the preconception period through pregnancy, the postpartum period, and breast-feeding. Consistency in the guidance provided by different members of the healthcare team is essential to minimize duplication of activities and avoid confusing the client.

ELEMENTS OF BASIC NUTRITION CARE

Basic nutrition care encompasses the following services that should be available to all women before, during, and after pregnancy:

- Early identification of nutrition risk factors
- Provision of health maintenance activities such as education about pregnancy weight gain or breast-feeding
- Implementation of common interventions.

Nutrition assessment encompasses anthropometric data; laboratory values; past and current medical, pregnancy, and social history; and dietary intake patterns. Reassessment should be completed each trimester of pregnancy unless other nutrition concerns arise. The Public Health Nutrition Practice Group of the American Dietetic Association (1993) has developed quality assurance and quality improvement criteria for the nutritional care of pregnant and postpartum women and adolescents to supplement the guidelines from the IOM (1992a). These guidelines can be used to ensure that any program is providing adequate nutrition services.

PRECONCEPTIONAL CARE

For some conditions and nutrition-related behaviors, the risk of an adverse pregnancy outcome can be reduced with early intervention. The overall objective of nutrition care during the preconception period is to assist women in achieving appropriate body weight-for-height and in following healthful dietary patterns that will optimize chances for a favorable pregnancy outcome. Such assessment before conception allows the woman to implement constructive actions to improve her health. Assessment and remedial action may decrease the likelihood or severity of adverse pregnancy outcomes. For situations that may require long-term changes or treatment, such as substance abuse or severe eating disorders, it is desirable to delay conception until nutrition status improves.

CONDITIONS FOR EARLY INTERVENTION

Chronic disease: diabetes mellitus, hypertension, human immunodeficiency virus, tuberculosis
Dietary patterns: strict vegan diet, inadequate intake
Behaviors/habits: alcohol use, cigarette smoking, illicit drug use

PRENATAL NUTRITION

The value of nutrition intervention in ensuring adequate dietary intakes and appropriate weight gains has been well documented (Krueger and Scholl, 2000). The process begins with basic nutrition assessment, which encompasses measurement of stature and weight, determination of hemoglobin values, and assessment of dietary practices. Abnormal findings may indicate the need for nutrition education or counseling. In some instances in-depth assessment and specialized nutrition care may be necessary.

Assessing Weight-for-Height

Extremes of maternal body weight increase the risk of an adverse pregnancy outcome. Recommendations for gestational weight gain are based on weight-for-height as determined by pregravid BMI. As described in Chapter 2, BMI can be calculated using the following formula:

$$\text{BMI} = \text{weight (kg)/height}^2\text{ (m)}$$

For example Melissa, the woman in the example at the beginning of the chapter, was 165 cm (65 in) tall and weighed 52 kg (115 lb) before conception and had a prepregnancy BMI of 19. That value would be recorded on the prenatal weight gain chart (Figure 4-13) at zero weeks of pregnancy. Because Melissa is somewhat underweight, her recommended weight gain would be 28 lb to 40 lb. Throughout pregnancy Melissa's weight is plotted on the weight-gain chart. Her pattern of weight gain should approximate that shown for underweight women along the dashed line at the top of the chart.

Laboratory Tests

Requirements for iron increase during pregnancy to support fetal and placental growth and expanded maternal blood volume. Daily supplementation with 30 mg of ferrous iron is recommended for all pregnant women by the twelfth week of gestation. Analysis of hemoglobin or hematocrit is used routinely for screening for anemia. If those levels are low, a measurement of serum ferritin to confirm the diagnosis of anemia is appropriate. If anemia is present, supplements containing 60 mg to 120 mg of ferrous iron and copper and zinc are recommended until hematologic values return to acceptable levels.

Assessment of Dietary Patterns and Related Habits

Box 4-6 illustrates a nutrition questionnaire that a woman can complete before she meets with the healthcare provider. It addresses factors that affect the nutrition status of the mother, such as resources available to obtain an adequate diet, typical food intake, and eating behaviors. Information

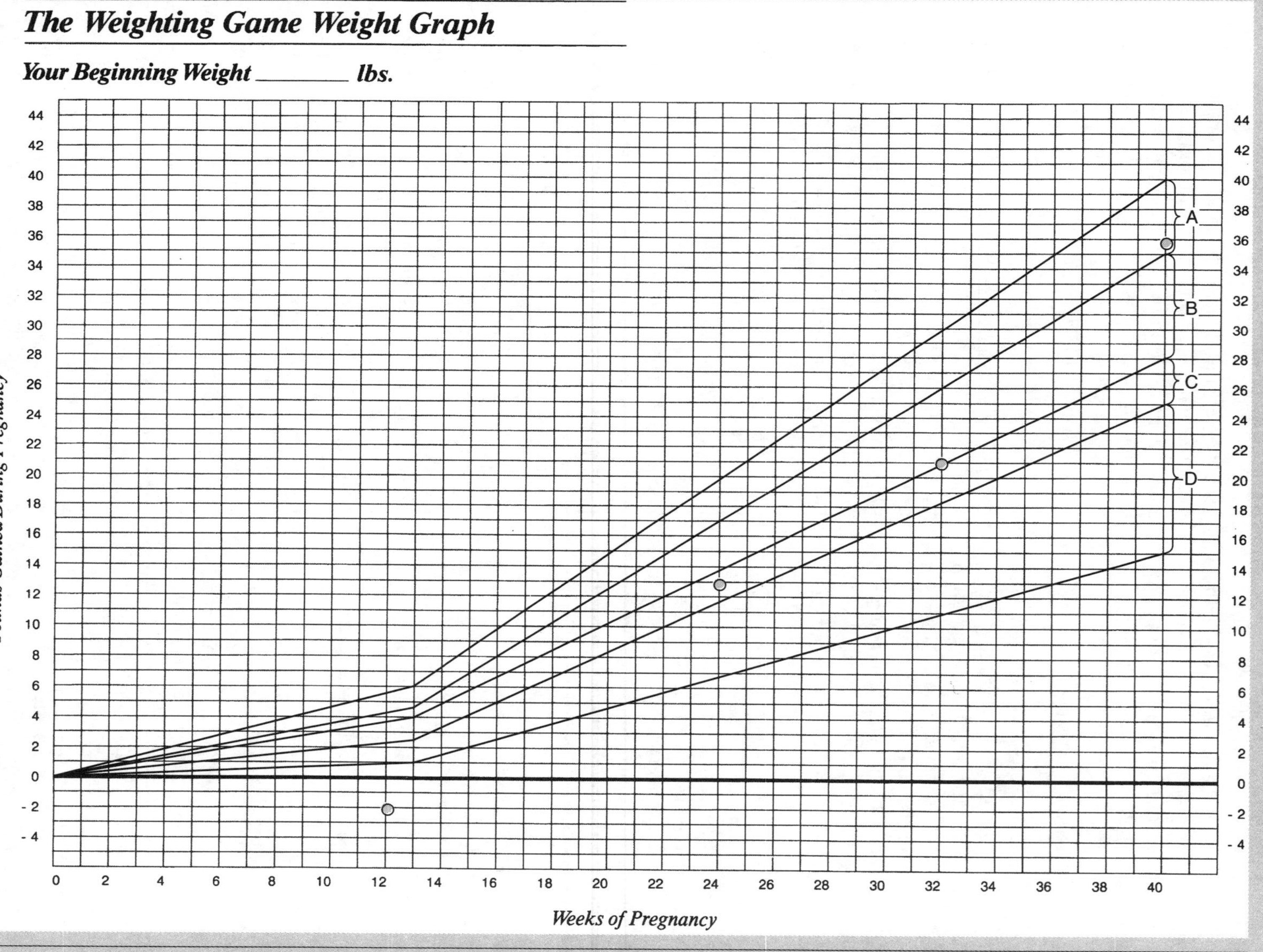

Figure 4-13 Melissa's weight gains, as plotted on the recommended weight gain during pregnancy based on maternal BMI chart (see Figure 4-11). For a woman with a BMI between 19.8 and 26, weight gain should be in the B-C range (26-35 lb). For the underweight woman (BMI <19.8) weight gain should be in the A-B range (28-40 lb). The overweight woman (BMI >26) should gain in the D range (15-25 lb). *(Chart only from the National Dairy Council: Great beginnings: the weighting game graph, Rosemont, IL, 1991, National Dairy Council. Courtesy of NATIONAL DAIRY COUNCIL (R). Adapted from the National Academy of Sciences: Nutrition during pregnancy, Washington, DC, 1990, National Academy Press.)*

Box 4-6 Nutrition Questionnaire

What you eat and some of the lifestyle choices you make can affect your nutrition and health now and in the future. Your nutrition can also have an important effect on your baby's health. Please answer these questions by circling the answers that apply to you.

EATING BEHAVIOR

1. Are you frequently bothered by any of the following? (Circle all that apply)
   Nausea   Vomiting   Heartburn   Constipation
2. Do you skip meals at least 3 times a week? No Yes
3. Do you try to limit the amount or kind of food you eat to control your weight? No Yes
4. Are you on a special diet now? No Yes
5. Do you avoid any foods now for health or religious reasons? No Yes

FOOD RESOURCES

6. Do you have a working stove? No Yes
   Do you have a working refrigerator? No Yes
7. Do you sometimes run out of food before you are able to buy more? No Yes
8. Can you afford to eat the way you should? No Yes
9. Are you receiving any food assistance now? (Circle all that apply): No Yes
   Food stamps   School breakfast   School lunch
   WIC   Donated food/commodities   CSFP
10. Do you feel you need help in obtaining food? No Yes

FOOD AND DRINK

11. Which of these did you drink yesterday? (Circle all that apply):
    Soft drinks   Coffee   Tea   Fruit drink
    Orange juice   Grapefruit juice   Other juices   Milk
    Kool-Aid   Beer   Wine   Alcoholic drinks
    Water   Other beverages (list) ____________
12. Which of these foods did you eat yesterday? (Circle all that apply):
    Cheese   Pizza   Macaroni and cheese
    Yogurt   Cereal with milk
    Other foods made with cheese (such as tacos, enchiladas, lasagna, cheeseburgers)
    Corn   Potatoes   Sweet potatoes   Green salad
    Carrots   Collard greens   Spinach   Turnip greens
    Broccoli   Green beans   Green peas   Other vegetables
    Apples   Bananas   Berries   Grapefruit
    Melon   Oranges   Peaches   Other fruit
    Meat   Fish   Chicken   Eggs
    Peanut butter   Nuts   Seeds   Dried beans
    Cold cuts   Hot dog   Bacon
    Cake   Cookies   Doughnut   Sausage
    Chips   French fries   Pastry
    Other deep-fried foods, such as fried chicken or egg rolls
    Bread   Rolls   Rice
    Noodles   Spaghetti   Tortillas   Cereal
    Were any of these whole grain? No Yes
13. Is the way you ate yesterday the way you usually eat? No Yes

LIFESTYLE

14. Do you exercise for at least 30 minutes on a regular basis (3 times a week or more)? No Yes
15. Do you ever smoke cigarettes or use smokeless tobacco? No Yes
16. Do you ever drink beer, wine, liquor, or any other alcoholic beverages? No Yes
17. Which of these do you take? (Circle all that apply):
    Prescribed drugs or medications
    Over-the-counter products (such as aspirin, Tylenol, antacids, or vitamins)
    Street drugs (such as marijuana, speed, downers, crack, or heroin)

gained from the questionnaire and a follow-up interview form the basis for dietary assessment.

If assessment of the woman's dietary pattern reveals major nutrient deficiencies, nutrition education or individualized counseling should be initiated (see Chapter 3). Nutrition counseling should build on the woman's strengths and reinforce the positive aspects of her diet while promoting small behavioral changes with positive reinforcement. Except for iron, nutritional needs can be met by selection of a variety of foods to meet the recommended servings consistent with the Good Food Guide (see Figure 4-12). Women who have inadequate resources or skills to ensure an adequate diet should be referred to food assistance programs (discussed in the Application in Chapter 5) that provide improved access to food or assistance in learning basic food preparation practices. If after counseling a mother with inadequate nutrient intake is resistant to dietary changes, a multivitamin and mineral supplement may be prescribed. Women should be cautioned against taking self-prescribed supplements because that can create nutrient imbalances or excesses.

Promotion of Breast-Feeding

Research related to a mother's decision to breast-feed is generally made before delivery. Recommendations from healthcare professionals universally support breast-feeding for the health of the infant and mother. However, breast-feeding is a learned behavior and most new mothers require support for initiating and supporting the process. In particular there is a lower incidence of breast-feeding among racial minorities. In Puerto Rican women breast-feeding initiation was more likely for those who received breast-feeding counseling (Perez-Escamilla et al., 1998).

Follow-Up Visits

Follow-up prenatal visits are used to evaluate changes in behavior in response to nutrition counseling from previous visits, to address problems perceived by the client, and to reinforce principles of sound nutritional practices and establish new activities or goals. At each visit the woman is weighed and the weight is recorded on the prenatal weight gain chart to assess her progress throughout pregnancy. If weight gain deviates substantially from recommendations, dietary assessment and counseling may need to be initiated or reinforced.

The client is monitored throughout pregnancy. Visits are typically scheduled as follows:

1-27 weeks' gestation	every 4 weeks
28-35 weeks' gestation	every 2 weeks
36-40 weeks' gestation	weekly

POSTPARTUM NUTRITION

The traditional emphasis of counseling in the postpartum period has been on breast-feeding. In addition basic nutrition services for a postpartum woman should focus on replenishing nutrient stores and returning to prepregnancy weight by promoting sound nutrition practices. Postpartum nutrition counseling and education can be a positive influence on the long-term food habits and health of the mother and her family. Establishment of healthy dietary practices is important in preparation for a later pregnancy.

SPECIALIZED CARE

Special nutrition services may be necessary for some high-risk pregnancies. For a woman with hypertension (National High Blood Pressure Education Working Group on High Blood Pressure in Pregnancy, 2000), for a metabolic disorder such as diabetes mellitus (Jovanovic, 2000) or phenylketonuria, nutrition care may require detailed assessment, counseling for complex dietary modification, careful monitoring, and extended follow-up. Specialized nutrition care may also be necessary for women with health conditions that compromise dietary intake or nutrient use and those with poor intake. Life-style habits that include cigarette smoking and substance abuse increase nutrition risk and women with such habits may require specialized nutrition care (Walker and Wilging, 2000).

REFERENCES

Carver KP and Moss NE: The effect of WIC and Medicaid in infant mortality in the United States, Am J Public Health 88:1354, 1999.

Institute of Medicine: Nutrition during pregnancy and lactation: an implementation guide, Washington, DC, 1992a, National Academy Press.

Institute of Medicine: Nutrition services in prenatal care, ed 2, Washington, DC, 1992b, National Academy Press.

Jovanovic L: Medical nutrition therapy in pregnant women with pregestational diabetes mellitus, J Matern Fetal Med 9:21, 2000.

Kogan MD et al.: Relation of the content of prenatal care to the risk of low birth weight, JAMA 271:1340, 1994.

Krueger PM and Scholl TO: Adequacy of prenatal care and pregnancy outcome, J Am Osteopath Assoc 100: 485, 2000.

Moss NE and Carver KP: The effect of WIC and Medicaid in infant mortality in the United States, Am J Public Health 88:1354, 1999.

National High Blood Pressure Education Working Group on High Blood Pressure in Pregnancy: Report, Am J Clin Obstet Gynecol 183:S1, 2000.

Perez-Escamilla R et al.: Prenatal and perinatal factors associated with breast feeding initiation among inner-city Puerto Rican women, J Am Diet Assoc 98:657, 1998.

Rush D et al.: Longitudinal study of pregnant women, Am J Clin Nutr 48:439, 1988.

Public Health Nutrition Practice Group of the American Dietetic Association: Quality assurance/quality improvement criteria for nutritional care of pregnant and post partum women and adolescents, Atlanta, 1993, U.S. Department of Health and Human Services, Public Health Services, Centers for Disease Control and Prevention, Division of Nutrition.

U.S. Department of Health and Human Services: Healthy People 2010: national health promotion and disease prevention objectives, Washington, DC, 2000, U.S. Department of Health and Human Services.

Walker LO and Wilging S: Rediscovering the "M" in "MCH": maternal health promotion after childbirth, J Obstet Gynecol Neonatal Nurs 29:229, 2000.

CHAPTER

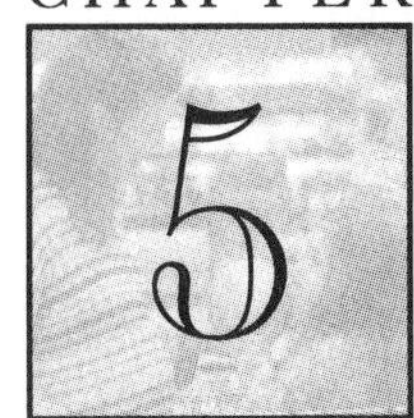

High-Risk Pregnancy

Chapter Outline

Tasha was looking forward to celebrating her sixteenth birthday. Her best friend had turned 16 last year and Tasha had a good time at her party, meeting her boyfriend Damon. But today she woke up feeling sick. She vomited all morning and had an upset stomach throughout the day. The party was no fun, her friends asked her what was wrong, and Damon said she was "no fun to be with." The nausea and vomiting continued for the next couple of weeks. It felt better if she didn't eat, so she skipped eating all day and ate only in the evenings when she felt better. She made many excuses to her grandmother, who was accustomed to Tasha's having a big appetite. When she missed her period for the second time, Tasha had to admit that she could be pregnant. When her home pregnancy test showed that she was indeed pregnant, she still couldn't believe it and she really didn't know what to do. When she told Damon, he insisted that the baby couldn't be his. He stopped calling her and wouldn't talk to her when she called him. She was afraid to tell her grandmother. She'd be so disappointed. Finally Tasha told her best friend. Her friend suggested that she talk to the teacher in their school who worked with a program for pregnant teens. Tasha went to see her the next day. The teacher counseled her about the importance of getting prenatal care using the resources available to her, explained how she could adapt her schoolwork during her pregnancy, and she told her what to expect after the birth of the baby. She also counseled Tasha to tell her grandmother immediately. As Tasha had expected, her grandmother was furious, but when she calmed down she made an appointment for Tasha at an adolescent clinic at the city hospital as suggested by the teacher. Five weeks later Tasha and her grandmother visited the clinic.

In 1998 more than 28,000 babies born in the United States did not survive to see their first birthday—a rate of approximately 7 deaths for every 1000 live births (National Center for Health Statistics, 2000). When babies die it is most often because they are born prematurely and at a low birth weight (Mathews et al., 2000). Preterm babies who are small are 40 times more likely than are full-term babies to die in the first month of life. Those who do survive are at increased risk of mental retardation, growth and developmental problems, visual and hearing defects, **cerebral palsy, epilepsy,** learning difficulties, chronic lung problems, and abuse and neglect.

The progression and outcome of pregnancy are described in Chapter 4. Pregnancy is usually a serene time in a woman's life. However, in some instances, maternal health status, psychosocial or economic factors, and life-style behaviors can complicate pregnancy. Each of the factors listed in Box 5-1 can constitute a risk for an adverse pregnancy outcome by compromising embryonic development, fetal growth, and maternal health. When two or more factors occur together the likelihood of a preterm birth, a low-birth-weight infant, and other unfavorable outcomes increases. In the United States 10% to 20% of the estimated 3.5 million pregnancies each year fall into the high-risk category.

Nutrition intervention through carefully planned care and monitoring can reduce the impact of risk factors on pregnancy outcome. Gravida, in whom the high-risk pregnancies discussed in this chapter occur, are mothers for whom nutrition management is appropriate.

Box 5-1 Factors That Contribute to High-Risk Pregnancy

MATERNAL FACTORS
Age—adolescent, older gravida
Low socioeconomic status
Non-Caucasian race
Marital status
History of poor obstetric outcome
Short interpregnancy interval
High parity

BODY WEIGHT
Underweight
Obesity
Poor weight gain

PRENATAL—COMPLICATED PREGNANCY
Hyperemesis gravidarum
Gestational weight gain
Multiple fetuses
Anemia

MATERNAL HEALTH PROBLEMS
Maternal hyperphenylalaninemia
Hypertensive disorders of pregnancy
Diabetes mellitus
Anorexia nervosa, bulimia nervosa
Human immunodeficiency virus

MATERNAL BEHAVIORS
Cigarette smoking
Alcohol use/abuse
Caffeine
Restrictive dietary patterns, e.g., vegetarianism

MATERNAL AGE

- *What are the risks of adolescent pregnancy for mother and infant?*
- *What are the social, psychologic, economic, and emotional concerns that influence nutrition status in adolescent gravida?*
- *What steps can be taken to reduce the risks associated with adolescent pregnancy?*
- *What are the maternal and fetal risks for gravida who are over 35 years of age?*
- *How can interventions, including nutrition intervention, improve pregnancy outcome?*

Perinatal mortality, low birth weight, and preterm births occur more frequently at the ends of the reproductive age spectrum. Very young adolescents (younger than 15 years of age) or mothers over 35 years of age are more likely to have low gestational weight gains, which is a major contributor to low birth weight. In addition each age group has specific characteristics or factors that increase risk for an adverse pregnancy outcome.

Adolescence

Tasha's story, which opened this chapter, is not unusual. In 1998 approximately one million teenagers became pregnant in the United States. Approximately 500,000 girls between 15 and 19 years of age gave birth, as did almost 13,000 adolescents younger than 15 years (Ventura et al., 1999). Rates of adolescent pregnancy and childbearing are decreasing in the United States, but rates are still much higher than other developed countries (Morbidity and Mortality Weekly Report [MMWR], 2001). Approximately 12% of all births are to adolescents. Although the ability to conceive is determined by biologic maturation, adolescent pregnancy can have profound health, social, psychologic, and vocational consequences for the teenager, her family, and her future.

A pregnant adolescent is likely to be unmarried and poor and to have unstable peer group relations. Adolescents are more likely to enter prenatal care late and have less-than-adequate care (Fraser et al., 1995). Young mothers have lower prepregnancy weights and less adequate gestational weight gains than do older women. Adolescent pregnancy is associated with reduced nutrient stores and inadequate intake (Story and Alton, 1995). In addition, early sexual activity is associated with a higher use of alcohol, tobacco, and drugs, which increases risk of a poor dietary intake, health problems, and inadequate healthcare (Hellerstedt, 2000).

Maternal Growth and Pregnancy

Although girls substantially increase height and weight before menarche, their growth continues for another 4 years to 7 years. Estimates of gains in stature and weight after the onset of menses range from 4.3 cm to 10.6 cm (2 to 4 in) and 6 kg to 8 kg (13 to 18 lb), respectively (Roche and Davilla, 1972). Thus a pregnant teenager who is within 2 years to 3 years of menarche may still be in a period of appreciable growth. Growth of the pelvic girdle also continues after menarche, but at a slower rate. Early maturation associated with pregnancy may result in a smaller pelvis and more difficulties with pregnancy and delivery because of **cephalopelvic disproportion.**

Risks of early delivery in mothers 16 years of age or older can be reduced with early and continuing prenatal care to ensure consumption of adequate energy and nutrients and attainment of recommended weight gains. In fact, for older adolescents, poor pregnancy outcome has a greater association with environmental and social conditions such as poverty, inadequate prenatal care, poor diet, and substance abuse than with young age. However, for young adolescents who give birth, perinatal outcomes are poorer than those of older adolescents even when they receive adequate prenatal care (Scholl et al., 1994). Infants of adolescents of young **gynecologic age,** who have not completed their own growth and development, are at greater risk for prematurity and low birth weight.

Growth of **gravida** of young gynecologic age may be masked by the tendency of women of all ages to measure slightly less in stature during pregnancy, probably as a result of vertebral compression. Scholl and Hediger (1993) demonstrated continued maternal growth in 50% of young primiparas and **multiparas** by measuring increases in length of the lower leg (knee height). In a recent study infants born to growing adolescents were approximately 130 grams lighter than those of nongrowing adolescents despite the fact that the growing adolescents gained almost 2.5 kg more weight during pregnancy (Scholl et al., 1994). This may result from reduced blood flow to the uterus and ineffective transfer of nutrients to the fetus (Scholl et al., 1997), representing a competition for nutrients between the mother and fetus and ineffective transfer of nutrients from lesser placental blood flow (Frisancho, 1985; Naeye, 1981).

Mothers who show gains in linear height during pregnancy also accrue additional body fat, almost exclusively during the third trimester, which is the period of most rapid growth by the fetus (Scholl et al., 1994). A larger percentage of gestational weight gain is retained in postpartum adolescents who experience growth during pregnancy when compared with nongrowing postpartum adolescents. Growing adolescents continue to deposit fat at the triceps and subscapular fatfold sites, whereas nongrowing gravida lose fat from these sites during pregnancy (Scholl et al.,

KEY TERMS

cerebral palsy: partial paralysis and lack of muscle coordination resulting from a malfunction of or damage to the brain

epilepsy: a disorder of the nervous system resulting from a temporary disturbance of the nerve impulses that may be manifested in convulsive seizures

cephalopelvic disproportion: a disproportionate maternal pelvic size and shape in relation to the fetal head

gynecologic age: current age minus age at menarche

gravida: a woman who is pregnant

multipara: a woman who has had two or more pregnancies

1997). Central body fat stores may be increased in postpartum adolescents who grow during pregnancy. Recently it was observed that **leptin** concentrations increase with gestation. However, concentrations were higher at both 28 weeks' gestation and postpartum in nongrowing teenagers and mature gravida than in growing adolescents (Scholl et al., 2001).

Consequences

Because pregnancy in young adolescents is associated with numerous environmental and lifestyle risk factors, it is difficult to differentiate the effects of those factors from physiologic maturity. Fraser and others (1995) examined the pregnancy outcomes of more than 134,000 singleton births of white **primigravida** between 13 years and 24 years of age. After adjustment for marital status, education, and prenatal care, the younger groups had a significantly higher risk of preterm delivery and low birth weight infants than did mothers who were 20 years to 24 years of age. A number of complications of pregnancy increase the risk for the teen mother. These include difficult labor and delivery and **pregnancy-induced hypertension** (see page 156) and infections.

The pattern of weight gain in young gravida also appears to be a significant factor in outcome. Infant birth weights of 3 kg to 4 kg in offspring of teenagers appear to be supported by a maternal weight gain of 1.4 kg to 2.3 kg (3 to 5 lb) during the first trimester and increases of approximately 0.5 kg (1 lb) per week thereafter until term.

Weight Gain Recommendations

Adolescents who are underweight at the time of conception and who gain inadequate amounts of weight during pregnancy are at greatest risk for the delivery of infants who are low birth weight or preterm. Appropriate weight gains for pregnancy are influenced by many factors, including pregravid weight and growth status, overall health status, and psychosocial and economic factors that influence behavior and health. Recommendations for specific levels of weight that should be gained have been controversial (Abrams et al., 2000). Until realistic new guidelines become available, it seems appropriate to use the Institute of Medicine (1990) recommended weight gains (based on pregravid Body Mass Index [BMI]) for pregnant adolescents (Table 5-1). The basis for these recommendations appears to have been reduction of the high incidence of low-birth-weight infants. The levels for young gravida represent the upper end of the ranges recommended for all women; the guidelines state that young mothers (gynecologic age less than 2 years) who are still growing may require higher weight gains during pregnancy than older adolescents or adults to achieve optimum birth weights of 3.5 kg to 4.0 kg (Institute of Medicine, 1990). Caution should be exercised because increased gains are associated with increased maternal weight and fat stores and their attendant long-term risks.

Table 5-1 RECOMMENDED GESTATIONAL WEIGHT GAINS FOR ADOLESCENTS

BMI	Weight Gain kg	Weight Gain lb
<19.8 (underweight)	14.0-18.0	35-40
19.8-26.0 (normal weight)	13.0-18.0	28-40
>26.0-29.0 (overweight)	8.0-11.5	18-25

Adapted from Institute of Medicine: Nutrition during pregnancy, Washington, DC, 1990, National Academy Press.

Maternal fat accretion usually occurs in the first two trimesters of pregnancy and some of that fat is mobilized in the final trimester. In contrast pregnant teenagers who are still growing continue to accumulate body fat after 28 weeks, resulting in larger weight gains. These gains appear to be related to failure to mobilize stored fat, as indicated by increased fatfold measurements postpartum. This pattern of fat accretion has been associated with decreased fetal growth and lower infant birth weights (Hediger et al., 1990). Despite this difference these still-growing teens had caloric intakes comparable with those of pregnant, nongrowing adolescents and mature women (Scholl et al., 1994).

Energy and Nutrient Needs

As discussed in Chapter 4, pregnancy increases the demand for energy, protein, and most vitamins and minerals. In young adolescents this increased need

Table 5-2 DIETARY REFERENCE INTAKES FOR VITAMINS AND MINERALS FOR PREGNANT AND NONPREGNANT ADOLESCENTS

Nutrient	Pregnant <19 years	Non-pregnant 14-18 years
Calcium, mg	*1300*	*1300*
Phosphorus, mg	**1250**	**1250**
Magnesium, mg	**400**	**360**
Fluoride, mg	*3*	*3*
Vitamin D, μg	*5*	*5*
Thiamin, mg	**1.4**	**1.0**
Riboflavin, mg	**1.4**	**1.0**
Niacin, mg	**18**	**14**
Vitamin B_6, mg	**1.2**	**1.9**
Folate, μg	**600**	**400**
Vitamin B_{12}	*2.6*	*2.4*
Pantothenic acid, mg	*6*	*5*
Biotin, μg	*30*	*25*
Choline, mg	*450*	*400*
Vitamin C, mg	**65**	**80**
Vitamin E, mg	**15**	**15**
Selenium, μg	**60**	**55**
Vitamin A, μg	**750**	**700**
Vitamin K, μg	*75*	*75*
Chromium, μg	*29*	*24*
Copper, μg	**1000**	**890**
Iodine, μg	**220**	**150**
Iron, mg	**27**	**15**
Manganese, mg	*2*	*1.6*
Molybdenum, μg	**50**	**43**
Zinc, mg	**19**	**9**

Adapted with permission from the Dietary Reference Intakes series, National Academy Press, Copyright 1997, 1998, 2000, 2001 by the National Academy of Sciences. Courtesy of the National Academy Press, Washington, DC.
RDAs are printed in bold type; AIs are printed in italics.

is superimposed on the already high demands of pubertal growth. Currently specific guidelines for energy and protein for pregnant adolescents do not exist. The Dietary Reference Intake (DRI) report on energy and macronutrients, to be release in 2002, will address these issues.

Energy needs depend on growth status, activity levels, body size, and the stage of gestation and will change throughout pregnancy. Levels greater than the additional 300 kcal per day recommended for gestation may be required to support greater weight gains for adolescents who begin pregnancy underweight. Increased protein requirements of gestation were discussed in Chapter 4. The Recommended Dietary Allowance (RDA) of approximately 46 g or 48 g per day is increased by 15 g, yielding approximately 60 g per day (National Research Council, 1989). Dietary studies of pregnant adolescents indicate that most teens who consume adequate energy tend to consume adequate protein (Giddens et al., 2000; Institute of Medicine, 1990). However, adequate protein may be a concern for adolescents who have inadequate energy intakes or those who follow vegan diets.

The new DRIs for vitamins and minerals have established a category for the pregnant adolescent (Institute of Medicine, 1997, 1998, 2000, 2001). The levels given in Table 5-2 include RDAs or Adequate Intakes (AIs) for mothers 18 years of age or younger and for nonpregnant teens age 14 years to 18 years.

Iron supplementation during pregnancy has been somewhat controversial regarding whether to supplement, how much to supplement, and how to supplement. Gestational iron needs for adolescents include the amounts required for maternal growth and the amounts needed to support fetal and placental tissue growth and increased red blood cell volume. According to the 1990 Nutrition Surveillance System data, the prevalence of iron deficiency anemia (based on the criteria in Table 4-3) in adolescents was 11%, 16%, and 37% in the first, second, and third trimesters of pregnancy, respectively (Beard, 1994). There is substantial evidence that maternal iron deficiency increases the risk of low birth weight and preterm birth (Allen, 2000). As for pregnant adults, the Institute of Medicine (1990)

KEY TERMS

leptin: a hormone secreted by the adipose tissue that seems to communicate the amount of adipose tissue to the brain; may play a role in increasing satiety and energy expenditure
primigravida: a woman in her first pregnancy
pregnancy-induced hypertension: increased blood pressure with onset during midpregnancy

recommends iron supplementation with 30 mg of elemental iron daily during the second and third trimesters of pregnancy. However, there are substantial side effects from iron supplementation that can decrease compliance, particularly in adolescents. If iron deficiency anemia develops, supplementation of 60 mg to 120 mg per day is recommended until anemia is resolved. A multivitamin and mineral supplement supplying 15 mg of zinc and 2 mg of copper is also recommended to prevent the additional iron from decreasing body levels of those minerals from impaired absorption (Institute of Medicine, 1990).

Calcium is transferred from the mother to the fetus at an average rate of 330 mg/day (Institute of Medicine, 1990). The 1998 DRI recommendation of 1300 mg has been determined as a level to promote attainment of peak bone mass and support fetal growth and development (Institute of Medicine, 1997). An intake of four to five servings of dairy products or their equivalent has been shown to approach the level needed. The Institute of Medicine (1990) recommends a supplement of 600 mg of elemental calcium (1.5 g of calcium carbonate) for adolescents with dietary intakes below 600 mg per day.

The American Dietetic Association (1994) emphasizes the importance of early, frequent, and continuous nutrition care in an interdisciplinary program specifically devoted to adolescents. Such care, which supports the unique biologic, psychosocial, developmental, and economic needs of the teen mother, will optimize the potential for a favorable pregnancy outcome.

Older Gravida

Concern about the primigravida 35 years or older has particular significance in the United States because the number of women aged 35 years to 49 years is increasing and more women are electing to delay childbearing, increasing the number of older mothers. Approximately 10% of births in the United States occur to women 35 years to 49 years of age.

Women 35 years and older have higher incidences of maternal and perinatal mortality, of low-birth-weight infants, and of both preterm and small-for-gestational-age infants (van Katwijk and Peeters, 1998). These data may be influenced by the fact that the incidence of births of multiple fetuses increases with age. Many medical conditions, such as cardiovascular and respiratory disorders, kidney disease, autoimmune disorders, obesity, **diabetes mellitus**, and tumors increase in frequency with advancing maternal age (Prysak et al., 1995). In fact the incidence of diabetes and hypertension increases almost linearly with age. Increased maternal mortality with age results mostly from increases in these underlying illnesses. Some obstetric complications in older gravida may also be related to the increased incidence of chronic diseases. For example the incidence of **placenta previa** and **abruptio placenta** increases with age and parity. These disorders may be related more to predisposing problems such as hypertension and smoking than to maternal age. Studies of pregnancy outcome in older women have not been able to control many important confounding variables such as substance abuse, life-style, cardiovascular fitness, obesity, or the use of medical care. However, today's older mothers may have fewer risks than previous generations because women who elect to delay childbearing tend to be better educated, to be in better general health, and to have more access to medical care.

Preconception management, including nutrition care, of the underlying disorders that complicate pregnancy in older gravida and careful control throughout gestation can reduce the risk of adverse outcomes. This management includes basic nutrition care (described in the Application at the end of Chapter 4) to ensure adequate dietary intakes to support fetal growth and maintenance of nutrition status and also specialized nutrition care to normalize blood glucose levels or control hypertension across the reproductive period.

SOCIOECONOMIC STATUS

- *What are the socioeconomic characteristics of a high-risk pregnancy?*
- *How does a woman's socioeconomic status influence pregnancy outcome?*

Infant mortality rates in the United States are higher than are those in many other developed countries. A number of interrelated socioeconomic factors contribute to the risk of an adverse pregnancy outcome. They include age, family income, social status, ethnicity, education, employment, marital status, and availability of healthcare and support systems. An important predictor of pregnancy outcome is gestational weight gain because it has a positive association with birth weight (Institute of Medicine, 1990). Some studies have used maternal weight gain as a surrogate to study nutrition adequacy related to pregnancy. Using data from the 1980 National Natality Survey, Hickey (2000) reported that the risk of low weight gain (less than 7.3 kg) increased almost twofold as the annual income fell from $30,000 to $9000. Similar observations have been made for weight gain and maternal education (Ventura et al., 1999).

Women of low socioeconomic status have a higher incidence of low-birth-weight and preterm infants than do affluent women (Jonas et al., 1992). This fact is important because even mildly preterm infants (34 to 36 weeks) and moderately preterm infants (32 to 33 weeks) are at 3 times and 6.6 times greater risk of death, respectively, in the first year of life than are term infants (Kramer, 2000).

A substantial portion of U.S. women of childbearing age consume diets that provide less than the recommended amounts of some micronutrients, especially calcium, iron, and zinc, which have been associated with the course and outcome of pregnancy. This observation applies to all women, but particularly to those who are at or below the poverty level. Scholl and colleagues (1997) have suggested that greater use of prenatal vitamin and mineral supplements may have the potential to reduce infant morbidity and mortality by decreasing the incidence of preterm and low-birth-weight infants.

Another confounding factor is marital status. Poor women are more likely to be unmarried and the risk of an adverse outcome is greater for women who have never been married and for those who are divorced or separated (Melnikow et al., 1991).

MATERNAL BODY WEIGHT

- *What are the risks of maternal obesity or underweight status to mother and fetus?*
- *How does nutrition intervention modify the risks of pregravid body weight?*

Prepregnancy weight has an effect on birth weight independent of maternal weight gain. As rates of overweight status and obesity have increased, there is growing concern about the effects on fetal outcome. Women who are obese or extremely underweight at the time of conception are at risk of increased mortality and morbidity for themselves and their infants. Nutrition assessment and intervention and modification of dietary and activity patterns can modulate weight gain for improved pregnancy.

Overweight and Obesity

Women who are overweight (BMI 26 to 29) or obese (BMI greater than 29) at the onset of pregnancy experience more complications than do mothers of normal weight. The greatest risk occurs with maternal body weights that exceed 135% of the reference weight or a BMI greater than 28 (Cnattingius et al., 1998; Naeye, 1979). The risks include a higher incidence of pregnancy-induced hypertension (Wolf, 1998), diabetes mellitus (American College of Obstetricians and Gynecologists, 1995), **thromboembolic disease,** and labor abnormalities and more inductions of labor and unscheduled cesarean sections (Cnattingius et al., 1998; Wolf, 1998). Infants of mothers with a high BMI are at increased risk for late fetal death

KEY TERMS

diabetes mellitus: a chronic disorder of carbohydrate and fat metabolism that is characterized by a relative lack of insulin
placenta previa: a placenta located in a lower position in the uterus than normal
abruptio placenta: premature separation of the placenta from the uterine wall
thromboembolic disease: a condition in which a blood clot obstructs a blood vessel

(greater than 28 weeks), early neonatal death (Cnattingius et al., 1998; Michlin et al., 2000), and **macrosomia,** a condition associated with greater risk of **shoulder dystocia** and maternal or infant morbidity (Institute of Medicine, 1990). Once they become pregnant obese women need careful monitoring for diabetes mellitus and hypertension (Allen, 2001).

Nutrition care of obese gravida must emphasize varied dietary intakes that are adequate in nutrients and provide sufficient energy to support fetal growth and sufficient carbohydrates to avoid ketosis. In general weight reduction during pregnancy is not recommended. For obese mothers weight gains of approximately 6 kg are associated with the lowest rates of infant mortality and birth weights between 3 kg and 4 kg (Naeye, 1979).

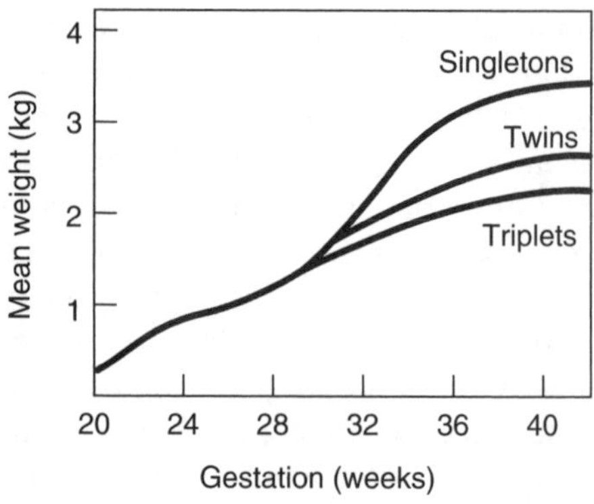

Figure 5-1 Mean fetal growth rates in singleton and multiple pregnancies. *(From MacLennan AH: Multiple gestation: clinical characteristics and management. In Creasy RK and Resnick R, editors: Maternal-fetal medicine: principles and practice, ed. 3, Philadelphia, 1994, WB Saunders.)*

Underweight

Women who have a low prepregnancy weight for their height have a greater risk of delivering a preterm (less than 37 weeks) infant and for delivering a small-for-gestational-age infant (Cnattingius et al., 1998; Hickey et al., 1997). They also have a higher incidence of complications such as antepartum hemorrhage, **premature rupture of the membranes,** and anemia (Edwards et al., 1979). The level of maternal body weight that constitutes increased risk may vary. For example an economically disadvantaged woman may have a higher risk of having a low-birth-weight infant although her body weight is greater than that of a middle-class woman (Mitchell and Lerner, 1989). Preconception and prenatal counseling, including referral to food assistance programs, can help women reduce risk by normalizing body weight before conception. For underweight women a weight gain of 12.5 kg to 18 kg (28 to 40 lb) is associated with improved birth weights and lower neonatal mortality rates (Institute of Medicine, 1990; Naeye, 1979).

> Judie and Bob had been married for 7 years. They wanted to start a family a couple of years ago, but had not successfully conceived. They consulted a fertility specialist at the university and were delighted when Judie became pregnant with twins. Judie watched her diet, exercised, and gained weight. By week 34 she had gained 40 pounds and was uncomfortable, had difficulty getting around, and experienced a lot of "heartburn." At 36 weeks an ultrasound revealed that one fetus was much larger than the other and a Cesarean-section was performed. They had two beautiful little girls who weighed 4.5 lbs and 8.2 lbs. The larger baby was able to go home within a couple of days, but her sister stayed in the neonatal intensive care unit for several more days.

MULTIPLE BIRTHS

- *What are appropriate birth weights for twin, triplet, and high-order pregnancies?*
- *How do the energy and nutrient needs of twin pregnancies and high-order pregnancies compare with those of singleton pregnancies?*

A similar scenario is played out thousands of times each year. A pregnancy involving more than one fetus is associated with low-birth-weight babies, preterm births, and higher perinatal mortality rates. For example twins make up less then 3% of U.S. births, but account for 21% of all low-birth-weight babies, 14% of preterm births, and 13% of deaths (Kogan et al., 2000). The greater the number of fetuses, the smaller the weight for each infant and the greater the risk of low birth weight (Figure 5-1). Multiple-fetus pregnancies are less likely to go to term. For example twin pregnancies are, on the average, 3 weeks shorter than singleton pregnancies and are associated with preterm delivery and low birth weight (Luke and Keith, 1992). Yet these infants are at low risk of dying, which reinforces the merits of ongoing prenatal care (Kogan et al., 2000), suggesting that some of the rise in preterm births is associated with twin and triplet births.

It is obvious that multiple pregnancies increase requirements for energy and nutrients. Weight gain should exceed that of singleton pregnancies because of greater increases in maternal, placental, and fetal tissue. A total weight gain of 16 kg to 20.5 kg (35 to 45 lb) has been recommended for twin pregnancies (Institute of Medicine, 1990). Pederson and others (1989) found that a weight gain of 22 kg (44 lb) was associated with optimal pregnancy outcome (birth weight greater than 2.5 kg and gestational age greater than 37 wk) in twin pregnancies. A weekly weight gain of approximately 0.75 kg (1.5 lb) during the second and third trimesters of pregnancy is advisable for a mother who is carrying twins. There is evidence that intrauterine growth is achieved earlier for twins than for singletons (Luke et al., 1993) and that the lowest morbidity may occur with delivery between 35 and 37 weeks. For triplet pregnancies the average length of gestation is 33 to 34 weeks (Brown and Carlson, 2000).

Appropriate weight gains for optimum growth of multiple fetuses and support of maternal health have not been defined. Recommendations for optimizing pregnancy outcome include liberalized weight gains, reduced physical effort, and early, comprehensive prenatal care. Although the data are limited Brown and Carlson (2000) suggest weight gains for triplet pregnancies of about 50 lbs at a rate of gain of approximately 2.5 pounds per week by 23 weeks of gestation. A recent study comparing the outcome of pregnancy with twins and triplets, with mothers matched for age and obstetric characteristics, revealed that triplets had significantly lower mean birth weight (1596 g versus 2317 g), more frequent preterm delivery, and a longer hospital stay (Ziadeh, 2000). A mother's early weight gain is critical for multiple fetuses because sufficient early intrauterine growth is more crucial for multiple-fetus pregnancies than for singleton pregnancies. First-trimester weight gain of 4 lbs to 6 lbs may be beneficial (Brown and Carlson, 2000).

HEALTH CONDITIONS OF THE MOTHER

Hyperemesis Gravidarum

- *What are the implications of hyperemesis gravidarum for mother and fetus?*
- *What are appropriate intervention strategies for severe cases of hyperemesis gravidarum?*

As discussed in Chapter 4, many pregnant women experience some nausea and vomiting during early pregnancy. Hyperemesis gravidarum is a nutritionally debilitating condition characterized by **intractable** vomiting that develops within the first 22 weeks of gestation. It is estimated that hyperemesis gravidarum develops in about 0.5 to 10 women per 1000 pregnancies (Ling and McCluskey, 1996). In the United States 50,000 pregnant women are hospitalized for hyperemesis each year (Signorello et al., 1998). The etiology of hyperemesis gravidarum is unknown. High levels of estrogen circulating in the woman's bloodstream have been considered a likely culprit. In addition progesterone, adrenal hormones,

KEY TERMS

macrosomia: birth weight greater than 4000 g
shoulder dystocia: abnormal delivery from difficulty in delivering the shoulders of the fetus through the birth canal after the head has emerged
premature rupture of the membranes: rupture of fetal membranes before the onset of labor
intractable: not easily managed

and human chorionic gonadotropin (HCG) have all been implicated, yet none has been positively linked to hyperemesis. Other factors under investigation include changes in taste perception (Sipiora et al., 2000), high dietary fat (Signorello et al., 1998), supplements with vitamin B_6, and psychosomatic factors.

Hyperemesis gravidarum can result in weight loss, dehydration, electrolyte imbalance, and metabolic abnormalities. There are limited data relating this condition to pregnancy outcome. Loss of more than 5% of pregravid weight has been associated with significant fetal growth restriction (Snell et al., 1998). A recent study from Oslo, Norway found that birth weight of the offspring of mothers treated for hyperemesis was associated most strongly with maternal weight gain during pregnancy (Vilming and Nesheim, 2000). The hyperemetic woman who has little or no dietary intake because of nausea and vomiting must meet her energy needs by breaking down or metabolizing body fats and proteins. Use of fat in the absence of carbohydrate intake can result in the formation of ketone bodies and ketonemia that may impair neurologic development in the fetus.

Perinatal nutrition assessment and management are appropriate, particularly if nausea and vomiting persist beyond the first trimester. If fluid and electrolyte imbalances occur or if weight loss exceeds 5% or is accompanied by ketonemia, hospitalization may be indicated. Treatment includes intravenous (IV) fluid and sodium, potassium, chloride, lactate/bicarbonate, and glucose replacement to correct electrolyte imbalance, prevent ketosis, acid/base imbalance, hypovolemia, and ketosnemia (Snell et al., 1998). When nausea and vomiting resolve, oral intake is slowly introduced as small, frequent meals of foods low in fat and high in carbohydrate, with solid and liquid foods consumed at different times.

For the small number of women who do not respond to the gradual progression to an oral diet, enteral or parenteral feeding is instituted. Enteral feeding of commercial formula via tube into the stomach has been shown to be efficacious in treatment of hyperemesis. In many cases the nausea and vomiting dissipate with this treatment. If enteral intake remains impossible, parenteral nutrition can be instituted in the hospital setting. Total parenteral nutrition (TPN), which provides all energy and nutrient needs by IV infusion, has been successful in supporting maternal weight and fetal growth. Duration of such therapy may be a few days or weeks, depending on the severity of the condition. Mothers can be maintained as inpatients until they are stable and then discharged to the home with TPN support from a home care service.

Maternal Hyperphenylalaninemia

- *How does an elevated maternal blood level of phenylalanine increase fetal risk?*
- *Why is hyperphenylalaninemia a public health concern?*
- *What is appropriate prenatal nutrition intervention for hyperphenylalaninemia?*

Phenylketonuria (PKU), an autosomal recessive inborn error of phenylalanine metabolism, affects approximately 1 in 17,000 Caucasians each year (deFreitas et al., 1999). It results from the absence of the liver enzyme, phenylalanine hydroxylase, which is required for the first step in the catabolic pathway of phenylalanine (Figure 5-2). The deficiency of this enzyme results in an increase in the level of phenylalanine in the blood and the accumulation of other metabolites in body fluids and excreted in the urine. Restriction of phenylalanine has long been the primary treatment modality for individuals with PKU during infancy and childhood when brain growth is most rapid. Treatment needs to begin shortly after birth to prevent mental retardation and hyperactivity. Phenylalanine intake is restricted to the amount required for protein synthesis. This limit is accomplished by restriction of natural food protein to an amount that meets phenylalanine requirement. As seen in Figure 5-2, tyrosine is incorporated into all body protein and is a precursor of melanin for skin pigment and the neurotransmitters dopamine and norepinephrine. Normally tyrosine is a nonessential amino acid synthesized from phenylalanine. If phenylalanine is to be restricted, tyrosine becomes an essential amino acid and must be provided in the diet.

A major component of the dietary treatment is a protein substitute formula that provides es-

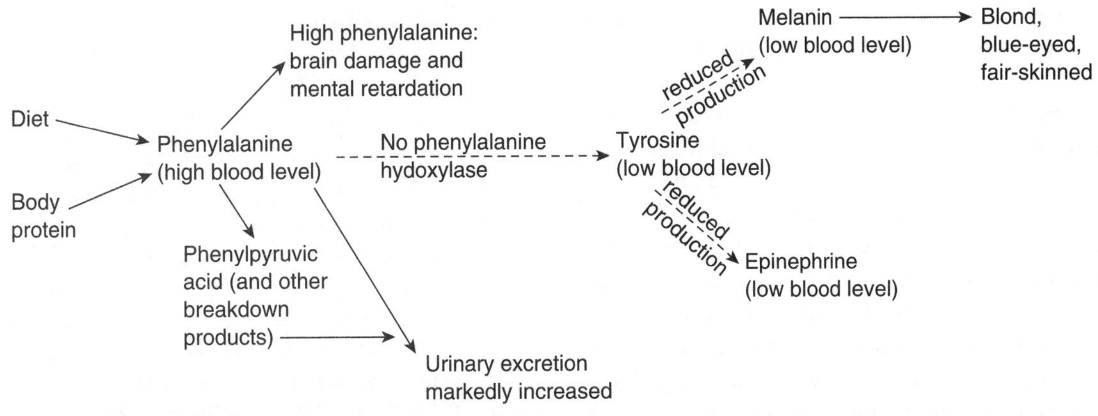

Figure 5-2 Metabolic pathway of phenylalanine. *(From Bolander VB: Sorensen and Luckmann's basic nursing: a psychophysiologic approach, ed 3, Philadelphia, 1994, WB Saunders.)*

sential amino acids (except phenylalanine) and additional tyrosine to meet needs for synthesis of body proteins and other essential body compounds. It is important that the tyrosine supplement be distributed throughout the day to maintain blood levels of tyrosine to support protein synthesis (van Spronsen et al., 2001).

If the enzyme block is mild and blood phenylalanine levels are only somewhat elevated, the individual is said to have hyperphenylalaninemia. Because blood levels of these individuals may be below what would cause damage, infants and children with this form of the disorder may not require restriction of dietary phenylalanine.

Newborn screening for PKU is required in most states and has resulted in prevention of the effects of PKU. Ironically successful treatment of PKU in infants has created new challenges in pregnancy and childbearing. There are approximately 2000 to 4000 girls and women with normal intelligence of childbearing age in the United States who were diagnosed with hyperphenylalaninemia and did not require treatment or with PKU and had treatment discontinued at an early age (Platt et al., 1992). There is probably a similar number of women with unknown hyperphenylalaninemia. All of these women have elevated phenylalanine levels in their plasma that are not detrimental to them, but the levels are sufficiently high to damage a fragile developing embryo and fetus. Effects of uncontrolled maternal hyperphenylalaninemia include microcephaly, mental retardation, **congenital** heart disease, and facial abnormalities (Levy et al., 1996).

Only 1 in 120 infants of these women actually have the autosomal inborn error PKU and that diagnosis is made after birth. The real issue is the damage caused to the embryo or fetus because maternal blood levels are excessive. There is no question that the appropriate intervention is to maintain the blood levels of phenylalanine at the same level as that of normal (nonPKU) gravida from conception to delivery. However, treatment at any time during pregnancy may reduce the severity of developmental and cognitive impairment. The international, longitudinal Maternal PKU Collaborative Study followed 253 children of women with PKU and hyperphenylalaninemia to age 4 years (Waisbren et al., 2000). At the end of 4 years the researchers found that delayed development in offspring of women with PKU is associated with poor maternal metabolic control before or early in pregnancy. At 4 years of age offspring of mothers who did not comply with treatment or who began the diet late had lower scores on tests of language, memory, and quantitative abilities in general (Koch et al., 1999). Motor skills and behavior were less affected.

KEY TERMS

congenital: signifying a condition present at, and usually before, birth

This study reinforced the importance of beginning the dietary treatment before pregnancy for true success.

Guidelines for nutrition care appear in Box 5-2. The diet relies on a formula product low in phenylalanine and adequate in tyrosine and other nutrients for most of its protein. The formula is supplemented in foods low in phenylalanine. The diet is highly restrictive and the mother will require specialized nutrition counseling and follow-up to promote compliance. Compliance with nutrition care is monitored by measuring blood levels of phenylalanine and tracking gestational weight gain.

Box 5-2 Guidelines for Prenatal Nutrition Care in Women with Hyperphenylalaninemia

- Develop a diet plan to maintain serum phenylalanine levels between 2 mg/dL and 6 mg/dL or lower prior to conception and throughout pregnancy.
- Meet recommended levels for protein, phenylalanine, vitamins, and minerals.
- Provide sufficient energy to maintain the recommended patterns of weight gain.
- Limit intake of phenylalanine to an amount needed to maintain recommended serum levels using the following:
  Phenylalanine-free formula product
  Foods low in phenylalanine, to provide a minimum of 200 mg of phenylalanine as a baseline, with the addition of more foods to maintain blood levels
- Provide sufficient tyrosine to maintain serum levels in the normal range.
- Assist the mother in planning a diet to meet the dietary guidelines.
- Assist the mother with food shopping, selection, and preparation.
- Monitor blood levels of phenylalanine and tyrosine.
- Monitor weight gain.

Hypertension during Pregnancy

- *What is pregnancy-induced hypertension and what are its implications?*
- *What is the potential role of nutrition in prevention or treatment of hypertension during pregnancy?*

Human pregnancy is normally characterized by systemic vasodilation and modest hypotension, but hypertensive disorders of pregnancy affect approximately 5% to 8% of all pregnancies. Hypertension is a major risk factor for maternal and perinatal morbidity and mortality (Roberts, 2000). Hypertensive disorders include hypertension, preeclampsia, eclampsia (Box 5-3), and preexisting (chronic) hypertension. Gestational hypertension is characterized by an abnormal rise in blood pressure that usually develops after the twentieth week of pregnancy. In the majority of affected gravida, hypertension is mild and the pregnancy is uncomplicated.

Preeclampsia

Preeclampsia, the most common hypertensive disorder of pregnancy, is characterized by a blood pressure of 140/90 mm Hg, **proteinuria,** edema, and one or more of the following: **hypovolemia, hypoalbuminemia,** and disturbances in liver function, kidney function, or blood coagulation (Magann and Martin, 1995). If the condition progresses to eclampsia, life-threatening convulsions and coma can occur.

Preeclampsia is associated with increased risk of abruptio placenta, maternal renal failure, and cerebral hemorrhage (Sibai et al., 1998). It is the major cause of maternal, fetal, and perinatal morbidity and mortality (Naeye, 1979; National Center for Health Statistics, 1994).

The symptoms are newly developed hypertension with proteinuria or edema, or both, usually during the third trimester. The syndrome involves reduced placental perfusion often secondary to abnormal implantation and maternal endothelial dysfunction. Evidence indicates that the endothelial dysfunction is caused by oxidative stress secondary to the poor placental perfusion (Roberts, 2000). It can end in eclampsia with severe and potentially fatal seizures. Although the cause of preeclampsia is not yet understood, several risk factors are nutrition related: maternal obesity, diabetes, chronic

Box 5-3 Hypertensive Disorders of Pregnancy

PREGNANCY INDUCED HYPERTENSION
(blood pressure ≥140/90 mm Hg)

GESTATIONAL HYPERTENSION
Blood pressure elevation detected for the first time after midpregnancy

PREECLAMPSIA
Pregnancy specific syndrome observed after 20th week
(blood pressure ≥140/90 mm Hg)
Significant proteinuria
May have: headache, abdominal pain

ECLAMPSIA
Preeclampsia plus seizures
Convulsions usually occur after midpregnancy

CHRONIC HYPERTENSION
(blood pressure ≥140/90 mm Hg)
Blood pressure elevation predated pregnancy
Increased risk for superimposed preeclampsia (25% risk)
Preterm delivery, fetal growth restriction or demise
Abruptio placentae

Adapted from Report of the Working Group on Research on Hypertension During Pregnancy. Am J Obstet Gynecol 2000 183:S1-SA22.

hypertension, hyperhomocysteinemia, and possibly antioxidant status.

Although the cause of preeclampsia is unknown, it often occurs in primigravida, particularly African-American, low-income women who lack prenatal care and are younger than 20 years of age or older than 35 years of age, or in women with chronic hypertension or kidney disease (Umans and Lindheimer, 2001).

Management of preeclampsia. The only cure for preeclampsia is the termination of pregnancy. If the diagnosis of preeclampsia is suspected, bed rest or hospitalization allows monitoring of mother and fetus and may reduce the likelihood of convulsions. Treatment of mild preeclampsia is aimed at relief of symptoms and prescription of drugs to regulate blood pressure and prevent convulsions. Delivery may be indicated, regardless of gestational age, if severe hypertension persists after 24 hours to 48 hours of treatment or if there is evidence of progressive kidney or liver dysfunction or signs of eclampsia.

Role of diet in preeclampsia. The diet for any pregnant woman must supply sufficient energy to achieve recommended weight gain and adequate amounts of protein, vitamins, and minerals. In preeclampsia, adequate dietary protein is essential because of protein loss in the urine and reduced levels of serum proteins. Restoration of serum protein levels is important in correction of hypovolemia.

Over time various dietary components have been discussed in relation to the development, prevention, or treatment of preeclampsia. For over two decades sodium or salt restriction was recommended for prevention and treatment, undoubtedly because of the rapid fluid retention. It is now apparent that the sodium retention of preeclampsia is not related to dietary intake and it is undesirable to restrict sodium.

In the last decade epidemiologic data have suggested an inverse correlation between dietary calcium and the incidence of hypertension in diverse populations (Viller and Belizan, 2000) and have shown that women with preeclampsia excreted lower amounts of urinary calcium (Seely et al., 1992). Studies of calcium supplementation have reported lowered blood pressure in pregnant and nonpregnant women (Knight and Keith, 1992), particularly in women who had low calcium losses. A review of 14 randomized controlled trials involving more than 2500 women who received calcium supplements in the range of 375 mg to 2000 mg reported significant reductions in

KEY TERMS

proteinuria: the presence of more than 5 g of protein in the urine in 24 hours
hypovolemia: low blood volume
hypoalbuminemia: low blood levels of the protein albumin

systolic and diastolic blood pressure and a reduction in development of gestational hypertension and preeclampsia (Bucher et al., 1996). A later metaanalysis of many of the same trials revealed that the risk of preeclampsia was more reduced in populations with low-calcium diets (Allen, 2001), making it possible that women and teenagers consuming very low amounts of dietary calcium may benefit from calcium supplementation during pregnancy. This beneficial effect remains to be proven. On the other hand the multicenter Calcium for Preeclampsia Prevention Trial, which included 4589 pregnant women, found no significant effect of a 2000 mg/day supplement on blood pressure or pregnancy-induced hypertension (Levine, 1997). It therefore appears to be too early to formulate recommendations for calcium supplementation to prevent hypertension in pregnancy. Look for more new research on this topic.

Diabetes Mellitus

- *Why does diabetes mellitus increase the risk of an adverse pregnancy outcome?*
- *How do pregestational diabetes and gestational diabetes (GD) differ?*
- *What are the principles of nutrition care for women with diabetes during pregnancy?*

Diabetes mellitus is a chronic disorder of carbohydrate and lipid metabolism in which blood levels of glucose and lipids are elevated. This abnormal metabolism results from a relative lack of insulin—either too little insulin is secreted or the insulin that is secreted is not effective. In addition diabetes is associated with chronic systemic complications, which, over time, can affect the retina, kidneys, nerves, and cardiovascular system. The most common classifications of diabetes mellitus are type 1, or insulin-dependent, diabetes mellitus (IDDM); type 2, non–insulin-dependent diabetes mellitus (NIDDM); and GD, an intolerance to carbohydrates of varying severity that is first recognized in pregnancy (Coustan, 1996). Treatment of diabetes requires a balance between the woman's dietary intake and the insulin produced by her pancreas or exogenous insulin, which must be administered to control blood glucose levels.

Metabolic Changes of Pregnancy

Maternal blood glucose concentration during pregnancy decreases about 20% compared with the nonpregnant state. Glucose is transported across the placenta to the fetus by **facilitated diffusion.** To spare glucose for fetal consumption, maternal metabolism increasingly uses alternative fuels. Several of the hormones that are synthesized by the placenta, such as human placental lactogen, estrogen, and progesterone, have antiinsulin activity and therefore can increase blood glucose levels. In addition placental enzymes promote breakdown of insulin. Under normal circumstances the pancreas adapts to these changes by increasing insulin secretion. If the pancreas does not respond to the metabolic alterations with increased insulin release, GD results (Tolstoi and Smith, 1999).

Pregestational Diabetes

Pregestational diabetes, usually type 1, is present before pregnancy and occurs in 0.2% to 0.8% of all pregnancies. A woman with type 1 diabetes requires exogenous insulin to control blood glucose levels and the metabolic changes of gestation may increase insulin requirements. If insulin is inadequate, **hyperglycemia** and ketosis result. If a mother is hyperglycemic, greater amounts of glucose pass to the fetus, causing hyperglycemia, which stimulates fetal insulin secretion. The excess insulin increases protein synthesis and lipogenesis, promoting macrosomia, and may impair development of the lungs and cardiovascular and nervous systems (Jovanovic-Peterson and Peterson, 1996).

Adverse outcomes of pregnancy in mothers with diabetes are related to elevated blood glucose levels. Normalizing maternal glucose levels through diet, multiple insulin injections, or both has produced significant improvement in infant mortality rates and other adverse outcomes (Coustan, 1992).

Preconception counseling is important to assist the mother with insulin-dependent diabetes in avoiding wide fluctuations in blood glucose levels before pregnancy and maintaining steady levels throughout gestation. Therefore the goals of dietary management for a woman with type 1 diabetes are to maintain **normoglycemia** and to promote weight gain appropriate for pregravid BMI (see Table 4-1). The diet should consist of frequent small feedings designed to avoid **postprandial** hyperglycemia and preprandial fasting ketosis.

Three to five injections of insulin per day to coincide with food intake may be needed to maintain normoglycemia. The total amount of insulin administered daily is based on the week of gestation and the woman's pregnant body weight.

Gestational Diabetes

Occurring in 3% to 5% of all pregnancies, GD usually has an onset late in the second trimester (American Diabetes Association, 1996). Carbohydrate tolerance is normal before gestation and usually returns to normal after delivery. Regardless of the form, diabetes that is untreated or poorly regulated during pregnancy increases the risk of maternal and fetal mortality and morbidity (Rudge et al., 2000). The effects of GD on pregnancy outcome are usually limited to those associated with hyperglycemia in the latter half of pregnancy. Gestational diabetes is characterized by higher fasting and postprandial plasma concentrations of glucose, amino acids (especially branched chain), and lipids (fatty acids and especially triacylglycerol). It may be an extreme manifestation of the normal insulin resistance of pregnancy, or it may reflect a predisposition to type 2 diabetes (Butte, 2000). The Diabetes in Early Pregnancy Trial found that postprandial, but not fasting, concentrations of plasma glucose predicted birth weight (Jovanovic-Peterson and Peterson, 1996). To improve insulin sensitivity and reduce infant macrosomia, the American College of Obstetricians and Gynecologists (1995) recommends lower energy intakes for overweight and obese pregnant women with GD, self-monitoring of glucose and urinary ketones, and exercise. Insulin therapy is needed if fasting blood glucose is greater than 90 mg/dL or if 1-hour postprandial glucose is greater than 130 mg/dL. Restricting energy intake of obese women with GD to between 1200 kcal/day and 1800 kcal/day reduced the prevalence of macrosomia to 6% compared with 23% in women with unrestricted intakes (Dornhorst et al., 1991). However, excessive restriction will lead to ketonemia, which should be avoided because it is potentially harmful to an infant's mental development (Rizzo et al., 1991).

Women with GD have a higher incidence of preeclampsia and operative delivery (Scholl et al., 2001) and an increased risk of developing overt diabetes later in life. Infants of mothers whose pregnancies are complicated by GD have a greater number of neonatal problems, including fetal macrosomia and associated birth injury and other neonatal morbidity, including **hypoglycemia, hyperbilirubinemia,** hypocalcemia, **polycythemia,** and major congenital **anomalies** (Hod et al., 1991). There are also links between maternal GD and macrosomia in the neonate and obesity and glucose intolerance in the offspring's childhood and later life (Coustan, 1992).

Screening and Diagnosis. Pregnant women should be screened for GD between the twenty-fourth and twenty-eighth week of gestation if one or more of the criteria outlined in Box 5-4 are met. If a mother shows any signs or symptoms of diabetes at any stage of pregnancy, testing for glucose intolerance should be performed. Rescreening at 32 weeks' gestation is recommended

KEY TERMS

facilitated diffusion: a carrier-mediated movement of gas, liquids, or solids across a membrane from a region of high concentration to one of lower concentration
hyperglycemia: elevated blood glucose levels
normoglycemia: blood glucose levels that remain within limits of persons with normal insulin response
postprandial: after eating
hypoglycemia: low blood glucose level
hyperbilirubinemia: *hyper,* increased; *bilirubin,* bile pigment from the breakdown of hemoglobin and other heme pigments; *emia,* in the blood
polycythemia: increase in the mass of red blood cells
anomalies: marked deviation from normal, especially congenital defects

Box 5-4 Criteria for Screening for Diabetes in Pregnant Women

- 25 years of age or older
- Younger than 25 years of age and obese
- Family history of diabetes in first-degree relatives
- From an ethnic or racial background at higher risk for diabetes:
  - Hispanic American
  - Native American
  - African American

If blood glucose in response to 50 g load is greater than 140 mg/dL, then a 100 g glucose, 3-hour oral glucose tolerance test is used to confirm diagnosis.

for women at increased risk for development of diabetes. The screening consists of administering a 50 g oral glucose load. If the plasma glucose level is 140 mg/dL or greater after 1 hour, then a 100 g, 3-hour oral glucose tolerance test (GTT) is performed in the fasting state to confirm the diagnosis of diabetes.

Treatment and monitoring. Women with GD who are able to maintain normal blood glucose levels (fasting levels less than 105 mg/dL; postprandial levels less than 120 mg/dL) during the remainder of their pregnancy have mortality and complication rates approaching those of nondiabetic women (Coustan, 1992; Fagan et al., 1995).

Minimizing fluctuations in blood glucose concentration and ensuring adequate weight gain are imperative to ensure favorable perinatal outcomes. Accomplishing these goals present a challenge because energy and nutrient requirements change across pregnancy. The Fourth International Workshop and Conference on GDM recommended that nutritional prescriptions be customized to account for a woman's body habitus, weight gain, and physical activity and suggested that prescriptions be modified as necessary to achieve the goals of nutritional therapy (Metzger and Coustan, 1998) (Box 5-5). Nutrition intervention is the cornerstone of therapy. If dietary management and exercise do not maintain recommended glucose levels, insulin may be administered. The pattern of multiple insulin injections recommended for women with type 1 diabetes is appropriate for a woman with GD. Self-monitoring of postprandial blood glucose allows the adjustment of insulin therapy, improving blood glucose values and glycemic control.

Box 5-5 Management of Gestational Diabetes Mellitus

Nutrition counseling goals

- Provide necessary nutrients and energy for fetal development and maintenance of maternal health.
- Maintain normal blood glucose levels (euglycemia).
- Prevent ketosis.
- Plan meals for distribution of glucose (food) intake.
- Achieve appropriate weight gain.
- Balance intake with exercise.
- If insulin is necessary, balance with dietary intake.
- Self-monitor blood glucose.

SUBSTANCE USE AND ABUSE DURING PREGNANCY

- *Does caffeine consumption constitute a risk for pregnancy outcome? Why or why not?*
- *What are the fetal effects of maternal cigarette smoking?*
- *Does nutrition or maternal nutrition status influence the effects of smoking?*
- *How does the amount and timing of alcohol use or abuse influence pregnancy outcome?*

Maternal Smoking

Approximately 30% of women of childbearing age are smokers. Although some pregnant women cease smoking and others decrease the number of cigarettes smoked each day, many women continue to smoke throughout pregnancy. It is difficult to define the effects of cigarette smoking during pregnancy because of the concurrence of other complicating risk factors including age, education, marital status, and use of alcohol and other drugs.

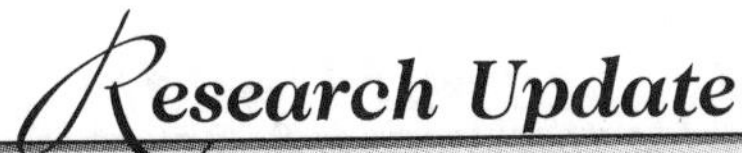

Research Update

Caffeine

Caffeine, one of a group of compounds called methylxanthines, is found in coffee, tea, cola and cocoa beverages, and chocolate-containing foods. Tea and cocoa also contain large proportions of the methylxanthines theophylline and theobromine, respectively. Caffeine is listed in the Code of Federal Regulations as a multipurpose food substance that is "GRAS": generally recognized as safe. It is a common additive in many nonprescription preparations such as cold tablets, allergy and analgesic preparations, appetite suppressants, and stimulants. Box 5-6 lists the caffeine content of common beverages, foods, and over-the-counter medicine preparations.

Box 5-6 Caffeine Content of Selected Foods and Drugs

COFFEE

Brewed (cup): 85 mg
Percolated (cup): 110 mg
Instant (cup): 66 mg
Instant, decaffeinated (cup): 3 mg

TEA

Brewed (cup): 46 mg
Instant (teaspoon): 32 mg

CARBONATED BEVERAGES

Cola (12 oz): 40-65 mg

CHOCOLATE

Cocoa, dry (1 tbsp): 10 mg
Hot chocolate (cup): 13 mg
Milk chocolate (1 oz): 6 mg
Semi-sweet chocolate (1 oz): 17 mg
Dark chocolate (1 oz): 20 mg
Chocolate powder for milk (1 tbsp): 10 mg
Chocolate ice cream (cup): 8 mg

NONPRESCRIPTION DRUGS

Anacin analgesic (tablet): 32 mg
Dristan (tablet): 16 mg
Excedrin (tablet): 65 mg
Triaminic (tablet): 30 mg

EFFECTS OF CAFFEINE

Caffeine can stimulate catecholamine release, which, in turn, stimulates the central nervous system; increases gastric acid secretion, heart rate, and basal metabolic rate; alters blood pressure; increases **diuresis;** and relaxes smooth muscle. Consumption of 500 mg to 750 mg of caffeine per day can result in restlessness, anxiety, irritability, agitation, muscle tremor, sensory disturbances (e.g., tinnitus), heart palpitations, nausea, or vomiting and diarrhea in some individuals.

For more than 30 years scientists have investigated the potential effect of caffeine on pregnancy course and outcome. The fact that the structure of caffeine resembles that of bases (such as adenosine) in nucleic acids has led to speculation that excess caffeine could have teratogenic effects. This potential effect is a concern because caffeine readily crosses biologic membranes, including the placenta, but is not effectively metabolized by the fetus.

FERTILITY AND MISCARRIAGE

Several researchers have explored the relationship between caffeine and infertility or delayed conception. One study reported that women whose daily caffeine consumption exceeded the amount in one cup of coffee (or three cans of cola) were less likely to conceive than were women who drank less caffeine. However, that study failed to control for age, frequency of intercourse, or life-style factors such as exercise, dietary habits, and stress. More recent studies have failed to establish a relationship between caffeine consumption and conception delay or infertility (Narod et al., 1991). Increased risk of first- and second-trimester spontaneous abortion in women consuming more than 150 mg of caffeine per day has been reported (Srisuphan and Bracken, 1986), but no increased risk was found by succeeding studies (Narod et al., 1991).

TERATOGENIC EFFECTS

In 1980 the Food and Drug Administration issued a statement that warned pregnant women to avoid caffeine-containing foods and drugs or to consume them only sparingly (Food and Drug

Continued

Research Update

Caffeine—cont'd

Administration, 1980). This warning was based on observations of teratogenic effects in offspring born to rats fed high doses of caffeine. Subsequent research confirmed a caffeine-birth defect connection, but only when pregnant rats ingested enormous amounts of caffeine—equivalent to the amount in at least 18 cups of coffee a day. Ever since a great deal of controversy and research on caffeine consumption during gestation has been generated. To date there is no convincing evidence that caffeine is associated with birth defects in humans (Nehlig and Debry, 1994). However, recent evidence has accumulated to suggest that elevated plasma homocysteine levels are related to adverse pregnancy outcome (see Research Update, Chapter 4, page 124). In 1997 a group of researchers who studied homocysteine and risk of cardiovascular disease in 15,000 men and women reported a positive association between coffee consumption and plasma homocysteine levels (Nygard et al., 1997). This is an intriguing but as-yet-unsupported extension of a potential role of caffeine in birth defects.

INFANT BIRTH WEIGHT

Caffeine and coffee consumption during pregnancy has been associated with a marginally increased risk of low infant birth weight (Caan and Goldhaber, 1989; Fenster et al., 1991). However, it is unclear if caffeine, coffee, or other characteristics of coffee drinkers (such as smoking, alcohol intake, poor dietary intake, or low weight gain) may be responsible for this effect (Godel et al., 1992).

MATERNAL EFFECTS

Although coffee is the major source of caffeine in the American diet, consumption of large quantities of other substances, particularly cola beverages, can substantially increase caffeine intake. Caffeine may influence the nutrition status of the mother by increasing the urinary excretion of calcium and thiamin and decreasing zinc and iron absorption (Institute of Medicine, 1990). In addition very large amounts of caffeine may produce **tachycardia** or increased blood pressure, interfere with normal sleep patterns, and cause gastric reflux associated with the heartburn common in late pregnancy.

The Food and Drug Administration (1980) recommends that pregnant women avoid or limit coffee intake during pregnancy. It also suggests that caffeine consumption should be limited to less than 300 mg/day. Reducing or eliminating dietary caffeine cannot harm the mother or her infant.

KEY TERMS

diuresis: increased excretion of urine
tachycardia: abnormally rapid heart rate

Pregnancy Outcome

Smoking during pregnancy has been linked to increased incidence of spontaneous abortion, particularly those that occur in the second trimester (Kolas et al., 2000). Over the last few decades studies have documented a **dose-related** fetal growth restriction in offspring of mothers who smoke (Figure 5-3). On average the birth weights of infants born to smoking mothers are approximately 150 g to 250 g lower than those of infants whose mothers did not smoke (Haug et al., 2000; Mitchell and Lerner, 1987).

Smoking during pregnancy is also associated with a dose-related increase in the incidence of preterm delivery (Kolas et al., 2000) and perinatal mortality (McDonald et al., 1992), probably from the greater occurrence of placenta previa, abruptio placenta, and premature rupture of the membranes in mothers who smoke. Maternal smoking is a major independent risk factor for sudden infant death syndrome (SIDS) (Poole et al., 2000). In addition children of mothers who smoke during pregnancy may have slight, but measurable, deficits in long-term physical growth

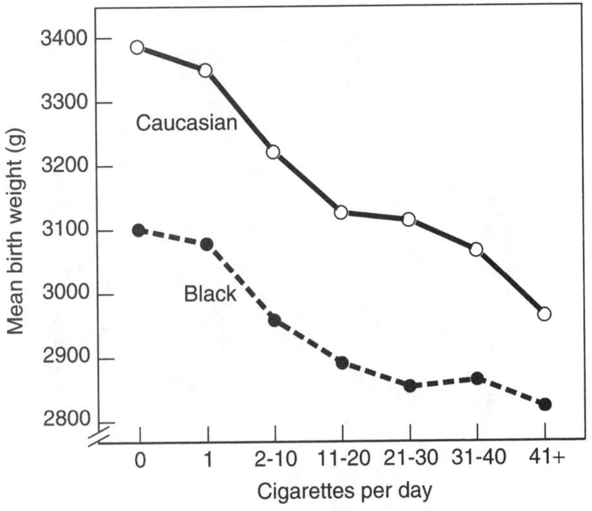

Figure 5-3 Dose effect of maternal cigarette use on infant birth weight. *(From Niswander KR and Gordon M: The collaborative perinatal study of the National Institute of Neurological Diseases and Stroke: the women and their pregnancies, Philadelphia, 1972, WB Saunders.)*

(Institute of Medicine, 1990), intellectual performance (Olds et al., 1994), and behavioral adjustment (Kallen, 2000; Weitzman et al., 1992).

The mechanisms by which cigarette smoking causes fetal growth restriction have not been established, but it is generally assumed to be from fetal **hypoxia** caused by increased carboxyhemoglobin levels. When carbon monoxide binds to the hemoglobin molecule, it is not readily displaced from that molecule, thereby decreasing available sites for oxygen binding. This finding is supported by observations that fetal body movements and fetal heart rate decrease 20 minutes after the mother has smoked a cigarette (Garcia et al., 1991).

Smoking is the single most important environmental influence on fetal growth and also the most readily modified. Mothers who smoke during one pregnancy, but do not during a succeeding gestation give birth to an infant with a higher birth weight the second time. Women who stopped smoking during the first trimester had little or no greater risk of having a low-birth-weight infant than did nonsmokers (McDonald et al., 1992). A recent study of 946 women who stopped smoking before week 32 of gestation found that they gave birth to infants whose measurements of head circumference and birth weight were indistinguishable from those of 9802 infants of nonsmokers. But the infants of women who ceased smoking still had a deficit in crown-heel length compared with the babies born to nonsmokers (Lindley et al., 2000). Although this study supports the value of smoking cessation even well into pregnancy, the best option is for mothers to abstain from smoking at the onset of pregnancy. However, smoking cessation programs for pregnant women have had inconsistent compliance (Kindrick et al., 1995; Rush et al., 1992).

Role of Nutrition

It has been suggested that the effect of smoking on infant birth weight is related to maternal nutrition status. Infants of obese mothers who smoke have birth weights similar to those of infants of normal-weight mothers who do not smoke. In addition increased maternal weight gain during pregnancy appears to counteract the growth-retarding effects of smoking (Rush et al., 1992).

Reports of dietary intakes of pregnant smokers have produced conflicting results. Haste and others (1991) reported that energy intakes were not significantly lower in smoking compared with nonsmoking gravida, but intakes of protein, vitamins, and minerals were lower. Smoking lowers serum vitamin C levels and additional vitamin C intakes are recommended for all smokers (Institute of Medicine, 2000). Exposure to tobacco smoke may increase the requirements for iron, zinc, and folate and decrease the availability of some nutrients. Multivitamin and mineral supplements are recommended for heavy cigarette smokers (Institute of Medicine, 1990).

KEY TERMS

dose-related: as the amount of use (e.g., number of cigarettes smoked) increases, the effect increases proportionately (e.g., decreased birth weight)

hypoxia: reduction of oxygen supply to tissues below physiologic levels

Box 5-7 Features of the Fetal Alcohol Syndrome and Alcohol-Related Birth Defects

GROWTH RETARDATION

Prenatal—low birth weight, microcephaly
Postnatal

NEUROLOGIC—DEVELOPMENTALLY DELAYED

Mental retardation
Learning disabilities—poor school performance
Behavioral disorders—hyperactivity, irritability, poor attention span
Speech difficulties—slow development
Sleep disorders—abnormal sleep/wake cycles
Hypotonia, poor sucking reflex
Tremor

CHARACTERISTIC FACIAL FEATURES

Eyes—short, palpebral fissures (eye openings)
Nose—short and upturned in early childhood
Midface—flattened, elongated
Mouth—thin vermilion of upper lip, cleft lip, small teeth
Ears—small, posterior rotation

CARDIAC DEFECTS

Atrial and ventricular septal defects

GENITAL ABNORMALITIES

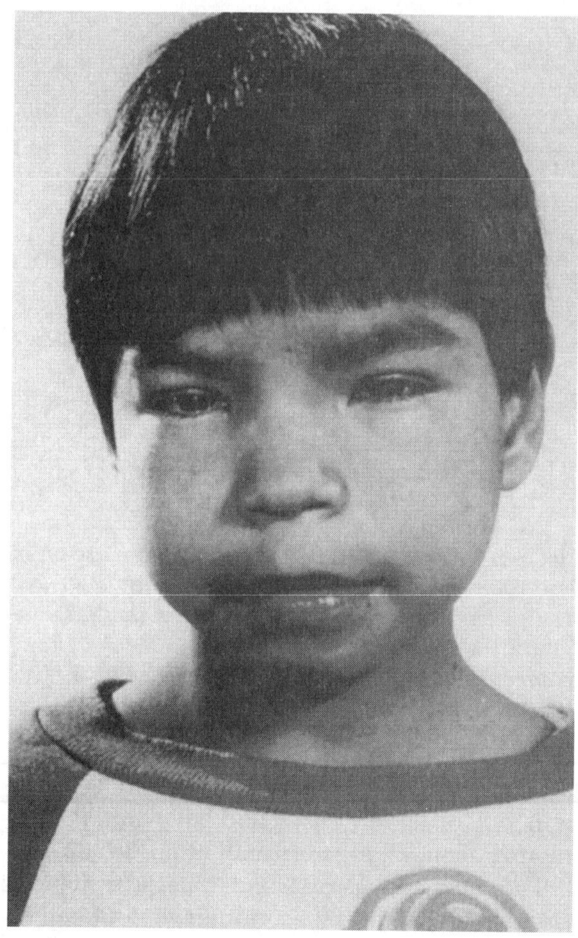

Figure 5-4 This 9-year-old boy has typical facial features of fetal alcohol syndrome. Note the widely spaced eyes, fat midface, short palpebral fissures, and thin upper lip. He has attention deficit disorder with hyperactivity and is mildly mentally retarded. *(From Moore KL and Persaud TVN: The developing human, ed 5, Philadelphia, 1993, WB Saunders. Courtesy Dr. A.E. Chudley, Children's Centre, Winnipeg, Canada.)*

Alcohol Abuse

Heavy alcohol consumption during pregnancy has potent teratogenic effects including prenatal and postnatal growth retardation and morphologic abnormalities—especially facial anomalies—and central nervous system, cardiac, and genitourinary system impairment. Recently alcohol exposure *in utero* has been linked to a variety of other neurodevelopmental problems (American Academy of Pediatrics, Committee on Substance Abuse and Committee on Children with Disabilities, 2000).

Fetal Alcohol Syndrome

The most severe form of effects of maternal alcohol abuse, fetal alcohol syndrome (FAS), is a cluster of these features observed in some offspring of women who abuse alcohol during pregnancy (Box 5-7). Figure 5-4 shows the typical facial appearance of FAS victims. FAS is estimated to affect 1 to 2 infants per 1000 live births and may account for as many as 20% of persons with mental retardation in developed countries.

First described in 1973, many cases of FAS have been documented in infants and young children. Follow-up of infants and children with FAS have described the long-term progression of the disorder into adulthood (Pykowicz et al., 1991; Spohr et al., 1993). Although characteris-

Maryann is 13 years old, but when her parents go out she needs a babysitter. She does not get phone calls from friends inviting her to go to the mall or to parties or just hang out. She loves to buy new clothes like other 13-year-olds, but she knows she does not look like other girls and sometimes that really upsets her. When she gets frustrated, she yells at her parents because she feels she is different and it's not fair.

Maryann's eyes are small and her ears are malformed. She has difficulty learning simple tasks, is poorly coordinated, and has a short attention span. Often her behavior is impulsive. Her mother says she is hyperactive and easily angered. According to her mother, she doesn't understand consequences and can't learn from her mistakes. She can repeat rules, such as don't go into the street, but she cannot remember or understand them. Maryann's life is the way it is because her birth mother abused alcohol both before and throughout her pregnancy.

Maryann was adopted when she was 5 months old. Her parents suspected something was wrong with her from the beginning. As a young infant she was very irritable and couldn't be soothed. She had difficulty eating and seldom slept through the night. Her growth was slow—she was at the fifth percentile on the growth charts for weight, height, and head circumference. By the time she was 3 years old, Maryann's short attention span and impulsive behavior had become more of a problem. She would repeatedly touch a hot stove, play with matches, or run into the street.

The diagnosis of FAS was made shortly before her fifth birthday. In many cases FAS is not formally diagnosed until the child enters school, when attention and learning problems become more apparent. If physical abnormalities are pronounced or the maternal history of abuse is known, the diagnosis may be made much earlier. In Maryann's case the signs were more subtle.

Maryann attends a neighborhood school, but is in a class for youngsters with severe behavioral handicaps. She has problems with learning, attention, memory, and problem solving. Education involves a lot of structure, repetition, and consistency. She does make slow progress, but backsliding is common.

tic facial features of FAS become less distinctive with time, short stature and microcephaly persist. Mental retardation also persists, with no improvement in IQ with age. Maladaptive behaviors such as poor judgment, distractibility, and difficulty recognizing social cues are common and may present the greatest challenge to management of the adult with FAS.

Alcohol-Related Birth Defects

Alcohol-related birth defects (ARBD) is a syndrome that can result in a variety of central nervous system dysfunctions and developmental difficulties in the absence of the distinctive physical appearance of FAS. The signs of ARBD may be observed at birth or later in development and symptoms include microcephaly, malformations of the heart and lungs, central nervous system problems such as tremors and decreased sucking, and minor physical abnormalities.

Alcohol-Related Neurodevelopmental Disorders

Alcohol-related neurodevelopmental disorders is a term used to describe other neurodevelopment problems that can result in central nervous system dysfunctions and developmental difficulties in the absence of the distinctive physical appearance of FAS. As many as 36,000 infants may be born each year with these more subtle fetal-alcohol effects.

Some infants exposed to alcohol during pregnancy show no physical evidence of either FAS or ARBD at birth, but they may have a wide range of cognitive disturbances, which become apparent as these children approach school age. These disturbances include shorter attention span and lower IQ than average, both of which have the potential for causing lasting learning and emotional problems.

Amount and timing of alcohol exposure. The mechanisms by which alcohol adversely affects fetal growth and **morphogenesis** have not been established. Alcohol readily crosses the placenta, so that the embryo or fetus is exposed to the same blood alcohol levels as the mother. Because the fetal organs are immature, the fetus may not metabolize or detoxify the alcohol as rapidly, resulting in prolonged exposure to alcohol during critical growth periods. Overall the fetal effects of alcohol are related to the quantity of alcohol consumed by the mother and her blood ethanol level. Approximately four drinks (one drink equals approximately 12 oz of beer, 4 oz of wine, or one cocktail) per day dramatically increase the risk of physical manifestation of FAS. Light drinking (one to two drinks per day) has not been reported to increase harm to the fetus. However, Jacobson and others (1993) reported that 13-month-old infants whose mothers consumed an average of 7 drinks per week while pregnant had very poor cognitive performance scores twice as often as those whose mothers abstained. Because the occurrence of ARBD is related to maternal blood alcohol levels, a pattern of drinking several drinks on several separate occasions may constitute increased risk, depending on timing and the level of fetal exposure.

A critical time for development of malformations is embryosis, often before recognition of pregnancy, when women may not even be aware of the risk. Effects of alcohol excess later in gestation are less severe, but Rossett and others (1983) maintain that the outcome of pregnancy can be improved substantially if alcohol abusers reduce alcohol intake even after conception.

KEY TERMS

morphogenesis: evolution and development of form as an organ or part of the body

Recommendations

A "safe" level of alcohol consumption during pregnancy cannot be defined because no one knows how much alcohol causes damage. The Surgeon General and the Food and Drug Administration recommend that pregnant women refrain from drinking alcoholic beverages during pregnancy. Many states require that warning notices regarding the risk of alcohol consumption during pregnancy be posted in establishments where alcoholic beverages are served. Warning labels are also required on containers of beer, wine, and hard liquor.

Role of Nutrition

Alcohol is directly toxic to the developing embryo and fetus. The development of FAS and ARBD are completely preventable—if a pregnant woman does not drink. A mother who abuses alcohol may also be undernourished because alcohol (7 kcal/g) replaces food and its nutrients. In addition alcohol reduces absorption and utilization of some nutrients. Undernutrition, especially in regard to protein and zinc, may enhance the effects of excess alcohol (Institute of Medicine, 1990). Nutrient supplements do not counteract the adverse effects of alcohol, but they may be needed to compensate for a poor diet and the effects of alcohol on nutrition status.

SUMMARY

Gestation is a period of rapid growth and development and a time of myriad physiologic adaptations by the mother to support the formation of a new human being. However, the road to the birth of a healthy baby is not always smooth. The issues described in this chapter illustrate how fragile the reproductive process can be and highlight the importance of nutrition in the changes that occur. Physiologic changes, health problems, and personal choices can create a less-than-favorable environment for reproduction. It is essential that the healthcare system and health providers offer education, counseling, programs, and assistance to optimize the reproductive experience for the mother and her fetus. Obviously nutrition is an integral part of these interventions. Nutrition assessment and intervention should encompass the whole reproduction process from preconception care through prenatal and postpartum periods to identify and change or ameliorate the impact of social, economic, physical, and behavior factors.

Nutrition intervention through carefully planned nutrition care and monitoring can reduce the impact of these factors on pregnancy outcome. The high-risk pregnancies discussed in this chapter are those for which nutrition management is appropriate.

Concepts to Remember

- A number of maternal characteristics, health conditions, and lifestyle factors, which may operate synergistically, can increase the risk of an adverse pregnancy outcome for infant and mother.
- Nutrition assessment and intervention can reduce or modify nutrition risk during the reproductive interval.
- Identification of risk and initiation of care before conception or early in pregnancy increase the effectiveness of nutrition intervention.
- Extremes of maternal age (particularly under 15 years or over 35 years) increase the risk of an adverse pregnancy outcome.
- Many sociodemographic characteristics of the mother, including education, income, marital status, and access to healthcare, can affect reproductive risk.
- Maternal health conditions such as obesity, hyperphenylalaninemia, diabetes mellitus, and hypertension, which may contribute to an unfavorable pregnancy outcome, can be modified by nutrition care.
- Use or abuse of cigarettes and alcohol is associated with adverse fetal outcomes.

REFERENCES

Abrams B et al.: Pregnancy weight gain: still controversial, Am J Clin Nutr 71:1233, 2000.

Allen LH: Anemia and iron deficiency effects on pregnancy outcome, Am J Clin Nutr 71:1280, 2000.

Allen LH: Pregnancy and lactation. In Present knowledge in nutrition, Washington, DC, 2001, ILSI Press.

American Academy of Pediatrics, Committee on Substance Abuse and Committee on Children with Disabilities: Fetal alcohol syndrome and alcohol related neurodevelopmental disorders, Pediatrics 106:358, 2000.

American College of Obstetricians and Gynecologists: ACOG technical bulletin. Diabetes and pregnancy, Int J Gynecol Obstet 48:331, 1995.

American Diabetes Association: Gestational diabetes mellitus, position statement, Diabetes Care 16:5, 1996.

American Dietetic Association: Position of the American Dietetic Association: nutrition care for pregnant adolescents, J Am Diet Assoc 94:499, 1994.

Beard JL: Iron deficiency: assessment during pregnancy and its importance in pregnant adolescents, Am J Clin Nutr 59:502S, 1994.

Brown JE and Carlson M: Nutrition and multifetal pregnancy, J Am Diet Assoc 100:343, 2000.

Bucher HC et al.: Effect of calcium supplementation on pregnancy-induced hypertension and preeclampsia: a meta analysis of randomized controlled trials, JAMA 275:113, 1996.

Butte NF: Carbohydrate and lipid metabolism in pregnancy: normal compared with gestational diabetes mellitus, Am J Clin Nutr 71:1256S, 2000.

Caan BJ and Goldhaber MK: Caffeinated beverages and low birthweight: a case control study, Am J Public Health 79:1299, 1989.

Caritis S et al.: Predictors of pre-eclampsia in women at high risk. National Institute of Child Health and Human Development Network of Maternal-Fetal Units, Am J Obstet Gynecol 179:946, 1998.

Cnattingius S et al.: Prepregnancy weight and the risk of adverse pregnancy outcomes, N Engl J Med 338:147, 1998.

Coustan DR: Gestational diabetes, Diabetes Care 15:716, 1992.

Coustan DR: Screening and testing for gestational diabetes mellitus, Obstet Clin North Am 23:125, 1996.

deFreitas O et al.: New approaches to the treatment of phenylketonuria, Nutr Rev 57:65, 1999.

Dornhorst A et al.: Calorie restriction for treatment of gestational diabetes, Diabetes 40:161S, 1991.

Edwards L et al.: Pregnancy in the underweight woman: course, outcome and growth patterns of the infants, Am J Obstet Gynecol 135:297, 1979.

Fagan C et al.: Nutrition management in women with gestational diabetes mellitus: a review by the ADA's Diabetes Care and Education dietetic practice group, J Am Diet Assoc 95:40, 1995.

Fenster L et al.: Caffeine consumption during pregnancy and fetal growth, Am J Public Health 81:458, 1991.

Food and Drug Administration: Caffeine and pregnancy, FDA Drug Bull 10:19, 1980.

Fraser AM et al.: Association of young maternal age with adverse reproduction outcomes, N Engl J Med 332: 1113, 1995.

Frisancho AR: Developmental and nutritional determinants of pregnancy outcome among teenagers, Am J Phys Anthropol 66:247, 1985.

Garcia LM et al.: Acute effects of maternal cigarette smoking on fetal heart rate and fetal body movements felt by the mother, J Perinat Med 19:385, 1991.

Giddens JB et al.: Pregnant adolescents and adult women have similarly low intakes of selected nutrients, J Am Diet Assoc 100:1334, 2000.

Godel JC et al.: Smoking and caffeine and alcohol intake during pregnancy in a northern population: effect on fetal growth, Can Med Assoc J 147:181, 1992.

Haste FM et al.: The effect of nutritional intake on outcome of pregnancy in smokers and nonsmokers, Br J Nutr 65:347, 1991.

Haug K et al.: Maternal smoking and birthweight: effect modification of period, maternal age and parenteral smoking, Acta Obstet Gynecol 79:485, 2000.

Hediger ML et al.: Rate and amount of weight gain during adolescent pregnancy: associations with maternal weight-for-height and birth weight, Am J Clin Nutr 52:793, 1990.

Hellerstedt WL: Economic, psychosocial and health risk associated with adolescent childbearing. In Story M and Stang J, editors: Nutrition and the pregnant adolescent: a practical reference guide, Minneapolis, 2000, Center for Leadership, Education, and Training in Maternal and Child Nutrition, University of Minnesota.

Hickey CA: Sociocultural and behavioral influences on weight gain during pregnancy, Am J Clin Nutr 71:1364S, 2000.

Hickey CA et al.: Low pregravid body mass index as a risk factor for preterm birth: variation by ethnic group, Obstet Gynecol 89:206, 1997.

Hod M et al.: Gestational diabetes mellitus: a survey of perenatal complications in the 1980s, Diabetes 40:74, 1991.

Institute of Medicine: Nutrition during pregnancy: weight gain and nutrient supplements, Report of the Subcommittee on Nutritional Status and Weight Gain During Pregnancy, Committee on Nutritional Status During Pregnancy and Lactation, Food and Nutrition Board, Washington, DC, 1990, National Academy Press.

Institute of Medicine: Dietary reference intakes for calcium, phosphorus, magnesium, vitamin D and fluoride, Washington, DC, 1997, Institute of Medicine.

Institute of Medicine: Dietary reference intakes for thiamin, riboflavin, niacin, vitamin B_6, folate, vitamin B_{12}, pantothenic acid, biotin, and choline, Washington, DC, 1998, National Academy Press.

Institute of Medicine: Dietary reference intakes for vitamin C, vitamin E, selenium and carotenoids, Washington, DC, 2000, National Academy Press.

Institute of Medicine: Dietary reference intakes for vitamin A, vitamin K, arsenic, boron, chromium, copper, iodine, manganese, molybdenum, nickel, silicon, vanadium and zinc, Washington, DC, 2001, National Academy Press.

Jacobson J et al.: Teratogenic effects of alcohol on infant development, Alcohol Clin Exp Res 17:174, 1993.

Jonas O et al.: The association of maternal and socioeconomic characteristics in metropolitan Adelaide with medical, obstetric and labor complications and pregnancy outcomes, Aust N Z J Obstet Gynaecol 32:1, 1992.

Jovanovic-Peterson L and Peterson CM: Vitamin and mineral deficiencies which may predispose to glucose intolerance in pregnancy, J Am Coll Nutr 15:14, 1996.

Kallen K: Maternal smoking during pregnancy and infant head circumference at birth, Early Hum Dev 58:197, 2000.

Kindrick JS et al.: Integrating smoking cessation into routine public prenatal care: the smoking cessation in pregnancy project, Am J Publ Health 85:217, 1995.

Knight KB and Keith RE: Calcium supplementation of normotensine and hypertensine pregnant women, Am J Clin Nutr 55:891, 1992.

Koch R et al.: The North American Collaborative Study of Maternal Phenylketonuria, Status Report 1999, Ment Retard Dev Dis Rev 5:117, 1999.

Kogan MD et al.: Trends in twin birth outcomes and prenatal care utilization in the United States, 1981-1997, JAMA 284:335, 2000.

Kolas T et al.: Smoking during pregnancy increases the risk of preterm births among parous women, Acta Obstet Gynecol Scand 79:644, 2000.

Kramer MS: The contributions of mild and moderate preterm birth to infant mortality, JAMA 284:843, 2000.

Levine RJ et al.: Trial of calcium to prevent preeclampsia, N Engl J Med 337:69, 1997.

Levy HL et al.: Maternal phenylketonuria: a metabolic teratogen, Teratology 53:176, 1996.

Lindley AA et al.: Effect of continuing and stopping smoking during pregnancy on infant birth weight, crown heel length, head circumference, ponderal index, and brain-body weight ratio, Am J Epidemiol 152:219, 2000.

Ling AMR and McCluskey S: Eating disorders associated with hyperemesis gravidarum, J Psychosomatic Res 40:231, 1996.

Luke B and Keith LG: The contribution of singletons, twins and triplets to low birth weight, J Reprod Med 37:661, 1992.

Luke B et al.: The ideal twin pregnancy: patterns of weight gain and discordancy and length of gestation, Am J Obstet Gynecol 169:588, 1993.

McDonald AD et al.: Cigarette, alcohol and coffee consumption and prematurity, Am J Public Health 82:87, 1992.

Magann EF and Martin JN: The laboratory evaluation of hypertensive gravida, Obstet Gynecol Surv 50:138, 1995.

Mathews TJ et al.: Infant mortality statistics from the 1998 period-linked birth/infant death data set, Natl Vital Stat Rep 48:1, 2000.

Melnikow J et al.: Characteristics of inner-city women giving birth with little or no prenatal care: a case control study, J Fam Pract 32:283, 1991.

Metzger BE and Coustan DR: Summary and recommendations of the fourth international workshop and conference on gestational diabetes mellitus, Diabetes Care 21(suppl 2):B161, 1998.

Michlin R et al.: Maternal obesity and pregnancy outcome, Isr Med Assoc J 2:10, 2000.

Mitchell MC and Lerner E: Factors that influence the outcome of pregnancy in middle-class women, J Am Diet Assoc 87:731, 1987.

Mitchell MC and Lerner E: Weight gain and pregnancy outcome in underweight and normal weight women, J Am Diet Assoc 89:634, 1989.

Morbidity and Mortality Weekly Report: National and state specific pregnancy rates among adolescents—United States, 1995–97, Mor Mortal Wkly Rep 49:605, 2001.

Naeye RL: Perinatal mortality rates of overweight, normal weight and underweight mothers as related to weight gain, Am J Obstet Gynecol 135:3, 1979.

Naeye RL: Teenaged and pre-teenaged pregnancies: consequences of the fetal–maternal competition for nutrients, Pediatrics 67:146, 1981.

Naeye RL and Friedman EA: Causes of perinatal death associated with gestational hypertension and proteinuria, Am J Obstet Gynecol 133:8, 1979.

Narod SA et al.: Coffee during pregnancy: a reproductive hazard? Am J Obstet Gynecol 19:157, 1999.

National Center for Health Statistics: Advance report of maternal and infant health data from the birth certificate, Monthly Vital Stat Rep 42(no. 11S):1, 1994.

National Center for Health Statistics: Infant mortality statistics shown variation by race, ethnicity and state, Natl Vital Stat Rep 49:28, 2000.

National Research Council: Recommended dietary allowances, ed 10, report of the Subcommittee on the Tenth Edition of the RDAs, Food and Nutrition Board, Commission on Life Sciences, Washington, DC, 1989, National Academy Press.

Nehlig A and Debry G: Potential teratogenic and neurodevelopmental consequences of coffee and caffeine exposure: a review of human and animal data, Neurotoxicol Teratol 16:531, 1994.

Nygard O et al.: Coffee consumption and plasma homocysteine: the Hordland Homocysteine Study, Am J Clin Nutr 65:136, 1997.

Olds DL et al.: Intellectual impairment in children of women who smoke cigarettes during pregnancy, Pediatrics 93:221, 1994.

Pederson A et al.: Weight gain patterns during twin gestations, J Am Diet Assoc 89, 1989.

Platt LD et al.: Maternal phenylketonuria collaborative study: obstetric aspects and outcome: the first six years, Am J Obstet Gynecol 166:1150, 1992.

Poole KA et al.: Effect of maternal smoking on ventilatory responses to changes in inspired oxygen levels in infants, Am J Respir Crit Care Med 162:801, 2000.

Prysak M et al.: Pregnancy outcome in nulliparous women 35 years and older, Obstet Gynecol 85:65, 1995.

Pykowicz A et al.: Fetal alcohol syndrome in adolescents and adults, JAMA 265:1961, 1991.

Rizzo T et al.: Correlations between antepartum maternal metabolism and child intelligence, N Engl J Med 325:911, 1991.

Roberts JM: Preeclampsia: what we know and what we do not know, Semin Perinatol 24:24, 2000.

Roche AR and Davilla GH: Late adolescent growth in stature, Pediatrics 50:874, 1972.

Rossett HL et al.: Treatment experience with pregnant problem drinkers, JAMA 249:2029, 1983.

Rudge MV et al.: Perinatal outcome of pregnancies complicated by diabetes and by maternal daily hyperglycemia not related to diabetes: a retrospective 10-year analysis, Gynecol Obstet Invest 50:108, 2000.

Rush D et al.: A trial of health education aimed to reduce cigarette smoking among pregnant women, Ped Perenat Epidemiol 6:285, 1992.

Scholl TO and Hediger ML: A review of the epidemiology of nutrition and adolescent pregnancy: maternal growth during pregnancy and its effect on the fetus, J Am Coll Nutr 12:101, 1993.

Scholl TO et al.: Maternal growth during pregnancy and the competition for nutrients, Am J Clin Nutr 60:183, 1994.

Scholl TO et al.: Maternal growth and fetal growth: pregnancy course and outcome in the Camden Study, Ann N Y Acad Sci 817:292–301, 1997.

Scholl TO et al.: Leptin and maternal growth during adolescent pregnancy, Am J Clin Nutr 72:1542, 2001.

Scholl TO et al.: Maternal glucose concentration influences fetal growth, gestation, and pregnancy complications, Am J Epidemiol 154:514, 2001.

Seely EW et al.: Lower serum calcium and abnormal calciotropic hormone levels in preeclampsia, J Clin Endocrinol Metab 74:1436, 1992.

Signorello LB et al.: Saturated fat intake and risk of severe hyperemesis gravidarum, Epidemiol 9:636, 1998.

Sipiora ML et al.: Bitter taste perception and severe vomiting in pregnancy, Physiol Behav 69:259, 2000.

Snell LH et al.: Metabolic crisis: hyperemesis gravidarum, J Perinat Neonat Nutr 12:26, 1998.

Spohr HL et al.: Prenatal alcohol exposure and long-term developmental consequences, Lancet 341:907, 1993.

Srisuphan W and Bracken MB: Caffeine consumption during pregnancy and association with late spontaneous abortion, Am J Obstet Gynecol 154:14, 1986.

Story M and Alton I: Nutrition issues and adolescent pregnancy, Nutr Today 30:142, 1995.

Tolstoi LG and Smith CL: Human Genome Project, Am J Diet Assoc 99:1421, 1999.

Umans JG and Lindheimer MD: antihypertensive therapy in pregnancy, Curr Hypertens Rep 3:392, 2001.

van Katwijk C and Peeters LL: Clinical apsects of pregnancy after the age of 38 years: a review of literature, Hum Reprod Update 4:185, 1998.

van Spronsen FJ et al.: Phenylketonuria: tyrosine supplementation in phenylalaine-restricted diets, Am J Clin Nutr 73:153, 2001.

Ventura SJ et al.: Declines in teenage birth rates, 1991-98: update of national and state trends, National vital statistics reports, vol 47, no 26, Hyattsville, MD, 1999, National Center for Health Statistics.

Viller J and Belizan JM: Same nutrient, different hypotheses: disparities in trials of calcium supplementation during pregnancy, Am J Clin Nutr 71:1375S, 2000.

Vilming E and Nesheim BI: Hyperemesis gravidarum in a contemporary population in Oslo, Acta Obstet Gynecol Scand 79:640, 2000.

Waisbren SE et al.: Outcome at age 4 years in offspring of women with maternal phenylketonuria. The Maternal PKU Collaborative Study, JAMA 283:756, 2000.

Weitzman M et al.: Maternal smoking and behavior problems of children, Pediatrics 90:342, 1992.

Wolf H: High prepregnancy body mass index: a maternal-fetal risk factor, N Engl J Med 338:147, 1998.

Ziadeh SM: The outcome of triplet versus twin pregnancies, Gynecol Obstet Invest 50:96, 2000.

APPLICATION

Healthcare and Nutrition Resources for Pregnant Women and their Offspring

When Lori was 27 years old, she was the single mother of boys ages 2 years and 4 years. Two years earlier when Lori was divorced, she was awarded custody and child support of $150 per week. That was barely enough to pay her rent, much less feed her children. A social worker advised her to apply for the Temporary Assistance for Needy Families Program (TANF). Qualifying for TANF also made her eligible for Medicaid, food stamps, and the Special Supplemental Food Program for Women, Infants, and Children, which together allowed her to "get by" and make sure the children got enough food. Over time Lori became discouraged and wanted to do something with her life. She applied for admission to a small community college and began to take classes one at a time. She was eligible for financial aid and, with some small scholarships and childcare allowances, she was able to manage school and her children. Today is graduation. Lori will receive an associate degree and already has a part-time position. Because she won't make very much money at first, she will continue to receive food stamps until she gets a full-time job. She can't wait to be on her own and is very grateful for the programs that made it possible.

Poverty creates a vulnerability that increases nutrition and health risk. Poor families are more likely to have inadequate diets than families with higher incomes. The primary goal of providing services for women is to improve their health and that of their children. Inadequate resources or skills may limit the ability of many women to obtain a sufficient quantity or quality of food or resources to access medical care.

Several government programs (Table 5-3) can help. For example TANF, which replaced the former Aid for Families with Dependent Children (AFDC) program, targets individuals and families who live at or near the **poverty level.** Other programs have more liberal income criteria, but are specifically designed for pregnant and lactating women and their infants and children who are considered at risk. With few exceptions, recipients must work after 2 years on TANF.

poverty level: a point defined by the federal government as a level below which people are at risk of being unable to obtain adequate food, shelter, and healthcare

HEALTHCARE PROGRAMS

Medicaid

Medicaid is a healthcare program for low-income individuals of all ages who lack the money or health insurance to pay for medical services. Eligibility criteria for Medicaid are determined by federal and state regulations. In general a family is considered financially eligible if the monthly income after allowable deductions is below 133% of the federally determined poverty level for that family size. Medicaid is available to families who are on TANF and to low-income pregnant women and their young children. Other individuals eligible for Medicaid include low-income people 65 years of age or older, adults and children who are blind or disabled, and people in nursing facilities who do not have enough income or resources to pay for the cost of their care.

Applicants must complete an application and be interviewed by a case worker regarding the need for medical assistance. Applicants are required to provide Social Security numbers, birth certificates, proof of income and assets, medical bills, and information about medical treatment. Medicaid recipients receive a medical assistance identification card that is renewed monthly. A current identification card is necessary to access medical services. Pregnant women who are eligible for Medicaid can get **Expedited Medicaid,** which makes them eligible for Medicaid very quickly. They have 60 days to provide documentation to ensure continued eligibility.

Expedited Medicaid: a category providing eligibility for Medicaid with only identification and proof of pregnancy

Women who qualify for Medicaid are often eligible for other food and nutrition programs and, if so, are encouraged to participate.

If a healthcare service is covered by Medicaid, there is no charge to the client. Medicaid pays for office visits or clinic visits (up to 24 medical visits in a calendar year), laboratory services, and prescription drugs. Pregnancy-related visits and well-child visits are not counted toward the 24-visit limitation. If a mother is already participating in Medicaid when she becomes pregnant, the medical care required during pregnancy, including regular checkups and the hospital stay during delivery, are covered financially. Medicaid is available to mothers who do not meet the eligibility requirements if the pregnancy is categorized as high risk. They can receive special services both prenatally and after the baby arrives.

Healthy Start

Healthy Start is a program established by Congress that extends Medicaid benefits to pregnant women with incomes up to 185% of the poverty level (Haas et al., 1993). This program provides

Table 5-3 Federal Programs That Assist Mothers and Their Infants and Children or Offspring

Program	Recipients	Benefits
Medicaid	All individuals with incomes <133% of poverty level	Total healthcare
Healthy Start (Medicaid)	Pregnant women with incomes <185% of poverty level; special high-risk pregnancies	Prenatal and postpartum care of infants and children
HEALTH CHEK (Medicaid)	Infants, children, and adolescents through 21 years	Health screening—vision, hearing, dental checks, and health education
Food stamps	All individuals with incomes <133% of poverty level	Increased food-buying power via stamps to be exchanged for food in food markets
Commodity distribution	Pregnant and postpartum women, infants, and children <6 years of age with household income ≤185% of federal poverty level	Monthly food package of fruits, vegetables, meats, infant formula, beans, and other foods as available
EFNEP*	Low-income (≤125% of federal poverty level) households with children under 19 years of age	Nutrition aides who provide nutrition education to homemakers
WIC†	Pregnant women, postpartum and lactating women, infants, and children up to 5 years of age	Direct food supplements, nutrition education, referral to health services

*Expanded Food and Nutrition Education Program.
†Special Supplemental Food Program for Women, Infants, and Children.

for regular medical care during and after pregnancy, delivery of the infant, regular check-ups for the new baby, medication prescribed for mother or child, vaccinations to prevent childhood disease, and routine care for the child. Coverage is extended to financially eligible pregnant mothers any time during their pregnancy until 60 days after delivery and to their children up through 8 years of age.

HEALTH CHEK

HEALTH CHEK is a preventive healthcare program for children and adolescents from birth through 21 years who are eligible for Medicaid. Four types of Early and Periodic Screening, Diagnosis, and Treatment (EPSDT) services are available through HEALTH CHEK: a complete screening physical examination including vision, hearing, and dental checks; assessment of growth and development; immunizations (polio, whooping cough, measles, mumps, diphtheria, and tetanus); and health education. Tests for tuberculosis, lead poisoning, anemia, sickle cell anemia, and other problems are completed as needed.

Food Stamp Program

The Food Stamp Program, initiated in 1964, is the cornerstone of the nation's food assistance programs. It is designed to help low-income people buy food they need for good health. All low-income households that have resources (aside from income) of $2000 or less are eligible. Eligibility is determined after application and certification by local public assistance or social services. The program increases the purchasing power of the eligible family by providing monthly allotments of coupons that can be used to purchase food at participating supermarkets. Monthly allotments are based on household size and income. The amount of the benefit received is based on the cost of the United States Department of Agriculture (USDA) **Thrifty Food Plan.** In most states food stamp benefits are delivered electronically to food stamp recipients' food stamp Electronic Benefits Transfer (EBT) accounts. The EBT can be used at a point-of-sale (POS) terminal in the checkout line the same way a credit card can be used.

Thrifty Food Plan: a food plan prepared by the USDA that tests specific types and amounts of food needed to achieve a nutritionally adequate diet at minimal cost. Costs of such a diet are published quarterly.

With the 1998 creation of a nutrition services staff, the federal Food and Nutrition Services (FNS) has refocused efforts toward nutrition and nutrition education. The FNS provides programs to increase the likelihood that all food stamp recipients can make healthy food choices based on the Dietary Guidelines and the Food Guide Pyramid.

Commodity Supplemental Food Program

The Commodity Supplemental Food Program (CSFP) was initiated to distribute **surplus food commodities** to individuals and federally supported organizations. Pregnant women, breastfeeding women, and other postpartum women, infants, and children below the age of 6 years with a household income equal to or less than 185% of the federal poverty level are eligible to receive food packages. The monthly benefits include fruits, vegetables, meats, infant formula, farina, beans, and other foods as available.

surplus food commodities: food products purchased by the federal government as part of agricultural programs, which are available for distribution

A federally funded program called Food Distribution Program on Indian Reservations distributes monthly food packages to American Indian households living on or near reservations. These packages contain a wide variety of canned or packaged foods.

A third food distribution program categorized under CSFP is the Temporary Emergency Food Assistance Program (TEFAP), which provides emergency supplies of dairy products and grains once a month and other staples quarterly. These products are available to households with incomes equal to or below 150% of the federal poverty level.

Cooperative Extension System—Expanded Food and Nutrition Education Program

The Expanded Food and Nutrition Education Program (EFNEP) was funded in 1969 through the USDA via the Agricultural Extension Service in each state. It is designed to teach low-income families the skills needed to select, purchase, and prepare a varied, adequate diet. Trained nutrition aides work directly with low-income homemakers (from households with incomes equal to or below 125% of the federal poverty level) and with children under 19 years of age who are considered at nutrition risk. The Cooperative Extension System is the predominant state-sponsoring agency contracted to develop and deliver Food Stamp Program education programs.

Special Supplemental Food Program for Women, Infants, and Children

The Special Supplemental Food Program for Women, Infants, and Children (WIC) was authorized by Congress in 1972 in Public Law 92-433, which added a new section to the Child Nutrition Act of 1966. It was developed to improve the health of pregnant and postpartum women, infants, and children up to 5 years old by providing supplemental foods, nutrition education and counseling, and access to healthcare services. Eligibility for the target population is determined by **income** and **residency criteria.** Program benefits are directed toward pregnant women and their children who are at nutrition risk based on the following criteria:

- Anemia
- Extremes of leanness or obesity
- Poor pregnancy history
- Dietary risks resulting from inadequate dietary patterns

income criteria: at or below 185% of the U.S. poverty level

residency criteria: residency in the area served by the WIC clinic as specified by the local agency

WIC serves approximately 45% of all infants in the United States and one in four new mothers.

Benefits-Supplemental Foods

By law, 80% of WIC funds must be expended on food benefits. Supplemental food is provided in the form of food packages delivered to participants or as vouchers for specific foods that can be exchanged for approved foods in a market. Food packages are tailored to meet the needs of the recipient, targeting specific nutrients frequently lacking in the diets of low-income individuals—protein, iron, calcium, vitamin A, and vitamin C. Except for infant packages, the food packages are provided to supplement the normal diet, not replace it.

WIC packages consist of the following:

- Iron-fortified infant formula
- Milk and cheese
- Eggs
- Iron-fortified adult and infant cereals
- Fruit and vegetable juices rich in vitamin C
- Dried peas or beans
- Peanut butter

To provide optimal nutrition and feeding for the infant, breast-feeding is promoted in the WIC program through education and support, but the mother is allowed to choose the feeding method. Breast-feeding women may receive benefits for up to 1 year postpartum, whereas nonbreast-feeding women are eligible for only 6 months postpartum. Approximately one third of WIC infants were being breast-fed at the time their mothers were discharged from the hospital compared with 64% of nonWIC infants.

The majority of the program's infants receive WIC food packages. The WIC program provides two separate food packages for infants, one for those up to 3 months of age and the other for those 4 to 12 months of age. The basic component of WIC food packages for infants is iron-fortified infant formula, which is a complete formula requiring only the addition of water to make it ready to feed the infant. After 4 months additional foods are provided.

WIC food packages for infants consist of the following:

- *0 to 3 months:* 40 oz concentrated liquid iron-fortified formula containing at least 10 mg iron/L and 67 kcal/100 mL

- *4 to 12 months:* Iron-fortified formula, iron-fortified infant cereal with a minimum of 45 mg of iron per 100 g of dry cereal, fruit or vegetable juice high in vitamin C

Nutrition Education

Nutrition education, an integral component of the WIC program, became mandatory in 1975. Local agencies are required to spend at least 16% of WIC administrative funds on nutrition education and counseling. A minimum of two education sessions must be provided to a mother receiving WIC supplements in each 6-month certification period. However, participants cannot be denied food supplements if they do not attend the education sessions. The education component addresses dietary needs of the recipients and often focuses on preparing WIC foods and incorporating them into the diet.

Referrals to Health and Social Service Agencies

The WIC funds are designated for foods and nutrition education. They may not be used to provide healthcare to participants. However, WIC providers must advise clients about available healthcare, accessible locations of healthcare facilities, how to receive healthcare, and why it is useful. In fact a major benefit of the WIC program may be a general improvement in the health of mothers and their children from increased access to healthcare as a result of the referral.

Effectiveness of the Program

Since its inception in 1972 the WIC program has grown steadily. In the fiscal year 1998 an estimated 7.4 million women, infants, and children received benefits at a cost of $4 billion (USDA, 2001). Because of the cost of the WIC program and the expectation that outcomes can be measured, much effort has been expended to document the effectiveness of the WIC program. The National WIC Evaluation (NWE) was a 5-year (1979 to 1984) study of pregnancy outcome of WIC participants compared with nonWIC women of similar backgrounds (Rush, 1986; Rush et al., 1988). Overall WIC participants were found to have a greater mean duration of gestation (1.4 days) and an increase in mean birth weight of 23 grams. The Third National Health and Nutrition Examination Survey (NHANES III) provides a nationally representative sample of WIC children between 1990 and 1994.

The WIC program is considered a cost-effective intervention program. The USDA estimates that, on average, every prenatal care dollar spent on WIC saves an average of $3 in later Medicaid costs (USDA, 2001). Numerous smaller studies have been conducted to evaluate the effect of WIC program participation on pregnancy outcome. Birth weight is considered the most significant predictor of subsequent short- and long-term health problems in neonates, such as respiratory difficulties and developmental disabilities. Most studies found a positive effect of prenatal participation in WIC on infant birth weight (Brown et al., 1996; Kotelchuck et al., 1994). Only a few studies have examined the effect of WIC participation on infants and children, mainly because criteria for success are difficult to determine and measure. Recently children participating in WIC were compared with other low-income children (<185% of federal poverty level) using data from NHANES-III, Comprehensive Child Development Programs (CCDP), and a nationally representative sample of children in the 1993 Panel of the Survey of Income and Program Participation (SIPP). The following is a summary of descriptive data of the children of WIC (Brown et al., 1996):

- Most (54%) live in poverty
- 25% are extremely poor
- 43% receive TANF and 60% receive food stamps
- 12% were low birth weight
- 33% of mothers smoked during pregnancy
- Average age of mothers at birth was 25 years

Studies have reported improved dietary intakes with WIC (Brown et al., 1996; Rush, 1986).

For millions of women, infants, and children, like Lori and her children, federal health and nutrition programs provide the safety net that decreases the risk of inadequate diets and promotes health. Increased referral of eligible pregnant women and their children to such programs will increase their effectiveness.

REFERENCES

Brown HI et al.: The impact of Women, Infants and Children Food Supplement Program on birth outcome, Am J Obstet Gynecol 174:1279, 1996.

Haas JJ et al.: The effect of providing health coverage to poor uninsured pregnant women in Masachusetts, JAMA 269:87, 1993.

Kotelchuck M et al.: WIC participation and pregnancy outcomes: Massachusetts statewide evaluation project, Am J Public Health 74:1086, 1994.

Rush D: National evaluation of the Special Supplemental Food Program for Women, Infants, and Children (WIC), vol I, summary, Washington, DC, 1986, United States Department of Agriculture.

Rush D et al.: National WIC evaluation: historical study of pregnancy outcomes, Am J Clin Nutr 48:412, 1988.

United States Department of Agriculture, Office of Analysis, Nutrition and Evaluation: WIC participant program characteristics, 1998. www.fns.usds.gov/oane/MENU/Published/WIC/FILES/PC98sum.htm; accessed July 7, 2001.

CHAPTER

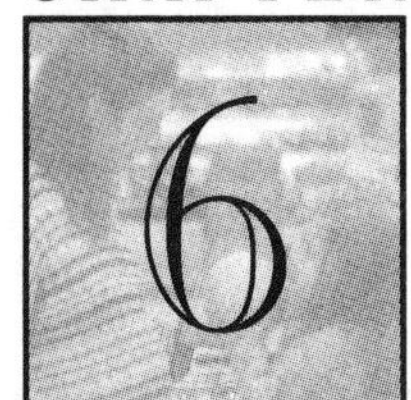

Lactation and Breast-Feeding

Kathryn A. Witt and Mary Ann Mihok

Chapter Outline

Daren and Joyce are expecting their first child in 5 months. Amid discussions of possible names, nursery decor, and childcare possibilities, they consider how to feed their infant. They learn that although both of them were bottle-fed, health experts now recommend breast-feeding. They wonder what breast-feeding is like. Is it easy or difficult? How will they be sure their infant is getting enough to eat? What will they do if Joyce needs to be separated from the baby at feeding time?

Many expectant parents wonder about breast-feeding, a natural relationship that has received increased attention as the unique composition of human milk and the benefits of breast-feeding have been discovered. To answer their questions parents look to family, friends, the media, and healthcare providers. Sometimes the information they receive is incomplete or inaccurate. It is vital that healthcare providers know the benefits of and techniques for breast-feeding and can communicate this important information with their patients.

ADVANTAGES OF BREAST-FEEDING

- *What health advantages does breast-feeding provide the infant?*
- *What constituents in human milk help provide health benefits for the infant?*
- *What advantages does breast-feeding provide the mother?*
- *What are the socioeconomic and environmental benefits of breast-feeding?*

Breast-feeding is acknowledged as the ideal method of feeding and nurturing infants, including premature and sick newborns, with rare exceptions (American Academy of Pediatrics, 1997). Experts on infant nutrition recommend breast-feeding, citing benefits for infants' health, growth, immunity, and development. Breast-feeding mothers benefit both in the immediate postpartum period and later in life. In addition breast-feeding provides economic and social benefits to the family, the healthcare system, the employer, and the nation (U.S. Department of Health and Human Services, 2000b).

In developing countries breast-feeding may mean the difference between life and death for the infant. Breast-feeding greatly reduces the incidence of diarrheal illness, particularly in environments with contaminated water and poor

Research Update

Are Breast-Fed Babies Smarter?

If you compared the Intelligence Quotient (IQ) scores of 500 6-year-old children who had been breast-fed with the IQ scores of 500 6-year-old children who had been formula-fed, it is likely that you would find that the breast-fed group had a higher average IQ score. A simple summary of this superficial observation would be that breast-fed babies are smarter. However, this study would not prove that breast-feeding itself caused the higher IQ in the breast-fed children.

A child's score on an intelligence test is influenced by many factors, which may differ between breast-fed and formula-fed individuals. Some of these factors are socioeconomic status, maternal age and intelligence, parental education, parent-child interaction, family size, parental smoking behaviors, and infant gestational age and birth weight. It is very difficult to separate the effect of breast milk or breast-feeding itself from these other variables. One way to account for these factors would be to randomly assign babies from similar families to be either breast-fed or formula-fed for a specified length of time and then to measure the intelligence of the children at specified ages. This is neither ethical nor practical. Therefore researchers investigating the relationship between breast-feeding and intelligence need to use other methods.

One popular approach to studying complex relationships such as intelligence and breast-feeding is to measure as many of the factors involved as possible and adjust for their effects statistically. These observational studies require large numbers of subjects and complex statistical analysis. In one recent study of this type the IQ of 323 children was measured at ages 4 years and 11 years. The children who had been breast-fed had higher IQ scores at both ages. After statistically adjusting for social class and education, the difference persisted, but when maternal IQ and parenting skills were added, the difference was no longer significant. The researchers concluded that the higher IQ in children who had been breast-fed was explained largely by genetic and socioenvironmental factors (Jacobsen et al., 1999).

In another recent paper the researchers used meta-analysis techniques to pool the results of 11 previous studies that used an observational design somewhat similar to that in the aforementioned study. These researchers found that the higher IQ observed in the children who had been breast-fed persisted even after statistical adjustment for socioeconomic and family differences. They also found a greater benefit for preterm than full-term infants and a greater benefit with longer breast-feeding duration (Anderson et al., 1999).

The conflicting conclusions of these two studies demonstrate the great difficulty of separating the effect of breast-feeding itself from the effect of other characteristics of families who choose to breast-feed their children. On the basis of the data available at this time, it is not possible to say whether breast-feeding itself is responsible for the higher IQ scores typically observed in children who have been breast-fed.

Another approach to this question is to investigate whether some component of breast milk supports improved cognitive development. The long-chain polyunsaturated fatty acids arachidonic acid (20:4 n-6; AA) and docosahexaenoic acid (22:6 n-3; DHA) are receiving much research attention for this reason. The DHA and AA are important components of the brain and are necessary for normal neurologic development. They are not present in the infant formula currently available in the United States, but they are present in breast milk in varying amounts depending on maternal stores and intake (Sanders, 1999). Although infants can synthesize DHA from alpha-linolenic acid (ALA), the amount of DHA in the brains of breast-fed infants is greater than that in the brains of formula-fed infants (Cunnane et al., 2000). The effects of increased infant DHA intake on cognitive development have been studied by comparing the development of infants receiving formula with and without DHA and AA. The results of these experiments are conflicting. One recent trial found a beneficial effect of adding DHA and AA to infant formula (Birch et al., 2000); another did not (Makrides et al., 2000).

Given the conflicts that exist in the scientific literature, how should a practitioner reply to questions about breast-feeding and intelligence? It is currently prudent to answer that, although a num-

Research Update

Are Breast-Fed Babies Smarter?—cont'd

ber of researchers have reported higher IQ scores in children who have been breast-fed, it is not yet clear whether the difference is from breast-feeding itself or some other characteristic of breast-feeding families. In the United States breast-milk provides an infant with more DHA and AA than does infant formula. These fatty acids are important for brain development, but supplementation trials have produced mixed results. It is too soon to say for sure whether or not breast-feeding causes improved intelligence; however, breast-feeding has many other benefits for both a mother and her infant. These benefits make breast-feeding the most intelligent feeding choice for almost all infants.

REFERENCES

Anderson JW et al.: Breast-feeding and cognitive development: a meta-analysis, Am J Clin Nutr 70:525, 1999.

Birch EE et al.: A randomized controlled trial of early dietary supply of long-chain polyunsaturated fatty acids and mental development in term infants, Dev Med Child Neurol 42:174, 2000.

Cunnane SC et al.: Breast-fed infants achieve a higher rate of brain and whole body docosahexaenoate accumulation than formula-fed infants not consuming dietary docosahexaenoate, Lipids 35:105, 2000.

Jacobsen SW et al.: Breastfeeding effects on intelligence quotient in 4- and 11- year-old children, Pediatrics 103:e71, 1999.

Makrides M et al.: A critical appraisal of dietary long-chain polyunsaturated fatty acids on neural indices of term infants: a randomized, controlled trial, Pediatrics 105:32, 2000.

Sanders TA: Essential fatty acid requirements of vegetarians in pregnancy, lactation, and infancy, Am J Clin Nutr 70:555s, 1999.

sanitation. Even in industrialized countries where the use of hygienic, scientifically formulated commercial substitutes for human milk is commonplace, breast-fed infants are less likely than are formula-fed infants to become ill and die. Breast-feeding is associated with reduced risks of gastrointestinal, respiratory, middle ear, and other infections and sudden infant death syndrome. Many studies suggest that later in life, individuals who were breast-fed are less likely to develop insulin-dependent diabetes, Crohn's disease, ulcerative colitis, lymphoma, allergic diseases, and other chronic digestive diseases (American Academy of Pediatrics, 1997). Recent studies indicate that breast-feeding promotes growth patterns resulting in less childhood obesity (Hediger et al., 2000; von Kries et al., 2000). Breast-feeding has also been related to possible enhancement of cognitive development (Anderson et al., 1999). There is strong evidence that most benefits to the infant occur to a greater degree with **exclusive breast-feeding.**

The health benefits of breast milk are related to its unique composition. The nutrient content of human milk is ideally suited for rapidly developing human infants. (Chapter 7 provides a description of the nutrient content of human milk.) Several nutrients, including iron and zinc, have been shown to be better absorbed from human milk than from cow's milk or a commercial formula (Institute of Medicine, Food and Nutrition Board, 1991).

KEY TERMS

exclusive breast-feeding: feeding a mother's breast milk to her infant as the only source of milk; no infant formulas or other milks are fed

In addition to these nutritional advantages, breast milk provides enzymes, hormones, and growth factors and a complex array of cells and compounds that prevent infection (see Tables 7-9 and 7-10) (Institute of Medicine, Food and Nutrition Board, 1991). The stomach of a newborn infant produces low amounts of acid and pepsin; thus the beneficial substances in breast milk are able to survive digestion. Most of these substances carry out their functions on the mucosal surface of the gastrointestinal tract, but some also cross the mucosal barrier (Wagner et al., 1996). These important nonnutritional benefits of breast milk are not available in commercial breast milk substitutes.

From the maternal perspective immediate postpartum benefits of breast-feeding are decreased risk of hemorrhage and iron-deficiency anemia. The uterus shrinks back to its prepregnant size more quickly. Ovulation and menstruation are suppressed for a longer period, especially in women who exclusively breast-feed, which lengthens the interval between births and conserves iron. Additionally the repeated intimate contact between mother and infant fosters maternal-infant bonding. Breast-feeding for longer periods (up to 2 years) and among younger mothers (in their early twenties) may reduce the risk of breast and ovarian cancers (U.S. Department of Health and Human Services, 2000b).

Breast-feeding brings economic benefits to the family through a savings of several hundred dollars over the cost of formula, even after accounting for the costs of breast pump equipment and additional food for the nursing mother (Montgomery and Splett, 1997). Because breast-fed infants have fewer illnesses, they require fewer physician visits, prescriptions, and hospitalizations; thus medical costs are lower. Maternal absenteeism from work is thereby less, resulting in employer cost savings and increased employee productivity (U.S. Department of Health and Human Services, 2000b). Breast-feeding contributes to environmental protection through decreased use of disposable materials associated with formula manufacture, home preparation, and packaging (Dermer, 1996).

BREAST-FEEDING RATES

- *How have breast-feeding rates in the United States changed in the past 2 to 3 decades?*
- *What is the current rate of breast-feeding in the United States?*

Breast-feeding rates in the United States have fluctuated over the past 50 years. After World War II rates declined, reaching a low of 22% of mothers initiating breast-feeding in 1972. Duration also dropped during this period (Institute of Medicine, Food and Nutrition Board, 1991). Trends in rates were reversed from 1972 until the early 1980s, with a peak in 1982 when 62% initiated breast-feeding and 30% continued to breast-feed at 6 months postpartum (Spisak and Gross, 1991). Rates fell again between 1982 and 1990 to 51.9% initiation and 17.6% still breast-feeding at 6 months (Ross Products Division of Abbott Laboratories, 1997). The decade of the 1990s saw a resurgence in breast-feeding rates and by 1998 64% of all mothers breast-fed during the early postpartum period and 29% were still breast-feeding at 6 months (U.S. Department of Health and Human Services, 2000a). The *Healthy People 2010* goal for breast-feeding is to increase the proportion of mothers who breast-feed in the early postpartum period to 75%, to 50% at 6 months, and to 25% at 1 year (U.S. Department of Health and Human Services, 2000a).

PHYSIOLOGY OF LACTATION

- *Describe the anatomy of the human breast.*
- *What hormones control milk production?*
- *How does infant suckling result in milk production and release?*
- *How is milk production sustained?*

Anatomy of the Mammary Gland

Human breasts consist of glandular tissue supported and protected by connective tissue and fat (Figure 6-1). The interior of the breast contains a system of 15 to 20 lobes that radi-

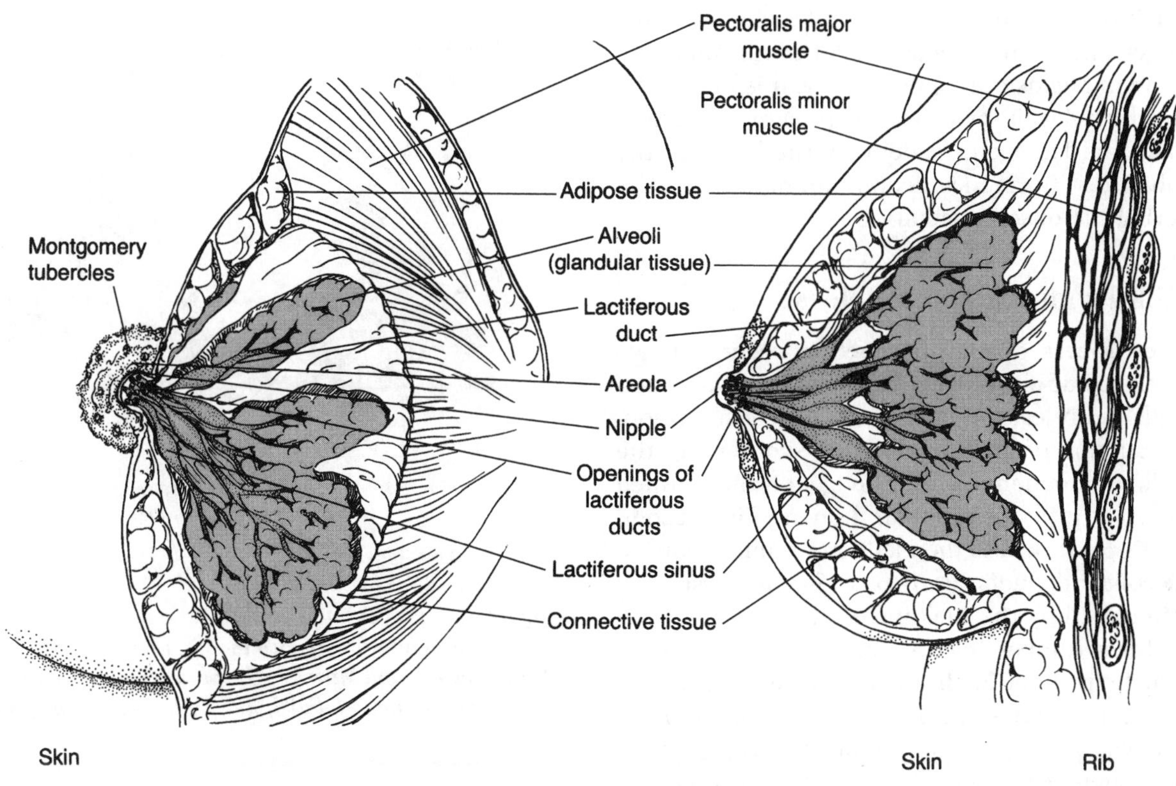

Figure 6-1 Anatomy of a mammary gland. *(From Gorrie TM, McKinney ES, and Murray SS: Foundations of maternal newborn nursing, Philadelphia, 1994, WB Saunders.)*

ate out from the nipple like the spokes of a wheel. Each lobe contains many **alveoli** that produce milk. The milk produced in the alveoli is transported toward the nipple by the **lactiferous ducts,** which are surrounded by muscle-like cells that can contract and help to push milk toward the nipple. Just below the **areola,** the circular pigmented area around the nipple, the lactiferous ducts widen into short lactiferous **sinuses.** Then the ducts narrow again and pass through the nipple. The areolar tissues contain bundles of smooth muscle that can stiffen the nipple, allowing a better grasp by the suckling infant. The areola also contains tiny raised areas called **Montgomery's tubercles,** which release secretions that lubricate the nipple and areola during lactation.

Breast Maturation

The breasts begin to develop at puberty, a process stimulated by estrogen and other hormones. The hormonal changes of pregnancy stimulate proliferation of the ducts and alveoli.

KEY TERMS

alveoli: small sac-like, milk producing, and secreting areas of the mammary glands
lactiferous ducts: small tubes through which milk flows
areola: a circular area of a darker color surrounding the nipple
sinuses: hollow cavities
Montgomery's tubercles: tiny raised areas around the nipple that secrete substances that lubricate and protect the areola and nipple

Additionally Montgomery's tubercles become larger and more noticeable. Although milk production begins during pregnancy, it is limited by the high levels of estrogen, progesterone, and placental lactogen. At delivery the levels of the inhibitory hormones decline dramatically, triggering the onset of lactation.

Milk Production and Release

The process of milk production occurs in two distinct but closely related stages: production of milk and release of milk for infant consumption. Production of milk involves the synthesis of the milk components and passage of the formed product into the alveolar **lumen.** The second stage, **let-down,** is the ejection of milk from the alveoli and ducts. Both of these processes are stimulated by the suckling of the infant.

Term human infants are born with reflexes that help them **latch on** and suckle effectively. When an infant's cheek is lightly brushed, he or she will open his or her mouth and turn toward the touch. This **rooting reflex** enables a mother to position her infant so he or she is able to grasp the areolar area in his or her mouth and exert pressure on the lactiferous sinus located underneath the areola. When an infant is properly latched on, his or her tongue and gums work together to push milk from the lactiferous sinus out through the nipple (Figure 6-2). Sucking and swallowing reflexes work together. The tongue and jaw suck milk from the breast and swallowing follows.

When an infant suckles, the hormones **prolactin** and **oxytocin** stimulate milk production and release (Figure 6-3). Prolactin, secreted by the anterior pituitary, stimulates the mammary alveolar cells to synthesize milk. Milk is secreted continuously into the alveoli, but it does not flow easily from the alveoli into the ductile system. Oxytocin, secreted by the posterior pituitary, causes the muscle-like cells around the alveoli to contract. The muscle contraction pushes the milk out of the alveoli and along the duct system where it is easily available to the nursing infant. The milk ejection or let-down reflex is sensitive to a variety of neurohormonal mechanisms. For example milk ejection can become inhibited by anxiety, stress, or fatigue in the mother. It can also become a conditioned response triggered by associations with nursing, such as the infant's cry.

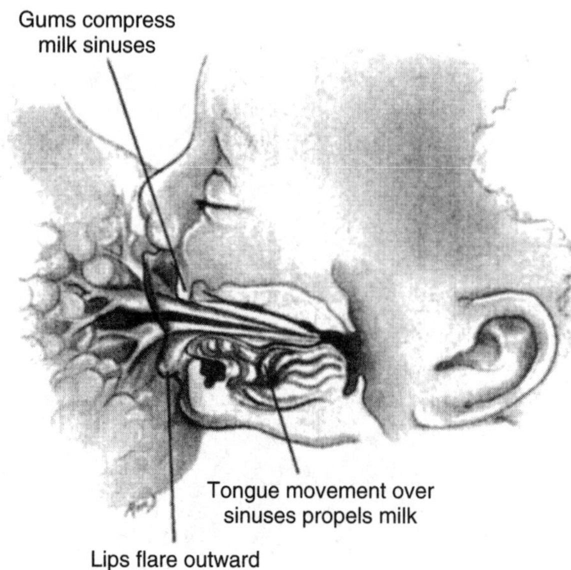

Figure 6-2 Proper latch on draws the nipple and most of the areola into the infant's mouth. *(From Gorrie TM, McKinney ES, and Murray SS: Foundations of maternal newborn nursing, Philadelphia, 1994, WB Saunders.)*

The fluid produced by the breasts changes during the course of lactation and within a feeding. Full lactation does not begin at **parturition.** During the first few days after birth, the breasts secrete a small amount of **colostrum.** Colostrum is higher in protein and lower in fat than mature breast milk and it is abundant in immune and protective factors. By the end of the first week postpartum, colostrum is usually replaced by increasing amounts of mature milk. This transition occurs more slowly in women breast-feeding for the first time.

Mature milk varies in fat content during the course of a single feeding. The **foremilk** released when an infant initially latches on to a breast is lower in fat than the **hindmilk** available later. To receive adequate calories, infants need to nurse long enough to receive the rich hindmilk.

Maintenance of Lactation

Suckling simulation and breast emptying stimulate milk production. When an infant is not able

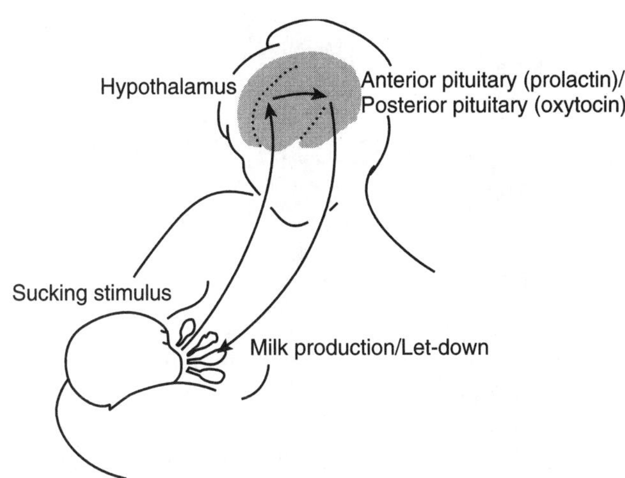

Figure 6-3 When the infant suckles, receptors in the nipple and areola send stimuli to the hypothalamus. The hypothalamus stimulates release of prolactin from the anterior pituitary, which stimulates milk secretion, and oxytocin from the posterior pituitary stimulates ejection of milk from the alveolus. *(From Worthington-Roberts BS and Williams SR: Nutrition in pregnancy and lactation, ed 5, New York, 1993, McGraw-Hill. Reproduced with permission of The McGraw-Hill Companies.)*

to nurse, manual expression of breast milk or a breast pump can be used to maintain or increase milk production. A mother who returns to work after breast-feeding has been established can successfully maintain lactation by a combination of nursing and manual expression or pumping. The expressed or pumped milk can be refrigerated and given to the infant in the absence of the mother. If milk is not regularly removed from a mother's breasts, the ability to continue producing milk is generally lost within a few weeks.

Lactation and Fertility

In many areas of the world, lactation is the primary means of spacing pregnancies. The higher prolactin level stimulated by regular breast-feeding helps to suppress menstruation and ovulation. The duration of **lactational amenorrhea** is typically 25 to 30 weeks, but this figure varies widely (Lawrence and Lawrence, 1999). It is shortened by the early addition of supplemental feedings or less frequent breast-feeding and is lengthened by the later addition of supplemental foods and extremely poor nutritional status of the mother (Lawrence and Lawrence, 1999). After menstruation returns ovulation may remain irregular for several months. However, it is worth noting that some women do become pregnant during lactational amenorrhea.

ENERGY AND NUTRIENT NEEDS OF LACTATING WOMEN

- *What factors influence the nutrient needs of breast-feeding women?*
- *How does the energy and nutrient intake of a breast-feeding mother affect milk production and composition?*
- *What is the effect of weight loss on lactation?*
- *How are the nutrient needs of a breast-feeding woman different from those of a woman who is not breast-feeding?*

Realizing that their diets are imperfect, many women worry whether the quality or quantity of

KEY TERMS

lumen: cavity or canal
let-down: the movement of milk from the alveoli through the duct system and lactiferous sinuses to the nipple
latch on: when nursing infants grasp the nipple and a portion of the surrounding areola in their mouths; a good portion of the areola should be grasped for successful suckling
rooting reflex: a reflex in which infants will turn and open their mouths toward the cheek that is brushed
prolactin: a hormone from the anterior pituitary gland that stimulates milk production
oxytocin: a hormone from the posterior pituitary gland that causes milk ejection and uterine contraction
parturition: the process of giving birth
colostrum: a milk-like fluid produced by the breast during the first days after parturition; precedes mature milk production
foremilk: lower-fat milk released at the beginning of a feeding
hindmilk: higher-fat milk released from the breast toward the end of a feeding
lactational amenorrhea: a lack of menstruation associated with breast-feeding

the milk they produce will be sufficient for their infants. It is reassuring to know that in the absence of severe malnutrition, the milk a mother produces will be adequate for her infant. In fact many women successfully meet the nutritional needs of twins by breast-feeding.

Breast milk production is a nutritionally demanding task. Possible sources for the energy and nutrients required for lactation are shown in Figure 6-4. The nutrients needed to produce breast milk can be drawn both from a woman's diet and from her nutrient stores. Additionally for some nutrients, adaptations such as enhanced intestinal absorption and reduced renal excretion help to meet the nutritional demands of breast milk production. The use of stored nutrients and these adaptations support adequate nutrition for the infant during times when a woman's dietary intake is low. However, when low dietary intake is combined with low nutrient reserves, nutritional problems in the mother or baby may result. Therefore adequate maternal nutrition is important during lactation to avoid depletion of maternal nutrient reserves and to promote the optimal nutrition status of both mother and child.

Determining the optimal nutrient intake for a breast-feeding woman is a challenge. Factors to be considered include the amount of a nutrient secreted in breast milk, changes in maternal nutrient stores, and adaptations such as increased absorption and reduced excretion. Unfortunately for many nutrients the information available at present is limited to a few studies of breast milk content. Therefore the recommended intake for most nutrients is derived by measuring the amount of the nutrient typically secreted in breast milk, determining how much additional dietary intake would be needed to supply that amount, and adding the additional dietary intake to the recommended intake for a nonlactating woman. When information about nutrient-conserving adaptations is known, it is used to modify the recommendation derived from breast milk losses. Complicating all of these calculations is the fact that breast milk nutrient losses vary with the volume of milk consumed by the infant, maternal dietary intake, and the stage of lactation. Nutrient losses even vary during the course of a single feeding.

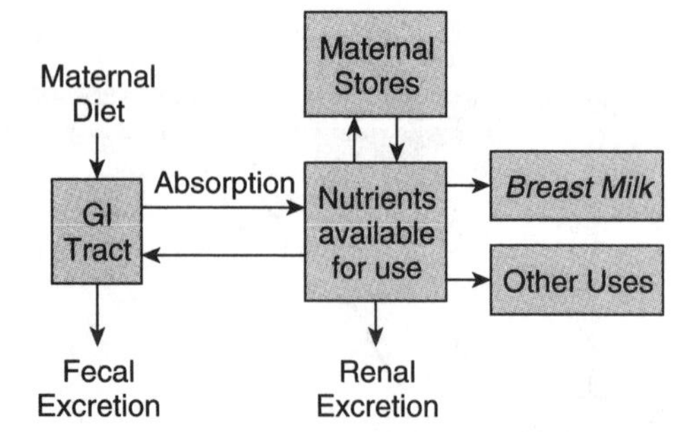

Figure 6-4 Sources of energy and nutrients for breast milk production.

As a result of the variability in nutrient losses over the course of breast-feeding, the 1989 Recommended Dietary Allowances (RDAs) include separate recommendations for the first and second 6 months of lactation. The newer Daily Recommended Intakes (DRIs) published thus far include only one recommendation for lactation. This recommendation is based on the average nutrient concentration in milk from healthy mothers who are not taking nutrient supplements and are exclusively breast-feeding. Exclusive breast-feeding is recommended for the first 4 to 6 months of an infant's life and the average volume of milk produced during this time is 780 mL per day. Women whose infants are partially breast-fed would have lower nutrient needs. Conversely women nursing twins would have much higher nutrient needs. Figure 6-5 shows the changes in nutrient needs thought to accompany lactation and Table 6-1 contains the recommended vitamin and mineral intakes for breast-feeding women.

Energy and the Energy-Providing Nutrients

Energy

The RDA for energy during breast-feeding is based on the calorie cost of breast milk production and the use of stored fat gained during pregnancy. The energy content of human milk is about 670 kcal/L to 700 kcal/L and the efficiency of converting the energy in a woman's diet to breast milk energy is thought to be about 80%. Therefore it costs about 850 kcal to produce a liter of milk (Dewey, 1997; National Research Council, 1989). The 1989 RDA

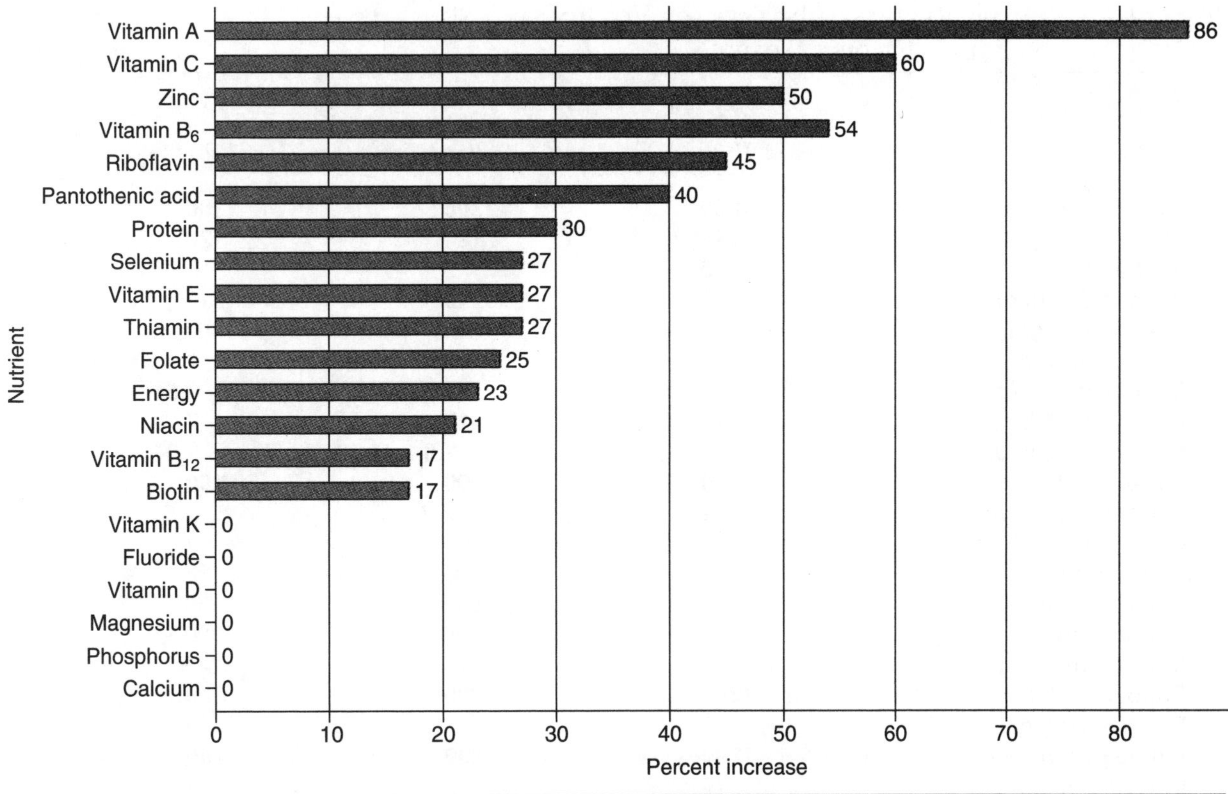

Figure 6-5 Increases in recommended nutrient intakes during exclusive breast-feeding.

for lactation is based on an average daily infant intake of 750 mL in the first 6 months and 600 mL during the second 6 months. With these volumes the additional energy needed for breast milk production is 640 kcal per day during the first 6 months of lactation and 510 kcal per day during the second 6 months. In the first 6 months it is assumed that 100 kcal per day to 150 kcal per day of this energy is derived from the 2 kg to 3 kg of maternal fat that is typically gained during pregnancy. With the use of stores factored in, the RDA for both the first and second 6 months of lactation is an additional 500 kcal per day, or a total intake of 2700 kcal per day (National Research Council, 1989).

The reported caloric intake of breast-feeding women is often below the RDA, prompting questions about the extent to which energy-conserving adaptations might help to sustain milk production when calorie intake is inadequate. Possible adaptations include declines in the basal metabolic rate, declines in the thermic effect of feeding, declines in physical activity levels, increases in the efficiency of milk production, and increases in the efficiency of muscular activity. Studies of lactation-induced changes in basal metabolic rate and the thermic effect of feeding have produced mixed results, suggesting that adaptations in these components of daily energy expenditure, if present, are small (Dewey, 1997). Physical activity levels appear to be slightly lower in lactating women, especially in the early postpartum period. However, the physical activity levels of breast-feeding women vary greatly, making it unwise to assume that all women are able to reduce their overall energy needs during lactation by reducing their physical activity level (Dewey, 1997). When the total daily energy expenditure of breast-feeding women is studied using the doubly labeled water technique, the daily caloric needs of breast-feeding women are found to vary from about 2500 kcal to 3300 kcal per day (Dewey, 1997). These results suggest that the RDA is a reasonable representation of the calorie needs of the average breast-feeding woman. The underreporting of

Table 6-1 DIETARY REFERENCE INTAKES FOR VITAMINS AND MINERALS FOR BREAST-FEEDING WOMEN

	Recommended Intake (RDA/*AI*)		
Nutrient	<18 yrs	19-30 yrs	31-50 yrs
Vitamin A (μg RAE/d)	**1200**	**1300**	**1300**
Vitamin C (mg/d)	**115**	**120**	**120**
Vitamin D (μg/d)	*5*	*5*	*5*
Vitamin E (mg/d)	**19**	**19**	**19**
Vitamin K (μg/d)	*75*	*90*	*90*
Thiamin (mg/d)	**1.4**	**1.4**	**1.4**
Riboflavin (mg/d)	**1.6**	**1.6**	**1.6**
Niacin (mg NE/d)	**17**	**17**	**17**
Vitamin B_6 (mg/d)	**2.0**	**2.0**	**2.0**
Folate (μg DFE/d)	**500**	**500**	**500**
Vitamin B_{12} (μg/d)	*2.8*	*2.8*	*2.8*
Pantothenic acid (mg/d)	*7*	*7*	*7*
Biotin (μg/d)	*35*	*35*	*35*
Choline (mg/d)	*550*	*550*	*550*
Calcium (mg/d)	*1300*	*1000*	*1000*
Chromium (μg/d)	*44*	*45*	*45*
Copper (μg/d)	**1300**	**1300**	**1300**
Fluoride (mg/d)	*3*	*3*	*3*
Iodine (μg/d)	**290**	**290**	**290**
Iron (mg/d)	**10**	**9**	**9**
Magnesium (mg/d)	**360**	**310**	**320**
Manganese (mg/d)	*2.6*	*2.6*	*2.6*
Molybdenum (μg/d)	**50**	**50**	**50**
Phosphorus (mg/d)	**1250**	**700**	**700**
Selenium (μg/d)	**70**	**70**	**70**
Zinc (mg/d)	**14**	**12**	**12**

Adapted with permission from the following Institute of Medicine publications: Dietary reference intakes for calcium, phosphorus, magnesium, vitamin D, and fluoride (1997); Dietary reference intakes for thiamin, riboflavin, niacin, vitamin B6, folate, vitamin B12, pantothenic acid, biotin, and choline (1998); Dietary reference intakes for vitamin C, vitamin E, selenium, and carotenoids (2000); and Dietary reference intakes for vitamin A, vitamin K, arsenic, boron, chromium, copper, iodine, iron, manganese, molybdenum, nickel, silicon, vanadium, and zinc (2001). Washington, DC, National Academy Press.
RDAs are printed in bold type; AIs are printed in italics.
DFE, *Dietary Folate Equivalents;* NE, *Niacin Equivalents;* RAE/d, *Retinol Activity Equivalents*

food intake may account for some of the discrepancy between reported energy intake and theoretic energy needs, but more research in this area is clearly needed.

In affluent societies where excess body fat is a common health concern and a thin body shape is in fashion, women often want to know the effect of lactation on postpartum weight loss. Though weight change during lactation varies tremendously (some women gain weight), in general breast-feeding women lose weight slightly faster than their non–breast-feeding peers (Dewey, 1998; Janney, 1997). The average amount of weight lost during full lactation is 500 g per month (Dewey, 1997), which corresponds to the removal of 100 kcal to 150 kcal per day from fat stores assumed in the RDA calculation. Many women wish to lose weight faster than this rate and wonder if it is safe. In healthy women with adequate or high fat reserves, weight loss of up to 500 g per week (2 kg/month) by moderate dietary restriction, or a combination of diet restriction and exercise, does not appear to negatively affect lactation (Dewey, 1998; Lovelady et al., 2000). Increased prolactin levels may help to protect lactation when maternal energy balance is negative (Dewey, 1998). The risks of more rapid weight loss are unclear. Diets providing less than 1800 kcal per day make it difficult for a lactating woman to meet her nutrient needs (Institute of Medicine, Food and Nutrition Board, 1991) and in one small study, reduction of maternal energy intake to less than 1500 kcal per day for 1 week was associated with reduced infant milk intake the following week (Strode et al., 1986). Thus breast-feeding women with adequate energy stores can be reassured that moderate weight loss is compatible with lactation. However, they should be cautioned that severe caloric restriction or rapid weight loss is risky.

In developing countries where too often chronic undernutrition increases the risk of disease and death, a different question is of concern: whether providing food supplements to breast-feeding women increases milk production. This is a difficult question to study because variations in infant demand for milk (which is affected by the infant's size and health and by the use of supplemental feedings), food availability, necessary physical activity, maternal energy stores, and illness make the data very difficult to interpret. Studies conducted in rural Mexico, Gambia, India, Burma, and Guatemala have produced mixed results, suggesting that supplements may be more useful for severely undernourished women than for moderately undernourished women, resulting in increased milk volume, higher maternal weight, and a longer time before supplemental feedings are added (Dewey, 1997; Gonzalez-Cossio et al., 1998; Institute of Medicine, Food and Nutrition Board, 1991). These studies demonstrate both how complex and how hardy is the breast-feeding process.

Protein

The RDA for protein was calculated using a milk protein content of 11 g/L, with milk volumes of 750 mL per day during the first 6 months and 600 mL per day during the second 6 months, and 70% efficiency in converting dietary protein to breast milk protein. The resulting recommendations are an increase of 15 g per day during the first 6 months and 12 g per day during the second 6 months (National Research Council, 1989). More recently Dewey has suggested that these recommendations are likely to be low because they do not consider nonprotein nitrogen-containing compounds in breast milk (i.e., urea, choline, carnitine, creatinine, nucleotides, and others). When the loss of these compounds is considered, a recommended intake of an additional 18 g to 20 g of protein per day results (Dewey, 1997). In well-nourished women, the additional protein needed for lactation appears to be obtained from the diet, not by a decrease in lean body mass (Motil et al., 1998). Protein intakes do not appear to significantly affect milk volume, but severe protein restriction may alter the breast milk content of some nitrogen-containing compounds (Dewey, 1997; Lawrence and Lawrence, 1999).

Carbohydrate and Lipid

With the current available data it is difficult to determine specific guidelines for carbohydrate and lipid intake during lactation. On average a lactating woman secretes about 56 g of carbohydrate (mainly lactose) and 32 g of lipid per day in her milk (Blundell et al., 1999). A diet providing adequate energy with 15% to 30% of the energy from fat and 50% to 60% of the energy from carbohydrate should provide adequate carbohydrate and lipid.

The sources for milk fat include synthesis in the mammary gland, the maternal diet, and maternal stores. Dietary alterations do not appear to affect the amount of fat in the milk, but women with low fat stores appear to secrete milk with a lower fat content (Institute of Medicine, Food and Nutrition Board, 1991). Additionally the type of fatty acids consumed by a woman appears to influence the type of fatty acids secreted in her breast milk. A topic of great interest currently is the influence of a woman's intake of linoleic and alpha-linolenic acids and the longer-chain fatty acids that can be synthesized from these two essential fatty acids, especially docosahexaenoic acid (DHA) and eicosapentaenoic acid (EPA) (Makrides and Gibson, 2000; Sanders 1999). The DHA and EPA appear to be important for the development of the central nervous system and retina. The research update in this chapter provides more detail on this topic.

Calcium and Related Nutrients

Calcium

The amount of calcium secreted in breast milk is approximately 210 mg per day (Institute of Medicine, Food and Nutrition Board, 1991). This calcium appears to be obtained primarily by a net removal of calcium from **trabecular bone** and by a reduction in the amount of calcium excreted in the urine. Surprisingly the efficiency of intestinal calcium absorption does not increase and additional dietary calcium does not prevent the bone loss that occurs during lactation or influence the calcium content of breast milk (Institute of Medicine 1997; Prentice, 2000). Because of these adaptations, the Adequate Intake (AI) for calcium during lactation does not differ from that of a nonlactating woman.

Fortunately after weaning or the resumption of menstruation, the efficiency of dietary calcium absorption increases and renal calcium conservation continues so that bone mineral content is restored, typically by 6 months after weaning (Institute of Medicine, 1997; Prentice, 2000). Though adaptations in calcium metabolism enable women to meet the demands of lactation without an increase in dietary calcium, calcium intake before and during lactation remains a concern. Several cases have been reported in which women developed osteoporosis during lactation. Risk factors for this rare condition include poor general nutrition, low calcium intake, and a family history of osteoporosis (DiGregorio et al., 2000).

Phosphorus and Magnesium

A lactating woman loses approximately 90 mg to 120 mg of phosphorus and 9 mg to 26 mg of magnesium in milk daily. Although these minerals are studied less often than calcium, the available evidence suggests that like calcium, the phosphorus and magnesium needed for milk production are obtained through bone resorption and reduced urinary excretion. Serum values of phosphorus are generally higher in lactating women than in nonlactating women and serum magnesium values are uninfluenced by lactation (Institute of Medicine, 1997). Thus the DRIs for these minerals are the same for lactating women as they are for nonlactating women.

Vitamin D

The amount of vitamin D secreted in breast milk is small and varies with maternal vitamin D intake (Specker, 1994) and with exposure to sunlight (Greer et al., 1984a). The AI and Tolerable Upper Intake Level (UL) for vitamin D during lactation are the same as those for nonlactating women; however, attention to the vitamin D status of lactating women is warranted. Rickets has been observed in the breast-fed infants of vitamin D-deficient women (Daaboul et al., 1997). Conversely potentially harmful levels of vitamin D have been reported in the breast milk of a woman taking very high doses (i.e., 2500 μg/day) of supplemental vitamin D (Greer et al., 1984b).

Fluoride

The amount of fluoride secreted in breast milk is very small and is not significantly affected by maternal fluoride intake. Thus the RDA and UL for fluoride during lactation are the same as those for nonlactating women.

B Vitamins and Choline

Thiamin, Riboflavin, and Niacin

The breast milk content of these vitamins varies with maternal intake (Institute of Medicine, Food and Nutrition Board, 1991). To calculate the additional amount needed during lactation, the average amount of each vitamin secreted in breast milk (i.e., 0.16 mg thiamin, 0.3 mg riboflavin, and 1.4 mg niacin per day) is adjusted upward to account for increased energy needs and the efficiency of use by the body (Institute of Medicine, 1998). Compared with the RDAs for nonlactating women, the RDAs for lactation are 0.3 mg higher for thiamin, 0.5 mg higher for riboflavin, and 3 mg higher for niacin.

Vitamin B_6

The vitamin B_6 concentration in breast milk varies with maternal intake and averages 0.13 mg/L in the milk of well-nourished mothers. This amount represents a daily loss of 0.1 mg. The efficiency of transfer of this vitamin from the diet to breast milk appears rather low. To ensure an adequate breast milk concentration, the RDA for lactation is 0.7 mg higher than that for nonlactating women. The UL for vitamin B_6 is the same as that for nonpregnant, nonlactating women. Very high doses of vitamin B_6 have been reported to have an antilactogenic effect. Therefore lactating women should avoid vitamin B_6 intakes over the UL (Institute of Medicine, 1998).

Folate

Breast milk folate levels do not appear to vary greatly with maternal intake, except in the case of severe maternal deficiency. The folate content of breast milk is about 0.85 μg/L, yielding a daily output of 664 mg per day. The increase in the RDA for folate during lactation (i.e., 100 μg) is substantially greater than milk losses because of the low bioavailability of folate from food. Maternal folate levels decline during the postpartum period in both lactating and nonlactating women, but whether this represents a loss of maternal stores, the discontinuation of prenatal vitamin supplements, or some other factor is unclear (Institute of Medicine, 1998).

Vitamin B_{12}

The average vitamin B_{12} content of breast milk from well-nourished mothers is 0.42 μg/L, resulting in a typical daily loss of 0.33 μg. The RDA for lactation is 0.4 μg higher than that for nonlactating women. Women with a poor vitamin B_{12} status from a low intake or poor absorption may produce milk with an inadequate vitamin B_{12} content, placing their infant at risk for a vitamin B_{12} deficiency (Institute of Medicine, 1998).

Pantothenic Acid, Biotin, and Choline

The breast milk content of pantothenic acid increases with maternal intake, with an average value of 2.2 mg/L, or 1.7 mg of pantothenic acid in a daily milk output of 780 mL. The AI for lactating women is 2 mg higher than that for nonlactating women. Biotin appears to be actively transported from maternal plasma to milk because milk concentrations are much higher than maternal plasma concentrations. Measurements of breast milk biotin concentrations vary widely and reflect maternal intake and maternal plasma values, with a typical value of 6 μg/L. To calculate the AI, 5 μg is added to the AI for nonlactating women (Institute of Medicine, 1998). Human milk contains about 160 mg choline/L found as choline itself and choline-containing compounds such as phosphocholine, phosphotidylcholine, and sphingomyelin. This combination represents a loss of 125 mg per day in 0.78 L milk. Thus the AI for choline during lactation is 125 mg greater than that for nonlactating women (Institute of Medicine, 1998).

Antioxidant Nutrients

Vitamin C

The typical daily loss of vitamin C in breast milk is 40 mg per day and the RDA for lactating women is 45 mg higher than that for nonlactating women. Women consuming less than 100 mg per day may produce milk with a lower vitamin C content and as maternal intake of vitamin C increases beyond 200 mg per day, the excess vitamin C appears to be excreted primarily in maternal urine, not breast milk (Byerley and Kirksey, 1985; Institute of Medicine, 2000).

Vitamin E

Most of the vitamin E in mature breast milk is alpha tocopherol (Institute of Medicine, Food and Nutrition Board, 1991). A lactating woman secretes about 4.9 mg of alpha tocopherol per liter of breast milk, which is about 4 mg per day. Therefore the RDA for lactating women is 4 mg higher than the RDA for nonlactating women. A recent research study suggests that the vitamin E content in the breast milk of women who smoke is significantly lower (Ortega et al., 1998). Whether increased dietary vitamin E would help to counteract this difference is unknown.

Selenium

The amount of selenium secreted in mature breast milk varies with maternal intake. An average woman in North America loses about 14 μg

> **KEY TERMS**
>
> **trabecular bone:** bone with a spongy or meshlike internal structure found in the vertebrae and joints

per day in her milk and the increase in the RDA for lactation is 15 μg (Insitute of Medicine, 2000).

Vitamins A and K

Vitamin A

The vitamin A in breast milk mainly takes the form of retinyl esters, although a variety of carotenes are present, particularly in colostrum. The amount of vitamin A in breast milk varies with maternal intake and vitamin A status (Haskell and Brown, 1999) and decreases during the course of lactation (Institute of Medicine, Food and Nutrition Board, 1991). The vitamin A content of mature breast milk is typically about 670 μg/L, resulting in maternal losses of about 523 μg per day (Institute of Medicine, Food and Nutrition Board, 1991). To replace the vitamin A secreted in milk, the RDA for lactating women is 600 μg higher than that for nonlactating women (Institute of Medicine, 2001).

Vitamin K

Breast milk contains only about 2 μg/L of vitamin K, representing daily losses of 1.2 μg to 1.5 μg per day, an amount easily replaced by typical diets. The RDA for vitamin K during lactation is the same as that for nonlactating women (Institute of Medicine, 2001). Although the milk vitamin K levels of women with low vitamin K intakes are improved by supplementation, even the milk of women with a high intake of this vitamin from food or supplements may not contain sufficient vitamin K to ensure adequate vitamin K status of an infant (Institute of Medicine, Food and Nutrition Board, 1991).

Iron, Zinc, and Iodine

Iron

Iron losses during lactation (0.13 to 0.3 mg/day in breast milk) are smaller than menstrual iron losses (0.5 mg/day). Because amenorrhea is typical in exclusively breast-feeding women, the RDA for iron during lactation is less than that for nonlactating women (Institute of Medicine, 2001). Maternal iron status does not appear to influence the breast milk iron content (Institute of Medicine, Food and Nutrition Board, 1991).

Zinc

Typical daily zinc losses in breast milk are 1.2 mg per day (Institute of Medicine, Food and Nutrition Board, 1991). Zinc is not well absorbed; however, it may be conserved during lactation by an increase in the efficiency of zinc absorption (Fung et al., 1997) and a reduction in the amount of zinc excreted in the urine (Klein et al., 1995). The RDA for zinc during lactation is 4 mg higher than the RDA for nonlactating women. The zinc content of breast milk decreases over the course of lactation, but supplemental zinc does not seem to influence milk zinc concentrations (Chierici et al., 1999).

Iodine

The iodine content of breast milk parallels worldwide maternal iodine intake. In the United States where iodine intake is high, the breast milk contains about 178 μg iodine per liter. In northwestern Zaire where iodine deficiency is prevalent, breast milk contains about 20 μg iodine per liter (Institute of Medicine, Food and Nutrition Board, 1991). The RDA for lactation is based on maternal milk losses in the United States and is 140 μg higher than the RDA for nonlactating women.

Electrolytes

Sodium and Potassium

Milk losses of sodium and potassium are approximately 135 mg per day and 375 mg per day, respectively. These increases are easily met by usual dietary intakes and breast milk levels are not influenced by maternal nutrition (Institute of Medicine, Food and Nutrition Board, 1991). Therefore a separate minimum requirement for these nutrients during breast-feeding has not been established (National Research Council, 1989).

Fluid

Lactating mothers have been encouraged to drink 2 L to 3 L of fluid each day. Records of dietary intakes of lactating women indicate that total fluid intake, including food and beverages, typically falls in this range (Stumbo et al.,

1985). A number of investigators have demonstrated that milk output is unrelated to fluid consumption and that increased fluid consumption does not result in increased milk production. In fact forced fluid consumption beyond thirst may reduce milk production (Duskieker et al., 1985; Duskieker et al., 1990; Institute of Medicine, Food and Nutrition Board, 1991). However, lactating women should be encouraged to be alert for and respond to thirst (Lawrence and Lawrence, 1999).

DIETARY RECOMMENDATIONS FOR LACTATING WOMEN

- *Which nutrients are likely to be low in the diets of lactating women in the United States?*
- *Describe the recommended number of servings from each food group during lactation.*
- *What guidelines for consumption of alcohol and caffeine, smoking, and physical activity are appropriate during lactation?*

Adequacy of Typical U.S. Diets

The nutritional adequacy of a diet is related to both energy intake and nutrient density. Although little information is available on the nutrient intake of lactating women, it appears that a varied, balanced diet that meets a woman's energy requirements usually provides adequate vitamins and minerals to support lactation. Women who consume a nutrient-dense diet and who meet the RDA for energy (i.e., 2700 kcal) are likely to approach or meet the RDA for all nutrients.

To estimate the nutrient intake of women with lower calorie intakes, the Committee on Nutritional Status during Pregnancy and Lactation calculated the average nutrient content per 1000 kcal of diets consumed by women in the United States from the Continuing Survey of Food Intakes of Individuals (Institute of Medicine, Food and Nutrition Board, 1991). Although these levels do not represent the intakes of lactating women specifically, they provide a general indication of the degree to which the typical diet of a women in the United States will meet the nutrient recommendations for lactation. With these calculations, at caloric intake levels of approximately 2200 kcal per day (the average reported caloric intake of lactating women), nutrients that are typically consumed in amounts less than the RDA are calcium and vitamin B_6. When intake levels fall below 1800 kcal, predicted intakes fall short of the RDA for the aforementioned nutrients and also for magnesium, thiamin, vitamin C, and selenium (Institute of Medicine, Food and Nutrition Board, 1991; Institute of Medicine, 1997; Institute of Medicine, 1998; Institute of Medicine, 2000; Institute of Medicine, 2001).

Because the RDAs are guidelines for intakes that include a wide margin of safety above requirements, it cannot be assumed that intake levels below the RDA are indications of deficiency. However, women who consume a low intake for a prolonged period increase their risk of deficiency. Additionally special attention should be paid to subgroups of women with nutrient intakes below those assumed in the calculations. Women with family incomes below the poverty level have a lower vitamin A intake; adolescents have a lower iron intake; and African-American women tend to consume less calcium, magnesium, and vitamin A (Institute of Medicine, Food and Nutrition Board, 1991). For these groups especially, attention to diet quality and quantity can help to ensure optimal nutrients for a mother and her infant.

Guidelines for Dietary Intake

Some women elect not to breast-feed because they do not wish to be subject to complicated dietary rules for breast-feeding. Because adequate milk quality and quantity is the result of both maternal diet and maternal stores, healthy diets during lactation vary considerably. General guidelines for dietary intake during lactation are given in Box 6-1. If more specific guidelines are needed, the Good Food Guide found in Figure 4-12 is appropriate for both pregnancy and lactation.

The nutritional needs of breast-feeding women should be met by a balanced, varied diet rather than by vitamin and mineral supplements. If dietary evaluation indicates a significant lack of

Box 6-1 Guidelines for Dietary Intake during Lactation

- Avoid diets and medications that promise rapid weight loss.
- Eat a wide variety of breads and cereal grains, fruits, vegetables, milk products, meats, or meat alternatives each day.
- Take two or three servings of milk products daily.
- Make a greater effort to eat vitamin A-rich vegetables or fruits often. Examples of foods high in vitamin A include carrots, spinach or other cooked greens, sweet potatoes, and cantaloupe.
- Be sure to drink when you are thirsty. You will need more fluid than usual.
- If you drink coffee or other caffeinated beverages, such as cola, do so in moderation. Two servings daily are unlikely to harm the infant. Caffeine passes into the milk.

Adapted from Suitor CW et al.: Nutrition care during pregnancy and lactation: new guidelines from the Institute of Medicine, J Am Diet Assoc 93:478, 1993.

important nutrient sources, mothers should be encouraged to select acceptable foods that will remedy the problem. If dietary counseling is ineffective in improving intake, however, the guidelines for improving nutrient intake, via supplementation described in Table 6-2 can be used.

Infant Reactions to Foods in the Mother's Diet

Foods consumed by a breast-feeding woman may alter the smell and taste of her milk. Although studies suggest that breast-fed infants exposed to a variety of odors and flavors from their mother's milk may be weaned more easily to solid foods, other evidence shows that some infants become colicky after their mothers consume certain foods, especially specific vegetables and fruits such as garlic, onion, other sulfur-containing vegetables, rhubarb, apricots, and prunes. Red pepper has been reported to cause dermatitis in breast-fed infants and cow's milk proteins from the mother's diet may be transferred to the infant, producing an allergic reaction (Lawrence and Lawrence, 1999). There is no evidence that all nursing mothers need to avoid these foods. Sensitivity to any maternal dietary component must be documented by the reversal of the infant's symptoms when the food is removed from the diet and confirmed with a repeat of symptoms when the food is reintroduced. There is no scientific basis for the widely held beliefs that gassy foods cause gas in a breast-fed baby or that chocolate should be avoided while breast-feeding.

MATERNAL BEHAVIORS

- *What are the consequences of caffeine and alcohol use during breast-feeding?*
- *What are the risks of smoking and drug abuse during breast-feeding?*

Caffeine and Alcohol

Maternal consumption of caffeine and alcohol may adversely affect the breast-feeding infant. When a nursing mother consumes large doses of caffeine (i.e., 6 to 8 cups of caffeine-containing beverages per day), caffeine can accumulate in the infant, causing irritability and wakefulness (Rivera-Calinim, 1987).

Alcohol is readily transferred to breast milk, with peak levels in milk at 30 to 60 minutes after maternal consumption. Daily intakes of more than 0.5 g ethanol per kg of maternal body weight (i.e., about 24 oz beer, 9 oz wine, or 2 to 3 oz hard liquor for a 125-pound woman) can reduce infant consumption of breast milk and may interfere with the milk let-down (Lawrence and Lawrence, 1999). Alcohol in breast milk may disrupt the infant's sleeping pattern. The effects of alcohol on infants' mental and psychomotor development remain under investigation (Lawrence and Lawrence, 1999). Breast-feeding women who consume alcohol should be counseled about the timing and volume of their alcohol intake.

Smoking and Drug Abuse

In addition to its deleterious effects on maternal health, smoking results in lower milk volume (Hopkinson et al., 1992) and the presence of

Table 6-2 Suggested Measures for Improving Nutrient Intake of Women with Restrictive Eating Patterns

Type of Restrictive Eating Pattern	Corrective Measures
Excessive restriction of food intake, i.e., ingestion of <1800 kcal of energy per day, which ordinarily leads to unsatisfactory intake of nutrients compared with the amounts needed by lactating women	Encourage increased intake of nutrient-rich foods to achieve an energy intake of at least 1800 kcal/day; if the mother insists on curbing food intake sharply, promote substitution of food rich in vitamins, minerals, and protein for those lower in nutritive value; in individual cases, it may be advised to recommend a balanced multivitamin–mineral supplement; discourage use of liquid weight loss diets and appetite suppressants
Complete vegetarianism, i.e., avoidance of all animal foods, including meat, fish, dairy products, and eggs	Advise intake of a regular source of vitamin B_{12}, such as special vitamin B_{12}-containing plant food products or a 2.6-μg vitamin B_{12} supplement daily
Avoidance of milk, cheese, or other calcium-rich dairy products	Encourage increased intake of other culturally appropriate dietary calcium sources, such as collard greens for African Americans from the southeastern United States; provide information on the appropriate use of low-lactose dairy products if milk is being avoided because of lactose intolerance; if correction by diet cannot be achieved, it may be advisable to recommend 600 mg of elemental calcium per day taken with meals
Avoidance of vitamin D–fortified foods, such as fortified milk or cereal, combined with limited exposure to ultraviolet light	Recommend 10 μg of supplemental vitamin D per day

nicotine in breast milk. Although no direct association between nicotine levels in the milk of heavy smokers and symptoms in the infant have been found, there is some evidence that breast-fed babies of smoking mothers have decreased growth and more respiratory infections (Lawrence and Lawrence, 1999). However, for women who are unable to stop smoking, breast-feeding is still advisable because the benefits of breast milk outweigh the risks associated with smoking (U.S. Department of Health and Human Services, 2000b).

The American Academy of Pediatrics states that amphetamine, cocaine, heroin, marijuana, nicotine, and phencyclidine hydrochloride (i.e., angel dust and PCP) are contraindicated during breast-feeding because these and other drugs of abuse are hazardous to both the mother and the nursing infant (American Academy of Pediatrics Committee on Drugs, 1994). Further study is needed to determine the likelihood that a breast-fed infant whose mother is using illegal drugs will develop withdrawal symptoms when breast-feeding is stopped.

BREAST-FEEDING BASICS

- *Suggest guidelines for the successful initiation of breast-feeding.*
- *What are some signs that breast-feeding is going well?*
- *What difficulties occasionally complicate breast-feeding and what can be done about them?*

Initiating Breast-Feeding

Although the production of breast milk is based on innate reflexes, breast-feeding behavior must be learned by both mother and infant. Almost all healthy women who want to breast-feed can do so, provided that they have adequate knowledge and support. Preparation for successful breast-feeding should begin during pregnancy, especially for a woman planning to breast-feed for the first time. Information about the breast-feeding process, what to expect, and where to get help if problems occur should be provided by a **lactation specialist.**

Newborn infants are ready to breast-feed. In fact they are alert, attentive, and able to begin breast-feeding the first hour after birth. Whenever possible, the first feeding should occur in the birthing room and the baby should remain with the mother throughout the recovery period. A tranquil, warm environment in the birthing room and reduced use of anesthesia during delivery facilitate a successful first feeding. Many hospitals and birthing centers have facilities and policies that promote early breast-feeding initiation. However, if medical intervention requires immediate separation, it should be remembered that early nursing is important, but not essential for successful breast-feeding.

During the first feedings, a new mother learns how to position herself and her infant for comfortable, successful feeding. Nursing infants may be placed in one of several positions (Figure 6-6). A lactation specialist can help a new mother and her infant practice these positions. Alternating positions can help alleviate fatigue and the potential for sore nipples. For all positions, it is important that the baby's body and head face the same direction.

KEY TERMS

lactation specialist: a person who has been specially prepared to teach women about breast-feeding and how to prepare for it; may be a physician, nurse, dietitian, or other healthcare professional trained as a lactation educator

Once the infant is comfortably positioned, he or she can latch on to the breast. To help the infant latch on, the mother supports her breast and gently squeezes the area behind her areola using a palmar or scissor grasp (Figure 6-7). Next she tickles the baby's lower lip with her nipple to stimulate the rooting reflex. When the infant opens his or her mouth wide, the mother pulls the baby in close so the baby's tongue extends under the nipple and draws the nipple into the mouth. A baby who is properly latched on draws both the nipple and much of the areola into his or her mouth.

When the infant is positioned and latched on correctly, the feeding experience should be pleasant. Occasionally the baby latches on to just the nipple, which results in very painful nursing. If the latch on is not comfortable, the baby's suction must be broken before the nipple is removed. This is done by slipping a clean finger into the corner of the baby's mouth. Most hospitals and birthing centers have a lactation consultant who can help with latch on difficulties. Once the baby is latched on and sucking, receptors in the nipple and areola send a neural message to the hypothalamus, which stimulates oxytocin release from the pituitary. Oxytocin stimulates milk let-down and uterine contractions. Let-down can be identified by the perception of uterine tightening and nipple tingling and by the infant's gulping. Anxiety and distraction interfere with this critical reflex. Therefore every effort should be made to ensure that new mothers are comfortable, rested, and relaxed. Mothers having difficulty with let-down while in the hospital or at home should contact a lactation specialist or other healthcare provider so that the problem can be remedied. For most women let-down is rapidly established and may occur in response to the infant's crying or other feeding cues.

Ensuring that the Infant Is Getting Enough Milk

Newborns should be nursed whenever they show signs of hunger, usually 8 to 12 times per day for 10 to 15 minutes on each breast. Babies who do

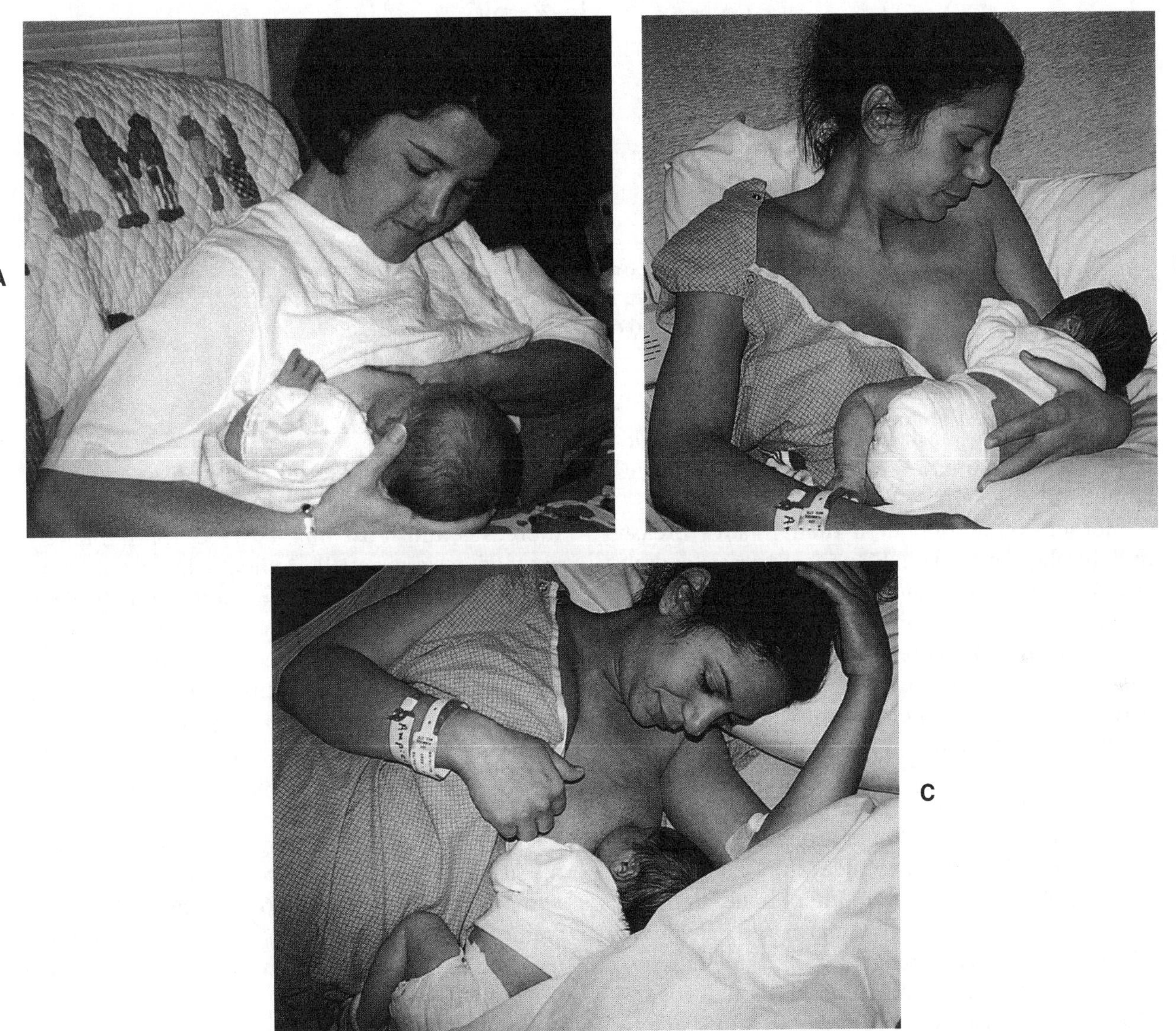

Figure 6-6 Positions for breast-feeding. **A**, cradle position; **B**, football position; **C**, side-lying position. *(B and C courtesy Marjorie Pyle, RNC, Lifecircle, Costa Mesa, Calif. A, B, and C from Lowdermilk DL, Perry SE, Boback IM: Maternity and women's health care, ed 7, St. Louis, 2000, Mosby.)*

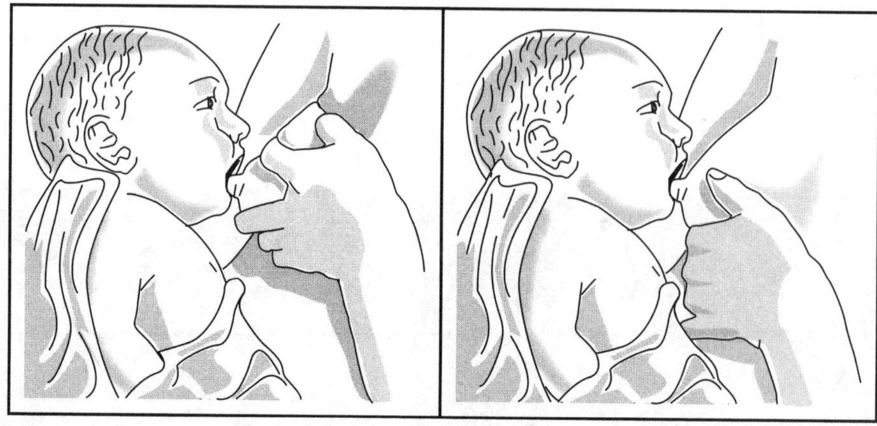

Figure 6-7 The breast may be supported using a palmar or scissor grasp. *(Drawn from Lawrence RA and Lawrence RM: Breastfeeding: a guide for the medical profession, ed. 5, St. Louis, 1999, Mosby.)*

not demand to be fed at least every 4 hours should be awakened to breast-feed, even during the night (American Academy of Pediatrics, 1997).

Mothers often wonder if their infant's breast milk intake is adequate. Signs that breast-feeding is going well include softening of the breasts after nursing; the observation that the infant gulps and slows the sucking pattern during the course of a feeding; a sleepy, relaxed feeling in the mother after feeding; and a content infant who has at least six wet diapers and three or four bowel movements per day by 5 days to 7 days of age (American Academy of Pediatrics, 1997). A baby who wants to nurse for a very long time (e.g., 30 minutes or more on each side) may not be getting enough milk and the mother should contact her lactation specialist (American College of Obstetrics and Gynecology, 2001). Supplements (i.e., water, formula, and glucose) should not be given to newborns who are breast-feeding unless there is a significant medical reason. Pacifiers, if used at all, should be reserved until breast-feeding is well established (Moore et al., 1998).

The American Academy of Pediatrics (1997) calls for evaluation of breast-feeding by a trained observer within 48 hours after delivery and again 2 to 3 days after hospital discharge. Infants discharged before 48 hours should be seen within 4 days of birth.

As the Infant Grows

As the infant grows and breast-feeding becomes well established, the interval between feedings increases and most infants need approximately six feedings per day. Periodically however, an infant will appear to be constantly hungry and nurse very frequently. This is typically the result of a growth spurt. The frequent nursing stimulates the increased milk production needed to meet the needs of the growing infant. In a few days milk production will have increased to meet the baby's needs and the feeding pattern will return to normal.

Exclusive breast-feeding provides sufficient nutrition to support optimal growth and development for the first 4 to 6 months and breast-feeding with weaning foods should be continued for at least 12 months (American Dietetic Association, 1997).

Overcoming Difficulties

Many mothers have some concerns or difficulties related to breast-feeding after they leave the hospital. Most problems can be resolved while continuing to breast-feed. If minor difficulties are unresolved, they may become major problems and can result in breast-feeding failure. It is important for new mothers to have someone to whom they can turn for assistance and support. The mother's obstetrician, pediatrician, or family physician is a logical choice if he or she is supportive of breast-feeding. Other sources include peer counselors or family members and friends who have successfully breast-fed. Many hospitals have lactation specialists who provide assistance and are available to new mothers after discharge. Support groups such as the La Leche League can provide information and moral support to a worried mother.

Sore Nipples

The most common cause of sore nipples is poor positioning and incorrect latch on. Correcting or changing feeding positions can help many cases of sore nipples. Additional measures include eliminating the use of irritating or drying soaps and ointments, avoiding the use of plastic-backed breast pads, and the application of therapeutic ointments. If the nipple becomes cracked or damaged, healing can be aided by leaving a few drops of milk to dry on the nipple after feeding (Lawrence and Lawrence, 1999). Sore nipples also may be from an infection, so a healthcare provider familiar with breast-feeding should be consulted for severe or persistently sore nipples.

Engorgement

When colostrum is replaced by mature milk, the breasts may become temporarily swollen. It is often difficult for the infant to latch on to the enlarged breasts. This results in a hungry, frustrated infant and painfully engorged breasts. **Engorgement** can be minimized by frequent nursing. When it occurs, applying cold packs to the breasts helps to provide some relief. Softening the breasts by a warm shower or by expressing or pumping a small amount of milk so the baby can latch on is helpful also. Engorgement is more likely in primiparas and usually resolves within a few days.

Separation

When mother and infant cannot be together, lactation can be maintained by manual expression or pumping of breast milk (Figure 6-8). The infant can be fed breast milk that has been expressed or pumped on previous occasions or commercial formula. Initially it may take several pumping sessions to produce the volume of milk required for a feeding. Breast milk can be refrigerated for 1 to 2 days or frozen for 3 to 4 months. Mothers who work can pump their milk at work so the infant can receive it in a bottle the next day. Alternatively an infant may receive commercial formula while the mother is at work and breast-feed while they are together.

Nipple Confusion

Some infants have difficulty switching back and forth between human and artificial nipples. Artificial nipples are less flexible and the tongue movements used to control milk flow from a bottle are different from those used in breast-feeding. To avoid nipple confusion it is best to avoid the use of artificial nipples in the first month of an infant's life, when breast-feeding is becoming established. If bottle feeding is needed after that time, most infants learn to switch back and forth successfully. If an infant rejects the artificial nipple, it may help if a caregiver other than the mother introduces the bottle.

Slow Growth

Occasionally breast-feeding gets off to a slow start. This is more likely with primiparas and may be from a variety of causes, including fatigue, stress, misinformation about appropriate breast-feeding practices, or a small and sleepy infant. Inadequate breast milk is a significant concern because it can rapidly result in life-threatening dehydration of the infant. Women and their infants are often discharged before their breast-feeding knowledge and skill can be thoroughly evaluated; thus it is important that breast-fed infants be evaluated several days after discharge to ensure that all is well and to provide guidance for questions and uncertainties. When breast-feeding is not progressing adequately, medical intervention is warranted. Instructing a mother to rest and nurse frequently and long enough usually resolves the

KEY TERMS

engorgement: temporary swelling of the breasts that occurs as mature milk secretion begins

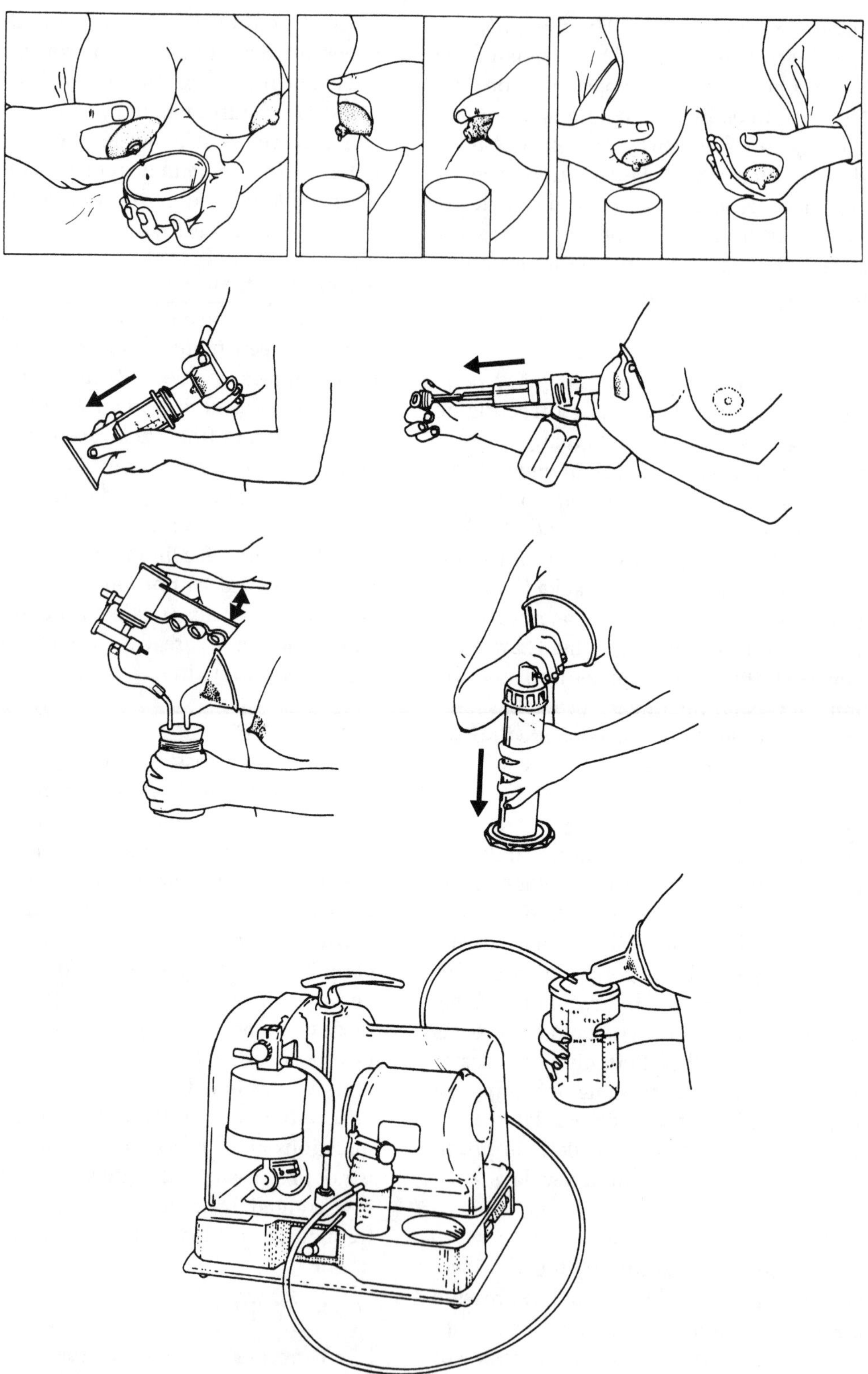

Figure 6-8 Manual expression of breast milk and breast pumps. *(From Worthington-Roberts BS and Williams SR: Nutrition in pregnancy and lactation, ed 4, New York, 1989, McGraw-Hill. Reproduced with permission of The McGraw-Hill Companies.)*

problem in a few days. In more severe cases a mother may be instructed to pump her breasts after her baby has finished nursing to provide additional stimulation for milk production.

Providing supplements of bottled commercial formula to the infant ensures an adequate nutrient intake, but often hampers breast-feeding. When an infant receives supplemental bottles, he or she nurses less frequently, reducing the sucking stimulation necessary to increase milk production. Nipple confusion may also result. If supplemental feedings are necessary, use of a supplemental nursing system (Figure 6-9) ensures adequate infant nutrition and promotes milk production without introducing nipple confusion. Supplemental nursing systems can be used to induce lactation in adoptive mothers or in birth mothers who initially chose not to breast-feed.

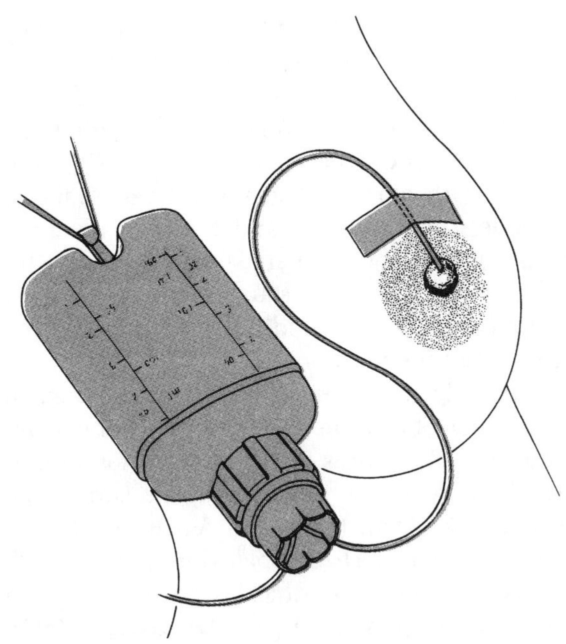

Figure 6-9 A supplemental nursing system helps stimulate milk production while providing nourishment to the infant. *(From Lawrence RA and Lawrence RM: Breastfeeding: a guide for the medical profession, ed 5, St. Louis, 1999, Mosby.)*

Plugged Ducts/Mastitis

Tenderness in one area of the breasts may indicate a plugged or blocked collecting duct. Application of warm and moist heat, breast emptying, and gentle massage of the tender area usually resolves the problem. If tenderness persists, the use of overly restrictive bras or clothing should be considered as a cause. If the tenderness is joined by redness, swelling, or fever, **mastitis** is a possibility and the mother should contact a physician.

Leaking Milk

Leaking milk can be a source of embarrassment or discomfort. Soft, breathable, washable, or disposable bra pads are available to absorb leaked milk. If let-down occurs in response to an infant's crying at a time other than feeding, gentle pressure on the nipples reduces the flow. This can be accomplished inconspicuously by crossing the arms across the chest.

CONTRAINDICATIONS TO BREAST-FEEDING

- *Describe the circumstances in which breast-feeding may be contraindicated.*

There are a few circumstances when breast-feeding is contraindicated. These are related to maternal health, medications, and personal habits that may influence the safety, composition, or availability of breast milk and to some disorders in the infant. Newborns with certain inborn errors of metabolism, such as **galactosemia, phenylketonuria,** or **primary lactase deficiency** cannot digest or metabolize one of the nutrients in human or cow's milk and require full or partial feeding of specialized formula or specially treated breast milk.

Most acute infectious diseases in the mother will not contraindicate breast-feeding. However,

KEY TERMS

mastitis: infection of the breast
galactosemia: lack of an enzyme required to convert galactose to glucose
phenylketonuria: a metabolic error in which the infant lacks an enzyme required to metabolize phenylalanine
primary lactase deficiency: genetic lack of the enzyme that digests lactose

women with untreated tuberculosis and human T-cell leukemia virus type 1 (HTLV-1) should not breast-feed because of the risk of infecting the infant (American Academy of Pediatrics, 1997; Lawrence and Lawrence, 1999). For women with chronic diseases such as diabetes mellitus, renal disease, and hypertension, the decision to breast-feed must be assessed with the physician on a risk-to-benefit ratio. Most women with these conditions do successfully breast-feed their infants.

Currently it is recommended that women in the United States infected with the human immunodeficiency virus (HIV) should not breast-feed because of the risk of transmission of the virus to the infant (American Academy of Pediatrics, 1997). It has been isolated from breast milk and is possibly responsible for person-to-person transmission (Lawrence and Lawrence, 1999). The role of breast-feeding in HIV infection is still being studied and advances in treatment may lead to changes in these recommendations in the future. In developing countries where safe and effective alternatives to breast-feeding are not available, the World Health Organization (1992) recommends that breast-feeding should be initiated regardless of HIV-1 serologic status of the mother.

The breast-feeding woman may safely use most prescribed and over-the-counter medications. However, breast-feeding should be avoided or discontinued if the mother needs to take radioactive isotopes, antimetabolites, or cancer chemotherapy agents (American Academy of Pediatrics, 1997). All medications must be evaluated by the physician on a case-by-case basis when a woman makes the decision to breast-feed. The risk of a small amount of a drug to a nursing infant compared with the benefits of being breast-fed should be carefully assessed. In the event that a drug is contraindicated, safer alternative drugs may be available (Lawrence and Lawrence, 1999).

Environmental pollutants such as dichlorodiphenyltrichloroethane (DDT), dioxin, polychlorinated biphenols (PCBs), and heavy metals such as lead and mercury have been found in breast milk, although no normal or abnormal values have been established (U.S. Department of Health and Human Services, 2000b). Women at high risk for these contaminants must carefully weigh the potential risk against the benefits of breast-feeding.

WEANING

- *At what ages are children typically weaned?*
- *How should weaning be accomplished?*

Weaning, the transition from exclusive breast-feeding to other sources of nourishment, is typically a gradual process. Children are weaned for varying reasons and at varying ages. In many developing countries children are normally breast-fed for 2 to 3 years. In fact the average worldwide age for weaning is 4.2 years (Lawrence and Lawrence, 1999). In the United States the American Academy of Pediatrics (1997) and other professional groups recommend that infants be breast-fed for at least 1 year (American Dietetic Association, 1997). In infants under 1 year of age, iron-fortified commercial formula should be used rather than cow's milk if breast-feeding is discontinued (American Academy of Pediatrics, 1997). The guidelines for adding solid foods to a breast-fed infant's diet are the same as those for a formula-fed infant (see Chapter 7).

When weaning an infant, decreasing breast-feeding slowly allows mother and infant to adjust to the change. Generally one feeding at a time is eliminated. After adapting to the change, another feeding is stopped, usually at the opposite time of day. Eventually one morning and one evening feeding remain. These feedings may be continued to provide nourishment and comfort if desired or they may be phased out. After breast-feeding has stopped completely, the breasts continue to be partially functional for about 1 month (Lawrence and Lawrence, 1999).

PROMOTING BREAST-FEEDING

- *What maternal characteristics and medical practices are associated with higher breast-feeding rates?*
- *When do parents decide whether or not to breast-feed?*

Although overall breast-feeding rates are increasing in the United States, the percentages of new mothers who initiate and continue breast-feeding are significantly lower among young women, women of ethnic minorities, low-income women, and not well-educated women. Factors that increase the likelihood that a woman will breast-feed include the woman's prenatal intention to breast-feed (Humphreys et al., 1998); support from family members, especially the infant's father (Bar-Yam and Darby, 1997); practice of health-enhancing behaviors (Pesa and Shelton, 1999); and breast-feeding knowledge (Susin et al., 1999). Maternal employment does not seem to be a detriment to the initiation of breast-feeding, but at 6 months the overall rate of breast-feeding in mothers working full-time (18%) is lower than the breast-feeding rate in mothers who are not working (29%) or who are working part-time (28%) (Ross Products Division of Abbott Laboratories, 1997).

Prenatal Counseling

When counseling an expectant family about their infant feeding decision, healthcare professionals should assess and consider cultural, social, and family acceptance factors and the mother's perceived value of breast-feeding versus bottle-feeding. Most parents make the decision regarding breast-feeding during pregnancy, so it is important to furnish complete information about the benefits of and techniques for breast-feeding and an evaluation of breast anatomy. The likelihood of breast-feeding success is much greater when women have confidence in their ability to breast-feed (Mihok, 1997). Perhaps most important in helping a woman to develop this confidence is to inform her of resources available after breast-feeding initiation for information, help with problems, and social support.

Initiatives and Resources for Breast-Feeding Promotion

Many government and nonprofit organizations have joined the effort to promote and support breast-feeding. The *Healthy People* goals, first published in 1978 and now set for 2010, establish national policy for the encouragement of breast-feeding. The Surgeon General's Workshop on Breast-Feeding and Human Lactation recommended several hospital practices now known as the "Ten Steps to Successful Breast-Feeding" adopted in 1991 by the United Nations' Baby Friendly Hospital Initiative (Box 6-2). The U.S. Department of Health and Human Services Office on Women's Health (2000b) has released a "Blueprint for Action on Breast-Feeding" that includes strategies for making breast-feeding as easy as possible and removing barriers that discourage breast-feeding. Among these strategies are culturally appropriate training for breast-feeding in health-profession schools, implementation of the "Ten Steps to Successful Breast-Feeding" by hospitals, worksite programs that facilitate breast-feeding after mothers return to their jobs, public education and support, and control of the marketing of breast milk substitutes. Box 6-3 lists national and international breast-feeding resources.

Regional resources include state and local health departments; state and local breast-feeding coalitions; Women, Infants, and Children (WIC)

Box 6-2 Practices for Successful Breast-Feeding Services at Hospital and Maternity Centers

- A written breast-feeding policy is communicated to all healthcare staff.
- Staff members are trained in the skills needed to implement the policy.
- Pregnant women are educated about the benefits and management of breast-feeding.
- Breast-feeding is initiated early.
- Mothers are taught how to breast-feed and maintain lactation.
- Use of any food or drink other than human breast milk is limited.
- Rooming-in is available.
- Breast-feeding on demand is practiced.
- Use of pacifiers and artificial nipples is limited.
- Breast-feeding support groups and services are fostered.

From U.S. Department of Health and Human Services: HHS blueprint for action on breast-feeding, Washington, DC, 2000b, U.S. Department of Health and Human Services Office on Women's Health.

Box 6-3 National and International Breast-Feeding Resources

ORGANIZATIONS

National

Academy of Breast-Feeding Medicine
PO Box 81323
San Diego, CA 92138
(877) 836-9947
http://www.bfmed.org

American Academy of Pediatrics
141 NW Point Boulevard
Elk Grove Village, IL 60009
(800) 433-9016
http://www.aap.org

National Center for Education in Maternal and Child Health
2000 15th Street North, Suite 701
Arlington, VA 22201
(703) 524-7802
http://www.ncemch.org

National Healthy Mothers Healthy Babies Coalition (HMHB)
121 North Washington Street, Suite 300
Alexandria, VA 22314
(703) 836-6110
http://www.hmhb.org

International

INFACT Canada (Infant Feeding Action Coalition)
6 Trinity Square
Toronto, ON M5G 1B1
Canada
(416) 595-9819
http://www.infactcanada.ca

International Baby Food Action Network (Organization consists of more than 150 groups worldwide)
http://www.ibfan.org

International Lactation Consultant Association (ILCA)
1500 Sunday Drive, Suite 102
Raleigh, NC 27607
(919) 787-5181
http://www.ilca.org

La Leche League International
1400 North Meacham Road
Schaumburg, IL 60173
(847) 519-7730
http://www.lalecheleague.org

Wellstart International
4062 First Avenue
San Diego, CA 92103
(619) 574-8163
http://www.wellstart.org

PUBLICATIONS

Lawrence RA and Lawrence RM: *Breast-feeding: a guide for the medical profession,* ed 5, St. Louis, 1999, Mosby.

Riordan J and Auerback K: *Breast-feeding and human lactation,* Sudbury, MA, 1999, Jones and Bartlett.

Journal of Human Lactation, the official journal of the International Lactation Consultant Association (ILCA), published quarterly.

offices; La Leche League chapters; and hospital-based lactation specialists. The WIC Program places a strong emphasis on breast-feeding, including provision of a food package for exclusively breast-feeding mothers. Many WIC clients have no experience or exposure to breast-feeding and need education and counseling to prepare for and sustain this practice. The WIC staff members are trained to provide the needed information and social support.

Concepts to Remember

- Lactation, the process by which the mammary gland produces and releases milk for the infant, is the natural extension of pregnancy. Successful lactation involves learning breast-feeding behaviors.
- Breast milk offers immunologic, nutritional, and psychologic advantages, yet only one half of mothers in the United States choose to breast-feed.

- Breast-feeding mothers require more energy, nutrients, and fluid than do their nonnursing peers. When nutrient intake is less than requirements, nutrients are usually removed from maternal stores to ensure adequate nutrition for the infant. To protect maternal stores and nourish the infant, a breast-feeding mother's diet should be rather nutrient-dense and she should be careful to drink when thirsty.
- Mothers are more likely to breast-feed successfully when they have accurate information; support from family, friends, and health professionals; and help with breast-feeding basics soon after the baby is born.
- Many breast-feeding difficulties can be prevented when breast-feeding is started in the delivery room, when mothers nurse their infants frequently and long enough, and when careful attention is paid to positioning and latch on.

REFERENCES

American Academy of Pediatrics: Policy statement: Breast-feeding and the use of human milk, Pediatrics 100:1035, 1997.

American Academy of Pediatrics Committee on Drugs: The transfer of drugs and other chemicals into human breast milk, Pediatrics 93:137, 1994.

American College of Obstetrics and Gynecology: Breast-feeding your baby, 2000. www.medem.com, accessed January 11, 2001.

American Dietetic Association: Position of the American Dietetic Association: promotion of breast-feeding, J Am Diet Assoc 97:662, 1997.

Anderson JW et al.: Breast-feeding and cognitive development: a meta-analysis, Am J Clin Nutr 70:525-535, 1999.

Bar-Yam NB and Darby L: Fathers and breast-feeding: a review of the literature, J Hum Lact 13:45, 1997.

Blundell JE et al.: Report of the IDECG working group on the modulating effect of stressors on the upper and lower limits of lipid and carbohydrate intake, Eur J Clin Nutr 53:S179, 1999.

Byerley LO and Kirksey A: Effects of different levels of vitamin C intake on the vitamin C concentration in human milk and the vitamin C intakes of breastfed infants, Am J Clin Nutr 41:665, 1985.

Chierici R et al.: Dietary supplements for the lactating mother: influence on the trace element content of milk, Acta Paediatr Suppl 88:7, 1999.

Daaboul J et al.: Vitamin D deficiency in pregnant and breast-feeding women and their infants, J Perinatol 17:10, 1997.

Dermer A: A campaign for breast-feeding, Top Clin Nutr 11:18, 1996.

Dewey KG: Energy and protein requirements during lactation, Ann Rev Nutr 17:19, 1997.

Dewey KG: Effects of maternal caloric restriction and exercise during lactation, J Nutr 128:386S, 1998.

DiGregorio S et al.: Osteoporosis with vertebral fractures associated with pregnancy and lactation, Nutrition 16:1052, 2000.

Duskieker LB et al.: Effect of supplemental fluids on human milk production, J Pediatr 106:207, 1985.

Duskieker LB et al.: Prolonged maternal fluid supplementation in breast feeding, Pediatrics 86:737, 1990.

Fung EB et al.: Zinc absorption in women during pregnancy and lactation: a longitudinal study, Am J Clin Nutr 66:80, 1997.

Gonzalez-Cossio T et al.: Impact of food supplementation during lactation on infant breast milk intake and on the proportion of infants exclusively breast-fed, J Nutr 128:1692, 1998.

Greer FR et al.: Effects of maternal ultraviolet B irradiation on vitamin D content of human milk, J Pediatr 105:431, 1984a.

Greer FR et al.: High concentrations of vitamin D_2 in human milk associated with pharmacologic doses of vitamin D_2, J Pediatr 105:61, 1984b.

Haskell MJ and Brown KH: Maternal vitamin A nutriture and the vitamin A content of human milk, J Mammary Gland Biol Neoplasia 4:243, 1999.

Hediger ML et al:. Early infant feeding and growth status of U.S.-born infants and children aged 4–71 months: analysis from the third national Health and Nutrition Examination Survey, 1988-1994, Am J Clin Nutr 72:159, 2000.

Hopkinson JM et al.: Milk production by mothers of premature infants: influence of cigarette smoking, Pediatrics 90:934, 1992.

Humphreys AS et al.: Intention to breast-feed in low-income pregnant women: the role of social support and previous experience, Birth 25:169, 1998.

Institute of Medicine: Dietary reference intakes for calcium, phosphorus, magnesium, vitamin D, and fluoride, Washington, DC, 1997, National Academy Press.

Institute of Medicine: Dietary reference intakes for thiamin, riboflavin, niacin, vitamin B_6, folate, vitamin B_{12}, pantothenic acid, biotin, and choline, Washington, DC, 1998, National Academy Press.

Institute of Medicine: Dietary reference intakes for vitamin C, vitamin E, selenium, and carotenoids, Washington, DC, 2000, National Academy Press.

Institute of Medicine: Dietary reference intakes for vitamin A, vitamin K, arsenic, boron, chromium, copper, iodine, iron, manganese, molybdenum, nickel, silicon, vanadium, and zinc, Washington, DC, 2001, National Academy Press.

Institute of Medicine, Food and Nutrition Board: Nutrition during lactation (report of the Subcommittee on Lactation, Committee on Nutritional Status during Pregnancy and Lactation), Washington, DC, 1991, National Academy Press.

Janney CA et al.: Lactation and weight retention, Am J Clin Nutr 66:1116, 1997.

Klein CJ et al.: A longitudinal study of urinary calcium, magnesium, and zinc excretion in lactating and non-lactating postpartum women, Am J Clin Nutr 61:779, 1995.

Lawrence RA and Lawrence RM: Breastfeeding: a guide for the medical profession, St. Louis, 1999, Mosby.

Lovelady CA et al.: The effect of weight loss in over-weight, lactating women on the growth of their infants, N Engl J Med 342:449, 2000.

Makrides M and Gibson RA: Long-chain polyunsaturated fatty acid requirements during pregnancy and lactation, Am J Clin Nutr 71:307S, 2000.

Mihok MA: An evaluation of the use impact of the enhanced food package for breast-feeding women in the Pennsylvania WIC Program, 1997 (unpublished).

Montgomery DL and Splett PL: Economic benefits of breast-feeding infants enrolled in WIC, J Am Diet Assoc 97:379, 1997.

Moore K et al.: New guidelines for breast-feeding, RN 61:36, 1998.

Motil KJ et al.: Lean body mass of well-nourished women is preserved during lactation, Am J Clin Nutr 67:292, 1998.

National Research Council: Recommended dietary allowances, ed 10, Washington, DC, 1989, National Academy Press.

Ortega RM et al.: Influence of smoking on vitamin E status during the third trimester of pregnancy and on breast-milk tocopherol concentrations in Spanish women, Am J Clin Nutr 68:662, 1998.

Pesa JA and Shelton MM: Health-enhancing behaviors correlated with breast-feeding among a national sample of mothers, Public Health Nurs 16:120, 1999.

Prentice A: Maternal calcium metabolism and bone mineral status, Am J Clin Nutr 71:1312S, 2000.

Rivera-Calinim L: The significance of drugs in breast milk, Clinical Perinatol 14:51, 1987.

Ross Products Division of Abbott Laboratories: Mothers' survey, 1997.

Sanders TAB: Essential fatty acid requirements of vegetarians in pregnancy, lactation, and infancy, Am J Clin Nutr 70:555S, 1999.

Specker BL: Do North American women need supplemental vitamin D during pregnancy or lactation?, Am J Clin Nutr 59:484S, 1994.

Spisak S, Gross SS: Second follow-up report: the Surgeon General's workshop on breast-feeding and human lactation, Washington, DC, 1991, National Center for Education on Maternal and Child Health.

Strode MA et al.: Effects of short-term caloric restriction on lactational performance of well-nourished women, Acta Paediatr Scand 75:222, 1986.

Stumbo PJ et al.: Water intakes of lactating women, Am J Clin Nutr 42:870, 1985.

Susin LR et al.: Does parental breast-feeding knowledge increase breast-feeding rates?, Birth 26:149, 1999.

U.S. Department of Health and Human Services: Healthy people 2010: national health promotion and disease prevention objectives (conference edition), Washington, DC, 2000a, U.S. Department of Health and Human Services.

U.S. Department of Health and Human Services: HHS blueprint for action on breast-feeding, Washington, DC, 2000b, U.S. Department of Health and Human Services Office on Women's Health.

von Kries R et al.: Does breast-feeding protect against childhood obesity?, Adv Exp Med Biol 478:29, 2000.

Wagner CL et al.: Special properties of human milk, Clin Pediatr (Phila) 35:283, 1996.

World Health Organization: Consensus statement from the consultation on HIV transmission and breast-feeding, J Hum Lact 8:173, 1992.

APPLICATION

Counseling for Breast-Feeding Success

In the early days and weeks of lactation, mother and baby learn the art of breast-feeding. Many new mothers need support or knowledge to help this process go well and occasionally infants have physical traits or behaviors that hamper progress. Therefore many hospitals and health clinics employ a lactation specialist. The lactation specialist is typically a health professional with interest and expertise in breast-feeding. Lactation specialists promote breast-feeding and provide assistance and support for nursing mothers and their babies. Their knowledge and skill can make the difference between a successful breast-feeding experience and lactation failure. In the following story a lactation specialist in a WIC clinic (Traci) helps a client (Laurie) establish a healthy breast-feeding relationship with her first child (Mark). Our story begins as the phone rings in Traci's office.

TRACI: Madison County WIC; may I help you?
LAURIE: Traci, this is Laurie. You talked to me about breast-feeding when I was in the clinic last month. I think there is something wrong with my milk. What should I do?
TRACI: Tell me what you're experiencing.
LAURIE: My baby, Mark, was born 4 days ago. Things went fine in the hospital. A nurse showed me how to hold him and help him latch on. He seemed very content and slept a lot. This morning when I got up my breasts were large and hurt. They feel awful. It hurts when I try to feed Mark and he cries and won't eat.
TRACI: How often did Mark nurse yesterday?
LAURIE: He slept a lot. I guess I fed him 6 or 7 times.
TRACI: Do you have a fever?
LAURIE: No, but my breasts feel like bricks! Do you know what is wrong?
TRACI: From what you are describing it sounds like your milk has come in. New moms often experience some temporary fullness or engorgement when this happens. When your breasts become too full it is difficult for Mark to latch on properly. He may be sucking on only your nipple. That hurts you and he won't get much milk so he cries.
LAURIE: So I shouldn't nurse him?
TRACI: No, the way to get over this problem is to get a little bit of the milk out of your breasts so he can latch on, then nurse him frequently so your breasts won't become so full. The problem usually clears up within a few days.
LAURIE: My breasts really hurt. What should I do?
TRACI: Try taking a warm shower, then express or pump a little milk out to soften your breasts. Do you have a pump?
LAURIE: Yes, I got one at the hospital.
TRACI: After you pump a little milk out, see if Mark can nurse. Remember to get some of the dark area around your nipple into his mouth, not just your nipple. Try feeding him every 2 to 3 hours during the day. You can put ice on your breasts between feedings to help reduce the swelling and help you feel more comfortable.
LAURIE: Ice? I'll try it.
TRACI: Good. Would you call me this afternoon, when it is convenient for you, to let me know how things are going?
LAURIE: Yes, I'll try. Bye. I'm going to go find the pump.
TRACI: Goodbye. Talk to you later.

That afternoon Laurie called back.

TRACI: Hi Laurie. Thanks for calling back. How are you doing?
LAURIE: Not great, but better. Mark was able to nurse after I pumped a little milk out. My breasts are still sore, but they're not as bad as this morning. Mark has nursed every 2 hours today. I don't like the ice, but it helps.
TRACI: It sounds like you are coping well. It might be a good idea to nurse once or twice during the night. That way your breasts won't get too full for Mark to latch on again.
LAURIE: Okay. I sure don't want that to happen again.
TRACI: You'll be glad to know that engorgement doesn't last long. I think you'll feel better tomorrow. Will you call me again?
LAURIE: Yes. Thanks. Bye.

The next day Laurie called.

TRACI: Laurie, thanks for calling. How are you and Mark doing today?

LAURIE: Well, I had to pump a bit this morning, but it's not nearly as bad. I don't think I'll need the ice today.
TRACI: Great. I'd continue to nurse at least every 3 hours during the day and once at night for a few days. You're over the hump!

The next week Laurie stopped in at the clinic.

TRACI: Hi, Laurie. Good to see you.
LAURIE: Hi. Mark just had his first check-up and I stopped in to say thanks. I also have a question. The doctor said he has gained 4 ounces. That doesn't sound like much to me for 10 days and my breasts don't feel so full anymore. Do you think that I have enough milk?
TRACI: Four ounces is a good weight gain for a 10-day-old. Babies lose a little weight after they are born. They usually are back up to their birth weight by about one week. Mark seems to be right on track. It's normal for the breasts to feel softer once you and Mark have gotten a feeding routine down. I'm glad you are both doing well.
LAURIE: Me, too. I was afraid I couldn't breast-feed, but now I feel like I can.
TRACI: Great. See you at Mark's next check-up.

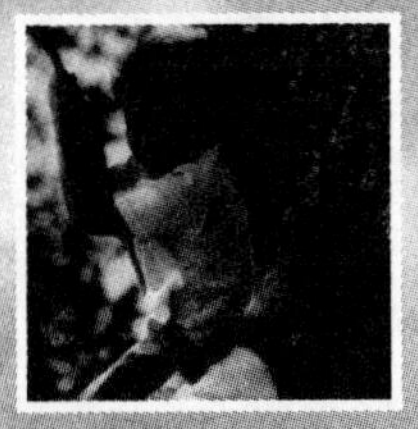

PART THREE

GROWTH AND DEVELOPMENT

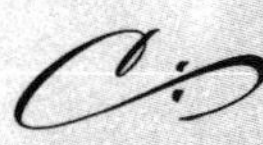

CHAPTER 7

Nutrition during Infancy

Chapter Outline

GROWTH AND DEVELOPMENT
ASSESSMENT OF NUTRITION STATUS
ENERGY AND NUTRIENT NEEDS
FEEDING INFANTS
NUTRITION-RELATED CONCERNS DURING INFANCY

Erin is a bright, active 1-year-old child and today is her birthday. She is celebrating by playing on her new swing set. With help she can climb to the top of the slide and sail to the bottom. She can sit on one of the swings, but someone has to push her. When the time comes, she will use both a spoon and her hands to eat cake and ice cream with enthusiasm. Last week at her medical check-up she weighed 9.1 kg (20 lb) and was 75.1 cm long (29.5 in). On the day she was born, 12 months ago, Erin measured 3.1 kg (6 lb, 8 oz) in weight and 50 cm (19.7 in) in length. By the time she was 5 months of age, she weighed 6.4 kg (14 lb) and was 64 cm (25 in) long.

Erin has changed dramatically in other ways as well. She started out almost totally dependent—she began with mostly visual exploration of her environment and nonspecific oral expression of her needs and progressed to maintaining eye contact, to cooing, to saying "da da" and "ma ma," and to using several words to communicate. She has progressed from holding her head up to rolling over, sitting up, crawling, standing, and walking short distances.

Erin's development is a typical example of the progressive growth and developmental changes that occur during the first year of life. These changes depend on many factors, including nutrition. As Erin moves into her second year she will grow more slowly, but will develop more skills, learn to interact with her environment, and develop more individuality and independence.

GROWTH AND DEVELOPMENT

- *What gains in length, weight, and head circumference can be expected for normal-term infants during the first year of life?*
- *How would you describe the velocity of growth during this period?*
- *How is growth measured and monitored?*
- *Describe the physical, neurocognitive, and psychosocial developmental changes that occur from birth to 1 year of age.*

At no time are extrauterine growth and development as rapid as during infancy. Although slow by comparison to the rate of fetal growth, gains during infancy are rapid in relation to those in the years that follow.

Physical Growth

Infancy is defined as the period of birth through 12 months of age. Differences in patterns of growth among individual infants are a function of genetic, hormonal, nutritional, and environmental influences. The mean birth weight of North American

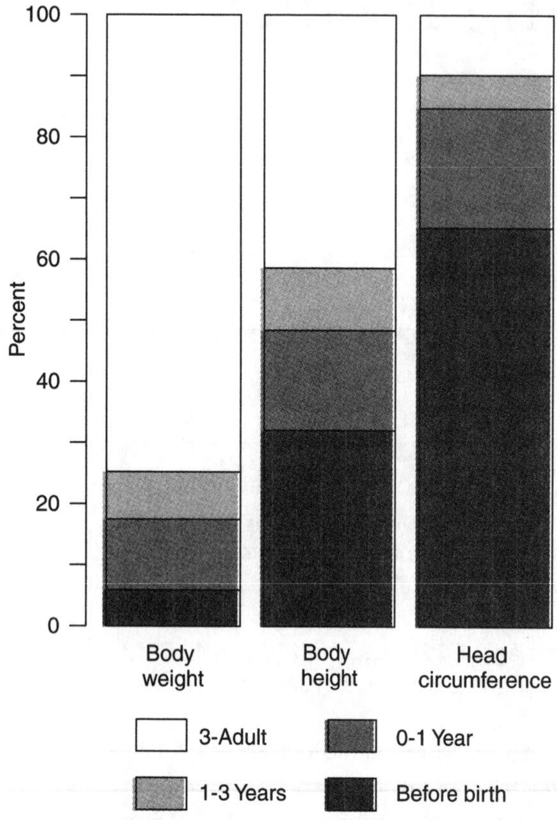

Figure 7-1 Growth in body parameters during development. *(From Valquist B: The young child: normal. In Jeliffe EF, editor: Human nutrition: a comprehensive treatise, vol 2: nutrition and growth, New York, 1979, Plenum Press.)*

infants falls between 3.0 kg and 3.4 kg (7 to 7.5 lb) and average birth length is approximately 50 cm (20 in) (Lowery, 1986). At birth the average head circumference is 33 cm to 35 cm (13 to 15 in), about one half the average adult size. Overall the full-term newborn male is slightly longer and heavier and has a larger head circumference than does the newborn female. As shown in Figure 7-1, body weight of the newborn is only approximately 5% of the eventual adult weight, but head circumference is almost 60%. These parameters increase substantially during early life. Although individual growth rates are rapid and highly variable during the first year, the infant generally triples her birth weight, gains about 50% in length, and gains approximately 30% in head circumference. In toddlerhood, or the second year of life, growth is much slower. Weight gain from 12 months to 24 months is approximately 2.5 kg (5.5 lbs) and height increases about 12 cm (4.5 in).

KEY TERMS

microcephaly: head circumference two or more standard deviations below the mean for age

Healthcare professionals are accustomed to plotting body measurements for infants on sex-specific growth charts for weight, length, weight-for-length, and head circumference. Growth charts from the National Center for Health Statistics (NCHS) Centers for Disease Control (CDC) in collaboration with the National Center for Chronic Disease Prevention and Health Promotion (CDC, 2000) developed to represent male and female infants and young children (aged 0 to 36 months) in the United States (see Research Update box). The charts are based on data collected from infants in five national health examination surveys and five supplementary data sources. These reference data for weight and recumbent length at various ages are used to compare the size of a particular infant to the reference population and identify infants with low or high weight or length for age. Growth charts for weight for age and length for age for boys and girls are in Appendix E2, E3, E4, and E5. Weight for length (Appendix E6 and E7 can be an indirect indicator of body fat accumulation, regardless of age. To some extent, growth of the skull parallels brain growth during the first 3 years of life and head circumference (Appendix E8 and E9) may reflect normality of brain development. **Microcephaly** usually suggests impaired development of the brain.

These growth charts do not consider genetic influences on infant size or individual growth rates and they may not be representative of infants from nonwhite populations. However, these charts are useful for tracking an individual infant's growth over time.

Interpretation of Growth Charts

The charts, or grids, (Figures 7-2 through 7-4) are divided at the third, fifth, tenth, twenty-fifth, fiftieth, seventy-fifth, ninetieth, ninety-fifth, and ninety-seventh percentiles. These percentiles

Text continued on p. 215

Research Update

Measuring Growth of Infants and Children

Growth charts are widely used as clinical and research tools to assess nutrition status, health, and general well-being of infants and children. Between 1977 and 2000 measurements of infants and children in the United States were charted on NCHS growth charts (NCHS, 1976). But in June 2000 those charts were replaced by the CDC growth charts that are presented in this text (CDC, 2000).

Growth charts are used extensively in private pediatric practice, public health clinics, and surveillance programs. Over time concerns about how representative the 1977 charts were for actual infants, children, and adults in the United States led to a reassessment and eventually a revision. Most of the questions about the 1977 charts centered on the concern that the infant charts were not representative of U.S. babies. The weights, heights, and head circumferences for infants were obtained from the Fels Longitudinal Study (Vital and Health Statistics, 2000). The Fels data were collected from 1929 to 1975 from a single longitudinal study of primarily formula-fed, white middle-class infants in a limited geographic area of southern Ohio. In addition to being a regional sample and not nationally representative, the Fels data were of concern because the observations were recorded at 3-month intervals (inadequate to present reference data at 1-month intervals used in the growth charts), the birth weights from 1929 to 1975 do not match recent national birth weight distributions, the difference between recumbent length and stature may have been too large (suggesting limitations in the recumbent length data), and the size and growth patterns of formula-fed infants do not represent growth patterns of combined breast- and formula-fed infants in the population (Victoria et al., 1998; WHO Working Group on the Growth of Reference Protocol, 1998).

The process for formulating revised, population-representative charts began in 1985 and involved representatives of many federal agencies, academic institutions with experience in child growth and growth charts, biostatistics, pediatric practice, and applied public health nutrition. The revised growth charts, developed to describe the size and growth of children in the United States, are based primarily on physical measurements taken as part of a series of national health examination surveys conducted by NCHS from 1963 to 1994. They include Cycles II and III of the National Health Examination Survey (NHES II and III) and three National Health and Nutrition Examination Surveys (NHANES I, II, and III). An important advantage of these data sets is the fact that the anthropometric data were obtained using standard pediatric procedures (Lohman et al., 1988).

To construct the revised charts, the national survey data were pooled with supplemental data to create a combined growth chart data set. Pooling data sets was required in part to obtain the necessary precision for calculating percentile distribution. In the growth chart data set, age was truncated to the nearest full month. Data were grouped by single month for age 1 month through 11 months, by 3-month intervals for age 12 months through 23 months, and by 6-month intervals from 24 months to 19 years. Statistical smoothing procedures were applied to the observed data to generate smoothed curves for selected percentiles and to generate parameters that can be used to produce additional percentiles.

The following are major features of revised charts:

- Development of BMI-for-age charts for children and adolescents
- Development of third and ninety-seventh smoothed percentiles for all charts
- Incorporation of data from five national surveys

The national survey data better represent the combined size and growth patterns of breast- and formula-fed infants in the general U.S. population (1971 to 1994) and replaced data for primarily formula-fed infants.

Another issue of concern in the use of the 1977 growth charts was the fact that the sample predominantly included white children. Differences in size and growth exist among the major racial and ethnic groups in the United States, but these variances appear to be small and inconsistent. Therefore the revised growth charts include all infants and children in the United States, regardless of race or ethnicity. The most important influences on growth potential appear to be economic, nutritional, and environmental factors (de Onis and Garza, 1997).

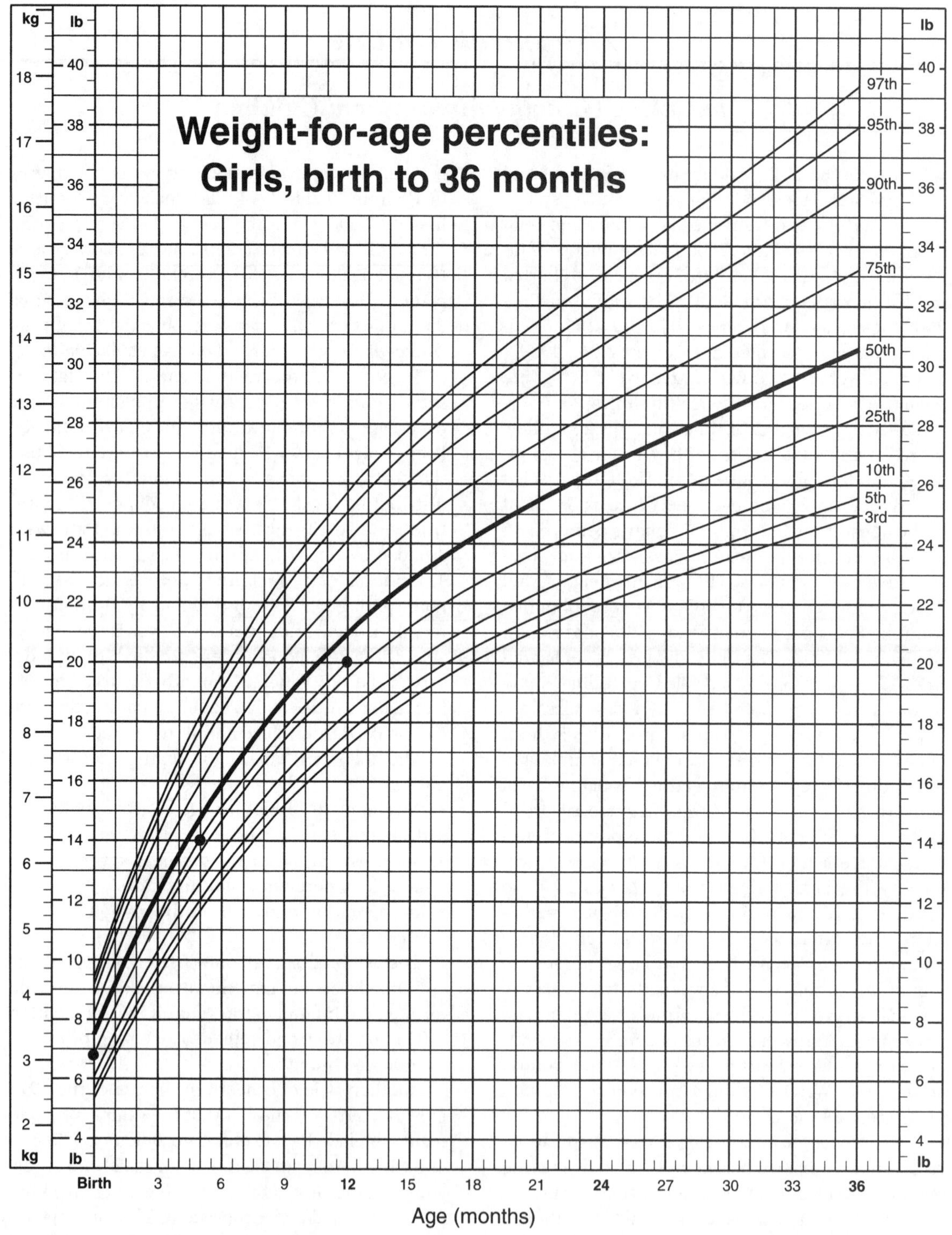

Figure 7-2 Erin's weight for age plotted on the weight-for-age percentiles for girls from birth to 36 months, CDC growth charts: United States. *(Growth chart only developed by the National Center for Health Statistics in collaboration with the National Center for Chronic Disease Prevention and Health Promotion, 2000.)*

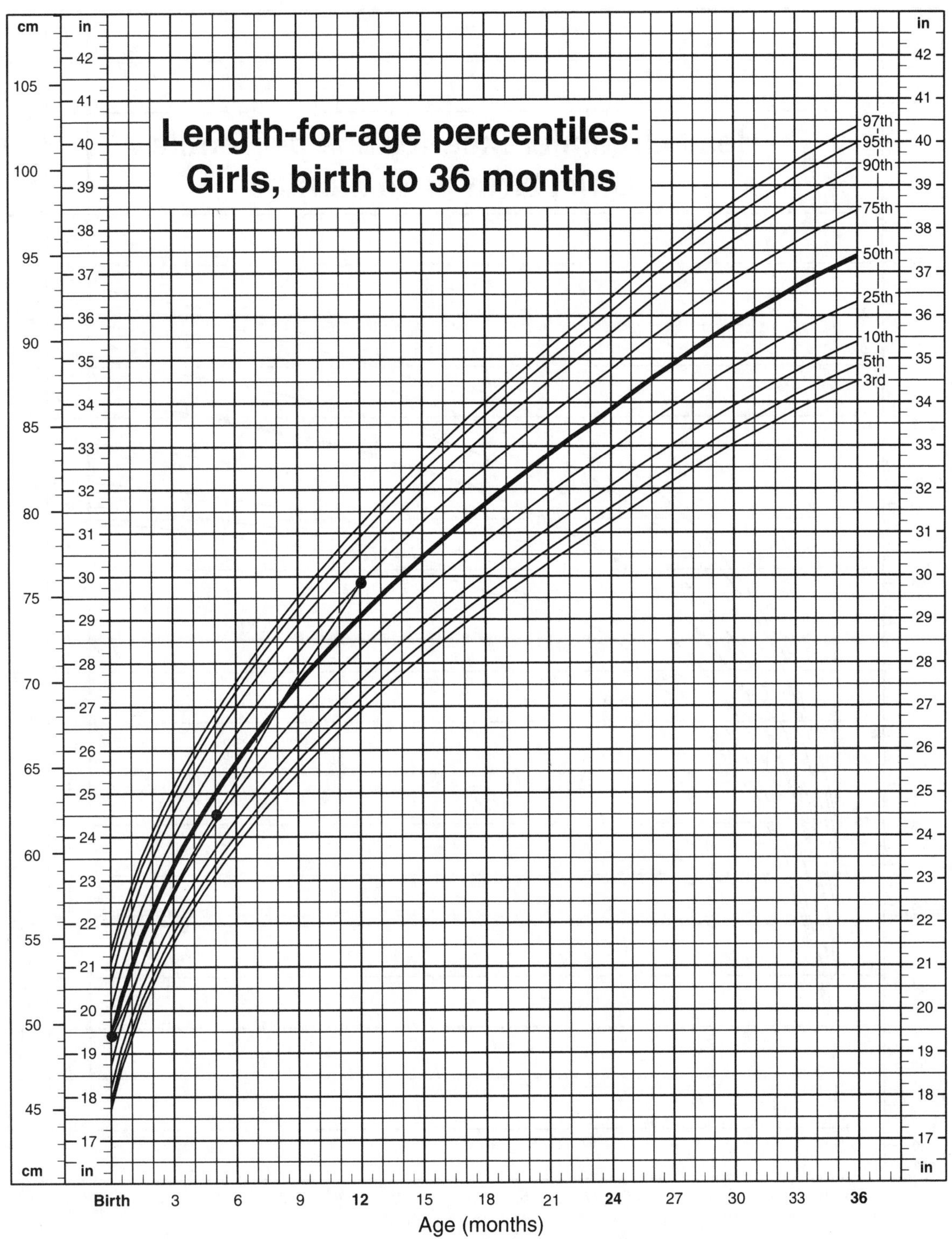

Figure 7-3 Erin's length for age plotted on the length-for-age percentiles for girls from birth to 36 months, CDC growth charts: United States. *(Growth chart only developed by the National Center for Health Statistics in collaboration with the National Center for Chronic Disease Prevention and Health Promotion, 2000.)*

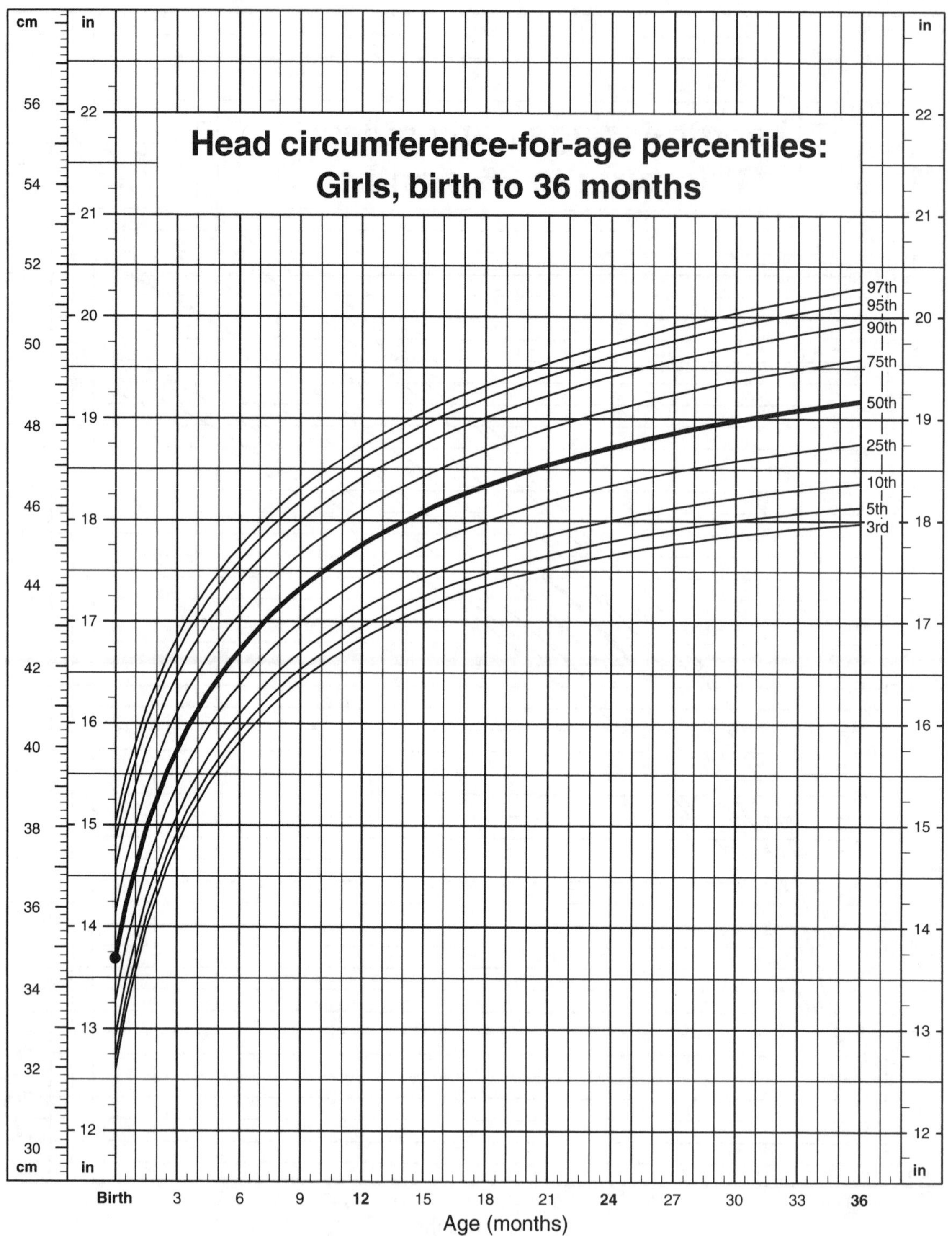

Figure 7-4 Erin's head circumference for age plotted on the head circumference-for-age percentiles for girls from birth to 36 months, CDC growth charts: United States. *(Growth chart only developed by the National Center for Health Statistics in collaboration with the National Center for Chronic Disease Prevention and Health Promotion, 2000.)*

represent the distribution of weight, length, and head circumference of the infants in the reference population. The percentile of an infant's weight, height, or head circumference is the point at which the age of the infant on the axis and the measurement along the abscissa intersect. For a true assessment of growth, measurements must be accurate (see p. 220-221). When plotted on the growth charts, Erin's birth weight of 3.1 kg (6 lb, 8 oz) and length of 50 cm (19.7 in) are at the twenty-fifth percentile and fiftieth percentile, respectively (see Figures 7-2 and 7-3). Erin's head circumference, 34.5 cm (13.6 in), is at the fiftieth percentile (see Figure 7-4).

Serial length, weight, and head circumference data are used to follow the growth of an individual infant, detect growth abnormalities, monitor nutrition status, and evaluate the effects of nutrition intervention. Erin's height, at the fiftieth percentile, indicates that 50% of the infants in the reference population were longer than Erin at birth. Her weight, at the twenty-fifth percentile, indicates that 75% of the reference infants were heavier. Percentile rankings for head circumference and weight-for-length are interpreted in the same fashion.

Successive measurements, plotted on growth charts, can be used to determine whether an infant is maintaining, reducing, or increasing his or her rate of growth compared with percentile channels or rankings. Such measurements give some indication of growth compared with the reference population by movement across the percentile ranking. For example an infant who, at 3 months, had a weight at the fifteenth percentile and at 6 months has a weight at the seventy-fifth percentile has gained weight more rapidly than might be expected. Although such a gain may be perfectly normal for that infant, it should trigger the attention of the healthcare professional to carefully assess factors contributing to such an unusual weight gain.

The 1977 NCHS growth charts were based on a population of bottle-fed infants. When compared with averages on the 1977 NCHS charts, breast-fed infants gain more rapidly early in infancy and less rapidly from 3 months to 12 months (Dewey et al., 1995). The new CDC growth charts are based on data from breast-fed infants and formula-fed infants (Binns et al., 1996; Victoria et al., 1998).

Velocity of Growth

An infant's length increases by approximately 2.5 cm (1 in) per month in the first 6 months. Gains then decrease to 1.2 cm (0.5 in) per month in the second 6 months. During the first month the average baby gains close to 1 kg (2.2 lb), or nearly 30 g (1 oz) per day. The monthly gain gradually declines and over the second 6 months the average increase is about 0.5 kg (1 lb) per month. Head circumference increases about 12 cm (4.7 in) from birth to age 1 year.

Although the NCHS charts allow assessment of changes in size of a specific infant relative to the reference population, such comparisons do not address the magnitude of the gains in length or weight in a specific time frame. Occasionally the **growth rate** can provide a more-accurate assessment of growth. Appendix E shows the fiftieth percentile of monthly increments in recumbent length and weight from birth to 12 months for the reference population from the Fels Longitudinal Study (Roche et al., 1989). These tables may be helpful in determining whether an infant's increases are occurring at an appropriate rate and in documenting increased growth in response to nutrition intervention in an undernourished infant.

Lampl and colleagues (1992) confirmed what mothers have known for years; that is, infants grow in spurts. These researchers measured infants up to 21 months of age and found that increases in length occurred in short-lived growth spurts of 0.5 cm to 2.5 cm (0.2 to 1.0 in) separated by periods of no apparent linear growth. Caution must be used in interpreting measurements of growth and growth velocity over short periods.

Development

As the brief description of Erin illustrated, dramatic developmental changes occur during the

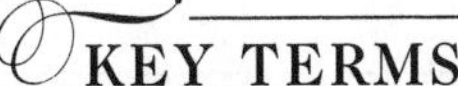

KEY TERMS

growth rate: growth increment divided by the time between measurements

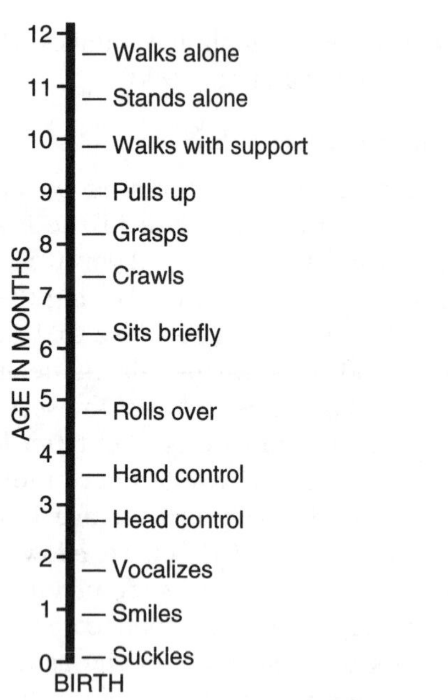

Figure 7-5 Behavioral development during the first year of life. *(From Guyton AC and Hall JE: Textbook of medical physiology, ed 9, Philadelphia, 1996, W.B. Saunders.)*

first year of life. Figure 7-5 highlights some major developmental changes and approximate ages at which they may occur. However, development is complex and encompasses neurodevelopment, cognitive and psychosocial development, and physical development. It is characterized by a progressive and irreversible sequence of events. Box 7-1 illustrates some of the characteristic developmental milestones of the first year of life. Because there is wide variation in the rate at which a normal infant progresses through these developmental stages, the ages at which each stage begins are approximate. Those given in the table represent the point at which 50% of infants have reached that stage.

Physical Development

Body proportions of newborn infants are sharply different from those of older infants, children, and adults. The head is relatively larger and the face is rounder. The chest tends to be rounded rather than flattened, the abdomen is more prominent, and the extremities are proportionally shorter.

Infancy is a period of substantial change in body composition. During the first few days of life a loss of fluid that averages about 6% of body weight occurs. With adequate dietary intake, birth weight is usually regained by day 10. The percentage of body weight that is fat increases from approximately 13% at birth to about 30% between 6 months and 9 months, then decreases to around 23% by 1 year of age (Butte et al., 2000) (Table 7-1) Protein, approximately 12% of body weight at birth, increases to about 15% by the end of the first year. As a percentage of body weight, fat-free body mass (lean body mass plus bone mass) decreases throughout infancy. This reduction results from the drop in water content from about 75% at birth to about 60% at 4 months of age and from a rise in body fat content.

In addition to the decline in the percentage of body weight that is water, there is a change in water distribution. At birth less than one half of body water is intracellular fluid (ICF), but that proportion increases to about two thirds as extracellular fluid (ECF) declines. Mineral content, about 3.3% of body weight, is mostly **osseous** and gradually increases to about 4.8% at age 18 years.

Growth of the human brain peaks at birth and during infancy. By the end of the first year, the brain has reached two-thirds of adult size. During infancy the first deciduous teeth erupt between 5 and 9 months of age. By 1 year of age most infants have between four and eight teeth.

Neurodevelopment

From the moment of birth, the term infant (gestation of 38 to 42 weeks) is able to fixate on objects visually and follow the movements of these objects. When infants are exposed to figures, they give preferential attention to those that resemble the human face. By 2 months of age a supine infant is able to follow an object as it is moved and attempts to make contact with an offered object.

At birth newborns can turn their head from side to side. By 4 weeks they can raise their head

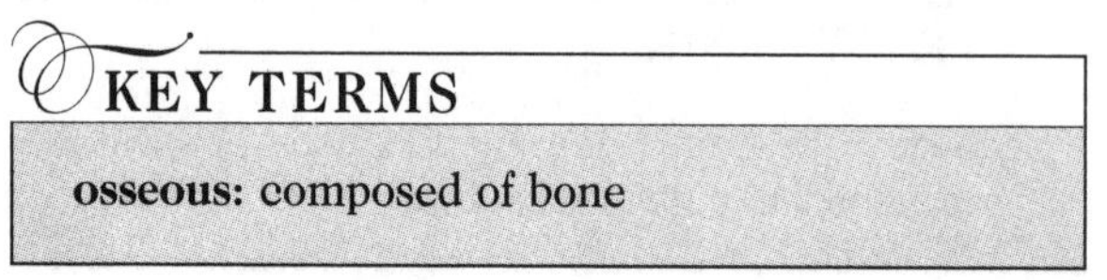
KEY TERMS

osseous: composed of bone

Box 7-1 Developmental Achievements during Infancy

4 WEEKS

Motor	
Gross	Poor control of head, neck, and trunk
Fine	Hands fisted
	Hands clench on contact
Adaptive	Regards object in line of vision only
	Follows to midline
	Drops toy immediately
Language	Vague indirect regard (receptive)
	Makes cooing sounds (expressive)
Personal/social	Stares indefinitely at surroundings
	Regards observer's face and diminishes activity

16 WEEKS

Motor	
Gross	Symmetric postures predominate
	Head steady in sitting
	Head lifted 90°; when on stomach, can support weight with straight elbows
Fine	Hands engage
	Reaches, grasps objects, brings to mouth
Adaptive	Eyes follow slowly moving object
	Waves arms on sight of toy
	Regards toy in hand and takes to mouth
	Regard goes from hand to object when sitting
Language	Laughs aloud
	Excites and breathes heavily
Personal/social	Responds to social overture with spontaneous smile or body movements
	Hand play with mutual fingering
	Pulls garment over face
	Anticipates food on sight

28 WEEKS

Motor	
Gross	Sits briefly leaning forward on hands
	Supports large fraction of weight in standing; rolls from back to front
	Bounces actively in supported standing
Fine	Has radial palmar grasp of toy
	Rakes at small pellet with whole hand
Adaptive	Rakes small object toward self
	Bangs and shakes rattle
	Transfers objects from one hand to other
	Uses sounds and gestures to communicate
Language	Talks to toys
Personal/social	Takes feet to mouth
	Reaches for and pats mirror image

40 WEEKS

Motor	
Gross	Sits steadily indefinitely
	Crawls, pulls self up to stand
Fine	Plucks pellet easily with thumb and index finger
Adaptive	Matches two objects in hands
	Index finger approach
	Spontaneously rings bell
Language	Says *mama* and *dada* with meaning
	Uses one other "word"
Personal/social	Waves "bye-bye" and does pat-a-cake (or other nursery trick)
	Feeds self cracker and holds own bottle

52 WEEKS

Motor	
Gross	Walks with one hand held
	Stands momentarily alone
Fine	Uses thumb and finger to hold small objects
Adaptive	Tries to build tower of two cubes
	Releases cube in cup (after demonstration)
Language	Two words besides *mama* and *dada*
	Gives toy on request or gesture
Personal/social	Offers toy to image in mirror
	Cooperates in dressing

From Hughes JG and Griffith JF: Synopsis of pediatrics, ed 6, St. Louis, 1984, Mosby.

Table 7-1 Body Composition of Reference Infants from Birth to 24 Months of Age

Age (months)	Weight (kg)	Fat		Fat-Free Body Mass	
		(kg)	%	(kg)	%
BOYS					
Birth	3.5	0.5	14	3.1	86
3	6.4	1.5	23	4.9	77
6	8.0	2.0	25	6.0	75
9	9.2	2.2	24	7.0	76
12	10.2	2.3	22	7.9	77
18	11.5	2.4	21	9.1	79
24	12.6	2.5	20	10.1	80
GIRLS					
Birth	3.3	0.5	15	2.8	85
3	5.7	1.4	24	4.4	76
6	7.3	1.9	26	5.3	74
9	8.3	2.1	25	6.2	75
12	9.2	2.2	24	7.0	76
18	10.8	2.4	22	8.4	78
24	11.9	2.4	20	9.5	79

Adapted from Fomon SJ et al.: Body composition of reference children from birth to age 10 years, Am J Clin Nutr 35:1169, 1982.

momentarily and at 2 months of age they can sustain that movement. At 5 months they can hold their head erect and steady. This accomplishment is followed shortly by the ability to roll over. At about the same stage infants can sit in an upright posture with support. By approximately 6 months of age, infants are able to change the orientation of their entire body to reach out toward a desired object.

Between 6 months and 9 months the grasp becomes clearly elaborated into movements involving the thumb and forefinger and by 9 months the thumb and forefinger can pick up a pellet with a pincer motion. In later infancy an infant's behavior becomes increasingly imitative. Nine-month-old infants can wave "bye-bye" or bring their hands together imitatively; at 12 months they may enter into very simple games with a toy such as a ball. By age 2 toddlers can run well, walk up and down stairs, and turn pages of a book singly.

Cognitive Development

Cognition. Infants become aware of their environment and respond in a variety of ways. **Cognition** begins with perception or comprehension of a question or problem, use of memory to determine if the problem resembles a past experience, and generation of ideas to bring about a possible solution. The final process is evaluation, as individuals measure the accuracy of their conclusions.

In the young infant there is little behavioral evidence of cognitive function, but evidence suggests that they make some perceptual (visual) choices when confronted with different patterns or objects. Later in infancy selective attention is given to familiar objects and anticipatory behavior is apparent as demonstrated by the infant quieting at the mother's approach. Another early indication of cognitive development may be curiosity and the exploration of surroundings and objects in the environment.

Cognitive development during the first 2 years of life is characterized by the appearance of repetitive activity that eventually becomes planned, indicating thinking before acting. Two major abilities that develop during this period are **object permanence** and **object recognition.**

Later cognitive development is reflected in the infant and toddler's efforts to manipulate the environment and imitate people.

Language

Infants are able to make repetitive vowel sounds by 6.5 months and can produce repetitive consonant sounds such as *ba ba* and *ma ma* by 8 months, although they do not necessarily associate these sounds with specific objects. By age 8 to 9 months, infants will be attentive to the sounds of their own names and they may knowingly use a few words by the age of 1 year. Toddlers will have a vocabulary of 50 to 75 words, or as many as 200, and will verbalize needs consistently.

Psychosocial Development

Visual, voice, and physical contact can elicit responses in the neonate. Bonding and attachment consist of those emotional ties and commitments that characterize the relationship between infants and significant persons in their environments to whom they turn for protection, nurturing, and love.

As early as 2 weeks to 6 weeks of age, infants can show that they are more comfortable with familiar persons than with strangers. In the early weeks patterns or rhythms of feeding and sleeping evolve, with the ability of infants to control their own state through self-stimulation, such as by finger-sucking or thumb-sucking. The interaction between the mother and the infant in the first weeks of life is initiated by the infant and becomes part of a growing and complex system of signals between infant and mother (or other caregiver). Through these communicative exchanges, emotional attachments are formed. In fact the consistency and promptness of the caregiver's response to the infant's behavior are more crucial to development than are caregiver's attempts to anticipate the needs of the infant. During the second year the child will play well with older children and imitate others through play.

All of these developmental changes are significant in the forming of the person each infant or toddler will be. But, as many pediatric and child development specialists have pointed out, nurturing of an infant is essential for development to occur. As T. Berry Brazelton, a prominent pediatrician, says, "Every baby needs a warm, intimate relationship with a primary caregiver over a period of years, not months or weeks" (Brazelton and Greenspan, 2000, p. 110).

ASSESSMENT OF NUTRITION STATUS

- *What are the methods of assessment most commonly used for infants and why?*
- *Describe anthropometric measurement of infants and how it is used in nutrition assessment.*
- *Why is accuracy of particular importance in measuring infants?*
- *What are the difficulties and advantages of determining dietary intakes of infants?*

The basic techniques of nutrition assessment described in Chapter 2 apply to infants. During this period of rapid growth emphasis is usually placed on growth and hematologic status, but clinical and dietary data are important components of a complete assessment.

Anthropometry

Growth changes are relatively large during the first year of life and monitoring the progression of growth via anthropometry is a primary tool of assessment. Recumbent length, weight, and head circumference are measured on every newborn and are repeated on successive visits to the clinic or physician's office. The keys to successfully monitoring an infant's growth are *accuracy* and *reliability* of each measurement (see Chapter 2). When an infant is evaluated in a healthcare setting, the most common reason for an

KEY TERMS

cognition: the means by which an individual accumulates organized knowledge of the world and the use of that knowledge to solve problems and modify behavior

object permanence: knowledge that objects continue to exist although not being perceived

object recognition: use of previously acquired information to identify an object

unexpected deviation in measurement is an error in technique. Measurements should be repeated, recorded, and plotted on growth charts immediately to reduce the chance of error. Growth measurements are plotted on standardized charts (such as the CDC charts in Appendix E) to allow comparison of an individual infant's values with statistical norms based on a representative population.

Recumbent Length

Recumbent length is measured with the infant in a supine position on a table equipped with a fixed headboard and a movable footboard that are perpendicular to the table surface. A measuring tape is secured along one or both sides of the table. Measurement of recumbent length in infants usually requires two individuals (Figure 7-6). To get an accurate measurement, the infant is placed so the crown of the head touches the headboard and the center line of the body is lined up with the center line of the measuring table. The shoulders and buttocks should be flat against the tabletop. One measurer standing behind the end of the table positions the head, ensuring that the baby does not change position, and checks that the body is aligned with the long axis of the table. The legs are extended at the hips and knees to lie flat against the tabletop. The arms rest against the sides of the trunk. The second measurer places one hand on the knees to ensure that the legs remain flat on the table and, applying firm pressure, moves the footboard against the soles of the feet. The length is recorded to the nearest 0.1 cm or ⅛ inch.

A very young or fussy infant may require gentle restraint to ensure adequate positioning. The more the positioning of an infant deviates from the guidelines, the lower is the reliability of the measurement.

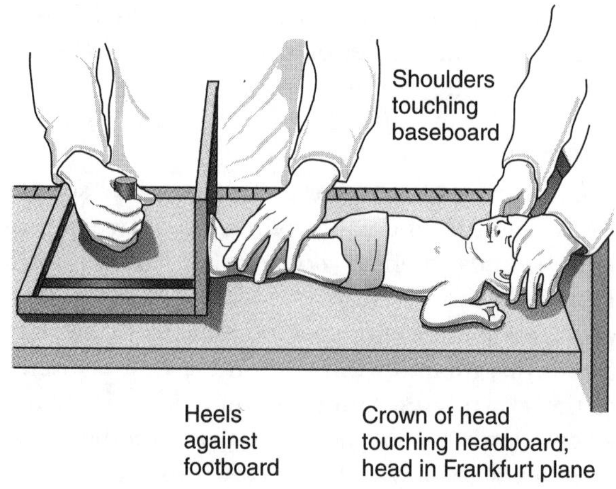

Figure 7-6 Measurement of recumbent length.

Weight

Infants can be weighed using a pan scale with a beam and moveable weights or with an electronic scale (Figure 7-7). The pan of the scale must be large enough to support an older infant or child up to about age 2 years. The scale must be leveled; if the infant is to be weighed with a blanket or diaper, the scale must be calibrated to zero with the blanket or diaper before the infant is weighed. The infant is placed on the scale so that the weight is distributed evenly on the pan. Weight is recorded to the nearest 0.1 kg or 0.25 lb while the infant is lying quietly. As with length, weight is recorded in tabular form and plotted on the growth chart. If an infant is restless or crying, it may be better to postpone the measurement and try again later when the infant is calmer.

Circumferences

In children younger than 36 months, head circumference is closely related to brain size and linear growth. Head circumference is measured with a flexible, nonstretch tape about 0.6 inches wide. The infant is seated on the lap of the mother or caretaker and the measurer positions the tape so that the zero end is on the front of the head. The tape is placed around the head with the ends overlapping so the zero mark on the tape is underneath the value to be recorded (Figure 7-8). The tape is placed just above the eyebrows so that the maximum circumference is measured. The tape must be in the same plane on both sides of the head. The tape is pulled firmly to compress hair and the measurement to the nearest 0.1 cm is recorded.

The length, weight, and head circumference should be recorded on the form and plotted on growth charts before the infant leaves the office

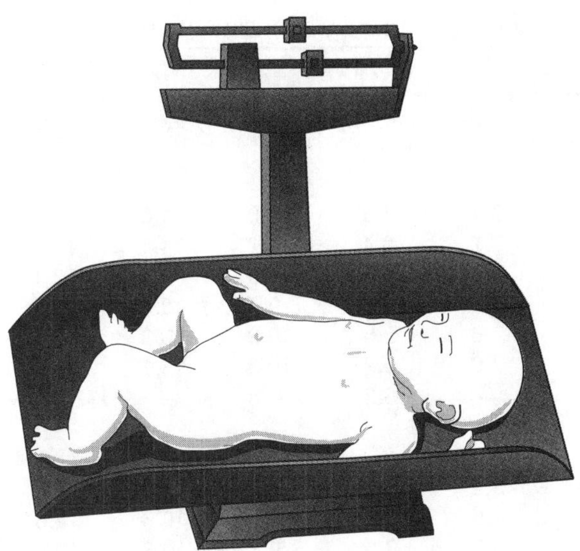

Figure 7-7 Pan scale with beam and moveable weights for weighing infants.

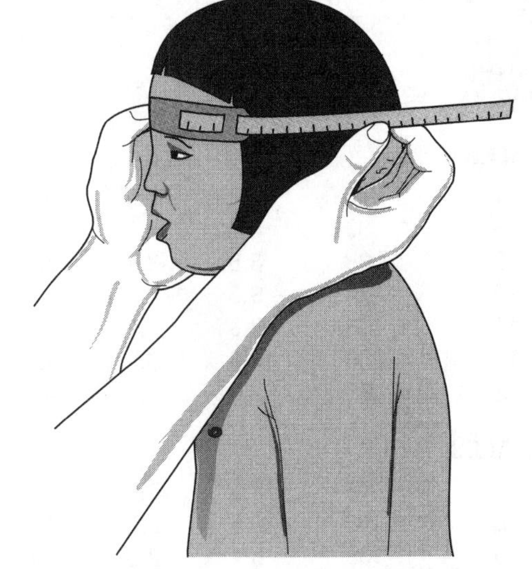

Figure 7-8 Measurement of head circumference.

or clinic. If a major discrepancy appears, the measurer can check the accuracy of the plotting and, if necessary, repeat the measurement in question.

Fatfolds

Estimation of body fatness using the fatfold measurement assumes that all components of the body maintain a relatively constant proportion, which is not true of early growth.

Fatfolds are not part of routine nutrition screening, but can be used to clarify nutrition status when weight-for-stature measures below the tenth percentile or above the ninetieth percentile. Triceps fatfold measurements have been completed on a population of infants 7 months to 13 months of age; percentiles appear in Table 7-2.

Biochemical Assessment

Blood and urine tests are not used extensively in the assessment of nutrition status of infants. If marginal nutrition status is suspected, biochemical assessment may be initiated using age-specific standards. In an outpatient or clinic setting, an estimate of iron status may be made using a small amount of blood obtained from a finger-stick to determine the hematocrit or hemoglobin level.

The Centers for Disease Control and Prevention recommends that infants and children aged 6 months to 5 years of age be screened for excess blood lead levels. Because infants or children most susceptible to lead toxicity are often those who are also at risk for iron deficiency, both measurements should be made.

Dietary Assessment

Breast-Fed Infants

It is assumed that breast-fed infants who have ample opportunity to nurse, have an adequate weight gain, and seem satisfied are receiving a sufficient quantity of milk to meet nutritional needs. Other indicators are at least one stool per day and six to eight wet diapers each day. If there is some question regarding the adequacy of the infant's milk intake, it may be necessary to question the mother in detail regarding the frequency and length of nursing periods.

Formula-Fed Infants

It is fairly simple to determine an infant's total formula consumption by measuring the amount in the bottle at the beginning of the feeding and

Table 7-2 TRICEPS SKINFOLD PERCENTILE VALUES FOR INFANTS 7 TO 13 MONTHS OF AGE

Age (months)	n	Mean	SD	Percentile 5th	10th	25th	50th	75th	90th	95th
MALES										
7	45	9.2	3.1	—	5.9	7.1	7.5	8.0	11.0	—
8	80	8.8	2.2	5.0	5.9	7.2	8.4	9.2	11.1	11.8
9	95	8.8	2.1	5.2	5.8	7.2	8.6	9.6	11.1	12.1
10	124	9.3	2.3	5.4	6.2	7.4	8.6	9.7	10.8	12.6
11	103	9.3	3.1	5.6	6.8	7.6	8.8	10.3	13.3	15.0
12	68	10.0	3.5	5.6	7.0	7.6	9.3	10.3	13.1	15.9
13	30	9.5	2.5	—	—	—	9.5	—	—	—
FEMALES										
7	46	8.2	2.5	—	3.0	5.2	7.5	9.0	11.0	—
8	88	8.6	2.7	3.0	3.5	5.5	7.5	9.3	10.8	12.0
9	109	8.4	2.5	3.7	4.2	5.6	7.5	9.2	10.8	12.0
10	120	8.7	2.3	3.9	4.6	5.8	7.7	9.5	11.1	13.3
11	95	9.4	3.5	4.4	5.0	6.0	8.3	9.7	11.1	13.8
12	70	9.2	2.7	5.2	5.4	6.4	8.9	10.2	11.1	12.3
13	27	9.5	1.9	—	—	—	9.2	—	—	—

From Ryan AS and Martinez GA: Physical growth of infants 7 to 13 months of age: results from a national survey, Am J Phys Anthropo 73:449, 1987.

subtracting the amount that remains in the bottle after the infant finishes nursing. The actual amount of formula that is fed can be compared with estimated requirements.

Supplementary Foods

Because someone is responsible for feeding the infant, that individual need only record the amount of a food offered (or the proportions in mixed foods such as cereal and milk) and the amount that remains at the end of feeding. After the quantities of breast milk, formula, and supplementary foods consumed have been determined, the infant's intake of energy and nutrients can be calculated from food composition data.

ENERGY AND NUTRIENT NEEDS

- *Compare and contrast the energy and nutrient needs of a term infant to those of an adult.*
- *Why do recommendations for energy and protein intakes per kilogram of body weight decrease after 6 months of age?*
- *Of which nutrients do term infants have body stores at birth?*

The rapid growth and major changes in body composition of infancy create high qualitative and quantitative demands for energy and nutrients. In fact an infant's requirements for many nutrients, per kilogram of body weight, are two or more times greater than are those of an adult. Obviously any inadequacy in intake will have measurable and potentially long-term effects on the infant's health and well-being.

Energy

The components of energy requirements of the healthy term infant are basal metabolic rate, the thermic effect of food, physical activity, maintenance, growth, and energy losses in urine and feces (Figure 7-9). The Recommended Dietary Allowance (RDA) for energy during infancy represents the sum of these expenditures.

The basal metabolic rate that constitutes the largest portion of the energy expenditure has been estimated as 48 kcal/kg to 55 kcal/kg per day (21 to 25 kcal/lb per day) and remains relatively constant during infancy. The energy required to maintain body temperature in the early ex-

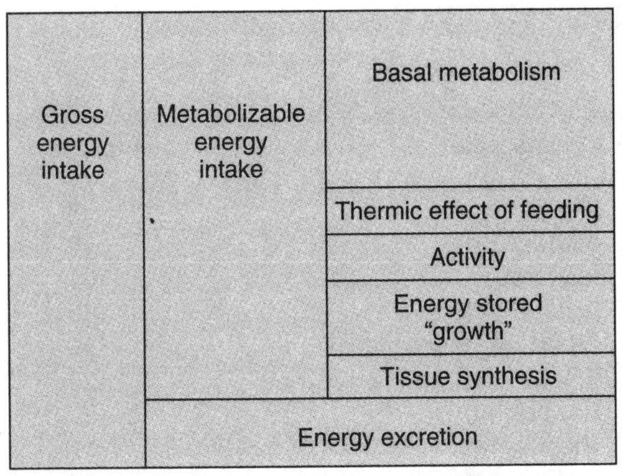

Figure 7-9 Components of energy expenditure. *(From Butte NF: Energy requirement during infancy. In Tsang RC and Nichols BL, editors: Nutrition during infancy, Philadelphia, 1988, Hanley & Belfus.)*

trauterine period is a significant component of this expenditure, but decreases with time. Growth, the second largest energy cost in early infancy, is the sum of the energy content of tissue synthesized and the energy cost of synthesis. The total cost of growth approximates 4 kcal/g to 6 kcal/g of tissue gained. The proportion of energy expended for growth decreases with time, especially after 6 months. The energy cost of physical activity is low in the neonate, but it increases as infancy progresses, offsetting the decreased expenditure for growth. The thermic effect of food is estimated at 5% to 10% of the energy intake, or approximately 4 kcal/kg to 5 kcal/kg per day. Energy lost in excretory products (urine and feces) is relatively small, but it is proportionally greater than that of adults.

Although energy needs per kilogram of body weight decline during the first year of life, total energy intakes increase with body size. For example the daily caloric recommendations for a female infant whose weight is at the fiftieth percentile on the CDC growth chart would begin at less than 400 kcal per day shortly after birth and increase to almost 1000 kilocalories over a period of 12 months (Table 7-3). Similar values for boys would be slightly higher because body weight at the fiftieth percentile is approximately 1 lb higher. Recommended Dietary Allowances (National Research Council [NRC], 1989) for en-

Table 7-3 Projected Daily Energy and Protein Intakes for a Female Infant

Age (mo)	Weight (kg)	Energy (kcal/day)	Protein (g)
Newborn	3.2	350	7
3	5.4	580	12
6	7.2	700	14
9	8.6	840	17
12	9.6	940	19

ergy during infancy are 108 kcal/kg of body weight for 0 to 6 months and 98 kcal/kg for 6 to 12 months. The Institute of Medicine is in the process of completing the Daily Recommended Intakes (DRIs) for energy and macronutrients.

Protein

Providing sufficient protein for the growing infant involves not only supplying an adequate quantity of protein, but also providing protein of high biologic value and an adequate amount of energy.

Protein Quantity

Protein requirements have been estimated in two ways: factorial estimates and intake levels of healthy breast-fed infants. A factorial estimate is the sum of protein required for growth and for replacement of inevitable losses of nitrogen in urine and feces (1 g nitrogen = 6.25 g protein). Factorial estimations yield a protein requirement of 1.98 g/kg per day during the first month of life, which decreases to 1.18 g/kg per day by 4 months to 5 months of age, then continues at that level to age 1 year (Fomon, 1991). Average protein intakes of breast-fed infants in developed countries are 2.04 g/kg per day in the first 3 months and 1.73 g/kg per day in the next 3 months (World Health Organization, 1985). The two estimates are quite similar when a margin of safety is added to factorial estimates. The RDAs for protein (0 to 6 months, 2.2 g/kg; 6 to 12 months, 2.0 g/kg) are based on the assumption that the protein consumed will be of the same quality as that in human milk (NRC, 1989). For the first 4 months, when such a protein provides 6.5% to 8% of total energy, protein intake will meet the requirements if the energy needs are met. If the protein is of lesser quality the amounts required will be greater. After 4 months to 6 months of age it may be necessary to add other foods to the breast milk or formula diet of the infant to meet protein needs. The approximate amounts of protein recommended for a female infant whose weight is at the fiftieth percentile on the CDC charts are shown in Table 7-3.

Protein intakes in excess of the body's need for maintenance and growth will not enhance growth or health. In fact excess amino acids require deamination in the liver so that the nonprotein portion can be used for energy. The liver must then convert the nitrogen portion to urea to be excreted by the kidney. Because the infant's ability to concentrate urine is limited, additional excretory products, such as urea from the catabolism of excess protein, require a larger volume of water and unnecessarily increase the workload of the kidney.

Protein Quality

Not all proteins are of equal biologic value or quality. Infants require nine essential amino acids in varying amounts (Table 7-4). Three additional amino acids, cystine, taurine, and tyrosine, have been referred to as conditionally essential or semiessential because they may be required by young infants under certain circumstances. For example tyrosine is produced in the body through enzymatic breakdown of phenylalanine. In some very young infants, the enzyme for this conversion may not be fully developed, therefore making a dietary source necessary. The quality of a protein depends on the amount of essential amino acids it contains in proportion to requirements. The composition of human milk is considered the reference pattern for human infants and serves as a guide for the formulation of human milk substitutes and supplementary feeding.

Adequate Energy Intake

Use of dietary amino acids for protein synthesis requires an adequate supply of energy. If kilocalories are inadequate, protein is used for energy and protein status suffers. Optimal growth cannot be maintained and, in severe cases, gains in length and weight slow or even cease.

Table 7-4 ESTIMATED AMINO ACID REQUIREMENTS FOR INFANTS 3-4 MONTHS OF AGE

Amino Acid	mg/kg/day
Histidine	28
Isoleucine	70
Leucine	161
Lysine	103
Methionine + cystine	58
Phenylalanine + tyrosine	125
Threonine	87
Tryptophan	17
Valine	93

Lipids

More than one half of the kilocalories in human milk come from fat. Dietary fat is a concentrated source of energy, a carrier of fat-soluble vitamins, and a source of essential fatty acids. Dietary essential fatty acids linoleic (18:2 omega-6) and alpha linolenic (18:3 omega-3) acid are precursors of the long-chain polyunsaturated fatty acids (LCPUFA) arachadonic acid (AA) (C24:4 omega-6) and docosahexaenoic acid (DHA) (C22:6 omega-3). During fetal growth the fatty acids are supplied through the placenta. Both DHA and AA function as precursors for eicosanoids, which include prostaglandins and leukotriene, that are components of numerous cellular signaling mechanisms, and are functionally important components of membrane phospholipids (Gibson and Makrides, 2000). Essential fatty acids and their metabolites are found in high concentrations in the phospholipids of all cells, especially in membranes of the brain and neural cells. Compared with cow milk, human milk is higher in polyunsaturated fatty acids, both omega-3 and omega-6 fatty acids, providing 6% of total kcal. The presumed daily requirement of linoleic acid is 2.7% of total calories (American Academy of Pediatrics, 1998).

A number of studies of preterm and low-birth-weight infants have demonstrated low biologic levels of essential fatty acids. To provide sufficient amounts for normal growth and development, formulas developed for these small babies are supplemented with LCPUFA. Recently there has been speculation on potential benefits of LCPUFA supplementation for term formula-fed infants.

Carbohydrate

Carbohydrate is a major contributor to energy intake and should be prominent in the diet of an infant. Lactose is the carbohydrate source in human milk and many cow-milk formulas. As infants begin to consume other foods, the percentage of calories obtained from carbohydrate increases as the proportion obtained from fat decreases. Approximately 20% to 25% of infants in the United States are fed lactose-free soy isolate formulas containing sucrose or corn syrup solids or a combination of both as carbohydrate sources (American Academy of Pediatrics, 1998).

Energy and Nutrient Recommendations

For the purposes of reporting reference intakes, infancy covers the period of birth through 12 months of age and is divided into two 6-month intervals. The first 6-month interval was not subdivided further because intake was considered to be relatively constant during this time. As infants grow, they ingest more food; however, on a kcal/kg of body weight basis the intake declines slightly. As growth velocity slows during the second 6 months, total daily nutrient needs on a body-weight basis may be less than those during the first 6 months of life, but total intake increases. After 12 months of age, Dietary Reference Intakes are grouped for 1 to 3 years. The age categories for DRI are 0 to 6 months, 6 to 12 months, and 1 to 3 years.

For a particular nutrient, average intake by full-term infants who are born to presumably healthy, well-nourished mothers and exclusively fed human milk has been adopted as the primary basis for deriving the Adequate Intake (AI) for most nutrients during the first 6 months of life (Institute of Medicine, 1998).

Using the human milk-fed infant as a model is consistent with the basis for estimating nutrient allowances for infants and supports the recommendation that exclusive human milk feeding is the preferred method of feeding for normal full-term infants for the first 4 months to 6 months of life. This recommendation has also been made by the American Dietetic Association (1997), the American Academy of Pediatrics (1997), and the Food and Nutrition Board report *Nutrition during Lactation* (Institute of Medicine, 1991).

For infants from birth through age 6 months, the AI value is the mean intake of a nutrient based on the average concentration of the nutrient from 2 months to 6 months of lactation. An average volume of 780 ml of milk per day has been reported from studies of full-term infants (Butte et al., 1984). Because there is variation in both of these measures, the computed values represent the mean. It is expected that infants will consume increased volumes of human milk as they grow.

There is no evidence for markedly different nutrient needs during the period of infants' growth acceleration and gradual weaning to a mixed diet of human milk and solid foods from ages 7 months through 12 months (Institute of Medicine, 1998). The basis of the AI values was the sum of the specific nutrient provided by 600 ml per day of human milk (Heinig et al., 1993) supplemented by the usual intakes of complementary weaning foods consumed by infants in this age category. The AIs and RDAs for micronutrients appear in Table 7-5.

One problem encountered in trying to derive intake data in infants is the lack of information on total nutrient intake from a combination of human milk and solid foods in the second 6 months of life. Most intake survey data do not identify the milk source, but the published values indicate that cow milk and cow milk formula were most likely consumed.

Calcium and Related Nutrients

Bone mineralization depends on several nutrients, including protein, vitamin D, calcium, phosphorus, and magnesium. Breast-fed infants retain approximately two thirds of the 240 mg of calcium in 750 mL of human milk, but retention from cow milk and commercial infant formulas is less than 50%. Recommended levels of calcium for formula-fed infants are 400 mg per day for the first 6 months and 600 mg for the second 6 months of life. The RDAs for phosphorus are based on a

Table 7-5 DIETARY REFERENCE INTAKES FOR MICRONUTRIENTS FOR INFANTS AND TODDLERS*

Nutrient/Day	0-6 mo	7-12 mo	1-3 yr
Calcium (mg)	*210*	*270*	*500*
Phosphorus (mg)	*100*	*275*	**460**
Magnesium (mg)	*30*	*75*	**80**
Fluoride (mg)	*0.01*	*0.5*	*0.7*
Vitamin D (μg)	*5*	*5*	*5*
Thiamin (mg)	*0.2*	*0.3*	**0.5**
Riboflavin (mg)	*0.3*	*0.4*	**0.5**
Niacin (mg)	*2*	*4*	**6**
Vitamin B_6 (mg)	*0.1*	*0.3*	**0.5**
Folate (μg)	*65*	*80*	*150*
Vitamin B_{12} (μg)	*0.4*	*0.5*	*0.9*
Pantothenic Acid (mg)	*1.7*	*1.8*	*2*
Biotin (μg)	*5*	*6*	*8*
Choline (mg/d)	*125*	*150*	*200*
Vitamin E (mg)	*4*	*5*	**6**
Vitamin C (mg)	*40*	*50*	**15**
Selenium (μg)	*15*	*20*	**20**
Vitamin A (μg)	*400*	*500*	**300**
Vitamin K (μg)	*2*	*2.5*	*30*
Chromium (mg)	*0.2*	*5.5*	*11*
Copper (μg)	*200*	*220*	**340**
Iodine (μg/d)	*110*	*130*	**90**
Iron (mg)	*0.27*	**11**	**7**
Manganese (mg)	*0.003*	*0.6*	*1.2*
Molybdenum (μg)	*2*	*3*	**17**
Zinc (μg)	*2*	*3*	**3**

Adapted with permission from the following Institute of Medicine publications: Dietary reference intakes for calcium, phosphorus, magnesium, vitamin D, and fluoride (1997); Dietary reference intakes for thiamin, riboflavin, niacin, vitamin B_6, folate, vitamin B_{12}, pantothenic acid, biotin, and choline (1998); Dietary reference intakes for vitamin C, vitamin E, selenium, and carotenoids (2000); and Dietary reference intakes for vitamin A, vitamin K, arsenic, boron, chromium, copper, iodine, iron, manganese, molybdenum, nickel, silicon, vanadium, and zinc (2001). Washington, DC, National Academy Press.
*RDAs are printed in bold type; AIs are printed in italics.

calcium-to-phosphorus ratio of 1.3 to 1.0 during the first 6 months and 1.2 to 1.0 for the second 6 months. The recommended intakes of 40 mg per day and 60 mg per day for magnesium for the first and second 6 months, respectively, are based on the average magnesium intake of breast-fed infants plus an allowance for variability in growth.

Human milk from a vitamin D-sufficient mother provides sufficient vitamin D for the infant. Vitamin D-deficient rickets has been reported in exclusively breast-fed infants of women with poor vitamin D status and women consuming vegan diets who did not receive vitamin D supplements (Dagnelie et al., 1990). Recently it has been observed that 30 infants and children diagnosed with nutritional rickets in two hospitals in North Carolina had been breast-fed and did not receive supplements of vitamin D. All were African American, leading the authors to recommend vitamin D supplementation for all dark-skinned breast-fed infants (Kreiter et al., 2000). Similar observations were made for toddlers and infants in Texas (Shah et al., 2000). The American Academy of Pediatrics (1998) recommends vitamin D supplements for breast-fed infants and its addition to formula products developed for infants.

The benefits of fluoride in early infancy are somewhat controversial because of the lack of evidence that fluoride supplements in the first 6 months alter the prevalence of dental caries in the secondary dentition. Unerupted teeth are being mineralized in later infancy, however;

so supplemental fluoride would be expected to have a beneficial effect during this period. The American Academy of Pediatrics (1998b) recommends evaluation of fluoride intake at 6 months of age and fluoride supplementation for 6 months to 3 years (0.25 mg/day) only when water fluoride content is less than 0.3 ppm. The AI for fluoride is 0.01 mg for infants from birth to 6 months, 0.5 mg for infants age 7 months to 12 months, and 0.7 mg for toddlers age 12 months to 24 months.

B Complex Vitamins

Thiamin, Riboflavin, Niacin, and Vitamin B_6

Thiamin, riboflavin, and niacin are essential coenzymes in energy metabolism. The AIs for these vitamins are based on the average content of breast milk. Vitamin B_6 functions as a coenzyme in the metabolism of amino acids, nucleic acids, and lipids. The AI levels are those provided in the milk of a mother who has adequate vitamin B_6 intake.

Folate and Vitamin B_{12}

As coenzymes, folate and vitamin B_{12} are essential for the synthesis of many body compounds. The newborn infant has small body stores of folate, which are rapidly depleted to meet the requirements for growth. An allowance for folate of 65 μg per day may be met adequately by human milk or cow milk. However, goat's milk contains only 10 μg of folate per liter and an infant fed goat milk requires a supplement to prevent megaloblastic anemia. Breast-feeding mothers with adequate serum vitamin B_{12} levels appear to supply sufficient vitamin B_{12} to their infants. However, a deficiency associated with irritability, anorexia, **failure to thrive** (FTT), and a long-term poor intellectual outcome has been reported in exclusively breast-fed infants of mothers who consumed a diet devoid of animal products and without vitamin B_{12} supplements (Graham et al., 1992).

Antioxidant Nutrients

Vitamin C

Vitamin C has several roles in human nutrition, the most carefully documented being the role in the synthesis and maintenance of collagen. The AI for vitamin C during early infancy (i.e., ages birth to 6 months) is 40 mg, which increases to 50 mg in the second half of an infant's first year. This level is based on the content of human milk plus an adequate margin of safety.

Viatmin E

Vitamin E (tocopherol) is required to protect a variety of body cells and compounds from oxidation. The AI for vitamin E for infants up to the age of 6 months is 4 mg per day, which reflects the tocopherol concentration of human milk. The level increases to 5 mg per day for infants age 6 months to 12 months. The AI for selenium during infancy is 15 μg and 20 μg for the first and second 6-month periods, respectively.

Vitamin A and Other Nutrients

The breast milk of a well-nourished mother contains 40 μg/dL to 70 μg/dL of retinol and a smaller amount of carotenoids (mainly beta carotene) that can be converted to retinol. A daily intake of 750 mL of milk provides the AI of 400 μg for infants from birth to 6 months and 500 μg for infants age 7 months to 12 months.

Iron

A term infant is born with an iron reserve of about 75 mg, which is sufficient to meet iron needs for the first 4 months to 6 months of life. Without an additional source, iron stores become depleted at about that time. For infants who are not breast-fed, the American Academy of Pediatrics (1998) recommends the use of iron-fortified formulas from birth to the end of the first year of life. Iron deficiency and the concomitant developmental delays and abnormal behaviors can be prevented in infants through the use of iron-fortified formulas or iron-fortified cereals with iron compounds of high relative

KEY TERMS

failure to thrive: deceleration of growth or growth failure from inadequate food intake or impaired food utilization; may be from psychosocial or physical factors

bioavailability and adequate vitamin C (Davidson et al., 2000).

Zinc

Zinc is an essential nutrient that functions in growth, reproduction, tissue repair, and cellular immunity. The AI for zinc of 2 mg per day for breast-fed infants is met from the approximately 2 mg of zinc obtained each day in breast milk. Formula-fed infants have greater needs from lesser bioavailability of zinc from formula. Although high amounts of dietary iron have been shown to reduce zinc absorption, the iron in fortified formulas does not appear to have a significant negative impact on zinc status (Institute of Medicine, 2001).

Vitamin K

The vitamin K status of the neonate is of concern for several reasons. First, the newborn has low plasma **prothrombin.** Second, human milk contains low levels of vitamin K (2 μg/L), and third, the intestinal microorganisms that synthesize vitamin K in adults are absent at birth and do not become fully active until later in infancy. Therefore exclusively breast-fed infants are at risk for development of fatal intracranial hemorrhage because of vitamin K deficiency. To prevent this problem, a prophylactic intramuscular injection of 0.5 mg to 1 mg vitamin K is recommended for all newborns (American Academy of Pediatrics, 1998). The AI levels are 2.0 μg and 2.5 μg, respectively, for the two age divisions during infancy: 0 to 6 months and 6 to 12 months, respectively.

Determining specific requirements for trace elements can be difficult because the effects of dietary inadequacies may be subtle and difficult to detect and because bioavailability can be influenced by many factors. In infancy this challenge is compounded by the movement of an infant from a single food source to a diet supplemented by a variety of foods, which may change the bioavailability of nutrients in milk.

Fluid and Electrolytes

Water

Infants have proportionally greater water requirements than adults because of their larger surface area per unit of body weight, their higher percentage of both body water and ECF, and their greater urine volume resulting from a lesser capacity of their kidneys to concentrate the **solute load.** Urea from protein metabolism, sodium, potassium, chloride, and phosphorus are major contributors to the renal solute load. A daily fluid intake of 1.5 mL/kcal of energy expenditure is adequate to meet the needs of infants. This figure corresponds to the water-to-energy ratio in human milk and commonly used infant formulas. Supplemental water generally is not indicated for healthy infants who are not yet receiving solid foods, except possibly during hot weather for formula-fed infants. When solid foods are introduced, additional water may be required from the greater renal solute load and water should be offered to the infant each day.

Infants younger than 6 months who are vomiting or have diarrhea are at risk for **hyponatremia,** particularly if they are fed fluids lacking sufficient sodium. Products containing water and electrolytes for rehydration are available in supermarkets. Hyponatremic seizures have been reported in infants fed excessive amounts of solute-free water (CDC, 1994). In addition to seizures, manifestations include altered mental status, hypothermia, and edema. Most commonly hyponatremia has been caused by giving excess tap water or overdiluting formula. In many instances this problem is from inadequate resources to purchase infant formula or a lack of knowledge about the potential dangers of feeding infants solute-free water. Sometimes bottled water products marketed as supplements for infants have been mistaken by parents and other caregivers as an affordable and appropriate feeding supplement or substitute for formula, resulting in hyponatremia. Labels of many of these products carry a disclaimer statement.

Sodium, Potassium, and Chloride

Estimated minimum requirements for sodium, potassium, and chloride are listed in Appendix A. Sodium, the major cation in ECF, is an important regulator of fluid volume. Chloride, the major inorganic anion in ECF, is essential for maintaining fluid and electrolyte balance. The major cation in ICF, potassium, is a necessary constituent of each body cell. As lean body mass increases, the need for potassium rises. Both human milk and commercial infant formula contain sufficient sodium, potassium, and chloride.

FEEDING INFANTS

- *What is the feeding relationship and why is it important to the health and well-being of the infant?*
- *What are the advantages and possible contraindications of breast-feeding?*
- *What adaptations or changes have been made in cow milk to make it suitable for infant feeding?*
- *Should regular cow milk be withheld from an infant until 1 year of age? Why or why not?*
- *Describe the basis for determining when and how supplementary foods should be given to an infant.*
- *Do nutrient supplements have a role in infancy? Why?*

Normal growth and development depend on the consumption of appropriate amounts and types of food. Breast milk or commercial infant formulas are usually the sole source of energy and nutrients during the first few months of life. Between 4 months and 6 months of age, supplementary foods are added to the diet and there is a gradual progression in the variety, quantity, and consistency of foods until soft table foods can be consumed at about 1 year of age. Recommendations for the introduction of solid foods depend on the individual infant's nutritional needs, physiologic maturation, and developmental and behavioral readiness for feeding (Dewey, 2001; Hendricks and Badruddin, 1992).

The Feeding Relationship

From the earliest moments of life, the infants depend on establishment of a social relationship for their nutritional needs and, thus, the maintenance of life and physiologic well-being. This relationship (Figure 7-10) not only provides energy and nutrients, but also supports an infant's development. Satter (1990) has characterized three stages of the feeding relationship between the infant and parents: homeostasis, attachment, and individualization. Homeostasis occurs in early infancy as extrauterine biologic functions stabilize and the infant increasingly interacts with the environment. The parents or primary caretakers facilitate development of the feeding relationship by responding promptly to hunger cues such as crying or fussing, calming the infant, and responding to his or her schedule and feeding capability.

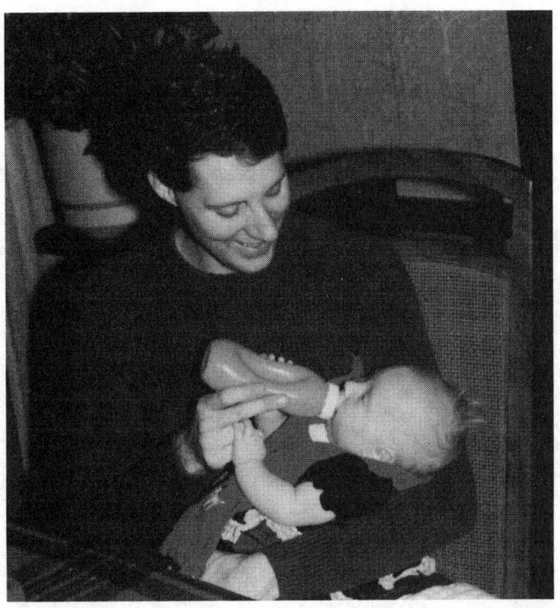

Figure 7-10 Infant feeding, both a nutritional and a social experience.

Attachment evolves from birth to about 4 months as infants achieve **affective** interactions with the parent. The caregiver maintains eye contact, smiles, speaks, and encourages the infant. The infant responds and takes the initiative in indicating readiness for the nipple and nursing. In fact infants may pause during nursing to socialize and then return to feeding (Figure 7-11). They may indicate satiety by falling asleep, smiling, drawing away from the nipple, and refusing reinsertion of the nipple.

KEY TERMS

prothrombin: protein for blood coagulation synthesized in the liver
solute load: amount of substances that must be dissolved in liquid (in this case, in urine)
hyponatremia: low blood levels of sodium
affective: relating to or influencing feelings or emotions

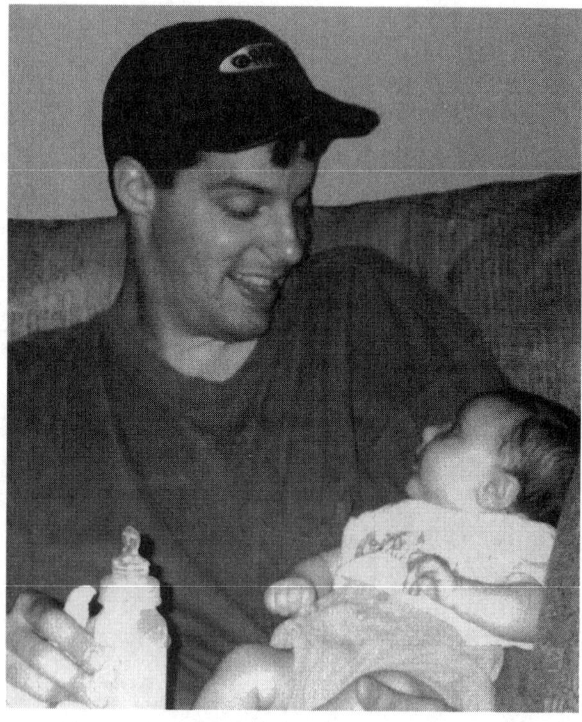

Figure 7-11 Pausing during feeding to socialize.

In the latter half of the first year and beyond, development is characterized by separation and individualization. With an increasingly complex sense of self, the infant struggles for autonomy and control. The ability to ingest an appropriate amount of food depends on a positive feeding interaction between the infant and his parents. Parents provide firm and caring support and direction in the development of eating habits and mastery of the feeding situation. The style and quality of caregiver-infant interactions have a strong influence on subsequent feeding behavior. Failure to establish this relationship results in inadequate intake, a major contributor to infant growth failure. Toward the end of the first year, parents and the infant develop a schedule and pattern in feeding as the intimate feeding relationship evolves into involvement in family meals.

Breast Milk

The physiology of lactation and the process of breast-feeding are discussed in Chapter 6. Breast-feeding is the universally recommended mode of feeding for early infancy. Health advantages associated with feeding breast milk include a nutritive composition uniquely suited to the human infant, bioavailability of nutrients, and the presence of growth factors, enzymes, hormones, a number of immune factors, and higher scores for cognitive development (Anderson et al., 1999). Breast-feeding is associated with reduced incidence and severity of certain infectious gastrointestinal and respiratory diseases, which may be the result of development of a breast milk-induced intestinal mucosal barrier against the penetration of harmful substances (Sheard and Walker, 1988).

Because the capacity of the stomach at birth is only about 7 mL, the amount of breast milk an infant can consume initially is limited. Gastric capacity increases rapidly, about tenfold in the first 2 weeks, when the infant is able to consume 2 oz to 3 oz per feeding. An outline of a typical amount and number of feedings of breast milk or formula is found in Table 7-6. Over time the feedings are characterized by greater volume and decreased frequency as solid foods begin to replace some of the energy and nutrients formerly obtained from milk.

Biochemistry of Human Milk

The nutrient content of human milk is variable. There are differences from one mother to another, across the stages of lactation, and even within individual feedings. Specific components in the milk may compensate for limited production of certain compounds by immature systems of the newborn. These include digestive enzymes, immunoglobulins, taurine, and specific long-chain fatty acids (Hamosh, 1992). Human milk is discussed in greater detail in Chapter 6.

Colostrum

The initial fluid released by the mammary gland, colostrum, is a thick, yellow, transparent fluid that is higher in protein and lower in fat than mature milk. The abundance of immune factors in colostrum also protects infants against viral and bacterial infections while their immune systems are still developing. After 3 days to 6 days colostrum evolves into transitional milk and by

Table 7-6 Typical Number and Volume of Feedings during Infancy

Age of Infant	Number of Feedings	Volume per Feeding
Newborn	6-10	60-90 mL (2-3 oz)
1 mo	6-8	90-120 mL (3-4 oz)
2-3 mo	5-6	150-180 mL (5-6 oz)
3-6 mo	4-5	180-210 mL (4-7 oz)
7-12 mo	3-4	210-240 mL (7-8 oz)

the seventh to fourteenth day, the change to mature milk has been completed, although protein levels remain high for the first month. Colostrum facilitates the passage of **meconium**, the infant's first stool, and contains the *Lactobacillus bifidus* factor, which facilitates the development of the protective *L. bifidus* bacteria in the gut of the young infant. These bacteria limit the growth of **enteropathogenic** organisms and promote the intestinal health of the breast-fed infant.

Mature Milk

The nutrient composition of human milk is listed in Table 7-7. Compared with cow milk, mature human milk has a slightly bluish, watery appearance. Its nutritional qualities are especially suited to the needs of the human infant.

Milk from adequately nourished mothers provides approximately 70 kcal per 100 mL of milk, digestible protein, fat, lactose, and adequate levels of vitamins and minerals. Except for fatty acids and vitamins, human milk appears to be relatively independent of the nutritional status of the mother. Maternal undernutrition is more likely to reduce the volume of milk produced than the quantity of a specific component. As illustrated in Table 7-8, the nutrients in milk have more than one function. Hormones and other bioactive compounds of human milk may aid in development, maturation, and functioning of the physiologic systems of the newborn (Ellis and Picciano, 1992).

Protein

The protein in human milk declines from about 2% in colostrum to 1.3% during the first month of lactation and then to about 0.9% to 1.1% (0.9 to 1.1 g/100 mL) in mature milk. In human milk whey proteins are dominant; alpha-lactalbumin makes up the largest single amount of protein in breast milk. Other major whey proteins are lactoferrin and the **immunoglobulin** secretory IgA (sIgA). Casein occurs in cow milk and forms large curds when exposed to acid in the stomach. Compared with cow milk, human milk has a low casein content (40% versus 80%) and forms small curds, which are easily digested.

Human milk contains all nine amino acids known to be essential for the human infant in proportion to requirements. In fact the **amino acid pattern** in human milk is used as the reference pattern for formulation of infant formula products (NRC, 1989). Compared with cow milk, human milk is higher in some amino acids that the young infant may not synthesize efficiently, such as cystine, tyrosine, and taurine. The enzymes required for the conversion of methionine to cysteine and phenylalanine to tyrosine develop late in the fetal growth period and may not be at full activity in the neonate, especially the preterm infant. Taurine is present in several body tissues, including fetal brain tissue and bile acids. Because the level is relatively high in human milk, it has been speculated that taurine is of significance in infant nutrition (Sturman, 1988).

Protective Factors

Human milk contains many factors that assist in protecting the infant from infections and viruses (Table 7-9). Many of these factors are relatively resistant to protein digestion and denaturation by the low pH in the stomach. Lactoferrin is an iron-binding protein in milk that reduces the amount

KEY TERMS

meconium: dark green mucilaginous material in the intestine of the newborn
enteropathogenic: *entero,* intestine; *pathogenic,* organism that can be harmful
immunoglobulin: serum globulins (proteins) that have antibody activity
amino acid pattern: the amount of individual amino acids present in relation to requirements

Table 7-7 NUTRIENT CONTENT OF COLOSTRUM, IMMATURE (TRANSITIONAL) AND MATURE HUMAN MILK, AND COW MILK PER DECILITER OF MILK

Nutrient	Human Milk			Mature Cow Milk
	Colostrum (1-5 days)	Transitional (Immature; 6-10 days)	Mature	
Energy (kcal)	67	72	74	70
Fat (g)	2.9	3.6	4.5	3.7
Lactose (g)	5.3	6.6	7.2	4.8
Protein (g)	2.7	1.6	0.9	3.3
Casein (g)	1.2	0.7	0.3	2.8
Lactalbumin (g)		0.8	0.3	0.4
Calcium (mg)	31	34	30	125
Phosphorus (mg)	14	17	15	96
Zinc (mg)	0.5	0.4	0.16	0.37
Iron (mg)	0.09	0.04	0.03	0.04
Vitamins				
A (IU)	296	283	240	303
Carotene (IU)	186	63	45	63
D (IU)			5	4
E (mg)	0.8	1.32	0.2	0.06
C (mg)	4.4	5.4	4.3	0.9
K (μg)			2.3	
Folacin (μg)	0.05	0.02	0.52	0.23
Niacin (mg)	0.075	0.15	0.20	0.085
Pantothenic acid (mg)	0.183	0.288	0.18	0.30
Pyridoxine (mg)			0.02	0.048
Riboflavin (mg)	0.029	0.033	0.035	0.16
Thiamin (mg)	0.015	0.006	0.014	0.042
Carnitine (mg)	1.1	1.6	1	2.1
Sodium (mg)	5	19	17	76
Potassium (mg)	74	63	53	152
Chloride (mg)	58	30	37	108
Magnesium (mg)	4.2	3.5	4	13
Iodine (μg)	6	—	6	11
Manganese (μg)	trace	trace	0.3	2.5
Selenium (μg)	—	—	2	4

Adapted from Geigy scientific tables, ed 7, Basel, Switzerland, Ciba-Geigy, Ltd.

of iron available to iron-requiring bacteria in the gastrointestinal tract. The bifidus factor, which promotes "friendly" bacteria, is unique to human colostrum and milk. The suckling infant can be protected by immunoglobulins present in human milk, including IgA, IgG, and IgM. IgA is produced in the mammary gland, but synthesis is probably triggered by **lymphoblasts,** which originate at maternal sites of pathogen exposure, usually the small intestine or respiratory tract.

The sIgA is the predominant immunoglobulin in human milk and specific IgA antibodies protect the infant's gastrointestinal and respiratory tracts from bacteria, viruses, parasites, and fungi and potentially allergenic macromolecules such

KEY TERMS

lymphoblasts: developing lymphocytes

Table 7-8 MULTIPLE FUNCTIONS OF THE MAJOR NUTRIENTS OF HUMAN MILK

Nutrient	Amount	Function
PROTEIN	**mg/dL**	
sIgA	50-100	Immune protection
IgM	2	Immune protection
IgG	1	Immune protection
Lactoferrin	100-300	Antiinfective, iron carrier
Lysozyme	5-25	Antiinfective
Lipase	10	Fat digestion
Lactalbumin	200-300	Calcium carrier
Casein	200-300	Carrier of calcium, phosphate, iron, zinc, and copper
CARBOHYDRATE	**g/dL**	
Lactose	5.5-6.0	Energy source
Polysaccharide	1.0-1.5	Prevent bacterial attachment to intestine
FAT	**g/dL**	
Triglyceride	3.0-4.5	
Long-chain polyunsaturated fatty acids		Brain and retinal function
Fatty acids (C12:0, C18:1, C18:2)		Antiviral, antiprotozoan, antibacterial

From Hamosh M: Human milk composition and function in the infant, Semin Pediatr Gastroenterol Nutr 3:4, 1992. Reprinted with permission of Decker Periodicals, Inc.

Table 7-9 PROTECTIVE FACTORS IN HUMAN MILK

Factor	Function
Antistaphylococcus factor	Inhibits growth of staphylococcal organisms
Bifidus factor	Stimulates growth of bifidobacteria, which antagonizes the survival of enteropathogens
Immunoglobulins: secretory IgA, IgM, IgE, EgD, and IgG	Act against bacterial invasion of the mucosa and/or colonization of the gut
Interferon	Inhibits intracellular viral replication
Lactoferrin	Iron-binding protein—decreases iron availability for bacterial multiplication
Lactoperoxidase	Kills streptococci and enteric bacteria
Lymphocytes	Synthesize secretory IgA
Lysozome	Enzyme that destroys bacteria by breakdown of cell wall
Macrophages	Synthesize lactoferrin, lysozyme; phagocytosis
Vitamin B_{12}–binding protein	Decreases availability of vitamin B_{12} for bacterial growth

as food proteins. Other host resistance factors include lysozyme, an antiinfective enzyme, and specific prostaglandins that protect the integrity of the epithelial cells that line the gastrointestinal tract. Lymphocytes in human milk produce the antiviral substance interferon. **Macrophages** in colostrum and mature milk produce **complement**, lactoferrin, lysozyme, and other immune factors.

Lipids

The lipid content of human milk is the major source of energy for the breast-fed infant, providing approximately 50% of the kilocalories in breast milk. The foremilk, that taken from the breast first, is relatively low in fat. Over a nursing period spanning 10 minutes to 20 minutes, the fat content gradually increases until the last milk (hindmilk) has a fat content two to three times that of the foremilk. It is important for a nursing session to be of sufficient length for the infant to consume the high-fat hindmilk for satiety and adequate energy for growth. The lipid in human milk is mostly triglyceride, but does include phospholipids, cholesterol, and other fats. Human milk contains more essential fatty acids and cholesterol than cow milk. Higher cholesterol levels may be important to the synthesis of the myelin (a fatlike substance) sheath around certain nerve fibers and may provide stimulus for development of enzymes for cholesterol degradation early in life. In addition to linoleic and alpha-linolenic acids, human milk contains the omega-3 fatty acids eicosapentanoic acid and DHA.

The fatty acid composition of human milk reflects the dietary intake of the mother. If a mother is in negative energy balance and increases mobilization of stored fat for milk synthesis, her milk will reflect the fatty acid composition of depot fat. Human milk contains several lipases, which may be the result of leakage from the mammary tissues. At least one, bile salt-stimulated lipase, is believed to contribute to fat digestion and may partially account for the greater digestibility of fat observed in breast-fed infants. The lipase in human milk may account for the fat breakdown that occurs in expressed breast milk that is refrigerated or frozen for later use.

Carbohydrate

The carbohydrate in human milk is lactose, which has a positive effect on calcium absorption. If an infant lacks the enzyme required to digest lactose, breast-feeding may be contraindicated or complicated by the need to provide some form of lactase activity.

Vitamins and Minerals

In general breast milk from healthy mothers contains all of the infant's needs for normal growth. The concentration of major minerals does not appear to be influenced by the mother's diet. The level of fluoride in breast milk is low and varies little, regardless of the level in the water supply. The content of most nutrients will be maintained in breast milk at the expense of maternal reserves. To a greater extent the vitamin content of human milk depends on maternal intake and stores. With poor tissue saturation and chronically low intakes, vitamin levels in human milk, especially levels of vitamins B_6, B_{12}, A, and D, can be reduced.

Infant Formula

Guidelines to Commercial Formulas

Commercially prepared infant formulas provide an acceptable alternative to breast-feeding. The major goal in preparing human milk substitutes is to formulate an acceptable product that is as nutritionally similar to human milk as possible. The nutrient content of breast milk and several major infant formula products is given in Appendix D. Guidelines for the minimum amounts of nutrients in commercial infant formulas were developed by the Committee on Nutrition of the American Academy of Pediatrics (American Academy of Pediatrics, 1998). The Infant Formula Act of 1980 (Public Law 94-359) gives the Food and Drug Administration the authority to regulate the composition, labeling, and quality assurance of commercial infant formulas sold in the United States. The act requires that all infant formulas distributed in the United States fall within the limits established by the American Academy of Pediatrics. Infant formulas may be purchased in ready-to-feed bottles (requiring only the addition of a nipple) or in concentrated liquid or powder preparations to be diluted with boiled or distilled water (Figure 7-12). These formulas are mixtures of proteins, carbohydrates, emulsified fats, vitamins, and minerals. Most standard infant formulas, like breast milk, have a caloric density of 20 kcal per ounce (70 kcal/100 mL).

Protein

The protein levels of most infant formulas range from 1.5 g/100 mL to 2.0 g/100 mL, which is sufficient to produce satisfactory growth in infants if their caloric intakes are adequate. Cow's milk protein is used in many infant formulas. In the stomach pasteurized cow's milk forms a large, firm curd that is difficult for the infant to digest. Therefore cow's milk-based formulas are heat treated to produce a smaller, softer curd. The major protein in cow's milk is casein with lesser amounts of whey, which resembles the protein in human milk more closely. The predominant whey protein is beta-lactoglobulin, which is more similar to the major protein in human milk, alpha-lactoglobulin, than is casein. The ratio between casein and whey proteins varies among formulas. Formula products with a higher ratio of whey:casein have the advantage forming a smaller curd in the stomach making them more digestible and they have an amino acid pattern similar to that of breast milk. Appendix D lists the content of major infant formula products.

For infants intolerant to milk protein other protein sources include soy protein and protein hydrolysates (protein partially digested by enzymatic hydrolysis). The hydrolysates are physically or chemically altered proteins, which makes them more digestible and less likely to induce an allergic response (American Academy of Pediatrics, 2000). The biologic value of soy protein is somewhat less than that of casein; therefore these formulas contain slightly greater concentrations of protein. Infants fed soy-based formulas have satisfactory growth and development. The bioavailability of minerals is lower with soy formula than milk-based formulas because of the presence of phytic acid in soy. Increasing the ascorbic acid content or reducing the phytate content improves iron absorption.

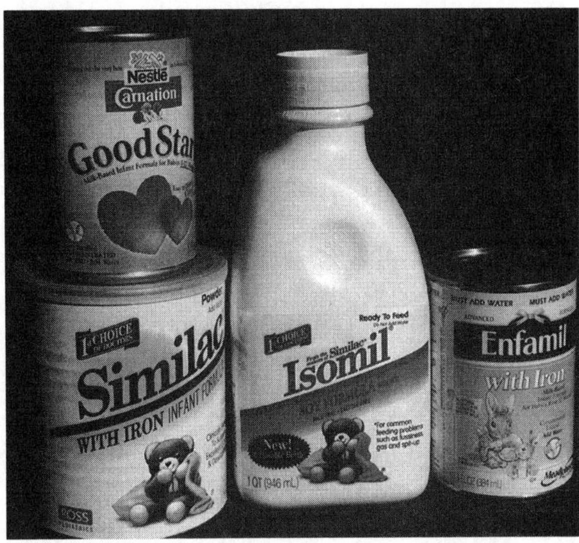

Figure 7-12 Infant formula products. Infant formula products include ready-to-eat forms in bottles, concentrated liquids, and powders.

Carbohydrate

Lactose, the carbohydrate source in most milk-based formula products, is present in those formulas in amounts similar to that of human milk (4 to 7 g/100 mL). Several formula products contain corn syrup, sucrose, and modified tapioca starch as their carbohydrate source. The lactose-free characteristic of these formulas makes them suitable for feeding infants with gastrointestinal problems that may result from primary or secondary lactase deficiency.

Lipids

In general, formulas contain 45% to 50% of their kilocalories as fat and the fatty acid profile is designed to be similar to that of human milk. To

KEY TERMS

macrophages: large cells that engulf bacteria and other foreign substances

complement: a complex series of enzymatic proteins occurring in normal serum that interact to combine with an antigen-antibody complex, producing lysis when the antigen is an intact cell; includes 11 discrete proteins, or 9 functioning components

accomplish this goal, butter fat of whole cow milk is replaced by a variety of vegetable oils, such as palm, soy, corn, coconut, and safflower. These oils, except coconut, are higher in polyunsaturated fatty acids and contain little or no cholesterol. They readily supply linoleic acid and some formula products also have omega-3 fatty acids added. The ideal fatty acid composition of cow milk-derived formulas is an area of intense research, particularly with regard to omega-3 and omega-6 fatty acids and their very-long-chain derivatives. Final recommendations for supplementation of these fatty acids in formulas for full-term infants await the results of ongoing clinical trials.

Vitamins

The vitamin content of most commercial infant formula products is similar to, or higher than, that of breast milk and thus is adequate to meet the requirements of normal healthy infants when they consume approximately 750 mL (26 oz) of formula each day.

Minerals

A calcium:phosphorus ratio of 1:1 to 2:1 is suggested for optimal calcium absorption during early infancy. There are both minimum and maximum levels for sodium, potassium, and chloride in formulas. Such levels are sufficient to meet growth needs of the infant without creating excesses to be excreted by the immature kidney. All formulas contain at least l mg/L of iron, but the American Academy of Pediatrics (1999) recommends that all formula-fed infants receive iron-fortified formulas that contain 10 mg/L to 12 mg/L or 6.7 mg/100 kcal to prevent iron deficiency. Despite early concerns about poor tolerance of supplemental iron, there is no evidence that these formulas cause more gastrointestinal problems, such as colic, constipation, diarrhea, or vomiting, than do unfortified formulas or that the higher level of iron significantly impairs absorption of other trace minerals (American Academy of Pediatrics, 1999).

Other Formula Products

Soy formulas were developed in the 1960s to meet the needs of infants who could not tolerate milk protein. The soy formula products on the market are also lactose-free, which has increased their use for refeeding after diarrhea, when lactase activity may be temporarily reduced. Today soy formulas constitute approximately 25% of the formula market (American Academy of Pediatrics, 1998). These formulas support growth rates equivalent to the rates observed in breast-fed and cow milk formula-fed infants (Hillman et al., 1988).

Breast-feeding has been recommended to prevent allergies or asthma (American Academy of Pediatrics, 2000). Breast-feeding alone cannot prevent these problems, but it may lower the risk by decreasing allergen exposure, strengthening the immune system, and preventing respiratory infections (Saarinen et al., 1999). Hypoallergenic infant formulas have been developed to supplement breast-feeding or to be used exclusively during infancy when symptoms of intolerance occur (American Academy of Pediatrics, 2000). The protein in hydrolysate formulas is partially digested to reduce the possibility of eliciting an immunologic response. They are also appropriate for feeding infants with gastrointestinal or hepatobiliary disease. Most of the formulas are lactose free. Disadvantages of the hydrolysate formulas include a poor taste from the presence of sulfated amino acids, greater cost, and high osmolality (American Academy of Pediatrics, 1998).

Supplementary Food

During the first few months of life, breast milk or iron-fortified infant formula alone provides optimal nutrition for the rapidly growing young infant. As physical and developmental capabilities mature, weaning is begun. Weaning is a developmental process in which semisolid foods are introduced and the composition and consistency of the diet are progressively advanced. Ideally by 12 months of age infants are eating a variety of foods from a mixed diet, with breast milk or formula as the main source of energy and nutrients. Patterns of introduction of supplementary foods should be based on the individual infant's nutrition needs, physiologic maturation, and development of feeding skills.

Nutrition Needs

By the time the infant is between 4 months and 6 months old, breast milk or infant formula can no longer meet nutritional needs to support growth. Supplementary foods are introduced initially to provide energy, protein, iron, vitamin C, and, eventually, other nutrients. By the end of the first year of life solid foods make up one third to one half of the infant's dietary intake.

Physiologic Maturation

At birth the kidney performs all its normal functions, but has limited ability to concentrate urine. The functional level of the kidney increases rapidly, so by 4 months of age, the increased solute load of solid foods can be handled if the foods are introduced gradually. Additional water should be offered to infants once they begin to receive solid foods.

Adequate enzyme activity and intestinal surface area are essential for efficient digestion and absorption of nutrients in solid foods. In the case of carbohydrate, disaccharidases to digest sugars are readily available at birth in term infants, but salivary and pancreatic amylase levels to hydrolyze starch are low and rise only as infancy progresses. Thus young infants have a limited ability to digest starch.

Newborns also have low levels of bile acids, pancreatic lipase, and colipase activity to digest and absorb triglycerides. Levels increase significantly during the first months of life and by 6 months of age, infants can absorb approximately 95% of dietary fat.

Successful adaptation of the infant to the extrauterine environment includes the development of a mucosal barrier against the penetration of harmful substances. At birth many of the intestinal defenses are passive or incompletely developed. Feeding breast milk not only limits the infant's exposure to pathogens and foreign proteins, but also provides the stimulus for development of active mechanisms that promote development of a mucosal barrier and eventual readiness for solid foods (Sheard and Walker, 1988).

Infant Feeding Skills

An infant's feeding skills define his or her developmental readiness to progress from nursing to a variety of new foods, textures, and feeding modes. Feeding depends on development of oral, hand-to-mouth, fine motor, body positioning, and communications skills. Table 7-10 outlines typical physical development and corresponding feeding behavior during the first year. As the table shows, by 5 months of age the tongue-extrusion reflex has disappeared and infants will accept semisolid foods placed on the tongue and move them to the back of the mouth for swallowing. Between 5 months and 7 months of age, infants will open their mouths when presented with a spoonful of food and take it from the spoon (Figure 7-13). By 7 months of age the tongue becomes more flexible and infants can swallow foods with small lumps. The ability to sit without support allows the infant greater ability to manipulate food and to interact during feeding. By 10 months infants make definite chewing movements and can take small bites of soft foods. As a pincer grasp develops, infants attempt self-feeding. By 1 year of age, most infants will accept a variety of foods from all the food groups, can finger-feed themselves many foods, and can drink from a cup using two hands.

Introducing Infants to Solid Foods

The introduction of solid foods to an infant's diet (sometimes called *beikost*) should begin

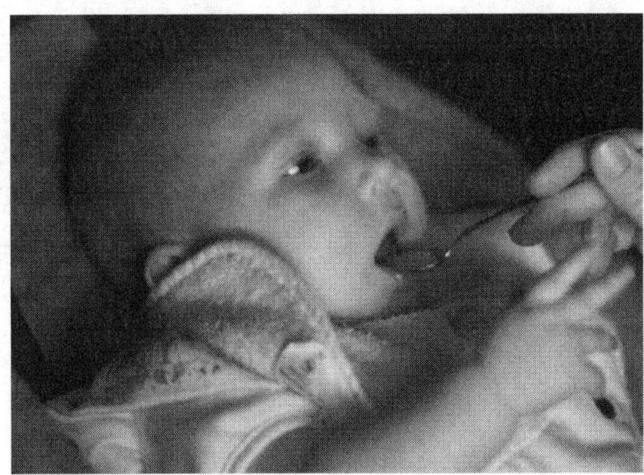

Figure 7-13 Adding supplemental foods to the milk diet of the infant depends on developmental readiness.

Table 7-10 DEVELOPMENTAL SEQUENCE GUIDE FOR NUTRITION AND FEEDING DURING INFANCY

Approximate Age	Motor Development	Oral Motor Skills Related to Eating	Self-Help/Social	Food and Appetite
Birth-1 month	Startle (Moro) reflex; minimal head control; hands fisted	Suck and swallow reflex; gag reflex; incomplete lip closure; lip movement in sucking; tongue thrust may be elicited	Looks at people	Breast milk or infant formula
2 months	Head bobs in supported sitting	Weaker suck and swallow reflex	Smiles at people; opens mouth while waiting for feeding	
3 months	Head stable; back rounded in sitting; holds toy placed in hands		Anticipates feeding	
4 months	Rolls over to back; head stable and tolerates propped sitting 10-15 min; bring toys to mouth	Tongue thrust present if spoon feeding attempted	Recognizes bottle	
5 months	Back straight in supported sitting; props self on forearms when in prone position; voluntary grasp	Tongue thrust reduced with spoon (may still be seen when cup drinking)	Mouth opens for spoon; brings hands to bottle	Strained, pureed, or blenderized food from spoon
6 months	Pushes up on extended arms in prone position; rolls both ways; briefly sits alone; reach and grasp	Good control with lips and tongue; beginning chewing motion (gumming food); drooling during mouthing	Holds, sucks, and bites cookie	Mashed food without lumps—plain crackers or cookies that are softened by saliva
7 months	Bears weight on legs when held; sits one minute alone; holds one object in each hand	Gag reflex is weaker; makes vowel sounds; attempts to use tongue to move lumps of food	Tries to finger-feed soft food	Mashed but lumpy food by spoon; easily chewed finger foods (large pieces)
8-9 months	Pulls to stand; transfers objects	Cup drinking with improvement in lip control; munching	Recognizes familiar names; fearful of strangers; babbles	Formula or breast milk recommended until end of first year, supplemented with other foods
10-12 months	Cruises, creeps; pincer grasp	Tooth eruption continues; chewing matures; little loss of liquid when cup drinking	Follows simple requests; gestures; plays pat-a-cake; begins to use a spoon	Continued addition of new food with easy-to-chew textures

Developed by Nutrition-Feeding Clinic Faculty, The Nisonger Center University Affiliated Program for Mental Retardation and Developmental Disabilities, The Ohio State University, 1980, Rev. 1995. Work supported in part by U.S. Department of Health and Human Services, Administration on Developmental Disabilities Grant #90DD032902 and Maternal and Child Health Bureau Grant #MCJ399155-04.

Table 7-11 SUGGESTED AGES FOR INTRODUCTION OF SOLID FOODS

Age	Appropriate Foods	Approximate Amount
0-4 months	Breast milk or iron-fortified formula*	23-29 ounces formula (6-8 feedings a day)
4-6 months[†]	Breast milk or iron-fortified formula*	26-32 ounces (4-6 feedings a day)
	Iron-fortified infant cereal	1-2 baby spoons 1-2 times a day
	Strained fruits and vegetables	1-2 baby spoons 1-2 times a day
7-9 months[††]	Breast milk or iron-fortified formula*	24-32 ounces (3-5 feedings a day)
		2-3 tablespoons 2 times a day
	Iron-fortified infant cereal	3-4 ounces a day
	Fruit juice (high in vitamin C)	2-3 tablespoons 2 times a day
	Strained vegetables	2-3 tablespoons 2 times a day
	Strained fruits	1-2 tablespoons 2 times a day
	Strained meats	1-2 tablespoons a day
	Breads, whole-grain or enriched	$^{1}/_{2}$-1 serving
10-12 months	Breast milk or iron-fortified formula*	24-32 ounces (3-4 feedings a day)
	Iron-fortified infant cereal	2-4 tablespoons 2 times a day
	Fruit juice (high in vitamin C) in a cup	3-4 ounces a day
	Chopped vegetables (table food)	3-4 tablespoons 2 times a day
	Chopped fruits (table food)	3-4 tablespoons 2 times a day
	Chopped meats (table food)	2-3 tablespoons 2 times a day
	Bread and bread products	$^{1}/_{2}$-1 serving a day

From Konstant LC et al.: Healthy mothers/healthy babies, Volunteer Instructor Guide, Columbia, Mo, 1985, The Curators of the University of Missouri.
*The American Academy of Pediatrics recommends iron-fortified formulas for all formula-fed infants.
†Infants consuming solid foods should be offered water daily.
††After 6 months of age, recommendations may be met by using combination foods.

with one single-ingredient food. That food should be given for 3 days to 5 days before another is added. Slow introduction gives the infant time to become adjusted to new tastes and permits parents to identify any negative reaction (allergy or intolerance) to a specific food. Repeated dietary exposure to the same food increases acceptance and behavior response to a new food (Sullivan and Birch, 1994). Table 7-11 outlines foods and amounts appropriate for most babies during the first year. Because iron reserves become depleted at 4 months to 6 months of age, iron-fortified infant cereals mixed with formula or breast milk are added first. The first cereal is usually iron-fortified rice cereal because it is the least **allergenic** cereal. Other cereals are introduced gradually, with wheat and mixed cereals added last. Single strained fruits, vegetables, meats, and egg yolks are other early food choices. Combination foods such as strained cereal with fruit, vegetables with meat, and meat-based dinners may be introduced after single-ingredient foods are well tolerated. Fresh, bottled, or frozen fruit juices are a good source of vitamin C and should be offered once the infant is able to drink from a cup. (See the Application at the end of the chapter.)

The first teeth begin to erupt at about 5 months to 6 months of age. Infants should be given foods that develop the ability to chew. Finger foods should be offered as infants develop

KEY TERMS

allergenic: having the potential to cause a negative reaction in the body from formation of an antibody in response to a foreign substance (antigen)

Table 7-12 SOME APPROPRIATE FOODS FOR INFANT SELF-FEEDING

Fruits	Soft, fresh or canned, unsweetened, such as bananas, peeled apples, apricots, peaches, or pears
Vegetables	Tender pieces of cooked vegetables such as carrots, potatoes, green beans, summer squash, yellow squash, sweet potatoes
Dairy	Cubes or slices of milk cheese, cottage cheese
Meat, Poultry, Fish	Small, tender pieces of cooked chicken, turkey, or white flaky fish without bones; ground meat such as meat balls, pieces of hamburger patty or meatloaf
Bread/Cereals	Toast, plain unsalted crackers, teething biscuits, individual cereal pieces
Other	Plain wafer cookies

hand and motor skills. Appropriate foods should be selected for ease of handling and chewing without increasing the potential for choking and aspiration (Table 7-12).

Over time a pattern of intake begins to evolve and gradually the infant's consumption of major nutrient sources centers around family meals, with snacks supporting the overall diet. Diet choices should emphasize foods in the Food Guide Pyramid. Strained and junior desserts and fruit-flavored drinks provide calories and few nutrients; therefore their use should be limited. Egg whites, a potential allergen, should be avoided during the first 12 months. In the second year self-feeding skills develop as toddlers become more independent (Figure 7-14).

Some foods are inappropriate for infants even toward the end of the first year. Babies and young children have difficulty swallowing foods such as popcorn, whole grapes, corn kernels, hot dogs, nuts, raisins, seeds, and potato chips. Unpasteurized honey should never be fed to infants because of the risk of **botulism.**

Supplements

Most healthy infants do not require nutrient supplements. The addition of supplemental foods at age 4 months to 6 months decreases the risk of nutrient deficiencies by diversifying dietary sources. Nevertheless about one third to one half of infants in the 6-month to 12-month age group are given nutrient supplements.

Nutrient supplements may be appropriate in some circumstances. Because the concentration of vitamin D in human milk is low and inconsistent, breast-fed infants may need supplemental vitamin D if the mother and infant have limited exposure to sunlight. Fluoride is considered essential in human nutrition to confer maximal resistance to dental caries. Fluoride supplements are recommended for infants over 6 months if the water supply contains fluoride at a concentration less than 0.3 ppm (American Academy of Pediatrics, 1998).

Full-term, exclusively breast-fed infants usually maintain adequate iron status during the first 6 months of life from mobilization of fetal iron stores and the high absorbability of the iron in human milk. After that time infants should receive additional iron. If breast-feeding continues, iron-fortified cereals should be added to prevent iron deficiency. Exclusively breast-fed infants of mothers who include no animal products in their diets may require a supplement of vitamin B_{12}. If the infant is weaned to a soy-based commercial infant formula, that formula will contain vitamin B_{12}.

NUTRITION-RELATED CONCERNS DURING INFANCY

- *What is nonorganic FTT and what are its causes?*
- *Iron deficiency is a public health problem in North America, but the incidence among infants and young children has been declining. Why?*
- *What is baby bottle tooth decay (BBTD)? How can it be prevented?*
- *Why is it important to decrease the potential for food allergies during infancy?*
- *Why are there concerns about chronic diseases during infancy and how should they be addressed?*

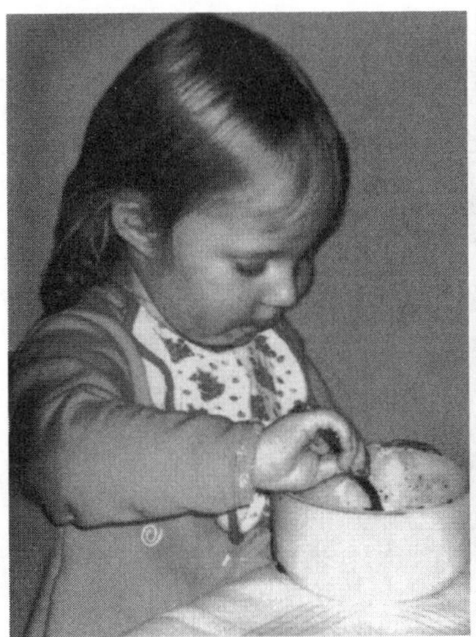
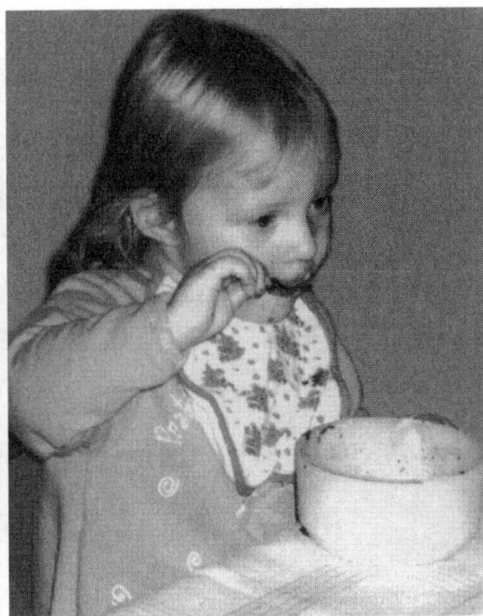
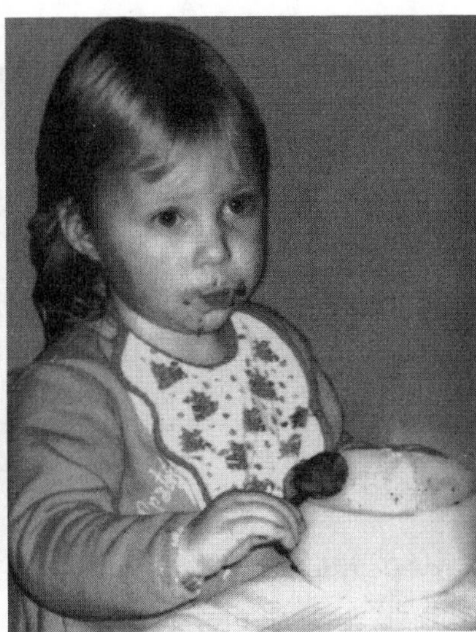

Figure 7-14 Toddler feeding skills.

Undernutrition

Failure to Thrive

Feeding is a process that requires the infant to indicate interest in being fed and the parent or caregiver to respond (Satter, 1990). When this process breaks down or when specific physiologic or metabolic disturbances in the infant interfere with food intake, FTT can occur. The term FTT is used to describe an infant or child who is failing to maintain growth above the third percentile for weight or height. The major characteristic of FTT is decreased growth rate. Body weight is affected more than linear growth, especially in infants. A small percentage of FTT infants may experience severe **wasting. Stunting** occurs less frequently, depending on the timing, duration, and severity of the nutritional inadequacy.

An infant may have a specific disease or disorder that leads to FTT (e.g., central nervous system damage, malabsorption, infections, or heart disease), which requires identification and medical intervention. However, most cases of FTT appear to be from factors that are primarily external to the infant. It is characterized by a syndrome of a low rate of gain in weight, length, or both, with social and developmental delays, abnormal behavior, and distorted caretaker-infant interactions. Two recent case control studies from the United Kingdom identified delayed weaning, diminished appetite, delayed progression to solid foods, and acceptance of fewer foods as characteristics of FTT.

The inadequate food intake and poor growth and development associated with FTT often occur in an environment of poverty, dysfunctional relationships, and inadequate education with a dearth of developmentally enriching experiences. It can be related to inadequate knowledge of nutrition and the feeding process and erroneous beliefs about infant needs. A disturbance in maternal-infant attachment or in separation and individualization by the infant may lead to food refusal. Counseling of parents and caretakers of FTT infants may require interaction among social workers, physicians, nurses, and dietitians to correct the disordered feeding relationship and to improve nutrition.

In breast-fed infants FTT may have a nutritional basis in an inadequate supply of maternal milk.

KEY TERMS

botulism: an often-fatal illness caused by the ingestion of food containing a toxin produced by *Clostridium botulinum* spores, which grow in improperly canned foods and honey

wasting: a deficit in weight relative to length

stunting: a deficit in length

Motil and others (1994) reported a case of a mother whose restricted fat intake appeared to result in "reduced lactation performance" and a decreased growth rate in her infant (Figure 7-15). One report described eight cases of FTT associated with infants' excessive consumption of fruit juice, which displaced more calorie- and nutrient-dense foods and also caused malabsorption from the large amounts of fructose and sorbitol consumed (Smith and Lifshitz, 1994). A recommendation of less than 12 ounces of juice per day is a reasonable quantity to provide nutrients while keeping sugar and food intakes adequate.

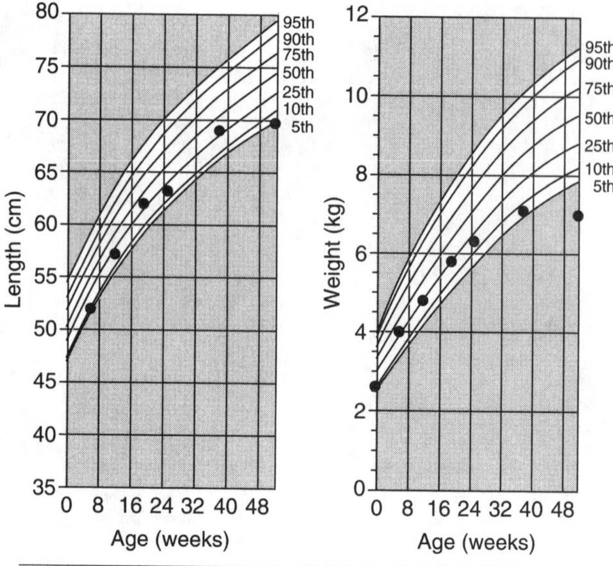

Figure 7-15 Length and weight measurements in a breast-fed infant with failure to thrive. *(From Motil KJ et al.: Case report: failure to thrive in a breast-fed infant is associated with maternal dietary protein and energy restriction, J Am Coll Nutr 13:203, 1994.)*

Iron Deficiency

Iron deficiency affects at least 20% to 25% of the world's babies. In the United States iron deficiency is most common in infants and children between 6 months and 3 years of age. Although iron deficiency in children has declined, the prevalence of anemia among low-income children in public health programs is 21% for 1 to 2 year olds and 9% for 2 to 3 year olds in the NHANES III (Looker et al., 1997). Decreases in iron deficiency have been related to increased use of iron-fortified formulas and iron-fortified cereals through participation in the Women, Infants, and Children (WIC) supplemental food program. But iron deficiency is still a significant problem for many older infants and young children and it is recognized as one of the priority concerns of *Healthy People 2010.*

Iron deficiency during infancy is associated with anorexia, irritability, and lack of interest in surroundings and it can eventually impair growth and development. Infants with iron deficiency perform more poorly on tests of mental and motor development than age-matched, iron-sufficient counterparts. Iron deficiency among infants causes substantial concern because behavior and learning deficits may persist even if iron deficiency is corrected. A 10-year follow-up study of infants who were treated for severe chronic iron deficiency and infants of good iron status found that children who were iron deficient as infants scored lower on measures of mental and motor function than the iron-sufficient comparison group. After control for background factors, there were still statistically significant differences in arithmetic achievement, written expression, motor functioning, and some cognitive processes (Lozoff et al., 2000).

Baby Bottle Tooth Decay

Primary teeth begin to erupt in a baby's mouth at about 4 months to 6 months of age. Formerly called the nursing bottle caries syndrome, BBTD is a form of rampant tooth decay that affects upper front teeth (incisors) and often the cheek surface of primary upper first molars (Figure 7-16). Occurring before the age of 2 years, BBTD has its origins in infant feeding practices, specifically with prolonged, inappropriate bottle feeding such as allowing an infant to fall asleep with a nursing bottle in his or her mouth.

The major dietary factor contributing to BBTD is liquids containing sugars, such as fruit juice and sweetened drinks, and milk and formula. Reduced flow of saliva during sleep permits extended exposure of the teeth to a solution that is fermented by plaque-forming microorganisms in

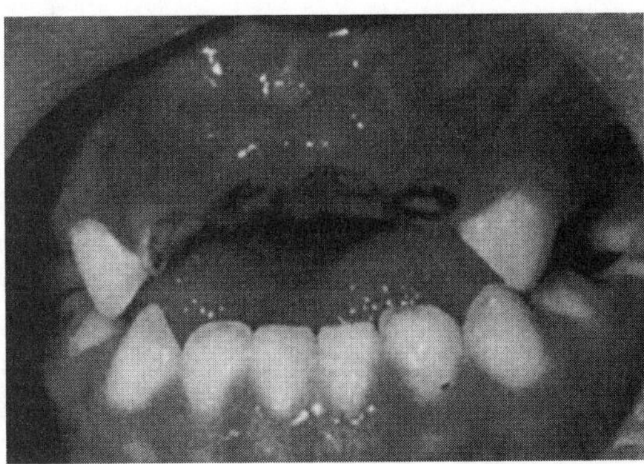
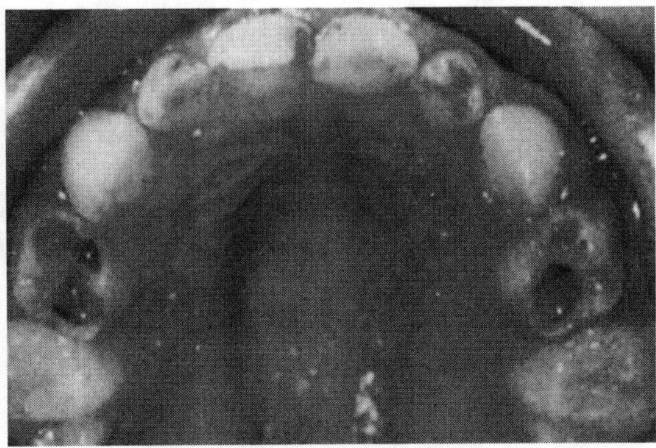

Figure 7-16 Baby bottle tooth decay. *(From Johnsen D and Nowjack-Raymer R: Baby bottle tooth decay [BBTD]: issues, assessment, and an opportunity for the nutritionist. Copyright © The American Dietetic Association. Reprinted by permission from Journal of the American Dietetic Association, 89:1113, 1989.)*

the mouth. The acid produced in this fermentation can damage the enamel layer of the newly erupted teeth and lead to dental decay.

The symptoms of BBTD are totally preventable. Contact of the teeth with baby bottle contents can be reduced by not using the bottle as a pacifier and not allowing the infant to fall asleep with a bottle in his or her mouth. A second part of prevention is reducing sugar content of beverages in the nursing bottle. Juices and liquids other than milk or formula should be offered in a cup. Prevention of BBTD is important because once decay occurs, treatment involves extensive and expensive restoration of teeth or extraction of teeth.

Allergic Reactions to Food

Food allergies and intolerances are discussed in the Application following Chapter 9. They are mentioned here because infant feeding practices involve introduction of food proteins, some of which may induce a food allergy in susceptible infants. Food allergy or hypersensitivity is an immune system-mediated response to dietary **antigens.** Antigenic constituents of cow milk protein, soy protein, or other solid foods may result in negative reactions such as hay fever, asthma, wheezing, vomiting, and dermatitis.

The process by which dietary antigens trigger an immune-mediated reaction is complex and incompletely understood. Factors that influence the immune response include genetic predisposition, the amount of antigen introduced, infant's age at the time of exposure to the antigen, maternal immunity, and development of the intestinal mucosal barrier. Determining that adverse reactions are, in fact, immune-mediated responses is often difficult, as is identifying infants at risk for the development of immune-mediated reactions to dietary antigens. Current indicators of risk are increased IgE (one of five classes of immunoglobulins or antibodies) concentrations in cord blood and a parental history of allergy.

Food allergies, particularly allergies to cow milk protein, can occur in some infants. Avoidance of food antigens may have a protective effect in the development of an allergy. Human milk and formulas based on hydrolysates of casein and whey protein are recommended for infants considered at risk for cow milk protein allergy. Delaying the introduction of solid foods until at least 6 months of age is recommended for these infants. Even greater care must be given in offering new foods gradually and in small portions. Several days should elapse between the introductions of each new food to allow time to recognize whether symptoms of sensitivity appear.

KEY TERMS

antigen: a foreign protein substance that, in the body, results in formation of an immune response such as antibodies

Development of Chronic Diseases

Obesity

Breast-fed infants gain weight more slowly than do formula-fed infants after the first few months of life. As a result it has been suggested that breast-feeding may prevent obesity, although no definitive evidence supports this theory currently. Also there is little evidence to support a link between excessive weight gain and formula feeding or the early introduction of solid foods.

The lack of a consistent effect of infant feeding practices on later development of obesity may be related to the many factors that contribute to obesity, particularly heredity and energy expenditure. For example Roberts and others (1988) found that rapid weight gain during infancy and overweight status at the age of 1 year were related to reduced energy expenditure and maternal overweight status rather than to infant dietary patterns. Body weight during infancy has little relationship to childhood or adult obesity. A study that investigated feeding practices of more than 300 infants and their relationship to two measures of adiposity—body mass index and the sum of fatfold thicknesses—at 4 years of age found no associations between the measures of adiposity and any of the infant feeding variables, duration of breast-feeding, or introduction to solids (Zive et al., 1992).

Cardiovascular Disease

In recent years high concentrations of low-density lipoprotein cholesterol (LDL-C) have been associated with the presence of fatty streaks in the aorta in pediatric autopsies (Berenson et al., 1998). This finding suggests that children with high cholesterol are predisposed to atherosclerosis and coronary heart disease (CHD). Many have suggested that early dietary intervention may retard this process. The American Academy of Pediatrics (1998) has stated that diets for infants and children under 2 years of age should not be restricted in kilocalories, fat, or cholesterol because of the importance of fatty acids and total energy intake in growth and development. Recommendations have instead taken a positive approach, involving feeding infants a variety of nutritious foods in response to their appetites. This decision not to recommend dietary restriction for infants was reinforced by reports showing that because of concern for subsequent risk of obesity or other health problems, some parents restricted their infants' dietary intakes to such an extreme that the infant or child developed FTT because the diet provided insufficient energy and micronutrients to support normal growth.

Studies of dietary interventions in children indicate that a low-saturated fat, low-cholesterol diet decreases serum LDL-C concentrations in 8- to 10-year-old children who were followed for 3 years without effects on growth and psychosocial health.

In a recent randomized, controlled trial, caregivers of 540 7-month-old infants were assigned to receive individualized counseling aimed at limiting the infants' saturated fat and cholesterol intake (Rask-Nissila et al., 2000). The caregivers of 522 infants were assigned to a control group that received the usual health education given to caregivers of young infants. At age 5 years 496 of the infants took part in neurologic and developmental testing. The diet low in saturated fat and cholesterol was associated with markedly reduced age-related increases in serum cholesterol concentrations, with neurologic development that was at least as good as that of children in the control group. The authors of this study concluded that the earlier the age at which serum cholesterol levels are decreased, the greater the decrease in incidence of CHD in adulthood. Although intriguing, these observations will require validation from other studies and follow-up studies of efficacy and potential long-term effects before major changes in dietary recommendations are likely to occur.

Concepts to Remember

- Infancy is a period of high nutritional need to support rapid growth and development.
- Infants will double their birth weight by 5 months and triple it by 1 year of age. Stature increases approximately 50% during the first 12 months of life.

- Per kilogram of body weight, the energy and protein needs of infants are more than twice those of adults.
- Because growth is rapid during infancy, nutritional status can be monitored by increases in weight, length, and head circumference.
- Because of rapid growth, infants are more vulnerable to nutritional inadequacies than other age groups.
- Breast-feeding is recommended for infants because of the nutritional and immunologic properties of human milk.
- Successful infant feeding depends on establishing a social relationship between the infant and mother or primary caregiver.
- During the first 4 months to 6 months of life, nutritional needs of infants can be met by breast milk or suitable infant formula. To meet nutritional needs after 4 months to 6 months, the breast milk or formula diet of the infant is augmented by supplementary foods, starting with iron-fortified infant cereals and gradually progressing to vegetables, fruits, and meats.
- Successful introduction of supplementary foods depends on the infant's nutritional needs, physiologic maturation, and developmental readiness.
- Undernutrition, either general or of a specific dietary component, requires prompt intervention to maintain normal growth and development.
- Concern regarding risk of chronic disease is balanced by attention to meeting energy and nutrient needs to support growth and development.

REFERENCES

American Academy of Pediatrics: Breastfeeding and use of human milk, Pediatrics 100:1035, 1997.

American Academy of Pediatrics, Committee on Nutrition: Soy protein for use in infant feeding, Pediatrics 101:148, 1998.

American Academy of Pediatrics: Pediatric nutrition handbook, ed 4, Elk Grove Village, IL, 1998, American Academy of Pediatrics.

American Academy of Pediatrics, Committee on Nutrition: Iron-fortification of infant formulas, Pediatrics 104:1, 1999.

American Academy of Pediatrics, Committee on Nutrition: Hypoallergenic infant formulas, Pediatrics 106: 346, 2000.

American Academy of Pediatrics, Vitamin K Ad Hoc Task Force: Controversies concerning vitamin K and the newborn, Pediatrics 91:1001, 1993.

American Dietetic Association: Position of the American Dietetic Association. Promotion of breast-feeding, J Am Diet Assoc 97:662, 1997.

Anderson JW et al.: Breast-feeding and cognitive development: a meta-analysis, Am J Clin Nutr 70:525, 1999.

Berenson CS et al.: Association between multiple cardiovascular risk factors and atherosclerosis in children and young adults, N Engl J Med 338:1650, 1998.

Binns HJ et al.: Growth of Chicago-area infants, 1985 through 1987, Arch Pediatr Adolesc Med 150:842, 1996.

Brazelton TB and Greenspan S: The irreducible needs of children, Cambridge, MA, 2000, Perseus Publications.

Butte NF et al.: Human milk intake and growth in exclusively breast-fed infants, J Pediatr 104:187, 1984.

Butte NF et al.: Body composition during the first 2 years of life: an updated reference, Pediatr Res 47:578, 2000.

Centers for Disease Control and Prevention: CDC growth charts: United States, Atlanta, GA, 2000, The Author.

Centers for Disease Control and Prevention: Hyponatremic seizures among infants fed with commercial bottled drinking water, MMWR 43:641, 1994.

Dagnelie PC et al.: High prevalence of rickets in infants on macrobiotic diets, Am J Clin Nutr 51:202, 1990.

Davidson L et al.: Iron bioavailability in infants from an infant cereal fortified with ferric pyrophosphate or ferrous fumarate, Am J Clin Nutr 71:1597, 2000.

de Onis M and Garza C: Time for a new growth reference, Pediatrics 100:1, 1997.

Dewey KG et al.: Growth of breast-fed infants deviates from current reference data: a pooled analysis of U.S., Canadian and European data sets, Pediatrics 96:495, 1995.

Dewey KG: The challenges of promoting optimal infant growth, J Nutr 138:679, 2001.

Ellis LA and Picciano MF: Milk-borne hormones: regulators of development in neonates, Nutr Today Sept/Oct 1992.

Fomon SJ: Requirements and recommended dietary intakes of protein during infancy, Pediatrics 30:391, 1991.

Food and Nutrition Board: Nutrition during lactation. Washington, DC, 1991, National Academy Press.

Gibson RA and Makrides M: n-3 polyunsaturated fatty acid requirements of term infants, Am J Clin Nutr 71:251S, 2000.

Graham SM et al.: Long-term neurologic consequences of nutritional vitamin B_{12} deficiency in infants, J Pediatr 121:710, 1992.

Hamosh M: Human milk composition and function in the infant, Semin Pediatr Gastroenterol Nutr 3:4, 1992.

Heinig MJ et al.: Energy and protein intakes of breast-fed and formula-fed infants during the first year of life and their association with growth velocity: the DARLING study, Am J Clin Nutr 58:152, 1993.

Hendricks KM and Badruddin SH: Weaning recommendations: the scientific basis, Nutr Rev 50:125, 1992.

Hillman LS et al.: Vitamin D metabolism, mineral homeostasis, and bone mineralization in term infants fed human milk, cow milk-based formula, or soy-based formula, Am J Dis Child 112:1302, 1988.

Institute of Medicine: Dietary reference intakes for calcium, phosphorus, magnesium, vitamin D and fluoride, Washington, DC, 1997, Institute of Medicine.

Institute of Medicine: Dietary reference intakes for thiamin, riboflavin, niacin, vitamin B_6, folate, vitamin B_{12}, pantothenic acid, biotin, and choline, Washington, DC, 1998, National Academy Press.

Institute of Medicine: Dietary reference intakes for vitamin C, vitamin E, selenium and carotenoids, Washington, DC, 2000, National Academy Press.

Institute of Medicine: Dietary reference intakes for vitamin A, vitamin K, arsenic, boron, chromium, copper, iodine, manganese, molybdenum, nickel, silicon, vanadium and zinc, Washington, DC, 2001, National Academy Press.

Kreiter SR et al.: Nutritional rickets in African American breast-fed infants, J Pediatr 137:153, 2000.

Lampl M et al.: Saltation and stasis: a model of human growth, Science 258:801, 1992.

Lohman TG et al.: Anthropometric standardization reference manual, Champaign, Il, 1988, Human Kinetics Books.

Looker AC et al.: Prevalence of iron deficiency in the United States, JAMA 277:973, 1997.

Lowery GH: Growth and development of children, ed 8, Chicago, 1986, Year Book.

Lozoff B et al.: Poor behavioral and developmental outcome more than 10 years after treatment for iron deficiency in infancy, Pediatrics 105:E51, 2000.

Motil KJ et al.: Case report: failure to thrive in a breast-fed infant is associated with maternal dietary protein and energy restriction, J Am Coll Nutr 13:203, 1994.

National Center for Health Statistics: NCHS growth charts, 1976. Monthly Vital Statistics Report, vol 25, no 3, suppl (HRA) 76: 1120, Rockville, MD, 1976, Health Resources Administration.

National Research Council: Recommended dietary allowances, ed 10, Washington, DC, 1989, National Academy Press.

Rask-Nissila L et al.: Neurological developments of 5-year old children receiving a low-saturated fat, low cholesterol diet since infancy: a randomized controlled trial, JAMA 284:993, 2000.

Roberts SB et al.: Energy expenditure and intake in infants born to lean and overweight mothers, N Engl J Med 318:461, 1988.

Roche AF et al.: Weight and recumbent length from 1 to 12 months of age: reference data for 1-month increments, Am J Clin Nutr 49:599, 1989.

Saarinen KM et al.: Supplementary feeding in maternity hospitals the risk of cow's milk allergy: a prospective study of 6209 infants, J Allergy Clin Immunol 104:457, 1999.

Satter E: The feeding relationship: problems and interventions, Pediatrics 117:S181, 1990.

Shah M et al.: Nutritional rickets in African American breast-fed infants, Texas Medicine 96:64, 2000.

Sheard NF and Walker WA: The role of breast milk in development of the gastrointestinal tract, Nutr Rev 46:1, 1988.

Smith M, and Lifshitz F: Excess fruit juice consumption as a contributing factor in nonorganic failure to thrive, Pediatrics 93:438, 1994.

Sturman JA: Taurine in development, J Nutr 118:1169, 1988.

Sullivan SA and Birch LL: Infant dietary experience and acceptance of solid foods, Pediatrics 93:271, 1994.

Victoria CG et al.: The NCHS reference and the growth of breast- and bottle-fed infants, J Nutr 128:1134, 1998.

Vital Health and Statistics: CDC growth charts: United States advanced data, No. 314, June 8, 2000, Centers for Disease Control and Prevention, National Center for Health Statistics.

WHO Working Group on the Growth of Reference Protocol: A growth curve for the 21st century: the WHO multicenter growth reference study, Geneva, 1998, World Health Organization.

World Health Organization: Energy and protein requirements: report of a joint FAO/WHO/UNU expert consultation, Technical Report Series 725, Geneva, 1985, World Health Organization.

Zive MM et al.: Infant-feeding practices and adiposity in 4-year-old Anglo- and Mexican-Americans, Am J Clin Nutr 55:1104, 1992.

APPLICATION

Foods for Infants: The Supermarket

In the early months of life the infant usually receives a diet consisting of human milk or a commercial formula product with a macronutrient and micronutrient composition that resembles human milk. Under the Infant Formula Act, the Food and Drug Administration regulates the composition, labeling, and quality assurance of commercial infant formula products. Safety and nutritional quality are ensured by requiring that manufacturers follow specific procedures in manufacturing infant formulas. To protect the highly vulnerable infant, these products are among the most highly regulated and controlled of all commercially available foods.

PREPARATION OF INFANT FORMULA

Manufacturers of infant formula provide directions for mixing their products with water and usually do not specify the source of water other than to indicate that the water should be safe to drink. In most situations it is safe to mix formula using ordinary cold tap water that is brought to a boil and boiled for 1 minute or as directed on the label. Some manufacturers sell bottled water labeled for use for infants. The water for infants must meet the same standards established for tap water by the Environmental Protection Agency. As with tap water, parents should boil bottled water 1 minute before mixing with infant formula.

In 1942 baby foods were classified as foods for special dietary use under the Federal Food, Drug, and Cosmetic Act. Under current labeling regulations, labels on foods designated for infants will use the Nutrition Facts format, but the information provided is different. See the sample food label on page 248. Serving sizes are based on average amounts that infants under 2 years of age would consume at one time. Because the current recommendation is that the fat content of an infant's diet should not be restricted, the label lists total calories and total fat, carbohydrate, sodium, and protein per serving, but not the distribution of calories from fat, saturated fat, or cholesterol content. The food label for infants (birth to 1 year) and children (under 4 years) lists percentages of the Daily Value for protein, vitamins, and minerals, but does not include daily values for fat, cholesterol, sodium, potassium, carbohydrate, and fiber because they have not been established for children under 4 years of age. Label information is designed to assist the parent or caregiver in making decisions about which foods to purchase to ensure a safe and nutritious diet for the infant.

Sometime around 4 to 6 months an infant will begin to show interest in solid foods. The milk or formula diet is gradually expanded to include single-ingredient foods, beginning with cereal, then moving on to fruits, vegetables, juice, and meats. Eventually the diet will include combination foods and selections from all food groups. An enormous variety of foods for infants are available in the market today. In fact a stroll down the aisle of any supermarket where baby foods are displayed reveals a confusing array of choices. Variety, balance, and moderation are as applicable to planning the infant's diet as they are to planning for older children and adults. Careful selection from available infant foods can provide nutritious, economical diets. Milk is the mainstay of the diet at this time and other foods are truly supplementary.

Most of the commercial infant food products available in the market today are designed to parallel current feeding recommendations. Textures range from strained to chunky. To assist consumers, foods designed for the first year of life are divided into stages first, second, or third. The designation is displayed on the label to guide the parent in selection of an appropriate level of foods.

Infants generally are ready for stage 1 foods when they have doubled their birth weight, have good control of head movements, can sit with support, and can swallow a spoonful of pureed

Nutrition Facts

Serving Size 1/4 cup (15 g)
Servings Per Container About 30

Amount Per Serving		
Calories 60		
Total Fat		1 g
Sodium		0 mg
Potassium		50 mg
Total Carbohydrate		10 mg
Fiber		1 g
Sugars		0 g
Protein		2 g
	Infants	Children
% Daily Value	**0-1**	**1-4**
Protein	7%	6%
Vitamin A	0%	0%
Vitamin C	0%	0%
Calcium	15%	10%
Iron	45%	60%
Vitamin E	15%	8%
Thiamin	45%	30%
Riboflavin	45%	30%
Niacin	25%	20%
Phosphorus	15%	10%

From FDA, USDA/USDHHS, Washington, DC.

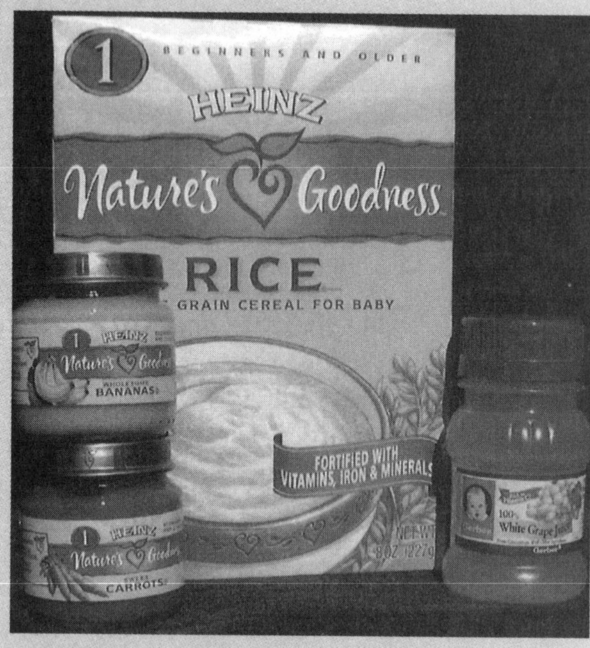

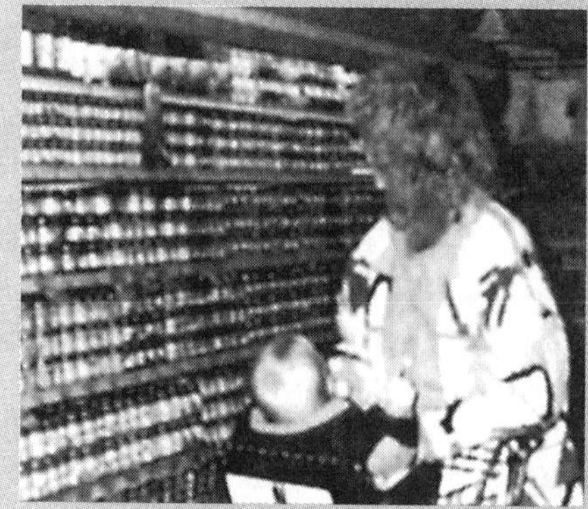

Photo credit: Mary Kay Mitchell.

food easily. Foods in stage 1, often referred to as "first foods," are single-ingredient foods. The first foods introduced are infant cereals, which are enriched with iron, thiamin, riboflavin, niacin, calcium, and phosphorus. Dry infant cereals do not need cooking. They are mixed with breast milk or formula to a semi-liquid consistency and fed from a spoon. As the baby learns to swallow, the cereal can be made thicker.

Some mothers introduce cereals before 4 months by making a thinner mixture and putting it in the nursing bottle. This practice is undesirable, however, because it is not necessary to meet the nutrient needs of most young infants and because it increases the potential for choking and for development of food allergies. Ready-prepared cereal in jars is available, but it is more costly than dry baby cereal and requires refrigeration after opening. Once cereals have been accepted and tolerated by the infant, other "first foods," single fruits and vegetables, are offered. These are usually packaged in 2.5-ounce jars.

Fruit juices enriched with vitamin C are usually offered as the infant adjusts to stage 1 foods. Juices for infants are available from single fruits and combinations of fruits and are categorized as stage 1, 2, or 3. Fruit juices should be unsweetened and should be offered from a cup.

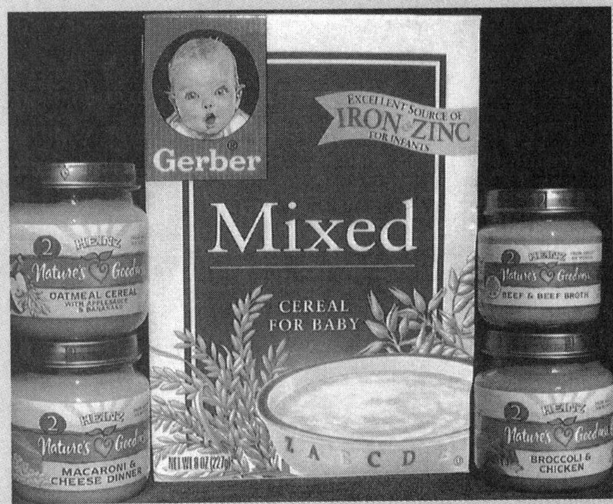

Four-ounce bottles are sold as singles or in six packs. Larger bottles ranging in size from 25 to 32 ounces are also available.

Introduction of stage 2 foods is appropriate when the infant has tried a variety of single-ingredient foods, sits well without support, eats easily from a spoon, and has begun to drink from a cup. The selection of foods designated as stage 2 is much larger. "Second" foods are to be offered to infants from about 6 months of age, after the infant has adapted to "first foods" in the diet. While these foods are still pureed or strained, they have a thicker consistency than "first foods" and, except for meats, are marketed in larger jars (usually 4 ounces). Stage 2 foods include single-item fruits and vegetables and combination foods such as cereals with fruit, mixtures of fruits, vegetables, and mixed dinners. Mixed dinners are available in a variety of food combinations, from turkey with vegetables to beef and macaroni. Strained meats for this stage are in 2.5-oz jars. Puddings and desserts are also available and may be appropriate to include in the diet occasionally. It should be remembered that throughout the first year of life, milk still constitutes a major portion of the diet.

Stage 3 foods are suitable for infants from about 9 months of age who sit alone easily, can handle finely chopped foods, can drink from a cup, and have begun some self-feeding. Foods at this stage include all the foods offered in stage 2, but in greater variety and combinations and, in some cases, in larger jars (6 ounces). The mixtures are more complex in consistency and require more chewing than stage 2 foods. Formerly such foods may have been called "junior" foods. Stage 3 foods may not be used for many older infants because the infant will move instead to mashed and finely chopped table foods. Table foods are suitable at this age if the consistency is such that the infant can gum and swallow them with ease and seasoning is moderate.

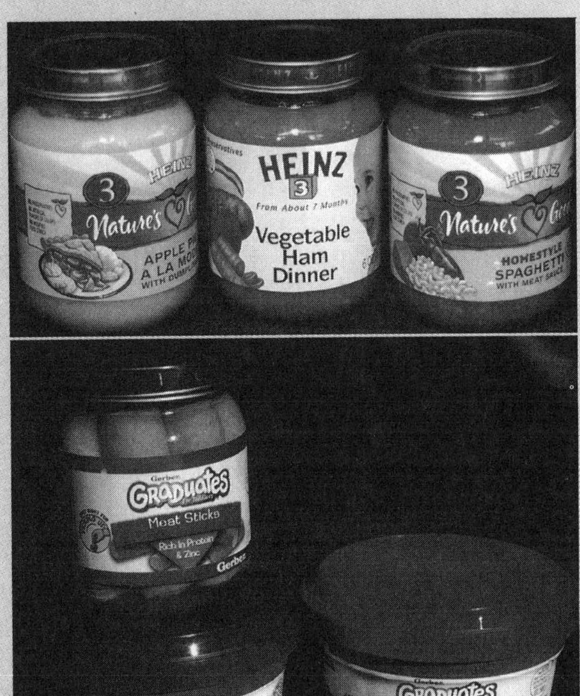

Additional food items, some more advanced than stage 3, are marketed under various names and may be convenient substitutes for table foods in late infancy and the early toddler period. The consistency of these products is appropriate for use of a spoon and the pieces are sized for easy chewing and swallowing. They may be in 6-ounce jars, and many come in 6-ounce containers with plastic replaceable lids. They are lower in salt, spices, and seasonings than similar adult foods. Once opened, these products need to be refrigerated promptly to control bacterial growth and should be discarded within 2 days if not used. Additional foods marketed for older infants include desserts, crackers, and finger foods.

Labels on infant food products must list all ingredients in the product. Virtually all infant foods are prepared without added sodium or monosodium glutamate, most are prepared without flavor or color enhancers, and many are prepared without added sugar. If any of these food additives are present, they must be listed on the label. Ingredients are listed on the product label in the order of greatest presence in the food. Therefore if water is the first ingredient listed on the label, as in the banana pudding, water is present in the greatest amount. The mixed dinner, often considered a protein source, has three ingredients, including water, that are present in greater quantity than beef, the protein source. This information on the label can assist parents in selecting foods of high nutrient value. It should be remembered, however, that similar foods can be prepared from the family's foods at lesser cost.

Commercial infant foods are a convenient, time-efficient, although somewhat costly, means to provide supplementary foods in the diet of the infant. If choices are made wisely, they can make a nutrient-dense contribution to the diet. Table 7-13 gives an example of such a menu for Erin at 8 months of age. The Nutrition Facts and the list of ingredients on the food label provide information to assist in selection of appropriate foods.

EXAMPLES OF LISTS OF INGREDIENTS ON FOOD LABELS

Stage 1: Carrots
Carrots and water

Stage 2: Macaroni and Cheese
Water, skim milk powder, enriched macaroni product, cheddar cheese, pasteurized milk, cheese cultures, salt, enzymes, vegetable color, and corn starch

Stage 3: Spaghetti
Tomato puree, water, beef, enriched macaroni product, rice flour, cheddar cheese, skim milk powder, onion powder, and spices

Table 7-13 TYPICAL INTAKE FOR AN 8-MONTH-OLD INFANT

Morning	3 tbsp mixed cereal with formula 1/2 jar of bananas (2 oz) Formula or breast milk
Midmorning	4-oz jar of peaches
Lunch	4 oz of chicken noodle dinner 2 oz sweet potatoes Formula or breast milk
Midafternoon	4 oz pear juice 3 crackers
Dinner	2.5 oz of turkey 4 oz of mixed vegetables 4 oz of applesauce Formula or breast milk
Before bed	Formula or breast milk

HOME PREPARATION OF INFANT FOODS

Home-prepared infant foods are an important alternative to commercially prepared foods. Using some of the regular family food can be convenient and economical and allows greater flexibility in altering food consistency. However, families that lack variety in their diets should be encouraged to supplement home-prepared foods with commercial foods to achieve a balanced diet. Home preparation of infant foods is not appropriate in homes that lack adequate facilities for refrigeration and freezing or those that have poor sanitation. Home-grown foods should not be prepared for infants if there is any question regarding the lead concentration of the soil in residential areas. Arrangements to test the lead content of soil can be made through the local health department.

Foods to be fed to infants can be prepared by steaming, roasting or broiling, microwave cooking, or boiling. Equipment for preparation can be as simple as a strainer and a blender or a baby food mill that can be used to achieve the desired consistency. If the family's foods are prepared with salt, spices, sugar, or fat, the infant's food should be prepared separately or the baby's portion removed from the family's food before seasonings are added.

Foods that are pureed, ground, or creamed can provide a medium for bacterial growth. Thus home-prepared infant foods need to be used promptly or stored immediately in the refrigerator or freezer. The practice of freezing infant-size portions in ice cube trays allows thawing of serving sizes when needed. Infant foods should be stored in the refrigerator no more than 2 days. Warming the food to a temperature for feeding creates an ideal environment for bacterial growth. Therefore only the amount the infant will consume at one meal should be warmed and this should be done just before serving. Any of the serving that is unused should be discarded.

Home preparation of infant foods can be time-consuming, but offers an economical way to provide nutritious meals that can be adapted to the developmental level and preferences of the infant. Care needs to be taken to prepare foods only under sanitary conditions and to provide a variety of foods for a balanced diet.

CHAPTER

The High-Risk Infant

Melody Thompson

Chapter Outline

McKenzie is 3 months old and weighs 1880 g (4 lb, 2 oz). She was born at 27 weeks' gestation and weighed 680 g (1 lb, 8 oz) at birth. Today she will be discharged home from the neonatal intensive care unit (NICU) at the regional medical center where she has been hospitalized since birth. Her parents have dressed her in a lacy, flowered doll dress and she smiles when the nurses wish her well as she leaves to go home. Her parents choke back tears as they express deep gratitude to the nursery staff. They have spent the three toughest months of their lives making almost daily trips to the hospital.

When McKenzie was born an extremely preterm infant, the odds were against her. But she was a fighter who kicked her little legs and twice grasped and removed the ventilator tubing that kept her alive. She remained on the ventilator for the first month of her life. During this time she was fed purified nutrients (parenteral nutrition [PN]) infused into one of her larger veins. McKenzie was also started on small quantities of her mother's milk, which her mom had pumped from her breasts. Eventually McKenzie was weaned from the intravenous (IV) nutrition and was fed fortified mother's milk by a tube threaded through her mouth and into her stomach.

McKenzie became strong enough to breathe on her own and then began the process of learning to eat on her own. She alternated nipple feeding and tube feeding until she had the maturity and endurance to stay awake and take all of her feedings by nipple. Her mom was also able to breast-feed her.

On her 3-month "birthday," McKenzie could maintain her temperature (while wrapped in a blanket) in a normal room environment. She was also able to breathe on her own and fully nipple- or breast-feed (without tube feedings). Her proud parents, nurses, doctors, and other healthcare team members were excited to see her "graduate" from the NICU and go home.

INTRODUCTION

- *Define the preterm, low-birth-weight infant and describe the factors that place this infant at high nutritional risk.*

Infants born before 37 weeks' gestation are considered to be preterm, or premature. Low-birth-weight (LBW) infants weigh less than 2500 g at birth (American Academy of Pediatrics/ American College of Obstetricians and Gynecologists, 1997). Being preterm and/or LBW is associated with an increase in morbidity and mortality compared with the statistics for a full-term, normal-weight infant. Thus preterm and LBW infants are considered "high-risk" infants. Advances in the technology of infant intensive care have allowed smaller and smaller infants to survive (El-Metwally, Vohr, and Tucker, 2000; Lemons et al., 2001). Thus birth weight categories have been further subdi-vided to define very-low-birth-weight (VLBW) infants as those weighing less than 1500 g and extremely-low-birth-weight (ELBW) infants as those weighing less than 1000 g (Anderson, 2000). Lower birth weight and younger gestational age are associated with higher medical and nutritional risk.

Infants who are preterm are often LBW, but these conditions do not necessarily occur together. Some infants are LBW because they did not grow properly *in utero*. These infants are small for gestational age (SGA) or have suffered intrauterine growth retardation (IUGR). For example a 40-week-gestation infant weighing 2300 g is the product of a mother who smoked 2 packs of cigarettes a day (maternal cigarette smoking can have a negative effect on fetal growth). This infant may behave like a mature infant, but have problems related to LBW. On the other hand preterm infants can be of normal birth weight. For example, a 36-week-gestation infant weighing 3500 g is the product of a diabetic mother. This infant is considered large for gestational age (LGA) and may have problems related to prematurity, but not to birth weight.

In the United States the incidence of prematurity is 11.6%. The incidence of LBW and VLBW are 7.6% and 1.45% of live births, respectively (Ventura et al., 2000). The rising incidence of prematurity and LBW in the United States is attributed to the rise in rates of multiple births associated with assisted reproduction technologies. Twins, triplets, and higher-order multiples are more likely to be preterm and LBW. Infants that are preterm, LBW, or both may require prolonged hospitalization before they are big enough, strong enough, and mature enough to be cared for at home.

NUTRITION RISK FACTORS

- *What factors put the preterm or LBW infant at high nutritional risk?*

Limited Nutrient Reserves

The majority of nutrient transfer and fetal weight gain occurs during the third trimester of pregnancy. At this time the fetus can gain 30 g daily. This transplacental transfer of nutrients is abruptly interrupted by preterm birth. A striking visual example of this phenomenon is the absence of subcutaneous fat stores in a tiny preterm infant (Figure 8-1). Fat is important for thermoregulation, organ support and insulation, storage of fat-soluble vitamins and essential fatty acids, and, most importantly, energy. Thus tiny infants are vulnerable to problems caused by inadequate fat stores. They need to be kept in incubators that help regulate their body temperatures. They need adequate supplies of fat-soluble vitamins and essential fatty acids. And they need exogenous energy sources to help preserve and build their small fat reserves.

Another good example of limited nutrient stores involves calcium. During the third trimester the placenta is pushing calcium into the fetus against a concentration gradient. Two thirds of bone mineralization occurs at this time. Thus an infant born early in the third trimester has undermineralized bones that may be susceptible to fractures unless an adequate mineral intake is ensured.

Increased Nutrient Needs

The increase in nutrient needs of high-risk infants relates to inadequate nutrient stores and rapid growth rates. For example, during the third trimester, the fetus receives 120 mg/kg to 150 mg/kg per day of calcium through the placenta (Krug, 2000). To approach this calcium retention rate, a preterm infant must ingest 200 mg/kg per day of calcium, which has an absorption rate of 50% to 70% (Yu, 1999). In contrast a full-term, normal-weight infant whose bones are adequately mineralized needs only 60 mg/kg of calcium per day. Adults need only 10 mg/kg to

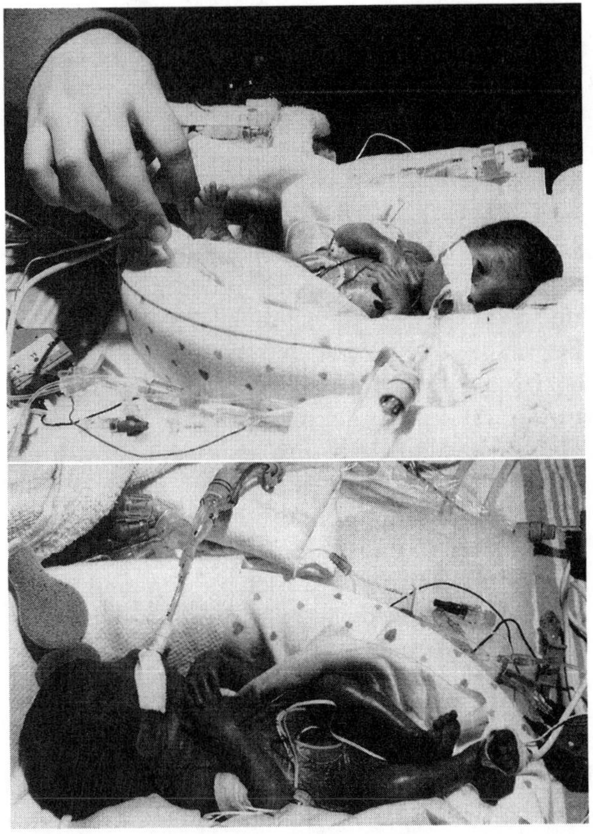

Figure 8-1 A 500 g infant. Note the absence of subcutaneous fat stores. *(Photo credit: Melody Thompson.)*

20 mg/kg of calcium per day. Providing this high calcium intake to high-risk infants poses clinical challenges to the medical team. Often these infants receive IV nutrition. Because there are limits to the solubility of minerals in IV solutions, infants are rarely able to receive the minerals they need by this route. When these infants are enterally fed, high-mineral formulas or supplements must be chosen.

Immature Alimentary Tract

Immaturities in the preterm infant's alimentary tract make it difficult to feed this infant by the enteral route. The infant's sucking and swallowing are immature and uncoordinated until approximately 34 weeks gestational age (Groh-Wargo, 2000a). The gastric capacity may limit the amount of formula that is tolerated. For example a 1500 g infant has a stomach capacity of only 3 mL at birth. By the end of the first week this infant's gastric capacity is 30 mL, or 2 tablespoons (Groh-Wargo, 2000a).

The motor function of the preterm infant's intestinal tract is underdeveloped. Peristaltic waves and segmentation do not propel the food bolus as effectively as they do in mature infants. There may also be enzyme and cofactor immaturities, which may limit digestion and absorption of nutrients. For example preterm infants have limited amounts of pancreatic lipase and one half of the bile acid pool that term infants have. This is thought to limit their ability to handle a normal intake of long-chain triglycerides (LCTs). Thus they are often fed diets containing medium-chain triglycerides (MCTs) (Yu, 1999).

Metabolic Immaturities

Adaptation to extrauterine life requires that high-risk infants regulate their own fluid, electrolyte, and glucose levels. Immature organs may limit their ability to do this effectively. The SGA infant, for example, may have hypoglycemia (low blood sugar) from inadequate glycogen stores. On the other hand the LGA infant also may have hypoglycemia because of the abrupt interruption in glucose supply with birth, resulting in relatively high insulin and low glucose levels. Both of these infants require an immediate source of glucose to correct low serum levels and prevent neurologic problems associated with prolonged or profound hypoglycemia (Cornblath and Ichord, 2000).

Medical Complications/Stresses

Some high-risk infants are born with or develop complications that have an effect on their nutritional status or nutrient needs. Some infants, for instance, are born with their intestines protruding through a defect in the abdominal wall. This condition is called gastroschisis. These edematous and malrotated intestines often function poorly and are too large to fit immediately into the infant's small abdominal cavity. The intestines are suspended in a plastic sheath until the swelling goes down and they fit comfortably in the abdomen. Meanwhile the infant must be fed completely by the IV route. Need for protein may be elevated by surgical stress and excess losses (Valentine, 2000).

Limited Diet

Infants depend solely on human milk or infant formula to meet their nutritional needs for the first 4 months of life. High-risk infants may require PN and human milk or formula. Having such a limited diet makes infants more vulnerable to nutrient deficiencies or toxicities. For example if the infant's sole source of nutrition is deficient in a nutrient (e.g., chloride, which occurred in several batches of infant formula in 1979), long-term development of that infant may be adversely affected (Roy III et al., 1996).

Inability to Seek Food

Infants are unable to obtain their own food; they depend on caregivers to recognize their needs and provide nourishment. This inability to supply their own needs for food when they feel the sensation of hunger puts infants at additional nutritional risk.

ASSESSMENT OF NUTRITION STATUS

- *What are the elements of nutrition assessment and how does each element apply to the high-risk infant?*

Nutrition assessment of high-risk infants involves the same elements as nutrition assessment of other populations; that is, it includes anthropometric, biochemical, clinical, and nutrient intake data. Assessment of the infant's gestational age and size is also important.

Determination of Gestational Age and Size for Age

Because the clinical problems of infants differ according to their gestational age and size for age, accurate estimation of gestational age is important. Several methods are used to determine gestational age. If the mother knows the date of her last menstrual period, this can be used to calculate the infant's gestational age. Because this method relies on the mother's memory, it may be subject to error.

Alternatively gestational age can be estimated by fetal measurements performed during ultrasound examinations early in the pregnancy. Measurements of fetal length, head diameter, or both are compared with established standards to assess the gestational age more accurately.

When the infant is born, physical and neuromuscular examinations are used to assess his or her maturity. For example muscle flexion is associated with maturity. The more flexed the posture of the infant, the more mature he or she is. Flaccid, extended posture is associated with extreme immaturity. Infants are scored on at least 12 physical and neuromuscular parameters. The summation of the scores correlates with a particular gestational age. This examination has been standardized for even very immature infants and is considered a reliable estimate of gestational age (Anderson, 2000).

To assess size for gestational age, the infant's weight, length, and head circumference measurements are plotted on an intrauterine growth chart (Figure 8-2). If birth weight is less than two standard deviations from the mean, the infant is classified as SGA. If the birth weight is greater than two standard deviations from the mean, the infant is classified as LGA (Anderson, 2000). Infants between these extremes are classified as appropriate for gestational age (AGA).

Anthropometric Assessment

Assessment of weight, length, and head circumference for high-risk infants involves the same techniques used for term infants (see Chapter 7). However, a few differences may be noted. For small infants requiring intensive care, the scale should be accurate to the nearest 5 g. Medical apparatus (e.g., ventilator tubing and IV tubing) must be supported while the infant is removed from the bed and placed on the scale for weighing. Some infants are too unstable to be moved from the bed to the scale. Bed scales are available that allow the infants to remain on scales in their beds for prolonged periods.

Small, plastic length boards are available to measure the lengths of tiny infants. As for larger

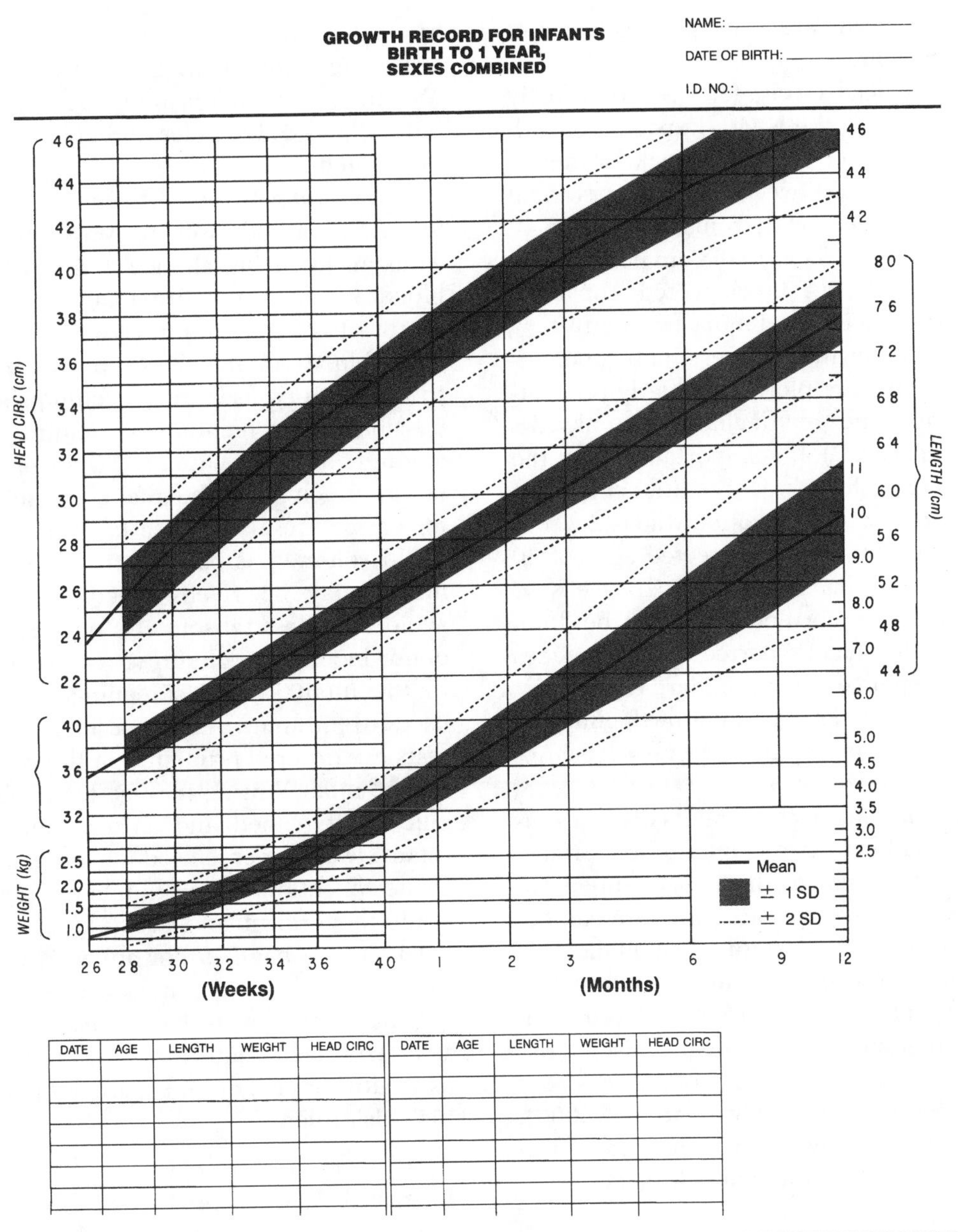

Figure 8-2 Intrauterine growth chart used to assess size for gestational age and to plot successive growth measurements. *(From Babson SG and Benda GJ: Growth graphs for the clinical assessment of infants of varying gestational ages, J Pediatr 89:814, 1976.)*

infants, two people are required to hold the infant's head and feet for accurate measurement. Measurement of head circumference is accomplished as for term infants (see Chapter 7).

High-risk infants are weighed at least once daily. Weight correlates with fluid status and growth. Small infants, like term infants, initially lose weight with diuresis of extracellular fluid. When fluid status stabilizes and they are given adequate calories, they gain weight with tissue growth. Normal weight gain is considered to be 10 g/kg to 20 g/kg per day (Catrine, 2000). Weight is one of the most important measurements in the NICU. Fluid, calorie, and many other nutrient needs are expressed in terms of the infant's weight.

Length and head circumference are usually measured weekly in the NICU. Expected growth in length is 0.8 cm to 1.1 cm per week for infants born at 28 weeks' to 40 weeks' gestation. Normal head circumference growth from 28 weeks' to 40 weeks' gestation is 0.5 cm to 0.8 cm per week. If abnormal head growth is suspected, the head circumference is measured more frequently.

To assess the infant's progress, anthropometric measurements are plotted regularly on postnatal or intrauterine growth charts (Ehrenkranz, 2000) (see Figure 8-2). It is important to plot the measurements at the correct gestational age. An infant born at 28 weeks' gestation who is 2 weeks old chronologically has a "corrected age" of 30 weeks' gestation. When the infant is 12 weeks, or 3 months, old, her corrected age will be "full-term." Once the infant's corrected age reaches term, it is acceptable to use standard Centers for Disease Control and Prevention growth charts to plot the infant's subsequent progress (see Appendix E).

Skinfold or fatfold measurements are not routinely performed in high-risk infants. The friable skin of tiny infants makes this measurement potentially invasive because skin puncture can occur. Variations in fluid status also make this measurement unreliable. The upper midarm circumference and the midarm circumference-to-head circumference ratio reflect muscle and fat stores and the relationship of these stores to brain growth, respectively (Catrine, 2000). Although not routinely taken, these measurements may be used for individual infants.

Biochemical (Laboratory) Assessment

The infant's initial laboratory measurements, if performed shortly after birth, reflect the mother's biochemical status. Over the first several days of life blood gases, blood count, and electrolyte measurements are performed in the laboratory to assess the high-risk infant's adaptation to the extrauterine environment. If the infant remains on IV nutrition, laboratory measurements are made several times weekly to monitor the safety and effectiveness of this therapy. Once the infant is stable and few changes are being made in the IV solutions, weekly biochemical assessments are made. Infants who are enterally fed have less frequent biochemical assessments.

An infant's blood volume is approximately 90 mL/kg of body weight (Moyer-Mileur, 2000). Thus an infant weighing 700 g will have a total blood volume of approximately 63 mL. Laboratory testing is minimized to preserve the infant's blood volume. When tests are performed the laboratory uses microtechniques whenever possible. Microtechniques require very small amounts of blood. Often NICU nurses keep track of how much blood the infant has had withdrawn for various tests. When a certain percentage of blood volume has been removed, a blood transfusion may be given. Blood transfusions are avoided unless absolutely necessary because donor blood can contain viruses that are passed to the infant. Blood screening procedures are used to minimize this possibility. Laboratory tests are ordered prudently in the NICU.

The infant's urine may be tested for pH, specific gravity, blood, and various metabolites. The infant's wet diaper is used for these spot-checks. Urine collections over a number of hours are difficult to perform and are seldom used in the NICU. Urine bags do not adhere well to immature skin, which is damaged in their removal, leaving abraded skin that is susceptible to infection. Thus tests requiring urine collections, such as creatinine-height index, are not performed for high-risk infants.

Clinical Assessment

Clinical assessment of the high-risk infant involves observing the infant's general condition. Clinical assessment can be supportive of laboratory and anthropometric data in determining the infant's state of hydration, for example. An infant suffering from **dehydration** can have sunken eyes and fontanelle, poor skin turgor, decreased urine output, increased urine specific gravity, and elevated laboratory values (hemoconcentration) and weight loss. An infant suffering from **overhydration** can have dependent edema; puffy hands, feet, and eyes; depressed laboratory values (hemodilution); and excessive weight gain. Clinical signs, observed in concert with other assessment parameters, can be used as a guide for adjusting the infant's therapy.

Feeding tolerance frequently is assessed clinically. The NICU nurse measures the infant's abdominal girth, checks the contents of the infant's stomach, records vomiting or emesis if it occurs, and records the characteristics of the infant's stools. These clinical observations are used to determine if the infant's feedings need to be halted or can be advanced safely.

Intake Assessment

Nutrient intake assessment can be qualitative and quantitative. **Qualitative assessment** involves evaluation of nutrient sources in relation to an infant's needs. Human milk and infant formulas contain a variety of nutrient sources. Lactose, the carbohydrate in mammalian milk, is common in many formulas, for example. Because an infant who has galactosemia cannot properly metabolize lactose or galactose, a lactose-free formula is indicated.

Quantitative assessment involves calculating the quantities of nutrients that the infant receives and comparing the results with recommended intakes. The infant's 24-hour intake is often used to perform calculations. Total intakes of fluid, calories, and protein are calculated. For parenterally fed infants, intakes of IV carbohydrate (glucose) and fat are calculated as well. With either enteral or PN, other nutrients may be calculated in addition, depending on the infant's particular problems. Computer programs are available to assist in calculating multiple nutrient intakes for infants who require intensive care (Thompson and Bamberger, 2000).

NUTRIENT NEEDS OF HIGH-RISK INFANTS

- *Why are the needs for fluid, energy, and protein greater for the high-risk infant than they are for the term, healthy infant?*

What constitutes optimal nutrient intake and growth in the high-risk infant is unknown and is the subject of some controversy. In 1998 the American Academy of Pediatrics reaffirmed its contention that the goal of nutritional care for preterm infants is to resume growth at an intrauterine rate (American Academy of Pediatrics Committee on Nutrition, 1998). Actual growth rates of LBW infants often fall short of this goal. Metabolic and excretory limitations of high-risk infants can preclude resuming intrauterine nutrient accretion and growth. Whether intrauterine-type growth is optimal or better than the slower growth customarily seen remains to be proved.

In the NICU, nutrient intakes and needs are often expressed as the amount of nutrient per kilogram of body weight per day rather than as the absolute quantity of the nutrient per day. This expression is necessary because the size of the infants in the NICU varies. A 500 g infant and a 4000 g infant may both require intensive care. The large infant weighs eight times more than the small infant and needs much larger quantities of nutrients. Each infant may grow on 110 kcal/kg per day. For the 500 g infant this is 55 kcal per day, whereas for the 4000 g infant, this is 440 kcal per day. Thus nutrient intakes and needs are often expressed *per kilogram* per day.

Fluid and Electrolytes

Fluid needs are quite variable for high-risk neonates. Fluids are lost through urine, stool, respiratory tract, and skin. Small infants lose much fluid (called **insensible water loss**) through their immature skin and respiratory

KEY TERMS

dehydration: a condition in which fluid output exceeds fluid intake

overhydration: a condition in which fluid intake exceeds fluid output

qualitative assessment: evaluation of nutrient sources

quantitative assessment: calculation of nutrient intake quantities and comparison with recommendations

insensible water loss: water lost through immature skin and respiratory tract

Table 8-1 APPROXIMATE FLUID REQUIREMENTS FOR LBW INFANTS

Birth Weight (g)	Transition (mL/kg/day)	Maintenance (mL/kg/day)
<1000	100	120-160
1000-2000	80	100-140
>2000	60	80-120

From Shaffer SG and Weismann DN: Fluid requirements in the preterm infant, Clin Perinatol 19:239, 1992. Used with permission.

Table 8-2 ESTIMATED CALORIC REQUIREMENT IN A TYPICAL GROWING PREMATURE INFANT

	kcal/kg/day
Resting caloric expenditure	50
Intermittent activity	15
Occasional cold stress	10
Specific dynamic action	8
Fecal loss of calories	12
Growth allowance	25
Total	120

tracts. They may need a lot more fluid per kilogram of body weight than a larger infant needs. Fluid needs in the first several days of life (transition) are lower than in the maintenance phase (Table 8-1). Like term infants, preterm infants lose weight (diuresis of fluid) initially after birth and start gaining after the first week, when adequate calorie intake is reached. A high-risk infant's immature kidneys do not conserve sodium and those of a mature infant do, so the premature infant's sodium needs are often higher than are those of a term infant. Chloride needs are similarly higher, but potassium needs are estimated to be the same as those of the term infant.

Energy

The high-risk infant needs energy to perform body functions and to grow. Categories of energy expenditure include basal metabolic rate (resting caloric expenditure), activity, cold stress, specific dynamic action (SDA), stool losses, and growth (Table 8-2). The average caloric need for the enterally fed high-risk infant is 120 kcal/kg per day. Because the parenterally fed infant does not use as many calories for activity, cold stress, SDA, or stool losses, the parenterally fed infant may need only 80 kcal/kg to 90 kcal/kg per day. As in other age groups, calorie needs differ among individuals and must be assessed for each patient in relation to that infant's growth and medical problems.

Because their digestive and absorptive mechanisms are immature, preterm infants benefit from receiving a variety of energy sources. As mentioned earlier in this chapter, preterm infants have a limited ability to digest and absorb LCTs. To compensate, MCTs are included in preterm formulas (PTFs) and human milk fortifiers. Mature intestinal lactase levels are not reached until term. Thus PTFs and human milk fortifiers contain glucose polymers (and lactose), which are readily hydrolyzed by brush border glucoamylase.

Protein

The high-risk infant needs protein to build and repair body tissues. Smaller infants need to accrete more nitrogen-containing tissue and thus have higher protein needs per kilogram than do larger infants. Infants who weigh less than 2000 g may need 3.5 g protein/kg per day or more (American Academy of Pediatrics Committee on Nutrition, 1998). Parenterally fed preterm infants need 2.5 g to 3 g protein/kg per day in the form of crystalline amino acids. In addition to essential amino acids, preterm infants, like term infants, fed by any route need exogenous sources of tyrosine, taurine, and cystine. If inadequate energy is supplied, protein will be broken down and used as an energy source. Thus enough calories must be provided as carbohydrate and fat to "spare" the protein.

Minerals and Vitamins

Because of their low nutrient stores and high needs for growth, high-risk infants often have mineral and vitamin needs that exceed those of

Table 8-3 GUIDELINES FOR SELECTED DAILY NUTRIENT INTAKES OF ENTERALLY FED PRETERM INFANTS

Nutrient	Recommended Intake
Protein	3-4 g/kg
Calcium	120-230 mg/kg
Phosphorus	60-140 mg/kg
Iron	2-6 mg/kg
Sodium	2-3 mEq/kg
Vitamin A	700-1500 IU/kg
Vitamin D	400 IU/d
Thiamine	180-240 μg/kg
Riboflavin	250-360 μg/kg
Vitamin C	18-24 mg/kg

Adapted from Groh-Wargo S: Recommended enteral nutrient intakes. In Groh-Wargo S, Thompson M, and Cox JH, editors: Nutritional care for high-risk newborns, Chicago, 2000, Precept.

term, normal-weight infants. Small infants have particularly high needs for the minerals (calcium and phosphorus) that provide structure for skeletal mass. Medications (diuretics and steroids) that are often used for sick infants can impair the retention of these minerals, making an optimal supply critical. Preterm infants' stores of iron, trace elements, and vitamins are depleted more quickly than are the stores of a mature infant. Clinical deficiencies of zinc and copper have been described in preterm infants (Groh-Wargo, 2000b). Sources of essential micronutrients must be ensured (Aggett, 2000; Greer, 2000). The American Academy of Pediatrics recommends providing at least 2 mg iron/kg per day by double birth weight or 2 months of age (American Academy of Pediatrics Committee on Nutrition, 1998). Little is known about the LBW infant's need for water-soluble vitamins. Supplemented parenteral solutions, fortified human milk, and PTF appear to provide adequate intakes. Suboptimal stores and poor absorption of fat-soluble vitamins increase the preterm infants' needs for vitamins A, D, E, and K. All are provided in fortified human milk, PTF, and PN supplemented with vitamins. Preterm infants, like term infants, are given an intramuscular injection of vitamin K at birth. Parenteral needs for minerals and vitamins often differ from enteral requirements. Intestinal absorption rates are considered in developing recommended enteral intakes (Table 8-3).

FEEDING THE HIGH-RISK INFANT

- *Describe the impact of physiologic development on the choice of feeding method for the high-risk infant.*
- *What are the unique features of fortified preterm human milk and PTFs?*

Physiologic Development

Although the fetus demonstrates sucking *in utero,* the preterm infant cannot effectively coordinate sucking, swallowing, and breathing until approximately 34 weeks' gestational age (Groh-Wargo, 2000a). Before that time the infant needs to receive tube feedings because the risk of aspiration with nipple feedings is too great. Preterm infants are given pacifiers during tube feedings to give them practice sucking and to promote the association of sucking with satiety. This is called **nonnutritive sucking** (Hafström and Kjellmer, 2000). Infants who engage in nonnutritive sucking interventions are able to bottle feed and are discharged from the hospital sooner than are infants who do not have this sucking practice (Pinelli and Symington, 2000). Nutritive sucking (taking formula from a nipple) often starts with one feeding daily. Preterm infants are capable of giving subtle cues to caregivers about their readiness to feed by mouth. Experienced NICU nurses recognize and respond to these cues. Eager sucking and swallowing that allows effective formula intake in a reasonable time indicates that the infant is ready for more nipple feedings daily. Poor sucking, poor state control (falling asleep during feeding), or poor autonomic control (loss of control in respiration, color, and/or heart rate) may mean that the infant is not ready to progress on an oral feeding regimen. This infant receives tube feedings to replace or supplement oral feedings as needed.

KEY TERMS

nonnutritive sucking: sucking on a pacifier

Research Update

Team Approach to Neonatal Nutrition Management

Because management of the nutritional care of high-risk infants occurs in the hospital, a team of professionals is involved. Key members of the team are physicians, nurses, and dietitians or nutritionists. The physician is responsible for writing orders that prescribe the nutrition care that the infant receives. The nurse implements the feeding orders (i.e., administers IV nutrition and enteral feedings) and notes the infant's reactions to feedings. The dietitian develops individual nutrition care plans and provides consultation to physicians and nurses on infant nutrient needs, product composition, and growth expectations (Thompson, 2000). The nutrition team can also include a clinical pharmacist, developmental therapist, and lactation specialist. These healthcare professionals work together to identify and provide optimal healthcare and nutrition to high-risk infants (Horbar et al., 2001; Rogowski et al., 2001).

Mode of Feeding

Parenteral

The medical conditions of high-risk infants often preclude enteral feeding immediately after birth. An IV of glucose in water is started to maintain fluid balance and to spare body tissues from being broken down for energy. When the infant has shown adequate urine output, usually within 24 hours, electrolytes are added to the glucose water IV solution. At this time or the next day all other IV nutrients are added to the solution. This is called PN. These nutrients are in forms (e.g., sterile, "predigested" forms) and quantities needed for infants. Prepackaged IV vitamins, minerals, and trace elements that meet the unique needs of high-risk infants are available. Pediatric crystalline amino acid solutions (the IV protein source) are available that contain the proper proportions of amino acids to meet high-risk infants' needs while reducing the risk of metabolic complications (Kalhan and Iben, 2000). Intravenous fat emulsions may be infused separately or added to the solution to provide a source of essential fatty acids and calories. These nutrients are combined under sterile conditions in the hospital pharmacy to provide a complete IV nutrient mixture for each infant. In many cases standard solutions that supply the same proportions of nutrients to all infants can be used. For infants with special needs, individual combinations of nutrients must be prepared. Investigators continue to define the unique parenteral nutrient needs of the LBW infant (Thureen and Hay, 2000).

Enteral

As mentioned earlier, high-risk infants receive enteral feedings by nipple or by tube. Traditionally, enteral feedings were withheld from high-risk infants for the first several weeks of life because their gastrointestinal (GI) tracts were thought to be too immature to handle feedings. Recent evidence shows that small-volume feedings are trophic to the infant's GI tract. If the infant is medically stable, this **minimal enteral nutrition** (also called gut stimulation or priming feedings) is started at 10 mL/kg to 20 mL/kg per day and is not advanced for the first week or two. Minimal enteral nutrition is associated with improved feeding tolerance, improved hormonal surges, and earlier intestinal maturation (McClure and Newell, 1999; Wessel, 2000). Early feeding also has beneficial effects on indirect hyperbilirubinemia, cholestatic jaundice, and osteopenia of prematurity. It is important to advance feedings slowly to avoid overwhelming the infant's digestive and absorptive capabilities because aggressive feeding advances can lead to intestinal disease such as neonatal necrotizing enterocolitis (NEC). The preferred feedings for high-risk infants are human milk and PTF.

Human milk. The benefits of human milk for the high-risk infant include superior digestibility and the presence of host resistance factors not available in current formulas (Atkinson, 2000). Nutrient composition of the milk of mothers who deliver preterm is different from the milk of mothers who deliver at term (Sapsford, 2000). Preterm mother's milk (PTM) is better suited to the preterm infant's needs than is term mother's milk (TM). The PTM contains higher amounts of protein and electrolytes than does TM, providing a bonus for high-risk infants who need more of these nutrients. However, PTM does not contain enough calcium and phosphorus to mineralize the bones of VLBW infants. These infants can develop osteopenia of prematurity and even fractured bones unless their mother's milk is fortified with minerals. Commercially available **human milk fortifiers** are added to PTM to enrich the mineral content and also to provide extra protein, calories, and vitamins. High-risk infants who are fed fortified PTM demonstrate improved growth (Reis et al., 2000) and tolerate fortified milk well (Moody et al., 2000). Although fortifiers are usually discontinued when the infant is discharged from the hospital, there is evidence that tiny infants may benefit from continued fortification at home (Wauben et al., 1998).

Although some NICUs accept donor milk, most prefer milk only from the infants' own mothers. Like donor blood, donor milk may contain viruses that can cause illness in the infant receiving the milk. Providing milk for her infant is a unique contribution that a mother can make to the care of her high-risk infant.

Preterm formulas. Formulas designed specifically for preterm infants are more suited to their nutritional needs than are standard term infant formulas. The PTF differs from term formula in nutrient sources and nutrient quantity. The protein in PTF (whey-predominant cow milk protein) is easier for the infant to digest and contains amino acids that preterm infants need. The PTF contains two sources of carbohydrate (lactose and glucose polymers) and two categories of fat (LCT and MCT). Because high-risk infants have immature intestinal tracts and may be unable to handle a full load of any one carbohydrate or fat, two of each are used. Each uses different enzymes and absorptive mechanisms, with a resulting increase in overall nutrient retention (Kien, McClead, and Cordero, 1998). Ongoing studies have implications for future modifications of PTFs (Morley, 1998). For example it remains unclear whether formula-fed preterm infants need exogenous sources of the long-chain polyunsaturated fatty acids present in human milk (O'Connor et al., 2001). These fatty acids are docosahexaenoic acid (DHA) and arachidonic acid (ARA). The American Academy of Pediatrics does not have specific recommendations for DHA and ARA in infancy and the FDA has not allowed their inclusion in U.S. preterm formulas.

Because high-risk infants have limited nutrient stores and high needs and can often tolerate only limited formula volume, PTF is highly fortified with nutrients. The protein, mineral, and vitamin content of PTF is higher than that of standard formula (Table 8-4). In practice, PTF is generally used for infants weighing less than 2000 g at birth. When the infant is well enough to go home, the formula is often changed to a preterm discharge formula. Preterm discharge formulas were developed in the 1990s because of the concern that term formula cannot meet the ongoing nutrient needs of high-risk infants. Some infants on term formula in follow-up have shown subclinical nutrient deficiencies, suggesting the continued need for nutrient-dense formulas following hospital discharge. Special preterm discharge formulas have promoted improved growth in high-risk infants at home during the first year of life (Cooke and Embleton, 2000). Two such formulas, Similac NeoSure (Ross Products Division, Abbott Laboratories, Columbus, OH) and Enfamil EnfaCare (Mead Johnson, Evansville, IN) are currently available

KEY TERMS

minimal enteral nutrition: small-volume feedings that are trophic to the gastrointestinal tract and help in its maturation

human milk fortifiers: nutrients added to boost the nutritional value of human milk for high-risk infants

Table 8-4 Selected Nutrient Comparison in 100 mL of Formula

Nutrient	Standard Infant Formula*	Preterm Infant Formula†
Protein	1.4 g	1.8-2.0 g
Calcium	53 mg	111-122 mg
Phosphorus	28-36 mg	56-68 mg
Iron	1.2 mg	1.2 mg
Sodium	0.7-0.8 mEq	1.1-1.3 mEq
Vitamin A	203 IU	845 IU
Vitamin D	41 IU	100-180 IU
Thiamin	54-67 μg	135-170 μg
Riboflavin	95-101 μg	200-420 μg
Vitamin C	6.1-8.1 mg	14-25 mg

*Ranges of nutrients contained in Similac with Iron 20, Ross Products Division, Abbott Laboratories, Columbus, OH and Enfamil with Iron 20, Mead Johnson Nutritionals, Evansville, IN.
†Ranges of nutrients contained in Similac Special Care with Iron 20, Ross Products Division, Abbott Laboratories, Columbus, OH and Enfamil Premature Formula with Iron 20, Mead Johnson Nutritionals, Evansville, IN.

in the United States. The American Academy of Pediatrics recognizes the benefit of preterm discharge formula for preterm infants for 9 months after hospitalization (American Academy of Pediatrics Committee on Nutrition, 1998).

Other formulas. Standard term infant formulas and protein hydrolysate formulas are not suited to the high-risk infant's needs. If these formulas must be used for prolonged periods, they require nutrient fortification. The use of soy-based formulas has been associated with osteopenia of prematurity because the minerals in soy formula are not as well absorbed as are the minerals in cow milk-based formulas. Even when it is supplemented with minerals, the use of soy formula in VLBW infants is associated with slower growth and lower serum protein status than that achieved with PTF. Soy formulas are not recommended for infants who weigh less than 1800 g at birth (American Academy of Pediatrics Committee on Nutrition, 1998).

Lactation management. The high-risk infant may be unable to breast-feed for a prolonged time. The mother who wishes to eventually nurse her infant will need to pump the milk from her breasts to establish and maintain a milk supply. Breast milk production follows the law of supply and demand. If the milk is removed from the breasts regularly, the body will produce more. Electric breast pumps are available, which effectively remove milk and assist in maintaining a milk supply over a prolonged period. Other methods of breast pumping (e.g., hand expression and manual pumps) are less effective for long-term pumping (see Figure 6-8, page 198) (Lawrence and Lawrence, 1999).

Expressed milk is placed in sterile containers, labeled, and stored in a refrigerator or freezer. This milk can be fortified in the NICU and fed (by tube or bottle) to the high-risk infant. Eventually the infant will be able to nurse directly from the breast. Because pumped human milk is not sterile and is a good growth medium for microorganisms, the milk may be cultured before it is fed to the infant (Lawrence and Lawrence, 1999). The milk can be contaminated by soiled pumping equipment or poor handwashing techniques. It is thus important to have policies and procedures for handling, storing, culturing, and feeding human milk in the NICU.

GROWTH AND DEVELOPMENTAL OUTCOME

- *What factors affect the high-risk infant's growth rate and developmental outcome?*

Several factors affect the high-risk infant's growth rate: birth weight, gestational age, nutrient intake, medical problems, home environment, and genetic potential. By definition LBW infants are smaller than average term neonates at birth. **Catch-up growth** may occur during the first 1 year to 3 years of life in infants without residual illness. Catch-up growth in head circumference usually precedes that in weight and length. Preterm infants who are appropriately grown for their gestational age are more likely to catch up eventually with their full-term peers than are SGA infants (McCowan et al., 1999; Theriot, 2000).

The feeding of human milk, PTF, or both confers developmental advantages to LBW infants compared with feeding of term formula. These advantages appear to persist into childhood.

Outcome studies are ongoing (see Application: Long-Term Outcome of Former LBW Infants).

MEDICAL/SURGICAL CONDITIONS COMPLICATING THE NUTRITIONAL MANAGEMENT OF HIGH-RISK INFANTS

- *What specific medical or surgical conditions complicate the nutritional management of high-risk infants?*

Hyperbilirubinemia

Hyperbilirubinemia (or jaundice) is a condition defined by high amounts of the pigment bilirubin in the blood. Bilirubin is produced from the breakdown of heme-containing proteins, particularly red cell hemoglobin. Hyperbilirubinemia is common in immature infants because their livers are not as capable of breaking down the bilirubin pigment as are the livers of term infants. Hyperbilirubinemia occurs more frequently in breast-fed than in formula-fed infants, for unknown reasons.

If too much bilirubin builds up in the bloodstream, it can cross the blood-brain barrier and cause mental retardation. Fortunately bilirubin can be changed to a water-soluble isomer by certain wavelengths of light. The infant receives phototherapy and bilirubin is then excreted in the infant's stool or urine.

Nutrition plays only a small, complementary role in treating hyperbilirubinemia. Feedings may be started or advanced to enhance intestinal movement and excretion of bilirubin. Breast-fed infants should continue to be breast-fed with an increase in the frequency of nursing (American Academy of Pediatrics Committee on Nutrition, 1998). If jaundice persists, interruption of nursing (i.e., feeding formula or alternating formula and breast-feeding) for 24 hours to 48 hours usually resolves hyperbilirubinemia related to breast-feeding (Hammerman and Kaplan, 2000). In the past water was given to infants with hyperbilirubinemia in an attempt to dilute the bilirubin concentration in the blood. Providing water supplements to breast-fed infants, however, has no impact on serum bilirubin levels (Gourley, 2000).

Respiratory, Cardiac, and Renal Problems

High-risk infants can have medical problems that involve their respiratory, cardiac, or renal systems. Often these infants may be sensitive to high fluid intakes, which make their conditions worse, leading to respiratory distress, congestive heart failure, or acute renal failure. These infants need alterations in their fluid and electrolyte intakes. They often have higher resting and total energy expenditures than do their healthy peers and they tire easily when eating. They may need nutrient- and calorie-dense formula or supplements to human milk (Premer and Georgieff, 1999).

Gastrointestinal Problems

Preterm infants are susceptible to a GI disease called neonatal NEC. This appears to be a multifactorial disorder associated with GI mucosal injury, possible GI infection, and the presence of enteral feedings. The diagnosis of NEC is associated with a high incidence of morbidity and mortality. Infants who have NEC or other GI problems may need to "rest" their intestines until they heal. Thus they receive PN during this time. When the intestines have healed, enteral feedings are gradually reintroduced (Price, 2000).

Bone Problems

Osteopenia of prematurity (decreased bone mass) can occur in infants with undermineralized bones, inadequate mineral intake, or excessive mineral losses. Treatment involves providing high intakes of calcium and phosphorus to mineralize the bones (Krug, 2000). These high

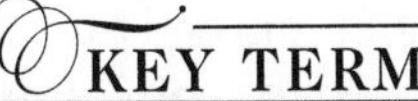

KEY TERMS

catch-up growth: growth at a faster-than-expected rate following a period of attenuated growth

levels are best supplied by fortified human milk or PTF. Adequate intake of vitamin D helps in calcium absorption and bone remodeling.

SPECIAL CONCERNS

- *Describe the impact of maternal substance abuse or human immunodeficiency virus (HIV) on the infant.*

Effects of Maternal Substance Abuse

Maternal substance abuse encompasses the use of alcohol, cigarettes, and/or illicit drugs during pregnancy. The effects on the fetus vary with the frequency and dose of the substance received and the stage of pregnancy in which the substance is used. Fetal effects can be caused directly by the substance itself or indirectly by maternal self-neglect. Because drug abuse, alcohol abuse, and cigarette smoking frequently coincide, it is difficult to isolate the effects of one substance from the other in studies of pregnant substance-abusing women.

Alcohol

Alcohol and its primary metabolite, acetaldehyde, are directly toxic to the developing fetus and are capable of producing abnormalities. Infants of mothers who drink heavily during pregnancy may be afflicted with fetal alcohol syndrome (FAS). The incidence of FAS is approximately one to two infants per thousand live births in the United States (American Academy of Pediatrics Committee on Nutrition, 1998) and includes physical and developmental abnormalities specific to infants with this condition. The infant is SGA and has microcephaly, postnatal growth deficiency, developmental delay, and distorted facial features. Adequate nutrition does not reverse the infant's growth delay. Children who are exposed to alcohol during the entire pregnancy demonstrate worse performance on developmental testing than do those exposed to alcohol during the first trimester only. Thus it behooves a mother to curtail alcohol consumption as soon as possible during pregnancy. Binge drinking during the first trimester, however, may be as dangerous to the fetus as steady exposure throughout gestation.

When compared with their peers, school-aged children with FAS have a lower intelligence quotient (IQ) and may have learning disabilities. Because no one knows how much alcohol during pregnancy is too much, alcohol use during pregnancy and when planning for conception is not recommended (American Academy of Pediatrics Committee on Nutrition, 1998).

Smoking

Cigarette smoking by pregnant women has been associated with an increased risk of spontaneous abortion, stillbirth, prematurity, and IUGR. Head growth of the infant is particularly affected. The degree of growth retardation is directly related to the number of cigarettes smoked (Källén, 2000). This growth failure may be irreversible in the postnatal period. The exact mechanism of the adverse effect of cigarette smoking on pregnancy is unknown (Pollack, Lantz, and Frohna, 2000). Smoking in the same room as the infant also increases the risk for sudden infant death (Klonoff-Cohen et al., 1995).

Illicit Drugs

Illicit drug use during pregnancy can have profound negative effects on the fetus. Infants who are exposed to drugs *in utero* are often growth-retarded and may be drug addicted at birth. The symptoms of neonatal withdrawal syndrome are primarily neurologic: jitteriness, restlessness, tremulousness, irritability, and hypertonicity. Alimentary tract symptoms include poor sucking and swallowing, vomiting, and diarrhea. Providing calorie and nutrient supplements; small, frequent feedings; and tube feedings when needed may help to attenuate problems with nutrition and growth.

Drug-exposed infants may have delayed postnatal growth, especially in head circumference. Small head size correlates with suboptimal developmental outcome, which may persist into high school (Eriksson, Jonsson, and Zetterstrom, 2000).

Human Immunodeficiency Virus

The HIV virus causes acquired immunodeficiency syndrome (AIDS). The most common cause of pediatric HIV infection is perinatal transmission from an infected mother. Maternal-infant transmission of HIV can be reduced with antiretroviral medication; antenatal HIV testing and counseling is therefore encouraged (Fernandez and McNeeley, 2000). Another rare cause is transmission of HIV in human breast milk (Black, 1996). A large, randomized, controlled trial concluded that the use of infant formula (rather than breast-feeding) for infants whose mothers are HIV positive prevents infant infections and is associated with improved HIV-free survival (Nduati et al., 2000).

Children with HIV infection who become symptomatic (develop AIDS) succumb to the disease more quickly than do adults. Symptoms of HIV infection in the pediatric population include generalized lymphadenopathy (swollen glands), hepatomegaly (enlarged liver), splenomegaly (enlarged spleen), failure to thrive (poor growth), diarrhea, and fever (Fernandez and McNeeley, 2000). Multiple nutritional deficiencies, particularly protein-calorie malnutrition, may develop. Malabsorptive disorders contribute to nutritional problems. Nutrition intervention may include protein-calorie supplementation and vitamin and mineral assessment and supplementation as needed. Tube feedings may be necessary if oral intake is insufficient; PN is indicated if the GI tract is nonfunctional (Olsen, Cutroni, and Furuta, 1999).

SUMMARY

The high-risk infant is usually preterm, LBW, or both. This infant is at high nutritional risk because of limited nutrient reserves, increased nutrient needs, immature alimentary tract, metabolic immaturities, medical complications or stresses, limited diet, and inability to seek food. Assessing the infant's nutrition status includes determination of gestational age and size for age; and anthropometric, biochemical, clinical, and intake assessments. Nutrient needs are usually higher for these infants than they are for term, normal-weight infants. Parenteral nutrition may be emphasized until physiologic maturity allows advancement to full enteral feedings. Pediatric parenteral products, fortified mother's milk, and PTFs are appropriate nutrient sources for high-risk infants. Infants who have appropriate size and weight for gestational age may catch up in growth to their term, normal-weight peers; SGA infants are less likely to catch up. Medical and surgical conditions complicate the nutritional management of high-risk infants. Maternal substance abuse (i.e., alcohol, cigarettes, and illicit drugs) has a negative impact on growth, development, and nutritional status of infants. Management of the high-risk infant's nutritional care is the responsibility of a team of health professionals.

Concepts to Remember

- The high-risk infant is usually preterm, low-birth weight, or both.
- Nutritional risk factors include limited nutrient reserves, high nutrient needs, physiologic and metabolic immaturities, medical complications, limited diet, and an inability to seek food.
- Nutrient needs are usually higher for these infants than they are for term, normal-weight infants.
- Pediatric parenteral products, PTFs, and fortified mother's milk are appropriate nutrient sources for high-risk infants.
- Growth in weight, length, and head circumference is the best measure of nutritional outcome.
- Maternal substance abuse has a negative impact on the growth, development, and nutritional status of infants.

REFERENCES

Aggett PJ: Trace elements of the micropremie, Clin Perinatol 27:119, 2000.

American Academy of Pediatrics/American College of Obstetricians and Gynecologists: Guidelines for perinatal care, ed 4, Elk Grove Village, IL, 1997, American Academy of Pediatrics.

American Academy of Pediatrics Committee on Nutrition: Nutritional needs of preterm infants. In Pediatric nutrition handbook, ed 4, Elk Grove Village, IL, 1998, American Academy of Pediatrics.

Anderson DM: Nutritional implications of premature birth, birth weight, and gestational age classification. In Groh-Wargo S, Thompson M, and Cox JH, editors: Nutritional care for high-risk newborns, ed 3, Chicago, 2000, Precept.

Atkinson SA: Human milk feeding of the micropremie, Clin Perinatol 27:235, 2000.

Black RF: Transmission of HIV-1 in the breast-feeding process, J Am Diet Assoc 96:267, 1996.

Catrine K: Anthropometric assessment. In Groh-Wargo S, Thompson M, and Cox JH, editors: Nutritional care for high-risk newborns, ed 3, Chicago, 2000, Precept.

Cooke RJ and Embleton ND: Feeding issues in preterm infants, Arch Dis Child Fetal Neonatal Ed 83:F215, 2000.

Cornblath M and Ichord R: Hypoglycemia in the neonate, Semin Perinatol 24:136, 2000.

Ehrenkranz RA: Growth outcomes of very low-birth weight infants in the newborn intensive care unit, Clin Perinatol 27:325, 2000.

El-Metwally D, Vohr B, and Tucker R: Survival and neonatal morbidity at the limits of viability in the mid 1990s: 22 to 25 weeks, J Pediatr 137:616, 2000.

Eriksson M, Jonsson B, and Zetterstrom R: Children of mothers abusing amphetamine: head circumference during infancy and psychosocial development until 14 years of age, Acta Paediatr 89:1474, 2000.

Fernandez AD and McNeeley DF: Management of the infant born to a mother infected with human immunodeficiency virus type 1 (HIV-1): current concepts, Am J Perinatol 17:429, 2000.

Gourley GR: Breastfeeding, diet, and neonatal hyperbilirubinemia, NeoReviews 1:e25, 2000.

Greer FR: Vitamin metabolism and requirements in the micropremie, Clin Perinatol 27:95, 2000.

Groh-Wargo S: Gastrointestinal development. In Groh-Wargo S, Thompson M, and Cox JH, editors: Nutritional care for high-risk newborns, ed 3, Chicago, 2000a, Precept.

Groh-Wargo S: Recommended enteral nutrient intakes. In Groh-Wargo S, Thompson M, and Cox JH, editors: Nutritional care for high-risk newborns, ed 3, Chicago, 2000b, Precept.

Hafström M and Kjellmer I: Non-nutritive sucking in the healthy pre-term infant, Early Hum Dev 60:13, 2000.

Hammerman C and Kaplan M: Recent developments in the management of neonatal hyperbilirubinemia, NeoReviews 1:e19, 2000.

Horbar JD et al.: Collaborative quality improvement for neonatal intensive care, Pediatrics 107:14, 2001.

Kalhan SC and Iben S: Protein metabolism in the extremely low-birth weight infant, Clin Perinatol 27:23, 2000.

Källén K: Maternal smoking during pregnancy and infant head circumference at birth, Early Hum Dev 58:197, 2000.

Kien CL, McClead RE, and Cordero L Jr: Effects of lactose intake on lactose digestion and colonic fermentation in preterm infants, J Pediatr 133:401, 1998.

Klonoff-Cohen HS et al.: The effect of passive smoking and tobacco exposure through breast milk on sudden infant death syndrome, JAMA 273:795, 1995.

Krug SK: Osteopenia of prematurity. In Groh-Wargo S, Thompson M, and Cox JH, editors: Nutritional care for high-risk newborns, ed 3, Chicago, 2000, Precept.

Lawrence RA and Lawrence RM: Breastfeeding: a guide for the medical profession, ed 5, St Louis, 1999, Mosby.

Lemons JA et al.: Very low birth weight outcomes of the National Institute of Child Health and Human Development Neonatal Research Network, January 1995 through December 1996, Pediatrics 107:e1, 2001.

McClure RJ and Newell SJ: Randomised controlled trial of trophic feeding and gut motility, Arch Dis Child Fetal Neonatal Ed 80:F54, 1999.

McCowan L et al.: Perinatal predictors of growth at six months in small for gestational age infants, Early Hum Dev 56:205, 1999.

Moody GJ et al.: Feeding tolerance in premature infants fed fortified human milk, J Pediatr Gastroenterol Nutr 30:408, 2000.

Morley R: Nutrition and cognitive development, Nutrition 14:752, 1998.

Moyer-Mileur L: Laboratory assessment. In Groh-Wargo S, Thompson M, and Cox JH, editors: Nutritional care for high-risk newborns, ed 3, Chicago, 2000, Precept.

Nduati R et al.: Effect of breastfeeding and formula feeding on transmission of HIV-1: a randomized clinical trial, JAMA 283:1167, 2000.

O'Connor DL et al.: Growth and development in preterm infants fed long-chain polyunsaturated fatty acids: a prospective, randomized controlled trial, Pediatrics 108:359, 2001.

Olsen LG, Cutroni R, and Furuta L: Pediatric acquired immunodeficiency syndrome. In Samour PQ, Helm K, and Lang CE, editors: Handbook of pediatric nutrition, ed 2, Gaithersburg, MD, 1999, Aspen.

Pinelli J and Symington A: How rewarding can a pacifier be? A systematic review of nonnutritive sucking in preterm infants, Neonatal Network 19:41, 2000.

Pollack H, Lantz PM, and Frohna JG: Maternal smoking and adverse birth outcomes among singletons and twins, Am J Public Health 90:395, 2000.

Premer DM and Georgieff MK: Nutrition for ill neonates, NeoReviews 20:e57, 1999.

Price P: Necrotizing enterocolitis. In Groh-Wargo S, Thompson M, and Cox JH, editors: Nutritional care for high risk newborns, ed 3, Chicago, 2000, Precept.

Reis B et al.: Enhanced growth of preterm infants fed a new powdered human milk fortifier: a randomized, controlled trial, Pediatrics 106:581, 2000.

Rogowski JA et al.: Economic implications of neonatal intensive care unit collaborative quality improvement, Pediatrics 107:23, 2001.

Roy S III et al.: Infant metabolic alkadosis and soy-based formula—United States, MMWR 45:985, 1996.

Sapsford AL: Human milk and enteral nutrition products. In Groh-Wargo S, Thompson M, and Cox JH, editors: Nutritional care for high-risk newborns, ed 3, Chicago, 2000, Precept.

Theriot L: Routine nutrition care during follow-up. In Groh-Wargo S, Thompson M, and Cox JH, editors: Nutritional care for high-risk newborns, ed 3, Chicago, 2000, Precept.

Thompson M: Perspectives on the neonatal nutritionist's role. In Groh-Wargo S, Thompson M, and Cox JH, editors: Nutritional care for high-risk newborns, ed 3, Chicago, 2000, Precept.

Thompson M and Bamberger JM: Computer use in neonatal nutrition information management. In Groh-Wargo S, Thompson M, and Cox JH, editors: Nutritional care for high-risk newborns, ed 3, Chicago, 2000, Precept.

Thureen PJ and Hay WW Jr: Intravenous nutrition and postnatal growth of the micropremie, Clin Perinatol 27:197, 2000.

Valentine C: Congenital anomalies of the alimentary tract. In Groh-Wargo S, Thompson M, and Cox JH, editors: Nutritional care for high-risk newborns, ed 3, Chicago, 2000, Precept.

Ventura SJ et al.: Births: final data for 1998, Natl Vital Stat Rep 48, 2000.

Wauben IPM et al.: Growth and body composition of preterm infants: influence of nutrient fortification of mother's milk in hospital and breastfeeding post-hospital discharge, Acta Paediatr 87:780, 1998.

Wessel JJ: Feeding methodologies. In Groh-Wargo S, Thompson M, and Cox JH, editors: Nutritional care for high risk newborns, ed 3, Chicago, 2000, Precept.

Yu VYH: Enteral feeding in the preterm infant, Early Hum Dev 56:89, 1999.

APPLICATION

Long-Term Outcome of Former Low-Birth-Weight Infants

Improvements in technology in neonatal intensive care have allowed smaller and sicker infants to survive the neonatal period (Lemons et al., 2001). What is the ultimate outcome of these preterm LBW infants? What affects this outcome? Can outcomes be modified by interventions?

Surveys of former preterm LBW infants have shown that they are more likely than their term, normal-weight peers to have problems with growth and development. Subnormal weight and length (below the third percentile) are typically observed in preterm, VLBW infants in the first year of life. Special preterm discharge formulas have promoted improved growth in high-risk infants at home during the first year (Cooke and Embleton, 2000). These children appear to catch up to their genetic potential in weight, height, and bone mineral density by 6 years to 8 years of age (Hack, Weissman, Borawski-Clark, 1996; Kurl et al., 1998).

Follow-up studies of former VLBW and ELBW infants have shown that 40% or more have neurodevelopmental impairment (Duvanel et al., 1999; Hack and Fanaroff, 1999; Hack et al., 2000; Kohlhauser et al., 2000; Piecuch et al., 1997). Factors that place these infants at higher risk for abnormal outcome include intracranial hemorrhage, chronic lung disease, social risk factors, recurrent hypoglycemia, and male sex. Preterm infants with NEC have an even greater risk of neurodevelopmental problems (Sonntag et al., 2000). Environmental influences appear to have a stronger impact than do genetic factors on the cognitive outcomes of preterm infants (Koeppen-Schomerus et al., 2000).

DOES ALTERING THE DIETS OF PRETERM, LOW-BIRTH-WEIGHT INFANTS AFFECT OUTCOME?

British investigators have explored the relationship of early diet (i.e., in the first month of life) to neurodevelopmental outcome (Lucas, 1998). Infants with LBW, fed PTF in the first month of life, scored significantly higher in developmental tests at 18 months of age than did those fed term formula in the first month. Male infants and SGA infants showed particularly striking advantages in mental and motor development if they had received PTF. Moderate developmental impairment was considerably more common in the group fed term formula. Infants fed PTF also showed a slight advantage in social maturity quotient. These same subjects were tested again at 7 and a half years to 8 years of age. Fourteen percent of those who had been fed PTF had low verbal IQ scores, whereas 31% of those fed term formula had low scores on the same tests. Again the difference was particularly striking in boys fed exclusively term formula, who had a 14.4 point disadvantage in overall IQ (Lucas, Morley, and Cole, 1998).

Follow-up studies in 7-and-a-half-year-old to 8-year-old former LBW infants demonstrate a significant improvement in IQ in infants who received their mother's milk compared with those who did not receive maternal milk (Lucas, 1998). The infants received the milk by tube, which eliminates the possibility that the act of breastfeeding itself conferred this advantage. There was a dose-response relationship between the proportion of mother's milk in the diet and subsequent IQ. These results persisted after adjusting for differences in maternal education and social class. Receiving mature donor human milk (as opposed to term formula) may also promote superior neurodevelopmental outcome in preterm infants.

Follow-up of infants involved in these intervention studies shows catch-up growth in weight, height, head circumference, and skinfold thickness to each child's genetic potential (by 7 and a half to 8 years) regardless of early diet group (Morley and Lucas, 2000). Children who had biochemical evidence of metabolic bone disease in the NICU, however, had long-term stunting persisting up to 12 years of age (Fewtrell et al., 2000). This finding supports the current practice of providing high-mineral diets to VLBW infants to prevent metabolic bone disease.

These initial outcome studies underscore the importance of early nutrition for LBW infants. Whether the positive influences of PTF and mother's milk are related to specific nutrients, nutrient ratios, or other components is unknown. Additional outcome studies are needed.

REFERENCES

Cooke RJ and Embleton ND: Feeding issues in preterm infants, Arch Dis Child Fetal Neonatal Ed 83:F215, 2000.

Duvanel CB et al.: Long-term effects of neonatal hypoglycemia on brain growth and psychomotor development in small-for-gestational-age preterm infants, J Pediatr 134:492, 1999.

Fewtrell MS et al.: Neonatal factors predicting childhood height in preterm infants: evidence for a persisting effect of early metabolic bone disease? J Pediatr 137:668, 2000.

Hack M and Fanaroff AA: Outcomes of children of extremely low birthweight and gestational age in the 1990's, Early Hum Dev 53:193, 1999.

Hack M, Weissman B, and Borawski-Clark E: Catch-up growth during childhood among very low-birth-weight children, Arch Pediatr Adolesc Med 150:1122, 1996.

Hack M et al.: Neurodevelopment and predictors of outcomes of children with birth weights of less than 1000g, Arch Pediatr Adolesc Med 154:725, 2000.

Koeppen-Schomerus G et al.: The interaction of prematurity with genetic and environmental influences on cognitive development in twins, J Pediatr 137:527, 2000.

Kohlhauser C et al.: Outcome of very-low-birth-weight infants at 1 and 2 years of age, Clin Pediatr 39:441, 2000.

Kurl S et al.: Determinants of bone mineral density in prematurely born children aged 6-7 years, Acta Paediatr 87:650, 1998.

Lemons JA et al.: Very low birth weight outcomes of the National Institute of Child Health and Human Development Neonatal Research Network, January 1995 through December 1996, Pediatrics 107:e1, 2001.

Lucas A: Long-term outcome trials of early nutrition on later health and development, Nestle Nutrition Workshop Series 40:181, 1998.

Lucas A, Morley R, and Cole TJ: Randomised trial of early diet in preterm infants and later intelligence quotient, Br Med J 317:1481, 1998.

Morley R and Lucas A: Randomized diet in the neonatal period and growth performance until 7.5-8 y of age in preterm children, Am J Clin Nutr 71:822, 2000.

Piecuch RE et al.: Outcome of extremely low birth weight infants (500 to 999 grams) over a 12-year period, Pediatrics 100:633, 1997.

Sonntag J et al.: Growth and neurodevelopmental outcome of very low birthweight infants with necrotizing enterocolitis, Acta Paediatr 89:528, 2000.

CHAPTER 9

Nutrition during Growth: Preschool through Preadolescence

Martha Orabella

Chapter Outline

Joyce walks in the door and puts a pot of water on to boil to make some noodles for dinner. She had placed several chicken breasts and a can of cream soup in the slow cooker this morning before she left for work. Although she only works two days a week, on work nights it is still a challenge to prepare something quick, easy, and reasonably healthy for dinner and, most importantly, something her three children will eat. Although Matt would love to have pizza every night and Jason always wants Chinese take-out, she is glad that her kids, for the most part, are very good eaters.

Joyce's son Matt is in second grade. He walks in the door and heads straight to the refrigerator to look for something to eat. Matt always likes to buy the school lunch because his friends buy it. Today he said the pizza was gross, so despite the snack of fruit juice and graham crackers at his after-school child care program, he is hungry. Joyce reminds him that dinner is just a few minutes away and asks him to unpack his backpack.

Matt is 50¾ in tall (seventieth percentile, according to the Centers for Disease Control [CDC] growth charts) and weighs 56 lb (seventy-fifth percentile). He is just about average size in his class. Matt has had a busy school year, learning to write in cursive and moving from easy reader books to chapter books. Tim, Joyce's husband, was pleased when they had to begin enforcing the "no books at the dinner table" rule because Matt enjoys reading so much. Matt loves to play soccer and takes gymnastics one night after school. He broke his arm last year on the playground practicing one of his gymnastics moves, but the doctor was not overly concerned because the break was not in a growth plate. Matt healed very quickly, wearing the cast for only 4 weeks. His parents try to make sure that he drinks plenty of milk to help build strong bones.

Joyce's older son, Jason, is 10 years old and in the fourth grade. He unpacks his backpack and cleans out his lunch bag. He doesn't like to buy the school lunch anymore. He used to buy it on pizza day and on grilled cheese and tomato soup day, but lately it just isn't enough food. He usually packs two sandwiches on days he has gym class.

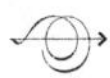

Jason has grown almost 3 in this year. He has always been tall for his age and he now is 57 in tall (ninetieth percentile CDC and weighs 74 lb (forty-fifth percentile). He has trouble finding pants that are long enough to cover his growing legs and yet slim enough to fit his small waist. It is hard to believe he was such a fat baby that he could barely crawl because of the size of his tummy. His pediatrician said not to worry about his weight when he was little as long as he was eating healthy foods and no one in his family was overweight. His parents now laugh to think how right she was.

Fourth grade has been a busy year with multiplication and long division in math and many long research projects in science and social studies. Jason stays busy with karate, which he practices 3 days a week. Next year Jason will leave the elementary school where he has been since kindergarten to attend the intermediate school. Jason will have to catch the bus almost an hour earlier next year. Joyce worries about what he will do for breakfast with the earlier start time. Jason is not a "morning person" and his mother always tries to make sure he eats something before school. Some of his friends eat breakfast at school, but Jason doesn't like the breakfast foods the school offers. They went through the instant breakfast drink mixed with milk phase, the bagel and cream cheese phase, and the peanut butter and jelly for breakfast phase this year. Joyce is always on the lookout for new breakfast ideas to try. Jason is excited about intermediate school because he will have a locker and can buy extra food such as juice, pizza, or potato chips at lunch next year.

Joyce's daughter Emily is 4 years old and has just started preschool this year. Emily just started to lose her "baby fat" this year and is really stretching out and getting taller without really gaining weight. She is 41 in tall (seventy-fifth percentile CDC) and weighs 42 lb (eightieth percentile CDC). She is always on the go between her gymnastics class, story time at the library, and preschool 2 half days each week. She loves to tell people that her favorite things about preschool are playing outside and the snack. Joyce is so pleased that they try different snacks at preschool. She likes to send baby carrots and ranch dip or corn chips and salsa on the days that they need to provide a snack.

Joyce asks what Emily had at the babysitter's for lunch today and she says, chicken nuggets and French fries. This is her standard response and would be her ideal lunch, but Joyce knows her sitter does not offer it every day.

Tim, Joyce's husband, walks through the door with a gallon of milk. Her family goes through 3 to 4 gallons of milk each week and it seems that they are always running to the store for milk. It is much easier having everyone drink the same kind of milk since Emily turned two and was able to transition from whole milk to 1% fat milk. Her pediatrician recommends that they use skim milk, but her kids don't like the taste of it. Joyce figures it is better for them to drink milk that they like than to have to fight with them to drink skim milk that they hate. She is careful to limit the amount of fat she cooks with and to not serve any fried foods at home.

Joyce has everyone wash their hands and then the children do their evening jobs of setting the table for dinner. Jason and Matt alternate handling the plates and silverware. Jason is much taller than his brother and can easily reach the plates in the cabinet. He grabs a smaller plastic plate for Emily and four dinner plates for the rest of the family. Matt grumbles about carrying the silverware, his least-favorite job, but he smiles when his dad reminds him that the only way they get dinner on the table is if they all work together. Matt grabs a smaller fork and spoon and a plastic cup with a lid for Emily. Emily loves to do her job and carefully places napkins next to each dinner plate.

Dinner is finally ready and everyone is hungry. They try to eat dinner together as a family each night, although Tim sometimes has to work late. Juggling homework, karate or soccer practice, and mealtime can make for some busy evenings. If soccer practice is early

Matt will sometimes just grab a sandwich before practice and then eat a late dinner when he gets home. Joyce tries to plan the meals for the week so that they can limit eating out and the use of take-out food. Sometimes they will make something really easy like soup and sandwiches for dinner or just pick up a pizza on the way home from soccer or karate practice. Joyce tries to have a fresh fruit and vegetable with dinner each night and insists that the kids drink milk with their meals. The kids love spaghetti, so they try to have that at least one night each week. Emily doesn't like anything mixed together and insists that her foods not touch each other on her plate. Emily did have a food jag last summer where all she would eat was grilled cheese for breakfast, lunch, and dinner, but luckily that lasted only about a week. Matt doesn't like hamburgers on the grill, but Jason will eat just about anything, even the salmon Tim likes to prepare on the weekends.

Since Jason and Matt started eating lunch at school, it is much harder for Joyce and Tim to know what the kids are actually eating. The school does send home a menu with the choices for the month, but just because it is served doesn't mean they will eat it. The school is very strict about not trading lunches or swapping food because several children have peanut or other food allergies. Matt is allergic to bees, so Joyce knows how scary allergic reactions can be.

During dinner the kids like to play the "best and worst" game. They have all come to enjoy the game, in which each person must share the best thing and the worst thing to happen to them that day. During the summer and when they have a free evening during the school year, Tim encourages the kids to have "kids cook" nights. Jason and Matt love to plan a meal and do as much of the shopping and cooking for dinner as is safely possible. Tim and Joyce have found the kids are much more likely to try foods if they had a part in purchasing or preparing them.

Dinner is a whirlwind of cutting up meat, serving second helpings, and sharing the day's events. It seems like they just sat down when it is time to clean up. Cleanup is a family effort and soon the dinner table becomes the homework table. Matt finishes his homework early and Tim helps him stir chocolate pudding on the stove to eat for an evening snack.

GROWTH

- *What are the characteristics of childhood growth?*
- *How does the growth of childhood compare with that of infancy?*
- *How is growth monitored?*
- *What changes in body proportion and composition occur during childhood?*

Children such as Jason, Matt, and Emily are all at different stages of growth and development and their eating habits can be as individual as are they. The period between toddlerhood and puberty is a time of tremendous change. Whereas an infant is totally dependent on a parent for feeding, toddlers are learning to self-feed and can exhibit quite strong likes and dislikes. Preschoolers are often so busy exploring their world that they do not wish to take time to eat. School-age children are influenced by their peers and advertising. They begin to eat meals away from home and the family has less influence on their food choices. Preadolescents are increasingly aware of their changing bodies and begin to develop a perception of peers and a society-oriented perception of self, including body image. Eating habits developed during this period lay the foundation of food behaviors for the rest of their lives.

Childhood growth can be divided into two periods: the preschol period and the school-age period. The preschool child is between the ages of 2 years and 6 years. The rate of growth during the preschool years, compared with infancy, is much less rapid. Whereas the birth weight of an infant can triple in the first year of life, it often takes a full year for the toddler to quadruple his or her birth weight. The school-age years, ages 6 years to 10 years in girls and 6 years to 12 years in boys, is often referred to as the latent growth period. This refers to the slow and steady growth rate preceding the prepubertal growth spurt that is typical for school-age years.

Heredity, hormones, and environment (including nutrition) influence the timing and pattern of growth and development during childhood. Growth patterns are highly individual, even erratic, with spurts in weight gain or growth in stature followed by periods of little or no growth. Therefore there can be wide variation in body size for children of the same age (Figure 9-1). Often parents will report that their child "grows out," or experiences a weight gain, before "growing up," or experiencing linear growth. Appetite and food intake can be quite variable and can parallel the erratic pattern of growth in healthy children.

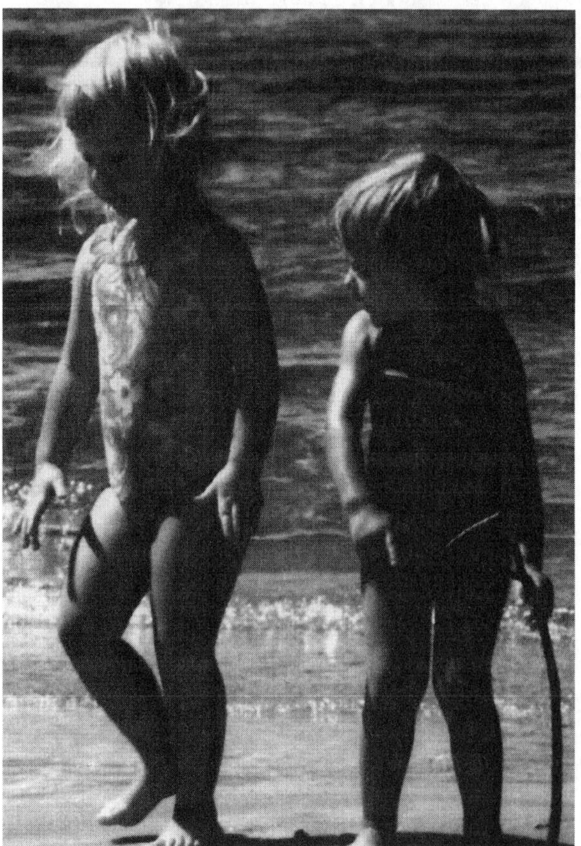

Figure 9-1 These 3-year-old cousins are the same age, but very different in size.

An Adequate Intake (AI) of energy, protein, and other nutrients is essential to maintain the health of a child and to support growth. Compromised growth is a significant, albeit nonspecific, indicator of inadequate nutritional intake.

Growth and Body Composition

The growth of a child is measured in terms of gains in stature and weight. The velocity of growth is much slower in children than in infants and toddlers. Approximate midpoint values for stature and weight by age from the National Center for Chronic Disease Control and Prevention 2000 growth charts for boys and girls from age 1 to age 12 appear in Table 9-1. The annual increments for weight change ranges from 2.5 kg (5 to 6 lb) per year for the second to third year of life to 2 kg (4.5 lb) per year between the ages of 3 years and 5 years. Increments in weight gain for the elementary school years average approximately 3 kg to 3.5 kg (7 lb) per year.

Height or linear growth changes follow a similar pattern and increase approximately 12 cm (5 in) during the second to third year and 6 cm to 8 cm (2.5 to 3.5 in) in school-age children until they begin the preadolescent growth spurt.

Growth of the brain does not continue the rapid increase seen in infancy, so head circumference is measured routinely only until the age of 36 months. A 12 cm increase in head circumference is typical in infancy, but the toddler experiences only an average 2 cm (0.75 in) increase in the second year of life. Although neuronal development continues into puberty, the brain has virtually reached adult size by 12 years of age.

Body composition remains relatively constant in preschool and school-age children. Total body water is approximately 60% to 65% of body weight by the time a child is 2 to 3 years of age and this percentage remains relatively constant into adulthood. The growth of new cells and the expansion of skeletal muscle brings a decrease in the extracellular fluid compartment to 20% to 25% of body weight and a similar increase in the intracellular fluid to 35% to 40% of body weight. The preschool or school-age child is thus less likely to suffer from rapid fluid shifts between intracellular and

Table 9-1 APPROXIMATE MIDPOINTS FOR STATURE AND WEIGHT OF CHILDREN ON THE 2000 CDC GROWTH CHARTS

Age (y)	Stature (cm) Male	Stature (cm) Female	Weight (kg) Male	Weight (kg) Female
1	76.1	74.6	10.4	9.5
2	87.5	86.2	12.7	11.9
3	96.5	95	14.4	13.9
4	102	101.1	16.2	15.2
5	109	108	18.2	18
6	115.2	115	21	20.5
7	121.5	121.8	23	22.8
8	127.4	127	25.5	26
9	133.4	133.8	28.1	28.6
10	138.5	138.2	32	33.5
11	143.3	144.8	36.2	37.6
12	149.8	151.7	41.1	41.8

Adapted from Vital and Health Statistics of the Centers for Disease Control and Prevention/National Center for Health Statistics: Advanced data: CDC growth charts: United States, No 314, Hyattsville, MD, 2000, NCHS.

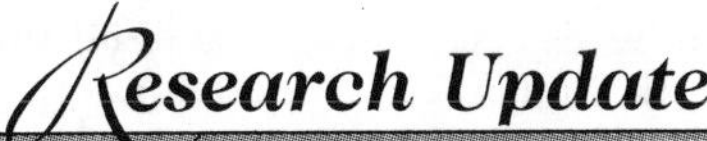

Research Update

Diarrhea in Children

Diarrhea, the passage of watery stools, is a common problem for children. It can emerge as an acute onset illness such as the flu or "tummy bug" and is usually of short duration, lasting 3 to 6 days if it is a viral illness. If not treated properly, diarrhea can lead to potentially dangerous dehydration. The American Academy of Pediatrics, in developing guidelines for the management of diarrhea, stated that approximately 9% of all hospitalizations in children younger than 5 years of age are from diarrhea (American Academy of Pediatrics Promotional Committee on Quality Improvement, Subcommittee on Acute Gastroenteritis, 1996). Children, however, with their increase in intracellular fluid, are less vulnerable to dehydration than infants. Diarrhea can also be the result of food intolerance. Lactose intolerance can result in gastrointestinal symptoms including abdominal discomfort, gas, cramping, or diarrhea following the ingestion of food substances (dairy products) containing lactose.

"Bubble gum" diarrhea can also occur when large quantities of bubble gum or sugarless gum or mints are consumed. Sugarless gum and mints frequently contain sugar alcohols, such as sorbitol, mannitol, or xylitol, which are poorly digested and can cause diarrhea.

The sugar alcohol sorbitol is also found in some fruit juices and excessive consumption of some fruit juices can cause diarrhea. Apple juice and pear juice naturally contain sorbitol. Citrus juices and grape juice contain little or no sorbitol. Not suprisingly prunes and prune juice contain the most sorbitol of any fruit, which contributes to their national laxative effect (American Academy of Pediatrics, 2001b).

Oral rehydration solutions (ORS) are used in oral rehydration therapy (ORT) and are special fluids made for the home management of diarrhea. These bottled, liquid solutions help to replace lost water and salts. Pedialyte (Ross Laboratories) and Enfalyte (Mead Johnson Nutritionals) and various generic or store brands are found in almost all pharmacies and some supermarkets. A recent study showed that children who were actually given oral hydration solutions when seeking medical care for acute diarrhea

Continued

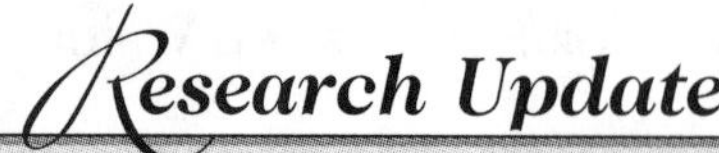

Diarrhea in Children—cont'd

were significantly less likely to need unscheduled follow-up visits and emergency room visits because of the illness than children who were just given information about the use of ORS (Duggan et al., 1999).

Although there are numerous home remedies for diarrhea, children with diarrhea who are not dehydrated should continue to consume age-appropriate diets. Antidiarrheal medications should not be used unless prescribed by a physician. Complex carbohydrates (e.g., rice, wheat, potatoes, bread, and cereals), lean meats, yogurt, fruits, and vegetables are usually well tolerated. The American Academy of Pediatrics recommends limiting fatty or fried foods and foods high in simple sugars such as sweetened tea, juice, or soft drinks (American Academy of Pediatrics, 2001a). The BRAT diet (consisting of bananas, rice, applesauce, and toast) has been a traditional home remedy for the treatment of diarrhea. Although these foods are usually tolerated, a diet restricted to these foods is low in protein, fat, and energy density and is not recommended.

extracellular compartment than an infant and is less vulnerable to dehydration. However, diarrhea in children creates a significant risk of dehydration (see the Research Update).

The percentage of weight as fat remains relatively constant throughout childhood, but fat-free body mass (i.e., skeletal muscle, bone, and soft tissue protein) increases. Girls are noted to have a higher percentage of weight as fat, but sex differences in fat and lean body mass do not become significant until puberty. By 10 years of age, lean body mass has reached approximately 17% in boys and 15% in girls. Mineral content increases gradually throughout childhood from less than 3.5% in infancy to 4.8% of body weight by the end of puberty.

DEVELOPMENT

- *Describe the typical physical, neurologic, cognitive, language, and psychosocial developmental changes of the preschool and school-age periods.*

The physical changes associated with childhood are readily apparent. The preschool and school years are also a time of rapid social, intellectual, and emotional growth.

Physical Development

As a child grows from toddlerhood, the subcutaneous "baby fat" is lost and the plump infant slowly evolves into a lean and muscular child. The protuberant (projecting) abdomen found in toddlers generally disappears by the fourth year. There is a general shifting in the accumulation and location of body fat so children of appropriate weight-for-height develop a slimmer appearance as childhood progresses. Body proportions change as limbs lengthen more than the trunk (Figure 9-2). The legs make up one half of the total body length of an adult, an increase from three eighths of the total body length of an infant.

Although the head does not continue to experience significant growth after infancy, there are significant changes in the facial configuration. The length of the skull increases and the face tends to grow proportionately more than the cranial cavity. The widening of the jaw accommodates the development of permanent teeth.

Bone Development

Bone is a living tissue with a matrix of collagen and protein that contains mineral salts, predominately calcium and phosphorus. Not only does it provide the physical support for the body, but it also serves as a storehouse of minerals. Roughly 99% of the total body calcium is found in the skeleton. The body can pull minerals from bone to maintain the necessary level of calcium in the blood. For proper bone formation to occur, there must be an adequate dietary intake of protein and minerals, espe-

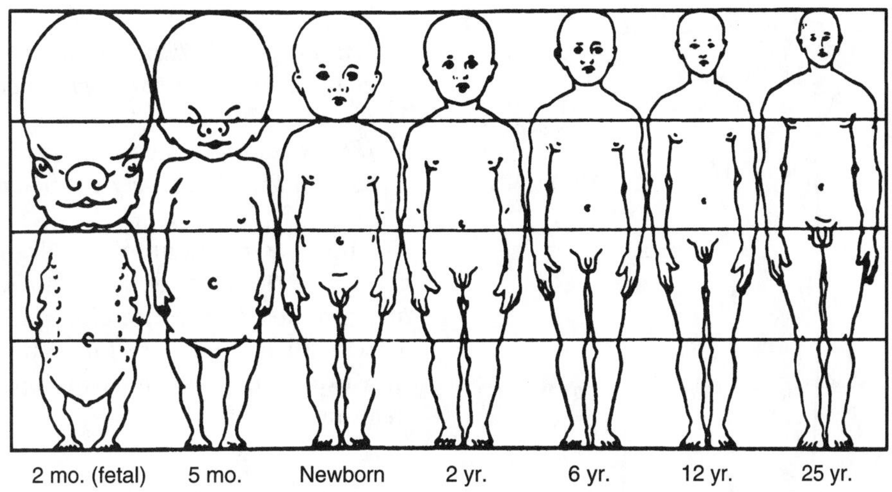

Figure 9-2 Body proportions change with growth and development. *(From Robbins WJ et al.: Growth, New Haven, 1928, Yale University Press. Copyright © Yale University Press.)*

cially calcium and phosphorus and other nutrients such as vitamin A, vitamin D, and fluoride.

During childhood bones experience steady growth. Growth in bone length occurs at the **epiphyseal plate,** a plate of actively growing cartilage (Figure 9-3). During bone growth the epiphyseal plate lays down new bone at the end of the **bone shaft** and the bone shaft lengthens. The outer shell of bone, **cortical bone,** grows by adding new tissue on the outer surface and resorbing tissue from the inner surface. Linear bone growth continues until the epiphyseal plates close after puberty.

Bone is in a constant state of flux. It is constantly remodeled or rearranged in response to the stress of body weight and exercise. The calcium in bone turns over at a rate of 100% per year in infants, but slows across childhood and adolescence to a rate of 18% per year in adults.

Psychosocial and Cognitive Development

The growth of children is not limited to physical change. The great change from a dependent toddler to an independent preteen is readily apparent to anyone observing children of different ages. A summary of the developmental achievements during the preschool years appears in Table 9-2.

As children grow, they move through various developmental periods. Newborns rely on automatic reflexes, such as sucking and rooting, to obtain food. Toddlers begin to have intentional interaction with the environment and begin to self-feed. Preschool children can begin to internalize thought processes. They can describe the color or shape of foods and form specific food acceptance patterns. Developmental skills of the preschool years progress sequentially, with naming and identifying skills between 2 years and 3 years; sorting and classifying starting at about 3 years and progressing between 4 years and 5 years; to ordering, sequencing, and comprehension (Debord, 1996).

As children begin to develop a more rational and systemic reasoning process they are able to realize the positive effect that nutritious foods can have on health. For the school-age child, mealtimes are quite social and food is no longer primarily used to satisfy hunger. As abstract thought

KEY TERMS

epiphyseal plate: area at the end of the long bone; during growth the epiphyses are separated from the main portion of bone by the cartilage of the epiphyseal plate and this space closes as maximum height is attained

bone shaft: the long, slender portion of bone between the wider ends

cortical bone: the outer layer of the bone

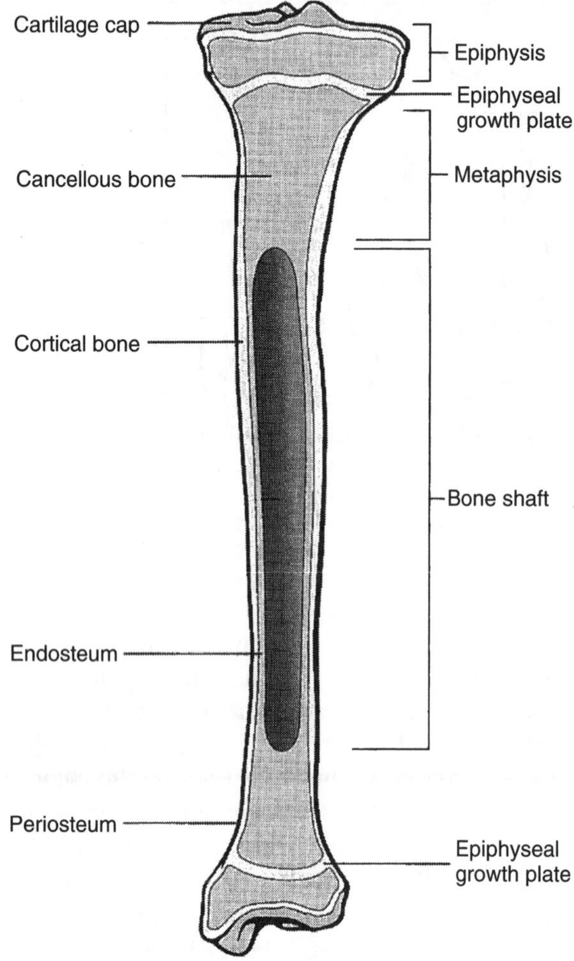

Figure 9-3 The long bone has a central part (shaft) and two terminal parts (epiphyses). The shaft of the bone consists of cancellous bone on the outside and trabecular bone on the inside. The epiphyseal growth plate allows bone lengthening. When the epiphyses close, linear growth ceases. *(From Applegate EJ: The anatomy and physiology learning system: textbook, Philadelphia, 1995, WB Saunders.)*

patterns expand, there is greater understanding of the chemistry and science of food.

ASSESSMENT OF NUTRITION STATUS

- *Describe the nutrition assessment techniques used for preschool and school-age children.*
- *What is the difference between wasting and stunting and how is this difference determined?*
- *How are growth charts used in nutrition assessment and in defining wasting, stunting, overweight status, and obesity?*
- *What special factors must be considered in the assessment of a child's dietary information?*

Nutrition assessment of children includes anthropometric, biochemical, clinical, and dietary measurements. Because children are constantly growing, it is important for a child's growth and nutrition status to be measured periodically by a healthcare professional.

Anthropometry

Weight and stature should be measured periodically and recorded on the appropriate growth chart. A single height or weight measure is not clinically meaningful. A growth pattern usually emerges after 2 years of age, with periodic measures falling in a channel, around the same percentile, on the growth chart. Individual children can experience periods of rapid growth or, conversely, periods of latent or little growth. These patterns are typical of normal childhood growth.

In 2000 the CDC and the National Center for Health Statistics (NCHS) revised the multipurpose growth charts developed in 1977 and released an analytic growth chart data set for infants (see chapter 7) and for children 2 years to 18 years of age that is representative of American children (Kuczmarski et al., 2000). Four growth indicators are charted for each sex: stature-for-age, weight-for-age, weight-for-stature, and body mass index (BMI)-for-age (see Appendix E). The charts were developed to describe size and growth of children in the United States (Kuczmarski et al., 2000). Data sets for the revised growth charts are based on physical measurements taken as part of a series of national health examination including the National Health Examination Surveys and the three National Health and Nutrition Examination Surveys (NHANES I, II, and III). The data were collected using standardized procedures for pediatric measurement. The revised growth charts are believed to be a better representation of the

Table 9-2 DEVELOPMENTAL ACHIEVEMENTS DURING THE PRESCHOOL YEARS

15 MONTHS	
Motor	
Gross	Toddles independently Crawls upstairs
Fine	Puts pellet into bottle
Adaptive	Builds tower of two cubes Puts six cubes in and out of cup
Language	Jargon Four to six words, including names Pats pictures in book
Personal-social	Says "thank you" or equivalent Points or vocalizes wants Hugs parents Throws objects in play or refusal
18 MONTHS	
Motor	
Gross	Walks, seldom falling; runs stiffly Sits in small chair and climbs into adult chair Hurls ball in standing position
Fine	Turns two or three pages of book at once
Adaptive	Builds tower of three or four cubes Imitates scribbling with a crayon Dumps pellet from bottle
Language	Ten words, names pictures Identifies one or more body parts Carries out one or two directions
Personal-social	Pulls toy on string Carries and hugs doll Feeds self in part, with spilling Seeks help when in trouble
2 YEARS	
Motor	
Gross	Runs well, no falling Walks up and down stairs, one step at a time Climbs, jumps
Fine	Turns pages of book singly
Adaptive	Builds tower of six or seven cubes Aligns cubes for train Circular scribbling
2 YEARS—cont'd	
Language	Three-word sentences; vocabulary of 50-75 words Carries out four directions with toy ("on the table," "on the chair," "to mother," "to me")
Personal-social	Verbalizes toilet needs consistently Helps undress Handles spoon well Listens to stories
3 YEARS	
Motor	
Gross	Alternates feet going upstairs Stands momentarily on one foot Rides tricycle
Fine	Holds crayon with fingers
Adaptive	Builds tower of nine or ten cubes Names own drawing Copies circle and imitates cross
Language	Counts three objects Gives action in picture book Knows full name and gender Obeys two prepositional commands ("on," "under," "over")
Personal-social	Feeds self well Puts on shoes and unbuttons buttons Knows a few rhymes or songs Plays simple games Plays "parallel" with other children
4 YEARS	
Motor	Walks downstairs alternating feet Hops on one foot Throws ball overhand
Adaptive	Draws human with two to four parts besides head Copies cross and square Counts three objects with correct pointing Imitates construction of five-cube bridge

From Hughes JG and Griffith JF: Synopsis of pediatrics, 6th ed, St. Louis, 1984, Mosby.

Continued

Table 9-2 DEVELOPMENTAL ACHIEVEMENTS DURING THE PRESCHOOL YEARS—CONT'D

4 YEARS—cont'd		**5 YEARS—cont'd**	
Language	Names one or more colors correctly	Personal-social	Follows three directions
	Obeys five prepositional commands ("on," "under," "in back," "in front," "beside")		Dresses and undresses without assistance
Personal-social	Tells a story, washes and dries face and hands, brushes teeth		Asks meaning of words
	Distinguishes front from back of clothes		Domestic role-playing
	Plays with several children	**6 YEARS**	
5 YEARS		Motor	Advanced throwing
Motor	Skips, alternating feet		Stands on each foot alternately, eyes closed
	Stands on one foot for several seconds	Adaptive	Knows right from left
Adaptive	Builds two steps with cubes		Draws human with neck, hands, and clothes
	Draws unmistakable human with body, head, etc.		Adds and subtracts within 5
	Draws triangle		Copies diamond
	Prints a few letters	Language	Composes a complex five- or six-word sentence
	Counts ten pennies correctly		Comprehends "if," "because," "why"
Language	Knows four colors	Personal-social	Ties shoelaces
	Five-word sentences		Differentiates morning and afternoon
	Descriptive comment on pictures		Knows right from left
			Increased interaction with peers

From Hughes JG and Griffith JF: Synopsis of pediatrics, 6th ed, St. Louis, 1984, Mosby.

racial and ethnic diversity of American children today.

New to the 2000 edition of the growth charts are charts for BMI-for-age percentiles for boys and girls ages 2 years through 20 years. A general indicator of body fatness, BMI can assist in classifying children as underweight, acceptable weight, overweight, or obese. For illustration growth in stature-for-age and growth in BMI-for-age for Jason, from the case presented at the beginning of the chapter, are charted in Figures 9-4 and 9-5, respectively. Jason's stature is consistently above the seventieth percentile (see Figure 9-4), indicating that he is taller than 74% of boys his age. However, his BMI (wt[kg]/ht[m]^2) is consistently around the twenty-fifth percentile, reflecting generally lean status (see Figure 9-5).

When a child is faced with inadequate nutrition, weight gain is compromised. In malnutrition there is an initial wasting or a loss of body weight. If energy and nutrient intake is not improved, stunting or compromised linear growth will occur. Wasting is defined as falling below the fifth percentile in weight-for-height. Stunting is diagnosed with a measurement lower than the fifth percentile in height-for-age. With growth charts weight-for-age is an indicator of acute short-term malnutrition. With a long-term inadequate dietary intake, growth is ultimately compromised. Thus height-for-age is an indicator of chronic undernutrition and growth failure. The weight-for-height growth chart is useful in that it helps to assess body weight in proportion to height, helping to identify children who are overweight or obese and also helping distinguish wasting or compromised growth from short stature or dwarfism.

If a lack of weight gain or a loss of weight occurs over time, the healthcare provider should evaluate the child more thoroughly, with a review that includes the child's living situation. A severe acute

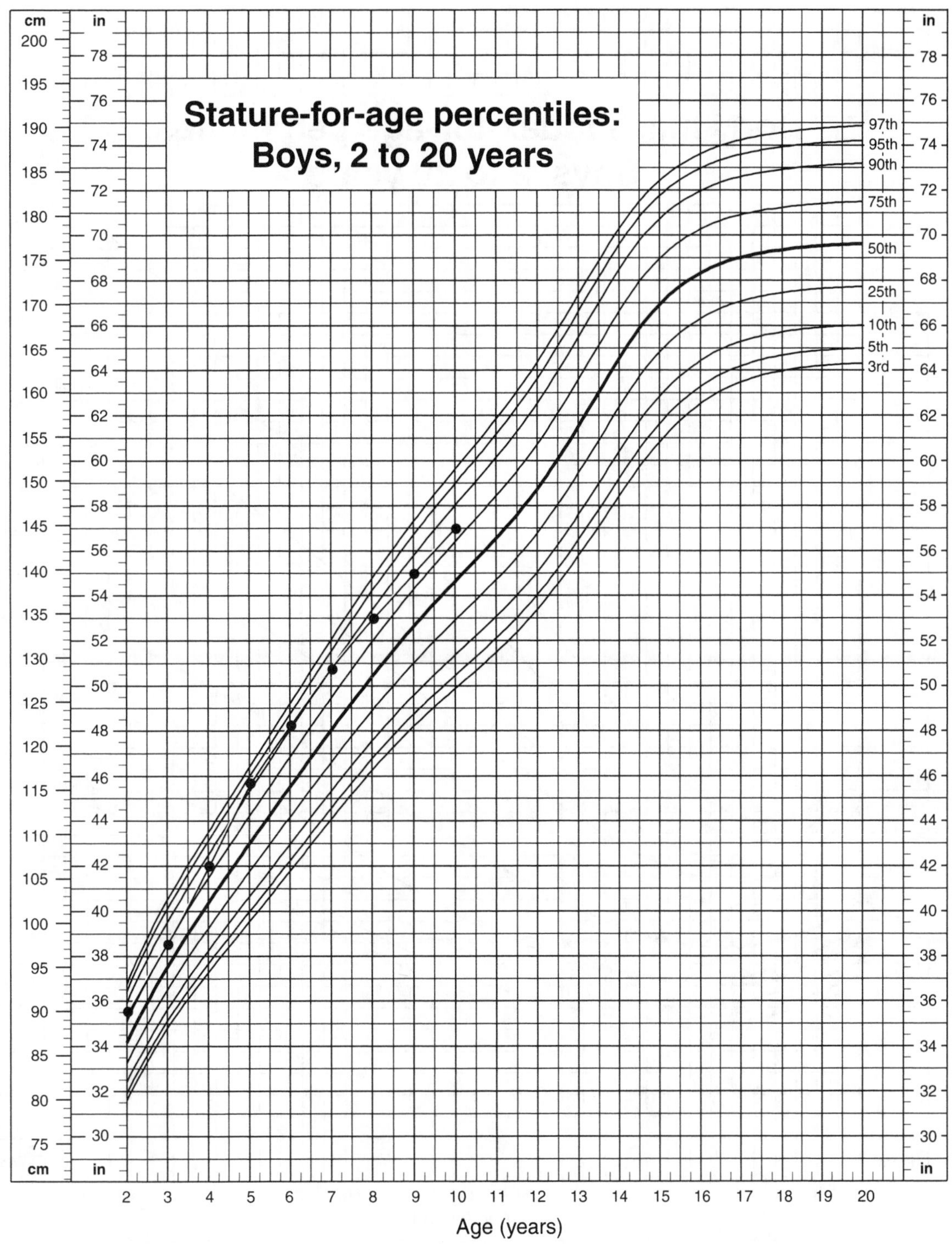

Figure 9-4 Jason's growth pattern charted as gains in stature on the stature-for-age percentiles for boys from 2 to 20 years, CDC growth charts: United States. *(Growth chart only developed by the National Center for Health Statistics in collaboration with the National Center for Chronic Disease Prevention and Health Promotion 2000.)*

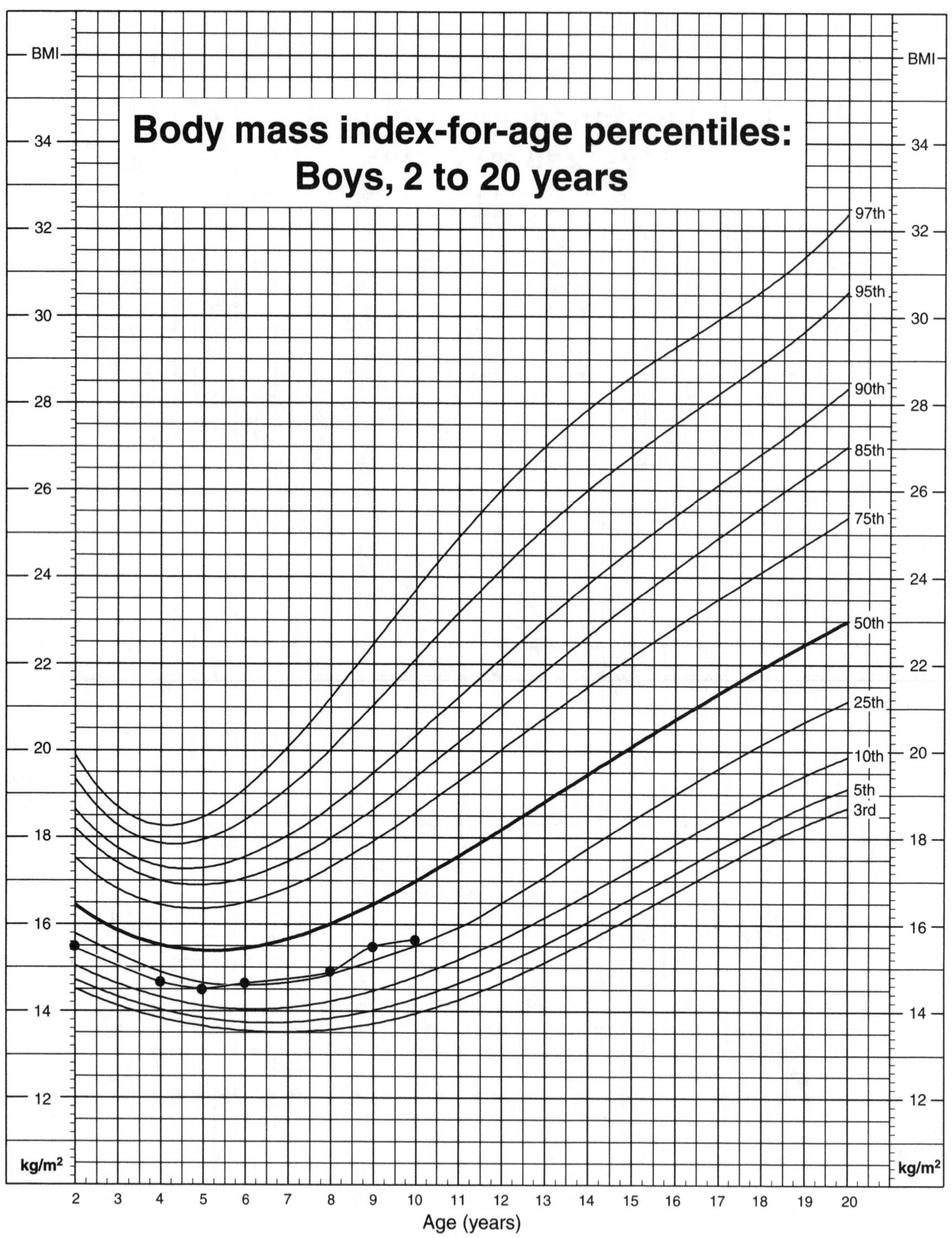

Figure 9-5 Jason's growth pattern charted as body mass index-for-age on the body mass index-for-age percentiles for boys from 2 to 20 years, CDC growth charts: United States. *(Growth chart only developed by the National Center for Health Statistics in collaboration with the National Center for Chronic Disease Prevention and Health Promotion 2000.)*

illness, an undiagnosed chronic illness, emotional stress, family problems, or financial problems can all compromise the nutrition status and, ultimately, the growth of the child. Failure to thrive is a combination of growth and development failure in the absence of underlying disease. It is usually the result of a combination of nutritional and environmental deprivation. Factors associated with failure to thrive include poverty, occurrence of infection, poor hygiene, poor caregiver-child relationships, and low family functioning.

Fatfold Measurements

Measurement of fatfold thickness can be useful in the assessment of body fat. Triceps and subscapular fatfold thickness measurements are the measurements most commonly used to assess energy reserves. Although fatfold measurements are not used routinely in the nutrition screening of healthy children, percentile values from NHANES data for triceps and subscapular fatfolds are available for comparison for various groups (see Appendices B2 and B3). Fatfold measurements are used increasingly to help estimate the body composition status of children at the ends of the weight-for-height percentiles—greater than the ninetieth percentile and thus at risk for obesity and less than the tenth percentile and thus at risk for wasting.

Biochemical Assessment

Laboratory measurements used for assessment of nutritional status are discussed in Chapter 2. Laboratory tests typically completed during well-child check-ups are usually quite limited. A urinalysis that tests a urine sample for protein, sugar, and ketone bodies may be done to screen for more serious medical problems. A simple finger stick that can measure the hematocrit, or packed cell volume, may be done. Healthcare providers try to limit routine or screening blood draws and more invasive biochemical assessments in typically needle-shy children.

Clinical Assessment

Although much of the assessment of nutrition status of children is done by the serial measurement of growth parameters, advanced stages of undernutrition are manifested in physical and, in a more subtle fashion, behavioral signs. Table 9-3 summarizes the clinical findings associated with undernutrition. It is important to note that the clinical changes appear more rapidly in undernourished children than in adults because of the higher nutritional demands of growth.

Dietary Assessment

Numerous tools are available to assist in the assessment of the dietary intake of children. A dietary record, 24-hour recall, and a food frequency questionnaire can help estimate and assess dietary intake (see Chapter 2). Obtaining accurate dietary information for young children requires cooperation of the parent or primary caregiver. For a child in daycare, preschool, or school, information is needed about the meals and snacks eaten away from home. Young children may be able to report what they ate at school, but they are seldom able to give accurate estimates of portion size. Snacks and beverages are frequently not reported, but can contribute a significant amount to the daily intake of a child.

For very young children it is important to assess feeding skill development. Interaction with the parent or caregiver at mealtime may also be observed. Many factors influence nutrient intake, such as psychosocial factors, all of which can affect the amount and types of foods eaten. Family eating patterns, food cooking and storage capabilities, feeding history, dentition or oral-muscular development, and food allergies or intolerances can affect the nutritional status of children.

As children reach the fourth or fifth grade, they may be able to report their food intake with some accuracy (Domel et al., 1994), but they typically have difficulty quantifying portion size, particularly in estimating how much they actually ate (Lytle et al., 1993). This age group is very receptive to nutrition and health education. Recent exposure to dietary information may bias a child's responses on dietary records or questionnaires. An accurate evaluation of food intake may require the use of multiple methods of dietary analysis.

Table 9-3 PHYSICAL SIGNS OF WELL-NOURISHED AND UNDERNOURISHED CHILDREN

	Well-Nourished	Undernourished
HAIR	Shiny, firmly in the scalp	Dull, brittle, dry, loose and falls out easily
EYES	Bright, clear, membranes pink	Pale membranes, spots, redness, slow adjustment to dim light
FACE	Good complexion	Off-color; scaly, flaky, cracked skin; lack of fat under the skin
GLANDS	No lumps	Swollen at front of neck, cheeks
SKIN	Smooth, firm, good color	Dry, rough, "sandpaper" feel, spotty, or sores
LIPS	Smooth, good color	Red, swollen, cracks at corners of mouth
TONGUE	Red, rough, bumpy	Sore, smooth, purplish, swollen
TEETH AND GUMS	No pain or cavities, gums firm, teeth bright	Missing teeth, bad color, decay; gums bleed easily, swollen, spongy
NAILS	Firm, pink	Spoon-shaped, brittle, ridged
MUSCLES AND BONES	Good muscle tone, posture; long bones straight	"Wasted" appearance of muscles; swollen bumps on skull or ends of bones; small bumps on ribs; bowed legs or knock-knees; pain
INTERNAL SYSTEM	Heart rate, rhythm, and blood pressure normal; normal GI function; reflexes, psychological development normal	Heart rate, rhythm, or blood pressure abnormal; liver, spleen enlarged; GI dysfunction; mental irritability, confusion; burning, tingling of hands, feet; loss of balance, coordination

Adapted from Christakis A: Nutritional assessment in health programs, Am J Public Health 63(Suppl)19, 1973. Copyright © American Public Health Association, Inc.

NUTRIENT NEEDS OF CHILDREN

- *How do the nutrient needs and energy needs for children differ from those of infants or adults?*
- *Why is it preferable to use weight or height rather than age as a reference to assess energy and macronutrient requirements?*
- *How do recommended levels for energy, protein, and micronutrients change across childhood?*
- *How much dietary fiber is appropriate for children?*
- *What nutrients are of special concern for American children?*

Children are constantly growing. Baby teeth are being lost and replaced with permanent teeth, bones are being built that will need to last a lifetime, and blood volume and muscle mass are steadily increasing. Because of childhood growth, albeit sporadic at times, there is a proportionally greater need for nutrient-dense foods in childhood than in adulthood. A child's nutritional needs are determined by several factors, including the child's size, sex, genetics, and rate of growth. Nutritional needs, dietary intake, and growth rate all vary greatly among children.

Table 9-4 Recommended Dietary Allowances for Energy for Children as Kilocalories per Day, Kilocalories per Centimeter, and Kilograms per Day

Age (y)	1-3	4-6	7-10
Reference Height (cm)	90	112	132
Reference Weight (kg)	13	20	28
Energy (kcal/day)	1300	1800	2000
Energy (kcal/kg)	102	90	70
Energy (kcal/cm/day)	15	16	15

Food and Nutrition Board: Recommended dietary allowances, ed 10, Washington, DC, 1989, National Academy of Sciences.

As discussed in Chapter 1, the Institute of Medicine is in the process of establishing Dietary Reference Intake (DRI) for energy and nutrients for children in the United States. At the time of this writing, the report of the DRI subcommittee on Energy and Macronutrients is not yet available. In this chapter the discussion of recommendations for energy and protein intakes reflects the currently used 1989 Recommended Dietary Allowances (RDAs) (Food and Nutrition Board, 1989). The new DRI values for vitamins and minerals for children are discussed on page 287-292.

Energy

Energy needs of children are as varied as children themselves. Total energy requirements are a function of the energy needed to support growth and development, the basal metabolic rate (BMR), physical activity, and the thermic effect of food. The BMR, the minimum amount of energy needed by the body at rest in the fasting state, is highest during periods of rapid growth. The BMR increases during growth with expanded lean body mass. In fact this higher heat production can help explain why children are seldom cold, even when adults feel a chill.

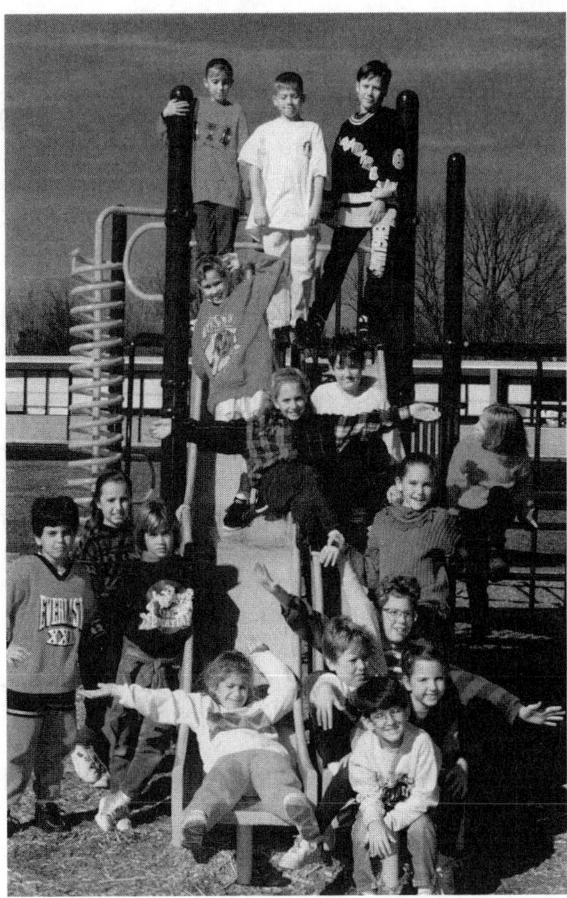

Figure 9-6 School-age children vary in size and grow at different rates.

The RDA for energy for children from 1 to 10 years of age appear in Table 9-4. It makes no distinction between boys and girls. Much of the information used to determine these recommendations was extrapolated from studies of adults (Food and Nutrition Board, 1989). During childhood energy intake must be sufficient to ensure adequate growth and to spare dietary protein from being used for energy. However, energy intake must not be excessive or overweight and obesity may result. Unfortunately American children are becoming less active and the number of children with excess body weight and fat is increasing concurrently (see page 303).

Because a child's growth is highly variable, age alone is not an adequate criterion for estimating energy needs. There is a tremendous difference in size of normal boys and girls at any age (Figure 9-6) and in development and needs within each of these age groupings. For example on the RDA chart, the energy recommendation for a child 4 years to 6 years of age is 1800 kcal. For a 5-year-old child who is 112 cm (44.1 in) tall, the reference height, this is an appropriate estimation of needs. However, there can be as much as a 10-in height difference in individual children of the same age. A 5-year-old child may have shorter parents and be 100 cm tall and thus require only 1600 kcal. Another 5-year-old child with taller parents might be 125 cm tall and thus require closer to 2000 kcal per day.

A more accurate way to estimate energy needs of children is to calculate kilocalories per cm of height or kilocalories per kg of body weight. This method is appropriate for children who are between the fifteenth and eighty-fifth percentile on the NCHS growth charts. For children whose measurements show them to be underweight (less than the fifteenth percentile) or overweight (greater than the eighty-fifth percentile), kcal per kg does not provide an accurate estimate of actual energy needs. As children grow energy needs decline when expressed per kg of body weight, but remain relatively constant when expressed per cm of height (see Table 9-4).

Protein

Children need an AI of protein to cover maintenance needs and to support optimal growth. For dietary protein to be used efficiently, a child must consume adequate energy so protein can be spared for growth needs. It is important to emphasize proteins of high biologic value, such as eggs, dairy products, meat, fish, poultry, or combinations of complementary vegetable proteins. An adequate energy intake allows the body to use the amino acids from dietary protein for protein synthesis.

Special attention must be given to children who consume diets that contain no animal proteins (high biologic value) (Sanders and Reddy, 1994). This is because plant proteins contain fewer essential amino acids in proportion to requirements than do animal proteins. Vegetarian diets that include dairy products can easily meet protein needs. If no animal proteins are included, attention needs to be given to combining proteins to provide essential amino acids and calcium and vitamin B_{12} intakes. Attention should also be given to children with multiple food allergies that limit food intake, children with medical conditions that increase their energy or protein needs or similarly limit their intake, and children who do not have access to diets adequate in energy and/or protein.

The RDAs (Food and Nutrition Board, 1989) for protein are presented in Table 9-5. Recommendations range from 16 grams per day at ages 1 year to 3 years to 28 grams per day at ages 7 years to 10 years. However, when considered in the context of body size, specifically height, protein recommendations range from 0.18 g/cm to 0.21 g/cm of height for children ages 1 year to 10 years. As children grow the need for protein per kg of body weight decreases from approximately 1.8 g/kg in early childhood to 1.2 g/kg in late childhood. As with energy, the most appropriate method for assessing the adequacy of an individual's intake is to evaluate the child's height, weight, and general state of health. The recommended levels of intake established for protein assume the diet contains a mixture of animal and plant proteins and sufficient energy to support protein synthesis (Food and Nutrition Board, 1989).

Table 9-5 Recommended Dietary Allowances for Protein for Children as Grams per Day and Grams per Centimeter per Day

Age (y)	1-3	4-6	7-10
Reference Height (cm)	90	112	132
Reference Weight (kg)	13	20	28
Protein (g/day)	16	24	28
Protein (g/cm/day)	0.18	0.21	0.21

From Food and Nutrition Board: Recommended dietary allowances, ed 10, Washington, DC, 1989, National Academy of Sciences.

Dietary Fat and Carbohydrate

In recent years attention has focused on the appropriateness of establishing guidelines for the intake of calories from fat in children. There have been reports of overzealous restriction of dietary fat associated with failure to thrive and abnormal myelin sheath development. However, with the growing incidence of childhood obesity and the public health concerns regarding the development of heart disease, recent research has focused on the impact of reduction of dietary fat on growth and development (Krebs and Johnson, 2000; Lauer et al., 2000).

The current dietary guidelines for children are consistent with those first proposed by the National Institutes of Health and the American Heart Association in 1985. It is recommended that after the age of 2 years, children should consume at least 20%, but no more than 30%, of energy from fat and that average saturated fat intake should be limited to less than 10% of energy (American Academy of Pediatrics Committee on Nutrition, 1998). This recommendation is based on the assumption that children younger than 2 years of age require a higher fat intake to support the rapid growth of infancy and toddlerhood. Several small studies have reported that children fed reduced-fat diets after 1 year of age experienced normal growth and development during the second year of life with lower blood lipid levels (Lytle, 2000; Olson, 2000). To date, few studies have assessed the long-term effects of such changes beyond the second year of life, but several research investigations are in progress.

There are numerous reasons for limiting dietary fat beginning with children over the age of 2 years (Williams, 1998). These include health benefits of a slower age-related increase in blood lipid levels in childhood, which is associated with reduced serum lipid levels in adulthood and thus reduced the risk of atherosclerotic disease (Washington, 1999). Lower fat intakes are less carcinogenic for some forms of cancer and, in particular, lower body weight. A child's diet can benefit immediately by replacing calorically dense fat with more nutritionally dense foods such as fruits and vegetables and low-fat dairy products, which will improve overall health. However, it has been suggested that dietary changes to reduce fat intake can result in increased consumption of "low-fat" or "fat-free" products, which may have higher levels of simple carbohydrates, increasing sugar intake (Dwyer, 2000).

Fiber

Dietary fiber is important, particularly for children, because it helps promote normal laxation (Williams et al., 1995). There is also evidence that fiber may reduce future risk of chronic diseases such as cardiovascular disease, some cancers, and adult-onset diabetes. The Conference on Dietary Fiber in Childhood concluded that the current dietary fiber intake of children in the United States was suboptimal (Saldanha, 1995). The Conference recommended that children increase their intake of dietary fiber by eating more fruits, vegetables, cereals, and other whole-grain products. Recommendations are for a fiber intake equal to or greater than their age plus 5 grams starting at age 2. Thus fiber intake should increase from 8 grams per day for a 3-year-old child to 25 grams per day by the age of 20. Examples of how to meet the fiber recommendations are shown for several ages in Table 9-6.

Vitamins and Minerals

Vitamins and minerals are essential for adequate growth and development. Vitamins function in numerous metabolic processes and, for many processes, vitamins are often interdependent on the energy and protein intake or levels of intake of other nutrients.

Although studies of food consumption of children in the United States and Canada indicate that intakes of some nutrients are likely to be low, overt signs of vitamin or mineral deficiencies are quite rare. Dietary intake studies of children indicate that calcium, iron, ascorbic acid, vitamin A, folate, and vitamin B_6 are commonly found to be below the recommended levels (Roberts and Hegman, 2000). Children who are at increased risk of having marginal intakes of some vitamins

Table 9-6 EXAMPLES OF FOODS TO MEET FIBER RECOMMENDATIONS FOR CHILDREN AT AGES 2, 6, AND 12 YEARS

2 Years		6 Years		12 Years	
Food	Fiber (g)	Food	Fiber (g)	Food	Fiber (g)
1 slice whole wheat bread	2	1 c Cheerios	3	Frosted Miniwheats	6
½ c cornflakes	1	1 raw carrot	3	10 dried apricots	3
1 banana	2	2 tbsp peanut butter	2	1 oz almonds	3
½ c applesauce	2	1 medium apple	3	2 c popped popcorn	2
Total	7		11		17

and minerals are those with anorexia, poor appetites, and poor eating habits; children who consume vegan diets; and children from low-income families (USDA Human Nutrition Information Services, 1986). Undernutri-tion does occur in certain circumstances. An estimated 11 million children in the United States experience food insecurity at some time each month (Taylor and Koblinsky, 1993; Wallman, 2000).

The DRIs, which include the RDAs and AIs, are those levels considered sufficient for growth and health. The DRIs are established for the life stage groups of children ages 1 year to 3 years, 4 years to 8 years, and 9 years to 13 years. Recommendations are separated based on a child's sex at age 9 years.

The DRIs are meant to be applied to groups and not to individual children. A reference height and weight are established for each age group. The DRIs for micronutrients appear in Table 9-7. An individual's intake of a given nutrient may be physiologically adequate for that person's specific needs, but may not meet the established level. The RDAs are set at levels that meet the needs of almost all (97 to 98%) individuals in a life stage group and the AIs are adequate for 50% of healthy individuals within a group.

Calcium

Recently the American Academy of Pediatrics Committee on Nutrition (1999) published a policy statement regarding the concern that children and adolescents are simply not getting sufficient calcium and it recommended a daily diet that includes milk, yogurt, cheese, and calcium-rich foods. The AI levels for calcium for children in the various age groups are given in Table 9-7. The DRI for calcium is only a guide because of the large variability in calcium requirements. The velocity of growth, the efficiency of calcium absorption, and the availability of other nutrients including phosphorus, vitamin D, energy, and protein influence calcium needs of individual children.

Children require calcium to maintain existing bone and to support the growth of new bone. Approximately 100 mg of calcium is retained as bone each day and this amount doubles and even triples during peak periods of adolescent growth (Matkovic, Fontana, and Tominac, 1990). The deposition of minerals in the bone tissue is a complex process that requires an adequate supply of protein, calcium, phosphorus, and vitamin D.

Recent research has focused on increasing bone mineral density during (see page 347) childhood and puberty to achieve peak bone mass. It is postulated that achieving maximum bone mineral density during these important periods of bone accretion will provide protection from osteoporosis later in life when bone resorption exceeds bone formation. Researchers recognize that factors in addition to calcium influence bone status. In children exercise also plays a crucial role in the development of bone density (American Academy of Pediatrics, 2001b).

In a critical analysis of pediatric calcium supplementation trials, Wosje and Specker (2000) reported that calcium supplementation resulted in increases in bone mineral density in children, primarily in cortical bone sites. The most apparent increase in bone mineral density was found in populations with low baseline calcium intakes. Unfortunately the increases in bone mineral density were not found to persist beyond the trial period of calcium supplementation. Welten

Table 9-7 DIETARY REFERENCE INTAKES FOR VITAMINS AND MINERALS FOR CHILDREN

Vitamin/Mineral	1-3 yr	4-8 yr	Females 9-13 yr	Males 9-13 yr
Calcium (mg)	*500*	*800*	*1300*	*1300*
Phosphorus (mg)	**460**	**500**	**1250**	**1250**
Magnesium (mg)	**80**	**130**	**240**	**240**
Vitamin D (μg)	*5*	*5*	*5*	*5*
Fluoride (mg)	*.7*	*1*	*1.6*	*1.9*
Thiamin (mg)	**.5**	**.6**	**.9**	**.9**
Riboflavin (mg)	**.5**	**.6**	**.9**	**.9**
Niacin (mg)	**6**	**8**	**12**	**12**
Vitamin B_6 (mg)	**.5**	**.6**	**1**	**1**
Folate (μg)	**150**	**200**	**300**	**300**
Vitamin B_{12} (μg)	**.9**	**1.2**	**1.8**	**1.8**
Pantothenic Acid (mg)	*2*	*3*	*4*	*4*
Biotin (μg)	*8*	*12*	*20*	*20*
Choline (mg)	*200*	*250*	*300*	**300**
Vitamin C (mg)	**15**	**25**	**45**	**45**
Vitamin E (mg)	**6**	**7**	**11**	**11**
Selenium (μg)	**20**	**30**	**40**	**40**
Vitamin A (μg)	**300**	**400**	**600**	**600**
Vitamin K (μg)	*30*	*55*	*60*	*60*
Chromium (μg)	*11*	*15*	*21*	*25*
Copper (μg)	**340**	**440**	**700**	**700**
Iodine (mg)	**90**	**90**	**120**	**120**
Iron (mg)	**7**	**10**	**8**	**8**
Manganese (mg)	*1.2*	*1.5*	*1.6*	*1.9*
Molybdenum (mg)	**17**	**22**	**34**	**34**
Zinc (mg)	**3**	**5**	**8**	**8**

Adapted with permission from the following Institute of Medicine publications: Dietary reference intakes for calcium, phosphorus, magnesium, vitamin D, and fluoride (1997); Dietary reference intakes for thiamin, riboflavin, niacin, vitamin B_6, folate, vitamin B_{12}, pantothenic acid, biotin, and choline (1998); Dietary reference intakes for vitamin C, vitamin E, selenium, and carotenoids (2000); and Dietary reference intakes for vitamin A, vitamin K, arsenic, boron, chromium, copper, iodine, iron, manganese, molybdenum, nickel, silicon, vanadium, and zinc (2001). Washington, DC, National Academy Press.
Bold type represents RDAs; italic type represents AIs.

and colleagues (1994) found that among children who participated in regular weight-bearing activity, the activity had a greater influence on peak bone mass than did dietary calcium.

It is apparent that to provide sufficient calcium for normal bone formation, children need to be encouraged to consume foods that are rich in calcium (Table 9-8). If a child does not consume dairy products, it will take substantial ingenuity to plan a diet that will provide adequate calcium. In such cases it would be appropriate to consider supplemental calcium.

Vitamin D

The human body can convert 7-dehydrocholesterol to vitamin D (cholecalciferol) when the skin is exposed to the ultraviolet rays of sunlight. Exposure to sunlight is variable with geographic location and the season (length of daylight). The amount of pigment in the skin also can affect the vitamin D status of an individual. Darker-pigmented skin blocks more of the sun's rays from being absorbed. Individuals with darker skin need a longer exposure to sunlight to produce an adequate amount of vitamin D. There has also been increasing concern about the detrimental effects of sunlight on the skin and the link to skin cancer. Use of sunscreen blocks not only potentially damaging ultraviolet radiation, but also the ultraviolet rays necessary for vitamin D formation.

The natural food sources of vitamin D include butter, cream, egg yolk, and liver. These foods

Table 9-8 APPROXIMATE CALCIUM CONTENT OF 1 SERVING OF SOME COMMON FOODS

Food	Serving Size	Calcium Content
Milk	1 cup	300 mg
White beans	½ cup	113 mg
Broccoli cooked	½ cup	35 mg
Broccoli raw	1 cup	35 mg
Cheddar cheese	1.5 oz	300 mg
Low-fat yogurt	8 oz	300-415 mg
Spinach cooked	½ cup	120 mg
Spinach raw	1-1½ cup	120 mg
Calcium-fortified orange juice	1 cup	300 mg
Orange	1 medium	50 mg
Sardines or salmon with bones	20 sardines	50 mg
Sweet potatoes	½ cup mashed	44 mg

Low-fat milk has comparable or greater calcium levels than whole milk.

are limited in most diets from reduced consumption of foods high in cholesterol and saturated fat. Almost all fluid milk is fortified with vitamin D. However, many dairy products made from skim milk such as yogurt, cheese, and cottage cheese may be excellent sources of calcium, but are not routinely fortified with vitamin D. Most fortified cereals provide 10% of the Daily Value for vitamin D, which, if consumed with one-half cup of vitamin D-fortified milk, will provide 25% of the Daily Value.

Vitamin D, 7-dehydrocholesterol, is activated in the kidney and the liver, forming 1,25 dihydroxy vitamin D. Thus vitamin D might be considered a prohormone. In its activated form, vitamin D has a major role in calcium absorption and metabolism. For children with limited exposure to sunshine, meeting the DRI for vitamin D from dietary sources becomes critical, particularly during the winter months.

Rickets associated with an inadequate intake of vitamin D was thought to be a disease of the mid1900s. Rickets can develop in children who receive an inadequate diet. It results when there is improper deposition of calcium phosphate and the bones thus lack the strength to support the weight of the body. Bowed legs, knock-knees, and various other skeletal abnormalities can result.

Because of rapid growth and bone formation, infants and young children are most vulnerable to vitamin D deficiency. Once thought to no longer be a problem in North America, rickets is again becoming a health concern. Several cases of rickets in infants and children have been reported (CDC, 2001).

Fluoride

Fluoride is a naturally occurring element. It has been shown to reduce the formation of dental cavities by up to 70%. The fluoride ion, when present at the tooth surface, acts to inhibit enamel demineralization and encourages calcium and phosphorus to leave saliva and remineralize the tooth. It also inhibits formation of dental plaque.

For children the optimal intake is 0.5 mg per kg of body weight (American Academy of Pediatrics Committee on Nutrition, 1998). This amount is provided in fluoridated water. Sodium fluoride is regularly added to drinking water supplies, usually as 1 part per million parts of water. Supplementation is recommended for children who have well water, drink filtered water, or live in areas where the water supply is not fluoridated.

Iron

Iron is needed to maintain hemoglobin concentration and to support growth. The preschool child is at high risk for iron deficiency anemia, especially from ages 1 year to 3 years (Looker et al., 1997). During periods of rapid growth, children experience an increase in the red cell mass and total body iron. Dietary requirements depend on the rate of growth, an individual's iron stores, and the efficiency of the absorption of iron from food sources. The DRI for iron (see Table 9-7) is based on the assumption that 10% to 15% of dietary iron is absorbed. Absorption of nonheme iron can be enhanced by the simultaneous consumption of foods containing vitamin C.

Iron deficiency is associated with an increase in the incidence of fatigue, decreased growth, and impaired resistance to infection. Iron deficiency also increases the risk of lead toxicity. Chronic iron deficiency in childhood may have long-term adverse effects on growth and development. Iron deficiency anemia has been associated with poor performance on infant development scales, poor performance on IQ and learning tasks in preschool children, and low educational achievement among school-age children. The mechanism by which low levels of iron affect learning and behavior is unclear. It has been suggested that iron deficiency causes a decline in hemoglobin concentration, resulting in reduced oxygen availability to the brain or decreased levels of iron-dependent neurotransmitter receptors

KEY TERMS

rickets: a disease associated with the malformation of bones from deficient deposition of calcium phosphate; usually the result of inadequate vitamin D activity in the body

Research Update

Lead Poisoning in Children

Lead poisoning, or plumbism, continues to be a significant public health concern in the United States despite the mandated removal of lead from gasoline and paint. The CDC reports that the blood levels in children have decreased significantly, approximately 80%, since the late 1970s (Lofgren et al., 2000). However, lead poisoning—a blood lead level equal to or greater than 10 μg/dL of blood—is estimated to currently affect more than 4% of preschool-aged children (Ellis, 2000). The CDC Childhood Blood Lead Surveillance (CBLS) team found that, in data reported from the surveillance programs in 19 states, the prevalence of lead poisoning decreased from 10.5% in 1996 to 7.6% in 1998 in children younger than 6 years (Lofgren et al., 2000). It noted concern that despite the decrease in the mean blood lead level in children, lead poisoning continues to be problematic. Some states reported blood lead levels indicative of lead poisoning in 14.9% of children studied (Ellis, 2000). It is significantly more prevalent in African-American children, children from low-income families, children who live in urban areas (Ellis, 2000), and those living in older housing (Lofgren et al., 2000).

Elevated lead levels are associated with damage to the central nervous system, kidneys, and blood production system and also with a decrease in intelligence quotient test scores. It is insidious because minute amounts of lead can impair a child's growth and cause irreversible damage to the nervous system. Unfortunately for many children, the physical symptoms of lead poisoning may be vague or absent until the lead accumulation reaches dangerously high levels.

Children are especially vulnerable to lead poisoning because they absorb lead more readily than do adults. Children also are at risk because of certain behaviors such as playing in lead-contaminated soil, chewing on lead-painted windowsills, or engaging in other hand-to-mouth activities with lead-contaminated items.

Prevention is the most important strategy for combating lead poisoning. A significant reduction in blood lead levels was noted with the removal of lead from gasoline and paint. Secondary prevention focuses on removing or preventing lead already in the environment from being consumed or absorbed. This includes interior dust abatement, use of high-efficiency particulate air (HEPA) vacuums,

Continued

Research Update

Lead Poisoning in Children—cont'd

soil abatement, and residential paint remediation. Family education that focuses on a safe water supply, avoiding use of lead-contaminated pottery and crystal, avoiding use of lead-contaminated medicines or natural remedies, and washing hands before eating is also important. Families are also counseled on the importance of an adequate diet that contains sufficient amounts of the key nutrients calcium, iron, and zinc.

ROLE OF DIET

The body handles lead by making use of existing metal nutrient transport systems. Consequently some nutrients may influence an individual's handling of lead, although exposure to excess lead results in high blood lead levels regardless of the adequacy of the diet. However, lead toxicity is more common in infants and children who are at nutritional risk, such as urban, economically disadvantaged, and nonwhite children. Lead uptake is greatly enhanced in the fasting state. Deficiencies of calcium, phosphorus, iron, zinc, or vitamin C may make children more susceptible to lead intoxication (Houston and Johnson, 2000).

Studies of animals and human infants have shown inverse relationships between the absorption and distribution of dietary calcium and levels of lead in the blood. It is thought that phosphorus and calcium may reduce lead toxicity (Mushak and Crocetti, 1996).

Iron deficiency anemia and high blood lead levels are likely to occur in the same child. At first it was assumed that lead caused microcytic anemia by impairing iron utilization. It is now recognized that iron deficiency and excess lead both impair hemoglobin synthesis (Yip et al., 1981). Iron deficiency may enhance lead poisoning because decreased iron in the intestine can allow absorption of a larger portion of ingested lead (Yip et al., 1981). Children with elevated blood levels should be screened for iron deficiency and treated properly.

The CDC, in response to the overall decline in lead poisoning, no longer recommends routine blood screening for lead levels for all children (Lofgren et al., 2000). They have, however, developed a screening protocol. It recommends universal screening in areas where at least 27% of houses were built before 1950 and in populations in which 12% or more of 1- and 2-year-old children have elevated blood lead levels (CDC, 1997). In other geographic areas, the CDC recommends that a screening questionnaire be given. Special attention should also be given to adopted foreign-born children who may have ingested significant amounts of lead before obtaining residence in the United States.

When a child is found to have significantly elevated blood lead levels, generally greater than 25 mg/dL, medical intervention is necessary. Chelation therapy is the use of various pharmaceutical agents that can be given orally, intramuscularly, or intravenously. They act to bind with lead and then the lead is excreted in the urine or in bile. For this therapy to be effective, special attention is concurrently given to reducing lead exposure.

in the brain (Wauben and Wainwright, 1999). Iron is essential for central nervous system functioning and is involved in the production and maintenance of myelin. It is also a component of many enzymes involved in neurotransmitter systems.

Children who had iron deficiency as infants may continue to perform poorly even when their iron status is improved (Hurtado et al., 1999). In older children with short-term iron deficiency, iron interventions that lasted for 2 months or more resulted in improvements in performance on one or more tests of cognitive processes (Pollitt, 1997). The importance of iron deficiency as a public health problem is indicated by the fact that a nutrition-related priority of the *Healthy People 2010* initiative is to reduce iron deficiency among young children.

Vitamin and Mineral Supplementation

Vitamin and mineral supplements are marketed specifically to preschool and school-age children. They are made in chewable animal or cartoon character shapes to facilitate ease in administration. It is estimated that up to 60% of children use vitamin and mineral supplements regularly or occasionally (USDA Human Nutrition Information Services, 1993). Supplement use declines as children get older.

The American Academy of Pediatrics does not recommend vitamin and mineral supplementation in healthy children who are consuming a well-balanced, varied diet, except for fluoride in unfluoridated areas and vitamin D in breast-fed infants. There is a concern that the use of vitamin and mineral supplements will foster complacency in parents, who may then cease to attempt to optimize the nutrient content of the child's diet. Vitamin and mineral supplements may not necessarily meet nutrient needs or make up for an otherwise inadequate diet. Calcium is a key nutrient in children's diets, yet vitamin and mineral supplements frequently do not contain enough calcium to meet the needs of children.

There is no risk for children from receiving a single vitamin and mineral supplement if it is given in the appropriate amount. Megadoses of vitamins or minerals, or anything greater than the age-appropriate DRI, should be avoided. Specifically, caution should be given to fat-soluble vitamins, because they can accumulate to toxic levels in the body.

NUTRITION AND ORAL HEALTH

- *Describe the role of nutrition in tooth development and prevention of dental disease.*

Oral health and good dentition are essential for the consumption of an adequate diet. Good nutrition is essential for maintenance of oral health. Inadequate nutrients for tooth formation can result in structurally weak teeth that are susceptible to injury and decay. Poor dietary habits can also contribute to tooth decay and periodontal disease.

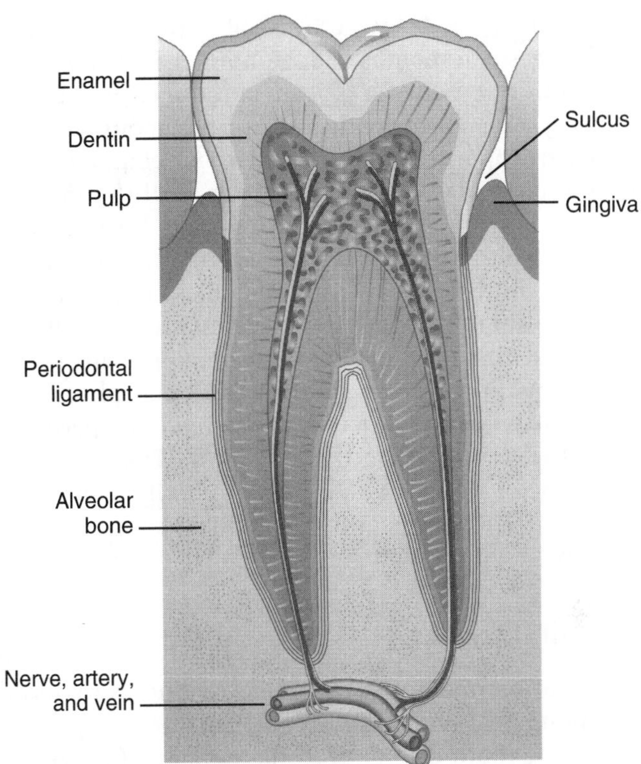

Figure 9-7 Parts of a tooth and its supporting structure. *(From Mahan LK and Escott-Stump S: Krause's food, nutrition, and diet therapy, ed 10, Philadelphia, 2000, WB Saunders.)*

Tooth Structure

Teeth are highly specialized structures of mineralized tissue that encase a highly vascular dental pulp and its ample supply of nerves (Figure 9-7). Dental enamel forms a hard protective coating over the tooth. Enamel consists mostly of calcium and phosphorus salts and other ions in a hydroxyapatite-like structure. Dentin has no vascular components but, compared with enamel, it is more readily permeable to fluids from blood through dentinal tubules. Overlying the dentin and the root of the tooth below the gums and alveolar bone is cementum, a bone-like connective tissue that assists in supporting the tooth. The support structures of the periodontium include the gingiva and the periodontal membrane that joins the root cementum to the alveolar bone.

Primary or baby teeth usually erupt between the ages of 6 months and 24 months. Permanent teeth erupt between 6 years and the early teenage years. The hard tissue of permanent teeth begins to form as early as birth, but completion of root formation does not occur until the midteens. During the preeruptive period, formation of a healthy tooth structure is fostered by adequate nutrition. Protein, calcium, phosphorus, magnesium, fluoride, and vitamins C and D are all essential for proper tooth formation. Saliva is supersaturated with calcium and phosphorus, the major minerals found in the hydroxyapatite of the dental enamel and dentin. The dental enamel is bathed with saliva, promoting continuous exchange of calcium and phosphorus, typically in equilibrium.

Dental Caries

Initiation of dental caries involves interactions among the susceptible tooth, cariogenic (promoting tooth decay) bacteria in plaque (a mass adhering to the enamel surface of a tooth, composed of a mixture of bacteria and fermentable carbohydrate), and a substrate. The substrate can be fermentable carbohydrates (monosaccharides and disaccharides and some cooked or processed starches) that are metabolized by the bacteria in plaque. The byproduct of that metabolism is organic acids. When the oral pH falls to about 5.7, the organic acids diffuse through the tooth surface, reaching susceptible surfaces where they dissolve calcium and phosphate. As mineral loss continues, the enamel actually breaks down, producing visible tooth destruction.

The ability of a food to be cariogenic is related to its ability to produce acid. Foods should be selected based on their nutritional contribution to the diet. It is, however, desirable to limit the frequency of consumption of sugary between-meal snacks or beverages high in simple sugars such as colas and fruit juices. Limiting snack frequency helps to limit the presence of fermentable carbohydrate substrate in the mouth. It is also wise to encourage tooth brushing after meals and snacks (American Dietetic Association, 1996). A program to avoid accumulation of plaque and prevent dental caries and periodontal disease is essential for good oral health. Regular brushing, consistent use of dental floss, and regular professional dental care should begin by 2 years of age.

FACTORS INFLUENCING FOOD INTAKE

- *Describe factors that influence dietary intakes of preschool and school-age children. How do they differ by age group?*

Poverty

Poverty is a significant risk factor threatening the health of children. In the United States, 18% of children under the age of 18 years live in a family whose income is below the poverty level (Wallman, 2000). Despite the availability of food and nutrition programs, economically disadvantaged children have a greater prevalence of short stature (Yip et al., 1993) and an increased risk of nutrient deficiencies (Drake, 1991; Taylor and Koblinsky, 1993). Studies have shown that poor households with children spend 32% of their income on food, compared with nonpoor families, who spend 16% of income on food (Lino, 1996).

In a survey that addressed household food security, children were asked if enough food and enough of the kinds of food they wanted were available. As responses moved from more food-secure to less food-secure, the mean level of energy intake for children fell and the levels of fat and saturated fat increased (Kennedy and Goldberg, 1995).

Family

Infants' rapid growth is reflected in their insistent demands for food. As infancy ends and toddlerhood begins, the slowed rate of growth is accompanied by a dramatic decrease in appetite. During early childhood growth is steady, but sporadic. Because a child's appetite ordinarily corresponds to rate of growth, food intake is often erratic. Parents may become concerned that their young child is not eating enough or insists on eating only one or two limited foods for each meal.

Such concerns can lead to unnecessary anxiety over the child's eating habits. The kitchen or dinner table can become a battlefield between the parent and the child. In reality, studies of daily intakes of children have found that despite a high degree of variability from meal to meal, overall energy and nutrition intakes were relatively constant (Birch et al., 1991; Shea et al., 1992).

Dietary habits are formed early in life. These eating patterns are often carried into adulthood. Dietary patterns are shaped by the available choices. Food patterns depend on food availability and cultural, environmental, and societal factors. Feeding young children is much more than just providing a variety of nutritious foods. A family must provide a social and emotional environment conducive to the enjoyment of food and the development of positive eating behaviors.

In the preschool years, parents usually determine what foods are available to children and how they are presented. The plain peanut butter and jelly sandwich that was previously refused by a 3-year-old child may become a favorite lunch when the bread is cut into a fun shape with cookie cutters. A child who dislikes sliced turkey may enjoy the same turkey rolled like an hors d'oeuvre with a pretzel stick. Simply providing low-fat ranch dressing for dipping makes carrots much more appetizing in a lunchbox.

Not surprisingly, there is a significant correlation between parents and young children in food preferences and attitudes toward food (Borah-Giddens and Falciglia, 1993). Although parents provide food to the child, it is the child who determines how much to eat, or even whether to eat. Allowing a child to make that decision, within limits, creates a structure that promotes positive eating habits (Birch et al., 1991).

Parents also have the responsibility to serve as good role models for eating habits. As part of the Framingham Children's Study, the development of excess body fat in children over a 6-year period was found to be influenced by parental eating habits. Parents who displayed high levels of **disinhibited eating** coupled with high **dietary restraint** raised children who had the largest increases in body fat. It is hypothesized that the parents, by binge eating and then strictly dieting, may unconsciously undermine their child's autonomy in food choices by imposing excessive control over the child's diet while at the same time modeling inappropriate eating behaviors (Hood et al., 2000).

Social and economic changes during recent decades have affected the American family significantly. There are more single-parent families, most of which are headed by women. In addition more women are employed outside the home, which influences family food patterns. In a dual-career family there may be less time available for food preparation and shopping and more meals may be eaten outside the home. An analysis of the nutrient contents of the diets of children 2 years to 5 years of age in the Nationwide Food Consumption Survey, however, found that maternal employment alone did not diminish the quality of the child's diet (Johnson et al., 1992). A survey of American families found that they are strongly committed to having dinner together. Forty-three percent of families with young children indicated they ate dinner together 7 days a week and another 28% said they ate together 4 to 6 times weekly (Food Marketing Institute and Better Homes and Gardens Magazine, 1995).

Peers

As children grow and begin to attend daycare, preschool, or school, people outside the home increasingly influence food choices. In the preschool or daycare setting, meal and snack times may provide an opportunity to expand a child's exposure to and acceptance of new foods. As children enter school, they become increasingly concerned with peer acceptance. Naïve is the parent who packs a child's lunch for school and assumes that lunch is what the child actually eats for lunch. The barter and trade system is thriving at school and other places where children gather. The peer group can have a great impact on food, snack, and beverage choices.

KEY TERMS

disinhibited eating: abandoning control of dietary intake in response to certain external cues

dietary restraint: tendency to restrict diet to control weight

Media and Advertising

The influence of television on a child can be incredible. Television reaches many children before they are capable of verbal communication. It has been estimated that the average child in the United States sees an estimated 30,000 television commercials per year (Coon et al., 2001). Preschool children usually are unable to discriminate between regular programming and commercial messages. They may watch commercials more closely than do older children. Because commercial messages are based on emotional and psychologic appeal and often promote products of questionable nutritional value, commercials may not support the development of positive eating habits. Approximately 60% of all advertising shown during children's programming is promoting food products (Sylvester et al., 1995) and even brief exposures to televised food commercials can influence a preschool child's food preferences (Borzekowski and Robinson, 2001).

Nutrition Knowledge and Education

The education level and nutrition knowledge of parents are important factors in determining foods available to their children. Young children are generally quite receptive to nutrition education. It is important that nutrition education and food-related activities be developmentally appropriate.

A 1997 conference on "How to Grow a Healthy Child" centered on environmental and sociological factors influencing children's eating behavior and nutritional status (Picciano, 1999). Emphasis was placed on the development of childrens' food acceptance patterns. The 1996 College of Nutrition Workshop addressing dietary guidelines for children concluded that messages to children about nutrition should be food based, not nutrient based. "Eat more carrots" is developmentally more appropriate for children than "Choose foods high in vitamin A." The need for more age specific and meaningful nutrition messages was stressed. Children, who are developmentally focused on the present and not the future, more easily relate to the specific message "Calcium builds strong bones" than to "The importance of calcium in the prevention of osteoporosis," a message that is not only abstract, but also focuses on health concerns several decades in the future.

The development of perceptions of health and attitudes toward food and eating behaviors begins very early in life. Educators may be underestimating the ability of young children to learn about food, nutrition, and health (Singleton et al., 1992). One group of researchers evaluated the health perceptions of 4- to 7-year-old children and the degree to which the children included food and eating behavior in their health perceptions. It was found that after participating in a 4-week home-based nutrition education program, the children in the experimental group significantly increased their perception that health and nutrition were related concepts compared with the control group (Murphy et al., 1995). After the education program the children's response to a question about what it means to be healthy included "eat the right foods" (82%), "big" and "strong" (27%), "exercise" (17%), and "not being sick" (8%). Preschoolers can have a basic understanding of the food pyramid. Young children are able to understand the general relationship of food and exercise to body fat and general health.

RECOMMENDATIONS FOR FOOD INTAKE

- *What developmental events mark progress in self-feeding?*
- *Why is it important to promote positive food habits in young children?*
- *What factors are important for overcoming neophobia?*
- *What influences the development of food acceptance patterns?*
- *What factors must be considered in planning vegetarian diets for children? What are the risks?*

In recognition of the unique nutritional needs of children, the U.S. Department of Agriculture (USDA) developed a Food Guide Pyramid for Young Children (USDA, 1999) (Figure 9-8). The pyramid is based on the actual eating patterns of young children from a USDA dietary analysis of children age 2 years to 6 years. The pyramid emphasizes variety and the message that there are no "good" foods or "bad" foods. A healthful

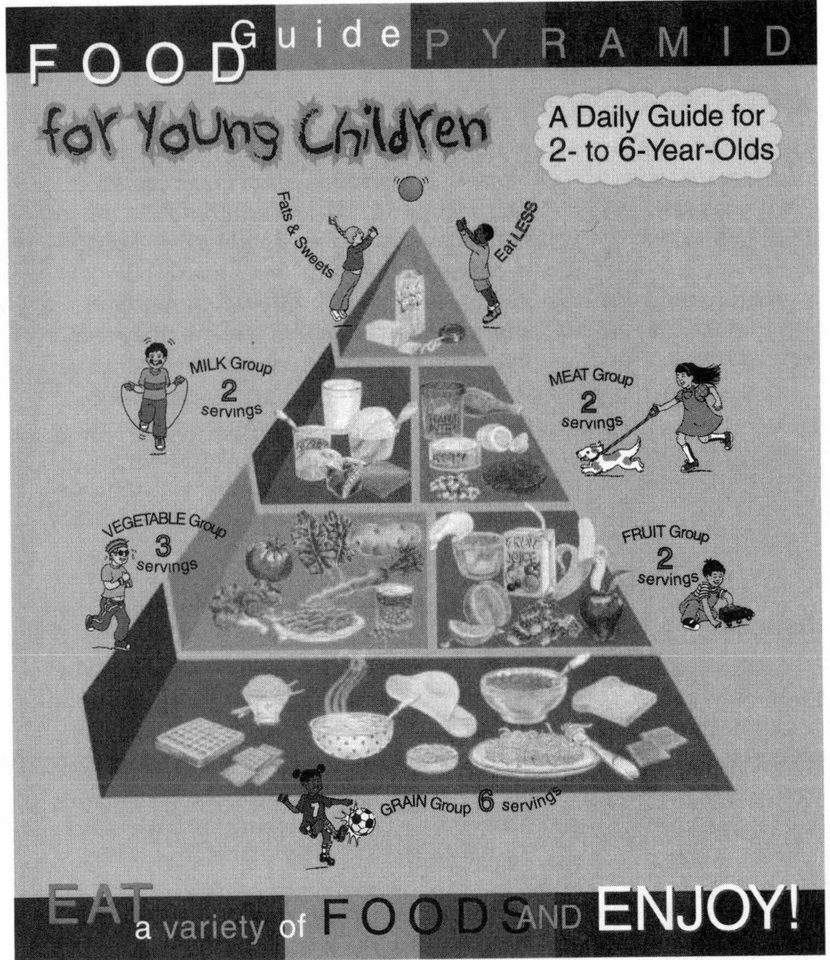
FOOD Guide PYRAMID
for Young Children
A Daily Guide for 2- to 6-Year-Olds
Fats & Sweets
Eat LESS
MILK Group 2 servings
MEAT Group 2 servings
VEGETABLE Group 3 servings
FRUIT Group 2 servings
GRAIN Group 6 servings
EAT a variety of FOODS AND ENJOY!

What counts as one serving?

Grain Group
1 slice bread
1/2 c cooked rice or pasta
1/2 c cooked cereal
1 oz ready-to-eat cereal

Vegetable Group
1/2 c chopped raw or cooked vegetables
1 c raw leafy vegetables

Fruit Group
1 piece of fruit or melon wedge
3/4 c juice
1/2 c canned fruit
3/4 c dried fruit

Milk Group
1 c milk or yogurt
2 oz cheese

Meat Group
2 to 3 oz cooked lean meat, poultry, or fish
1/2 c cooked dry beans, or 1 egg counts as 1 oz lean meat; 2 tbs of peanut butter count as 1 oz meat

Fats and Sweets
Limit kcalories from these.

Four- to 6-year-olds can eat these serving sizes. Offer 2- to 3-year-olds less, except for milk. Two- to 6-year-old children need a total of 2 servings from the milk group each day.

Figure 9-8 USDA Food Guide Pyramid for Young Children. *(From USDA Center for Nutrition Policy and Promotion, March 1999, Program AID 1649.)*

diet is built on a wide variety of all food types with a special emphasis on grain products, fruits, and vegetables. Children are shown actively playing around the food pyramid to symbolize that physical activity plays an important part in good health.

Feeding the Preschool-Age Child

Early in the preschool years, the child is developing self-feeding skills using large motor skills, a process that involves frequent spills and the use of fingers and hands. These somewhat messy behaviors are a normal part of the development and maturation of young children (Table 9-9). The shift from large motor to fine motor skills provides a greater precision in eating and marks a time when preschoolers can participate in supervised food preparation.

The preschool years are important in the development of positive attitudes toward food and learning to make food choices. An eating environment that is pleasant, both physically and emotionally, promotes this process. It includes a positive atmosphere with companionship and gentle guidance in fostering food-related behaviors.

A guide for types of foods and portion sizes appropriate for children age 1 year to 6 years appears in Table 9-10. Children require smaller portions than do adults, but will eat more frequently. An appropriate portion size in general is a tablespoon of each type of food for every year

Table 9-9 DEVELOPMENTAL SEQUENCE GUIDE FOR NUTRITION AND FEEDING DURING CHILDHOOD

Age (Approximate)	Motor Development	Oral Motor Skills Related to Eating	Self-Help/Social	Food and Appetite
12-24 mos	Walks; climbs; uses mature pincer grasp	Chews using rotary motion; uses refined cup drinking	Enjoys eating; uses words; uses refined spoon feeding skills; eats with family	Eats bite-size foods; has good appetite; should not be served foods associated with easy choking
24-36 mos	Runs; jumps; uses three-jaw chuck (finger) grasp; uses fork	Straw drinking; uses independent cup drinking	Uses phrases and sentences; negativism emerges; toilet training in progress	Growth slows with decrease in appetite; should not be served foods associated with easy choking
3-4 y	Hops; rides tricycle; uses static tripod (3-finger) grasp		Asserts independence; uses conversational body language; pours liquids	Picky eater; should not be served foods associated with easy choking
5-6 y	Rides bicycle; refines grasp to adult pattern; gains ability to use one upper extremity for one task and other for a different task		Beginning to use knife and fork for cutting; has acceptable table manners; peers becoming more important	Appetite more regular as rate of growth stabilizes; should be supervised eating foods associated with easy choking

Developed by Nutrition-Feeding Clinic Faculty, The Nisonger Center University Affiliated Program for Mental Retardation and Developmental Disabilities, The Ohio State University, 1980. Revised 1995. Work supported in part by U.S. Department of Health and Human Services, Administration on Developmental Disabilities Grant #90DD032902 and Maternal and Child Health Bureau Grant #MCJ399155-04.

of the child's age. More can be provided according to the child's appetite.

Because young children have a smaller capacity and variations in appetite, they need between-meal snacks. Snacks should be planned to provide nutrient-dense foods and timed so that they contribute to total nutrient intake, but do not interfere with meals. Preschool children prefer unmixed dishes with mild flavors at moderate temperatures.

Children age 3 years and younger are at greatest risk for choking on food. They need foods that can be easily handled with utensils or hands and close supervision while eating. The foods that most often cause choking are hot dogs, hard pieces of fruit or vegetables, peanut butter, popcorn, and nuts. Almost any food can cause problems with choking if the mouth is too full or if the child is running while eating.

Parents are often concerned when a toddler shows decreased interest in eating and even refuses favorite foods. Appetites may become erratic and unpredictable. Rejection of meats and vegetables is common. Children may refuse milk or may want to drink it to the exclusion of other foods. Often food jags, during which times the child may eat only a few foods or may want the same food meal after meal, characterize the preschool period. Most jags (such as a period of eating only peanut butter and jelly sandwiches) last only a few days or even weeks. When they are treated casually, they become passing food behaviors that are soon forgotten. However, placing importance on them may increase rather

Table 9-10 FOOD GUIDE FOR PRESCHOOL CHILDREN

	Suggested Portion for Age					
Type of Food	1 Year	2 Year	3 Year	4 Year	5 Year	Servings/Day
MILK, CHEESE, YOGURT						**TOTAL INTAKE** of 16-24 oz
Milk, yogurt	4 oz	5 oz	6 oz	6 oz	6 oz	
Cheese	½ oz	½ oz	¾ oz	¾ oz	1 oz	
PROTEIN FOODS						3-4
Meats, fish, poultry	½ oz	1 oz	1 oz	1 oz	1 oz	
Egg	1	1	1	1	1	
Cooked legumes	1 tbsp	2 tbsp	3 tbsp	4 tbsp	4 tbsp	
FRUITS						4-5
Fresh*	½ piece	½ piece	½ piece	¾ piece	¾ piece	
Canned	1-2 tbsp	2-3 tbsp	3-4 tbsp	¼ c	¼-½ c	
Juice	2 oz	2-3 oz	3-4 oz	4 oz	4 oz	
VEGETABLES						4-5
Dark green, leafy or yellow vegetable	1 tbsp	2 tbsp	3 tbsp	4 tbsp	5 tbsp	
Other	1 tbsp	2 tbsp	3 tbsp	4 tbsp	5 tbsp	
Raw*	—	2-3 pieces	2-3 pieces	few pieces	few pieces	
BREADS AND GRAINS						
Whole grain/enriched bread	¼ slice	¼ slice	½ slice	½ slice	½ slice	4-5
Cooked cereal	1 tbsp	2 tbsp	3 tbsp	⅓ c	⅓ c	
Dry cereal	2 tbsp	¼ c	⅓ c	½ c	½ c	
Rice/pasta	2 tbsp	2 tbsp	3 tbsp	⅓ c	⅓ c	

Adapted from McWilliams M: Nutrition for the growing years, New York, 1986, Wiley. Reprinted by permission of Prentice Hall, Upper Saddle River, NJ.
*Should be given to young children only when they can chew well.

than decrease such behaviors. Table 9-11 addresses solutions to some common feeding concerns in young children.

It is important for children to have control over their own food intake. Children should be encouraged to eat in response to hunger and satiety and not continue eating when they are full. Children who are allowed control over their food intake are significantly more aware of the role of foods in energy balance. They are more likely to make healthful food choices (Nestle et al., 1998). Pressure or rewards should not be used to get children to eat. Although the child may be forced to eat a given food, the long-term effects of such behavior may have a negative impact on food habits (Hood et al., 2000).

Feeding the School-Age Child

The period from 7 years to 12 years of age is one of slow, but steady, growth. As appetite increases, so does food intake. Most food-related behavior problems of the preschool years have been resolved. Older children develop more autonomy with eating and take the initiative in making changes, usually accepting a wider variety of foods. They make their own eating decisions, but parents still exert an influence in

Table 9-11 COMMON FEEDING CONCERNS IN YOUNG CHILDREN

Common Concern	Possible Solutions
Refuses meats	Offer small, bite-size pieces of moist, tender meat or poultry Incorporate into meatloaf, spaghetti sauce, stews, casseroles, burritos, pizza Include legumes, eggs, cheese Offer boneless fish (including canned tuna and salmon)
Drinks too little milk	Offer cheeses and yogurt, including cheese in cooking (e.g., macaroni and cheese, cheese sauce, pizza) Use milk to cook hot cereals; offer cream soups, milk-based puddings and custards Allow child to pour milk from a pitcher and use a straw Include powdered milk in cooking and baking (e.g., biscuits, muffins, pancakes, meatloaf, casseroles)
Drinks too much milk	Offer water if thirsty between meals Limit milk to one serving with meals or offer at end of meal; offer water for seconds If bottle is still used, wean to cup
Refuses vegetables and fruits	If child refuses vegetables, offer more fruits, and vice versa Prepare vegetables that are tender but not overcooked Steam vegetable strips (or offer raw if appropriate) and allow child to eat with fingers Offer sauces and dips (e.g., cheese sauce for cooked vegetables, dip for raw vegetables, yogurt to dip fruit) Include vegetables in soups and casseroles Add fresh or dried fruit to cereals Prepare fruit in a variety of ways (e.g., fresh, cooked, juice, in gelatin, as a salad) Continue to offer a variety of fruits and vegetables
Eats too many sweets	Limit purchase and preparation of sweet foods in the home Avoid using as a bribe or reward Incorporate into meals instead of snacks for better dental health Reduce sugar by one-half in recipes for cookies, muffins, quick breads, etc. Work with staff of daycare, preschools to reduce use of sweets

From Lucas B: Normal nutrition from infancy through adolescence. In Queen PM and Lang CE (editors): Handbook of pediatric nutrition, Gaithersburg, MD, 1993, Aspen.

terms of family food habits, availability of food, and food and health attitudes and expectations.

School-age children do not eat as often as preschoolers and are less dependent on between-meal snacks. The acceptance of a school lunch or a lunch packed at home is decided less by the foods themselves than by the preferences of peers. After-school snacks are almost universal. In the elementary school years, children increasingly assume responsibility for their own meals and snacks. Because of working parents and demanding schedules, many children are responsible for preparing their own breakfasts, packing their own lunches, getting themselves off to school, and finding snacks. Participation in organized sports and other after-school activities may reduce the frequency of family meals. In addition children in the early school years may share some of the responsibility for grocery shopping and even dinner preparation. As a result children are the targets of sophisticated advertising for a variety of food products.

Development of Food Acceptance Patterns

As children grow and develop, they must learn what to eat, when to eat, and how to eat it (Birch, 1998). The comparison of an active fourth grader eating lunch with friends (Figure 9-9) and a totally dependent infant taking a bottle of formula illustrates the amazing development of food acceptance patterns and food handling skills. It is important to note that food acceptance patterns are unique to each child and involve many factors, both learned and unlearned.

Neophobia is a normal, adaptive response and is thought by some experts even to be somewhat protective in delaying intake of some foods until tolerance or developmental readiness are appropriate. However, in extreme, neophobia can severely limit food acceptance and intake. Experience or familiarity with foods can overcome neophobia (Falciglia et al., 2000). A caregiver helping a small child transition to solid foods should continue to offer a new food a few times a week to increase the child's familiarity with the new food (Piner and Stallberg-White, 2000).

Family interactions and the eating environment have a great impact on a child's willingness to try new foods at any age and can affect a child's future eating habits. In a study involving 46 parent-child pairs through the Head Start program, parents' negative mealtime practices, such as hurrying children as they eat and requiring children to clean their plates, were associated with higher child weight-for-height, a possible indicator that a child may be overweight or obese in the future (Gable and Lutz, 2001). Similarly parents' healthful nutrition attitudes were associated with more pleasant mealtime experiences and fewer reported eating problems.

In older children the food choices and food behavior modeling of parents or adults can greatly influence food choices. A parent who refuses to eat green beans, but insists that a child eat them will generally have poor success. Coercive-feeding techniques rarely succeed and can interfere with a child's long-term ability to self-regulate energy intake (Birch, 1998).

Children should be involved in the selection or, as appropriate, preparation of a new food. A parent who sits with a child and joins the child in sampling the new food will make the introduction of new foods a much more pleasant and successful experience. Researchers, in studying child-feeding practices, have identified at least three child-feeding patterns: highly controlling parents may force-feed their child, or insist on the "clean plate club"; laissez-faire parents allow children to choose when and what to eat; and responsive parents set limits, but modulate the degree of parental control (Tibbs et al., 2001). Most

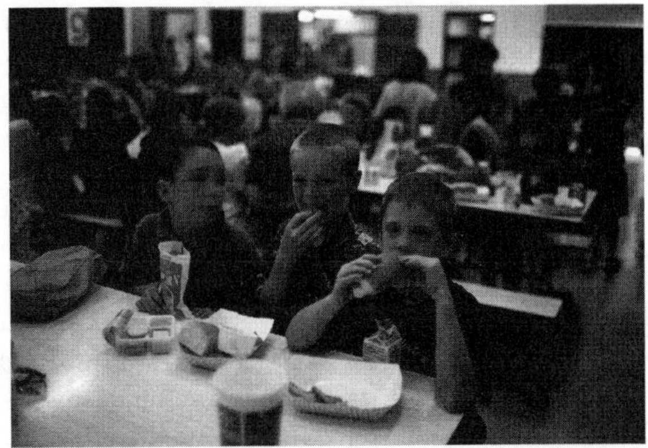

Figure 9-9 Boys eating in school cafeteria. *(From Getty Images.)*

nutrition experts believe that responsive parenting is important and that parents should model healthy dietary behaviors. Children should be given guidance as to appropriate food choices, but it is important that they have autonomy and independence in making food choices. However, parents may need to limit child-led snacking to encourage better intake at meals as noted by recent research in a study of 238 Mexican-American families that sought to prevent obesity (Kaiser, 2001). These researchers believed that it is important for a child to come to structured meals prepared to eat. Thus to be successful, child-led snacking needs to be limited.

Vegetarian Diets for Children

As the number of adults adopting vegetarian lifestyles increases, more children are also expected to become vegetarians (American Academy of Pediatrics Committee on Nutrition, 1998). Diets that sustain health in adult vegetarians are not necessarily appropriate for periods of rapid growth, however. The form of vegetarianism that is practiced determines the nutritional adequacy of the child's diet. The vegan diet, which excludes all animal products, may pose a risk for low intakes of protein, calcium, iron, zinc, riboflavin, and vitamins B_6 and B_{12}.

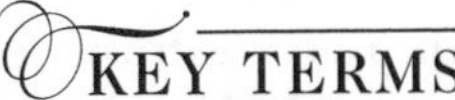

KEY TERMS

neophobia: the reluctance to accept new foods

One study that compared omnivore children with children who follow vegan-like diets reported decreased gains in structure and weight, but the differences were small (Dwyer, 2000). In that study limited food choices and the restriction of the number of meals and snacks may have reduced total food intake, especially for young children. Because of the high fiber content and low caloric density of a vegetarian diet and the smaller stomach capacity of children, a child may be unable to consume a sufficient volume of food to meet his or her needs (Sanders and Reddy, 1994). Caloric density can be improved by emphasizing cereals, nut butters, and legumes. Diets that include dairy products are generally more nutritionally adequate than strict vegan diets. Dairy products provide nutrients commonly lacking in the vegan diet and are more nutritionally dense.

With planning, vegetarian diets that include a variety of foods can provide all the nutritional requirements for growth (see the Application following Chapter 11). Use of calcium-enriched soy products that are fortified with vitamins B_{12} and D or similar products may be important in meeting nutritional needs.

UNDERNUTRITION

- *What factors contribute to the development of protein energy undernutrition?*
- *Describe the effects of undernutrition on growth and development.*
- *What is catch-up growth?*
- *How does short-term fasting influence cognition?*
- *Why is breakfast important for school performance? What nutrients are breakfast foods likely to contribute to the diet?*

Severe Undernutrition

With favorable conditions, a child will follow a genetically predetermined growth curve. However, growth retardation is the inevitable consequence of inadequate food intake. In developing countries growth retardation is primarily the result of a synergistic relationship between inadequate food intake and infection. In developed countries it is more frequently the result of inadequate absorption, chronic disease, psychologic stress, or nonorganic failure to thrive (see Chapter 7). The type, timing, and duration of the nutritional deficit determine the overall impact on an individual child's growth.

Successful nutrition rehabilitation depends on correcting the underlying condition and improving nutrient and energy intake. Initial dietary management begins with small, frequent feedings, with progressive increases in volume and concentration of nutrients. The term *catch-up growth* is used to describe the acceleration in growth that occurs when a period of growth retardation ends and favorable conditions are restored. Weight gain may occur at a rate several times faster than that of normal healthy children of the same age. The energy cost of weight gain can range from 10 kcal per gram of muscle gained to 2 kcal per gram of fat gained (Solomon, 1985).

Undernutrition and Cognition

Severe undernutrition rarely occurs in North America, but the impact of moderate undernutrition or inadequate food intake is a concern. Recent investigations have explored the subtle behavioral and cognitive consequences of inadequate intake and short-term fasting. Such studies are limited by the difficulty in measuring cognition and distinguishing the effects of nutrition from those of genetics and environmental factors.

Measuring Cognition

Most development in the human brain occurs prenatally and during the first 2 years of life. Cognition in infants has been measured using developmental scales, most commonly the Bayley Scales of Mental and Motor Development (BSMMD). These scales assume that the observed behavior is a reflection of intelligence or mental competence. For preschool and school-age children, IQ tests, learning tasks such as discrimination and oddity learning, and school achievement are used most often to estimate cognitive development.

Short-Term Fasting and Cognition

For decades it has been accepted that good nutrition has a positive effect on a child's ability to learn and that skipping a meal, especially breakfast, can have a negative impact on learning.

More recently carefully controlled experimental studies measured problem-solving performance of well-nourished 9- to 11-year-old children after they ate breakfast and after they skipped breakfast. When the children ate breakfast, they made fewer errors on tasks of picture identification, response to stimulus on a computer display, and arithmetic tests (Pollitt, 1995).

The acute effects of skipping breakfast involve the short-term physiologic changes associated with a diminished supply of nutrients to the brain. Under normal short-term fasting conditions, homeostatic mechanisms attempt to maintain blood glucose within physiologic ranges to maintain blood glucose levels. It may be that a decline (even within normal physiologic range) results in metabolic changes that influence cognition. A moderate elevation of blood glucose regulates a variety of brain functions, including memory and learning. Brain scans have shown that cognitive functions increase the rate at which glucose is metabolized and there is some evidence that moderate increases in blood glucose improve cognitive functioning in children (Hall et al., 1989). A proposed mechanism by which raised blood glucose levels may influence cognition is through the synthesis of acetylcholine, a neurotransmitter that has a well-established role in memory functions.

Researchers in Philadelphia and Baltimore public schools who offered a free breakfast program to all school children regardless of need found that program participation increased from approximately 15% to about 27% (Murphy et al., 1998). The children who increased their participation in the breakfast program had significantly improved their math and psychosocial scores and reduced their tardiness, absenteeism, and hyperactivity.

Such evidence led the 1995 International Symposium on Breakfast and Performance and Health to conclude that children who skip breakfast are less efficient in problem solving, have reduced recall of newly acquired information, and have decreased verbal fluency and creativity (Pollitt, 1995). The conferees encouraged the development of policies to promote recognition of the importance of breakfast and intervention programs to ensure that breakfast is available to children.

School feeding programs, funded by the USDA, were developed to combat hunger in school-age children. Research suggests that as many as 8% of children in the United States experience hunger and food insufficiency and that an additional 20% are at risk (Murphy et al., 1998). Although many children participate in the school lunch program, the USDA-supported school breakfast programs have been limited to schools with a high percentage of children receiving free and reduced-price lunches.

In Spain, Rosa and colleagues (1998) found that including breakfast enhanced the overall quality of the diet, particularly when breakfast provided at least 20% of the total daily energy intake and at least 200 ml of milk products were consumed.

When breakfast is skipped, the nutrients usually consumed at the breakfast meal are not recovered from intake during the remainder of the day (Nicklas et al., 1993). In an analysis of 10-year-old children participating in the Bogalusa Heart Study, a significant difference was found in the average daily vitamin and mineral intake pattern based on ready-to-eat (RTE) cereal consumption patterns. Children who ate cereal were found to have significantly higher mean daily intakes of vitamin A, Vitamin B_6, thiamin, niacin, riboflavin, vitamin B_{12}, vitamin D, folate, and iron (Nicklas et al., 1995).

Nonetheless examination of data from national surveys across all age groups indicates a decline in breakfast consumption. It is estimated that on any given day many school-age children skip breakfast (Pollitt, 1995). The USDA Center for Nutrition Policy and Promotion reported in 2000 that although 19% of children in low-income households do eat breakfast at school, many children simply do not eat breakfast (Food Institute Report, 2000). They estimated that 17% of children from low-income households and 16% of children from higher-income households do not eat breakfast at all.

CHILDHOOD OBESITY AND CARDIOVASCULAR DISEASE

- *What are the* Healthy People 2010 *recommendations related to nutrition for children?*
- *Why are there concerns about rapid weight gain in children?*

Obesity

In North America the incidence of obesity in children is at epidemic levels. The children of today have been nicknamed the "supersize" generation. This nickname reflects not only their choice of portion sizes at fast food restaurants, but also the size of their bodies. There has been an alarming increase in the rate of overweight (BMI >eighty-fifth percentile on growth charts) and obesity (BMI >ninety-fifth percentile) since the 1970s when national surveys such as NHANES began to assess the weight and height of children. Over this period, the prevalence of overweight doubled and obesity has increased by 50% in children 6 to 11 years and 12 to 17 years of age (Styne, 2001). Based on data from NHANES III, 13% of children and 14% of adolescents are overweight (NCHS, 2000). Overweight and obesity occur at disproportionately higher rates among African American, Native American, and Hispanic children (Crawford et al., 2001).

The etiology of obesity is a complex problem. Parental obesity is associated with obesity in children and adolescents (Tanasescu et al., 2000). An individual's weight reflects the long-term balance between energy intake and energy output. Energy intake is the food a person eats that is influenced by many factors. Atkin and Davies (2001) found no relationship between total energy, fat, or carbohydrate or protein intake and percentage of body fat in preschool children, suggesting that the established relationship between fat intake and body fat may develop over time. The food choices an individual makes can impact their overall energy intake.

Energy output includes the basal metabolic rate, the thermic effect of food, and the energy for growth and energy for activity. Obviously the most adaptable of these is the energy expended for physical activity. There has been much debate regarding the potential contribution of television and video games to the development of childhood obesity. It may be that excessive time spent with television and video games may contribute to the development of childhood obesity from decreased physical activity levels. Birch et al. (1984) observed that leaner children watch less television and are more physically active. Excessive television viewing promotes increased snacking, which is a lifestyle associated with obesity (DuRant et al., 1994).

It is difficult to know if the development of obesity in families is the result of nature vs. nurture. The recent focus for children is how to prevent obesity from developing because obese children tend to become obese adults. The age of onset of obesity is also important as an obese older child, age 15 to 17, is much more likely to be an obese adult than an obese child under the age of three (Whitaker et al., 1997). The probability that a child, especially a child younger than age 10 years, will become an obese adult also doubles if one or both parents is obese (Whitaker et al., 2000).

The influential role of parents and caregivers on the development of lifelong eating and activity patterns must not be underestimated. It is important that focus is placed on the development of healthful eating habits and the prevention of obesity. Parents must respect a child's appetite and not encourage overeating or the "clean plate club." This cueing in to the internal cues of fullness and satiety must be encouraged from infancy. Parents should not feel that a child must eat a designated amount of food or follow strict eating patterns. The best rule is to let hunger be the guide. It is counter productive to use food for nonnutritive purposes to comfort or reward children.

Obese children are at greater risk of developing cardiovascular disease and other chronic diseases. Childhood obesity is known to be associated with elevated levels of blood cholesterol. Obesity evaluation and treatment should begin as early as possible, but only when the family is ready for change. Clinicians should educate families about medical complication of obesity and involve the family and all caregivers in the treatment program (see Chapter 14). Treatment programs should institute permanent changes and not offer short-term diets or exercise programs aimed at rapid weight loss (Moran, 1999). The family should learn to monitor eating and activity and make small, gradual changes. Suggestions for parents to prevent excess weight or assist children in reducing the rate of weight gain are found in Box 9-1. A variety of experienced health care professionals can be involved with a weight management program and it is important that they encourage and empathize with, and not criticize, the overweight child and his or her family.

Cardiovascular Disease

Cardiovascular disease is the number one cause of death in the United States. Atherosclerosis is a life-long process that begins with fatty streak formation in childhood and adolescence and progresses to fibrous plaques leading to coronary heart disease (CHD) in adulthood. Many of the risk factors associated with CHD, such as diets high in total fat and saturated fat, obesity, hypertension, and lack of exercise, may originate in childhood. Evidence from long-term clinical trials of adults implicates elevated blood cholesterol levels in childhood in the eventual development of coronary artery disease (Freedman et al., 2001). It has been suggested that the cardiovascular disease process can be slowed or prevented by modifying risk-related behaviors early in life.

High blood cholesterol levels clearly play a role in the development of premature CHD in adults. Long-term clinical trials in adult populations have shown that lowering cholesterol levels reduces coronary risk and mortality from all causes. Because no longer-term studies of the relationship of blood cholesterol level measured in childhood to CHD in later life have been conducted, the relationship of childhood cholesterol levels to the atherosclerotic process has been inferred from less direct evidence (American Academy of Pediatrics Committee on Nutrition, 1998). This evidence includes observations that, compared with other countries, children and adolescents in the United States have high blood cholesterol levels and higher intakes of saturated fatty acids and cholesterol. Adults in the United States have higher rates of CHD morbidity and mortality. In autopsy studies signs of early atherosclerosis have been reported in children and adolescents and are related to high serum levels of total cholesterol (TC), low density lipoprotein-cholesterol (LDL-C), and low levels of high density lipoprotein cholesterol (HDL-C).

Children and adolescents with elevated serum cholesterol levels, particularly LDL-C levels, often come from families with a high incidence of CHD in adult relatives. These youngsters are more likely than are the general population to have high levels as adults.

Decreasing cardiovascular risk in children and adolescents involves management of body weight, increasing physical fitness, and measures to lower blood cholesterol levels. The American Academy of Pediatrics Committee on Nutrition (1998) recommends two complementary approaches for reducing blood cholesterol. A primary approach is to lower the average blood cholesterol levels in

Box 9-1 Habits to Decrease the Risk of Excess Weight Gain: Tips for Parents

Respect your child's appetite; children do not need to finish every bottle or meal.
Treat all foods equally; there are not good or bad foods.
Do not provide food for comfort or as a reward.
Limit where foods are eaten in your home, such as the kitchen or dining area.
Do not offer sweets in exchange for a finished meal.
Limit the amount of high-calorie, high-sugar, high-fat foods kept in the home.
Provide nutrient-dense snack foods of low caloric content.
Provide a variety of whole grains, fruits, and vegetables.
Provide ample fiber in the child's diet.
Skim milk may safely replace whole milk at 2 years of age.
Limit the amount of television your child watches.
Do not encourage eating while watching television.
Encourage play activities that increase physical activity.
Establish regular activities with your child such as walks, ball games, and other activities.

children and adolescents through population-wide changes in nutrient intake and eating patterns. These recommendations are reflected in the Dietary Guidelines for Americans (USDA and Health and Human Services, 2000) and *Healthy People 2010* objectives to increase to 75% of persons aged 2 years and older who consume no more than 30% of calories from total fat and less than 10% of calories from saturated fat. Data from NHANES III indicate that children and adolescents consume 34% of calories from total fat and 12% from saturated fat. After 2 years of age children should gradually adopt a diet that contains less than 30%, but at least 20%, of calories from fat over several days. Fat calories should be replaced with a wide variety of foods including more grain products, fruits, vegetables, low-fat milk products and lean meat, poultry, fish, or other protein-rich products. Such dietary changes can foster a healthier body weight and reduce obesity.

A second approach is screening to identify children and adolescents who are at increased risk of CHD as adults. These include persons with a family history of premature cardiovascular disease or have at least one parent with a high blood cholesterol level. The screening would include measurement of TC, LDL-C, and HDL-C. The dietary intervention above would be initiated. Success would be monitored in the physician's office or clinic setting and adjustments made as appropriate.

PROMOTING OPTIMAL NUTRITION FOR CHILDREN

- *What are appropriate dietary recommendations for children to promote long-term health?*

Childhood is a time of rapid physical growth and development, learning, and psychosocial development. These features are critical in defining guidelines for dietary intake (Williams, 1998). Childhood is also a time when individuals begin to establish eating habits and activity patterns that may discourage the development of chronic disease later in life. Evidence is accumulating that children are not little adults and that they have unique nutritional needs. The 2000 Dietary Guidelines target the general health population aged 2 years and older with a recommendation that after the age of 2. This guideline encourages children to make a gradual transition to a lower-fat diet with less than 30% of kilocalories from fat.

It is important to emphasize that the primary role of diet in childhood is to provide sufficient kilocalories and nutrients to support normal growth and development. Caution when restricting the fat intake of children must be exercised. Although dietary fat can be restricted safely to approximately 30% of kilocalories, care in planning is necessary to ensure an adequate energy and nutrient intake. This means including all food groups and making low-fat choices in each group, such as low-fat milk and fish, lean meats and poultry, and a wide variety of foods in moderation.

A sedentary lifestyle is also linked to the development of CHD and other chronic diseases. Regular physical activity results in substantial health benefits. In addition the actual energy expended allows larger amounts of food to be consumed with a decreased risk of obesity.

Concepts to Remember

- Childhood overall is a period of slow, steady growth, the rate of which is determined by genetic and environmental factors.
- In the short term, spurts and latent periods characterize childhood growth.
- Body size, body composition, and rate of growth and level of activity determine children's energy, and nutrient needs.
- Physical activity enables children to expend more calories and have more flexibility in energy and food intake.
- Dietary intake of children will vary greatly because of the day-to-day variation in the rate of growth, activity, energy, and nutrient needs.
- Undernutrition during childhood can slow the rate of growth and impair physical and cognitive development.
- Parents are responsible for offering developmentally and nutritionally appropriate foods. They should provide an environment that is conducive to the development of positive attitudes toward and acceptance of food that will influence long-term food habits.

- As children grow older, peers and other factors outside the home increasingly influence food preferences.
- Nutrition concerns of childhood center on ensuring a nutritionally adequate diet to support growth and to minimize the risk of chronic disease.
- Special nutrition and diet-related concerns include dental health, exposure to lead, and risk of childhood obesity and other chronic diseases.

REFERENCES

American Academy of Pediatrics Committee on Nutrition: Calcium requirements of infants, children and adolescents, Pediatrics 104:1152, 1999.

American Academy of Pediatrics Committee on Nutrition: Pediatric nutrition handbook, Elk Grove, IL, 1998 The Author.

American Academy of Pediatrics: Committee on nutrition cholesterol in childhood, Pediatrics 101:141, 1998.

American Academy of Pediatrics: Diarrhea and dehydration guidelines for parents, 2001a, http://www.aap.org.

American Academy of Pediatrics: The use and misuse of fruit juice in the diets of young children, Pediatrics 107:1210, 2001b.

American Dietetic Association: Position of the American Dietetic Association: oral health and nutrition, J Am Diet Assoc 96:184, 1996.

Atkin L and Davies P: Diet composition and body composition in preschool children, Am J Clin Nutr 72:15, 2001.

Birch LL: Development of food acceptance patterns in the first years of life, Proc Nutr Soc 57:617, 1998.

Birch LL et al.: Eating as a "means" activity in contingency: effect on young children's food preference, Child Dev 55:431, 1984.

Birch LL et al.: The variability of young children's energy intake, N Engl J Med 324:232, 1991.

Borah-Giddens J and Falciglia GA: A meta-analysis of the relation in food preference between parents and children, J Nutr Educ 25:102, 1993.

Borzekowski DL and Robinson TN: The 30-second effect: an experiment revealing the impact of television commercials on food preferences of preschoolers, J Am Diet Assoc 101:42, 2001.

Centers for Disease Control and Prevention: Screening young children for lead poisoning: guidance for state and local public health officials, Atlanta, GA, 1997, Centers for Disease Control and Prevention.

Centers for Disease Control: Severe malnutrition among young children: Georgia, January 1997-June 1999, MMWR Morb Mortal Wkly Rep 50:224, 2001.

Coon KA et al.: Relationship between use of television during meals and children's food consumption patterns, Pediatrics 107:E7, 2001.

Crawford PB et al.: Ethnic issues in epidemiology of childhood obesity, Pediatrir Clin North Am 48:855, 2001.

Debord K: Developmentally appropriate food and nutrition skills for young children, Virginia Cooperative Extension Pub No 348-651, 1996.

Domel SB et al.: Accuracy of fourth-and fifth-grade students' food records compared with school-lunch observations, Am J Clin Nutr 59:S218, 1994.

Drake MA: Anthropometry, biochemical iron indexes, and energy and nutrition intake of preschool children: comparison of intake at daycare centers and at home, J Am Diet Assoc 91:1587, 1991.

Duggan C et al.: Oral rehydration solution for acute diarrhea prevents subsequent unscheduled follow-up visits, Pediatrics 104:e29, 1999.

DuRant RH et al.: The relationship among television watching, physical activity and body composition of young children, Pediatrics 4:449, 1994.

Dwyer J: Should dietary fat recommendations for children be changed? J Am Diet Assoc 100:36, 2000.

Ellis MR: Lightening the lead load in children, Am Fam Physician 62:545, 2000.

Falciglia GA et al.: Food neophobia in childhood affects dietary variety, J Am Diet Assoc 100:1474, 2000.

Food Institute Report: Food marketing institute information, Washington, DC, 2000, Food Marketing Institute Information Service.

Food Marketing Institute and Better Homes and Gardens Magazine: Meal watch, summer 1995.

Food and Nutrition Board: Recommended dietary allowances, Washington, DC, 1989, National Academy of Sciences.

Freedman DS et al.: Relationship of childhood obesity to coronary heart disease risk factors in adulthood: the Bogalusa heart study, Pediatrics 108:712, 2001.

Gable S and Lutz S: Nutrition socialization experiences of children in the Head Start program, J Am Diet Assoc 101:572, 2001.

Hall JL et al.: Glucose enhancement of performance on memory tests in young and aged humans, Neuropsychologia 27:1129, 1989.

Hood MY et al.: Parental eating attitudes and the development of obesity in children. The Framingham children's study, Int J Obes Relat Metab Disord: 24:1319, 2000.

Houston DK and Johnson MA: Does vitamin C protect against lead toxicity? Nutr Rev 58:73, 2000.

Hurtado EK et al.: Early childhood anemia and mild or moderate retardation, Am J Clin Nutr 69:115, 1999.

Johnson RK et al.: Maternal employment and the quality of young children's diets: empirical evidence based on the 1987-1988 nationwide food consumption survey, Pediatrics 90:245, 1992.

Kaiser LL: Acculturation of Mexican-American mothers influences child feeding strategies, J Am Diet Assoc 101:542, 2001.

Kennedy E and Goldberg J: What are American children eating? Implications for public policy, Nutr Rev 53:111, 1995.

Krebs NF and Johnson SL: Guidelines for healthy children: promoting eating, moving, and common sense, J Am Diet Assoc 100:37, 2000.

Kuczmarski RJ et al.: CDC growth charts: United States. Advanced data from vital and health statistics, No 314, Hyattsville MD, 2000, NCHS.

Lauer RM et al.: Efficacy and safety of lowering dietary intake of total fat, saturated fat, and cholesterol in children with elevated LDL cholesterol: the Dietary Intervention Study in Children, Am J Clin Nutr 72 (5 Suppl):1332S-1342S, 2000.

Lino M: Income and spending of poor households with children, Fam Econ Nutr Rev 9:2, 1996.

Lofgren JP et al.: Blood lead levels in young children, United States and selected states, 1996-1999, MMWR Morb Mortal Wkly Rep 49:1133, 2000.

Looker AC et al.: Prevalence of iron deficiency in the United States, JAMA 277:973, 1997.

Lytle LA et al.: Validation of 24-hour recalls assisted by food records in third-grade children, J Am Diet Assoc 93:1431, 1993.

Lytle LA: In defense of a low-fat diet for healthy children, J Am Diet Assoc 100:39, 2000.

Matkovic V, Fontana D, and Tominac C: Factors that influence peak bone mass formation: a study of calcium balance and the inheritance of bone mass in adolescent females, Am J Clin Nutr 52:878, 1990.

Moran R: The evaluation and treatment of childhood obesity, Am Fam Physician 59:859, 1999.

Murphy AS et al.: Kindergarten students' food preferences are not consistent with their knowledge of the Dietary Guidelines, J Am Diet Assoc 95:219, 1995.

Murphy JM et al.: The relationship of school breakfast to psychosocial and academic functioning, Arch Pediatr Adolesc Med 152:899, 1998.

Mushak P and Crocetti F: Lead and nutrition: biologic interactions of lead with nutrients, Nutr Today 31:12, 1996.

National Center for Health Statistics: National Health and Nutrition Examination Survey CDC growth charts: United States, 2000, NCHS.

Nestle M et al.: Behavioral social influences on food choice, Nutr Rev 56:550, 1998.

Nicklas TA et al.: Breakfast consumption affects adequacy of total daily intake in children, J Am Diet Assoc 9:886, 1993.

Nicklas TA et al.: Total nutrient intake and ready-to-eat cereal consumption of children and young adults in the Bogalusa heart study, Nutr Rev 53:S39, 1995.

Olson RE: Is it wise to restrict fat in the diets of children? J Am Diet Assoc 100:28, 2000.

Picciano MF et al.: How to grow a healthy child: a conference report, Nutr Today 1:43, 1999.

Piner P and Stallberg-White C: "Pass the ketchup please": familiar flavors increase children's willingness to taste novel foods, Appetite 34:95, 2000.

Pollitt E: Does breakfast make a difference in school? J Am Diet Assoc 95:1134, 1995.

Pollitt E: Iron deficiency and educational deficiency, Nutr Rev 55:133, 1997.

Roberts SP and Hegman MB: Micronutrient shortfalls in young children's diets: common, and owing to inadequate intakes both at home and at child care centers, Nutr Rev 58:27, 2000.

Rosa M et al.: The importance of breakfast in meeting daily recommended calcium intake in a group of schoolchildren, J Am Coll Nutr 17:19, 1998.

Saldanha LG: Fiber in the diet of U.S. children: results of national survey, Pediatrics 96:S995, 1995.

Sanders TA and Reddy S: Vegetarian diets and children, Am J Clin Nutr 59:1176S, 1994.

Shea S et al.: Variability and self-regulation of energy intake in young children in their everyday environment, Pediatrics 90:542, 1992.

Singleton JC et al.: Role of food and nutrition in the health perceptions of young children, J Am Diet Assoc 92:67, 1992.

Solomon NW: Rehabilitating the severely malnourished child, J Am Diet Assoc 85:28, 1985.

Styne DM: Childhood and adolescent obesity: prevalence and significance, Pediatr Clin North Am 48:823, 2001.

Sylvester GP et al.: Children's television and nutrition: friend or foes? Nutr Today 30:6, 1995.

Tanasescu M et al.: Biobehavioral factors are associated with obesity in Puerto Rican children, J Nutr 130:1734, 2000.

Taylor ML and Koblinsky SA: Dietary intake and growth status of young homeless children, J Am Diet Assoc 93:464, 1993.

The Writing Group for the DISC Collaborative Research Group: Efficacy and safety of lowering dietary intake of fat and cholesterol in children with elevated LDL lipoprotein and cholesterol, JAMA 273:1429, 1995.

Tibbs F et al.: The relationship between parental modeling, eating patterns, and dietary intake among African-American parents, J Am Diet Assoc 101:535, 2001.

U.S. Department of Health and Human Services, Office of Disease Prevention and Health Promotion: Healthy People 2010, www.healthypeople.gov, 2001.

USDA and Health and Human Services: USDA Dietary Guidelines for Americans, ed 5, Washington, DC, 2000, Home and Garden Bulletin No 232.

USDA Human Nutrition Information Services: Nationwide food consumption survey. Continuing survey of food intakes by individuals: women 19-50 years and their children 1-5 years, 4 days, Washington, DC, 1986, CSFII Report 86-3.

USDA Human Nutrition Information Services: Food and nutrient intakes by individuals in the United States, 1 day, 1989. Nationwide Food Consumption Survey 1987-88, Washington, DC, 1993, MFCS Report 87-1-1.

U.S. Department of Agriculture: USDA unveils food guide pyramid for young children, www.usda.gov, 1999.

Wallman KK: America's children: key national indicators of well-being, 2000, Federal Interagency Forum on Child and Family Statistics, http://childstats.gov, 2000.

Washington RL: Cardiovascular medicine update: intervention to reduce cardiovascular risk factors in children and adolescents, Am Fam Physician 59:2211, 1999.

Wauben IPM and Wainwright PE: The influence of neonatal nutrition on behavioral development: a critical appraisal, Nutr Rev 57:35, 1999.

Welten DC et al.: Weight-bearing activity during youth is a more important factor for peak bone mass than calcium intake, J Bone Miner Res 9:1089, 1994.

Whitaker RC et al.: Predicting obesity in young adulthood from childhood and parental obesity, N Engl J Med 337:869, 1997.

Whitaker RC et al.: The relationship of childhood adiposity to parent body mass index and eating behavior, Obes Res 8:234, 2000.

Williams CL: Dietary fat and children's health. Nutrition and the life cycle, Nutr Today 33:144, 1998.

Williams CL et al.: A new recommendation for dietary fiber in childhood, Pediatrics 96:S985, 1995.

Wosje KS and Specker BL: Role of calcium in bone health during childhood, Nutr Rev 58:253, 2000.

Yip R et al.: Iron status of children with elevated blood-lead concentration, J Pediatr 98:922, 1981.

Yip R et al.: Trends and patterns in height and weight status of low income children, Crit Rev Food Sci Nutr 33:409, 1993.

APPLICATION

Food Allergies and Intolerances

Marion asks Tom to double check his backpack for his second grade field trip to the zoo. He checks that he has his lunch and his two ***Epi-Pens.*** *Tom is highly allergic to peanuts and tree nuts. As a toddler he had his first allergic reaction at a playgroup when he ate a bite of a peanut butter cookie. He began to salivate excessively and developed stomach cramps. He had hives all over his stomach and chest and began to wheeze and developed swelling of the tongue. Luckily Marion is a nurse and immediately rushed him to the local pediatrician. The doctor gave Tom a shot of* ***epinephrine*** *and admitted him to the hospital for observation.*

Although Tom is excited about the field trip, Marion always worries about him in a new or different situation. His school has a registered nurse in the building at all times and annual in-service education programs for all the teachers and staff on recognizing and treating allergic reactions. One of Marion's friends from the Food Allergy and ***Anaphylaxis*** *Network, a support group for families living with food allergies, has worked to have a peanut-free zone in her child's cafeteria. Although Marion worries about Tom in the lunchroom, she knows that Tom is very cautious about what he eats. The no-trading-food rule is strictly enforced. She doesn't want Tom to be unable to sit with his friends at lunch.*

Now that Tom is old enough it is much easier to ask about the ingredients in foods and use the Epi-Pen if necessary. Marion always makes sure he packs his lunch with "safe" foods and their house is peanut free and tree nut free. His brother, Alex, misses peanut butter sandwiches, but he can buy them at school or have them at a friend's house. Marion always buys a candy bar with nuts at work so she can enjoy it without the risk that it will contaminate any foods that Tom will eat.

Food allergies and intolerances are adverse reactions to food. There are various types of adverse reactions to foods, including the following:

- Food allergy from IgE mediated mechanism
- Food allergy not involving IgE, in which other immunologic mechanisms are implicated
- Nonallergic food intolerance (e.g., pharmacologic, metabolic, or toxic reactions to foods)
- Food aversions (symptoms are often nonspecific and unconfirmed by blinded food challenge)

Epi-Pen: the EpiPen Auto-Injector is a disposable drug delivery system with a spring-activated, concealed needle; it is designed for emergency self-administration to provide rapid, convenient first-aid for individuals sensitive to potentially fatal allergic reactions

epinephrine: a hormone that is a potent stimulator of the sympathetic nervous system; a powerful vasopressor; it increases blood pressure, stimulates the heart muscle, accelerates the heart rate, and increases cardiac output

anaphylaxis: an unusual or exaggerated allergic reaction, usually involving more than one organ system (skin or gastrointestinal, respiratory or circulatory system); can result in death if untreated

FOOD ALLERGY

A true food allergy is a response of the immune system in which an antibody, IgE, is produced. Antigens are any substances that are capable, under appropriate conditions, of producing an immune response. There are many potential food antigens, but most are prevented from entering the body by mechanisms in the gastrointestinal tract. If an antigenic molecule is ingested or absorbed, the antigen may reach immune competent cells that produce the antibody IgE, resulting in sensitization. Once a person becomes sensitized, a repeat exposure to that antigen can cause an allergic reaction.

True food allergies are estimated to affect between 1.4% (Bindslev-Jensen, 1998) to 2% (Sampson and Burks, 1996) of adults and 5% (Bindslev-Jensen, 1998) to 8% (Sampson and Burks, 1996) of children. The major culprits for food allergies are milk, eggs, soy, peanuts, tree nuts (e.g., cashews, walnuts), wheat, fish, and shellfish. It is estimated that these eight foods are responsible for 90% of the food allergic reactions (Koerner and Munoz-Furlon, 1998).

Many food allergies in children disappear as the child grows. Peanut allergy is almost never outgrown and must be considered a lifelong risk (Anderson, 1997). Some food allergies can be acquired later in life, especially the allergy to fish or shellfish.

The severity of allergic reactions can range from minor symptoms such as a runny nose to anaphylaxis. The most common symptoms include swelling of the lips, face, and tongue; itchy or watering eyes; rash or hives; throat tightness; a rasping cough; wheezing or asthma symptoms; abdominal pain; nausea; vomiting; and diarrhea (Figure 9-10). Peanuts, tree nuts, and shellfish can cause the most severe reactions of anaphylaxis and even death. It is thought that individuals with a combination of asthma and food allergies are the most likely to experience the severest reactions (Dietitians Face the Challenge of Food Allergies, 2000). An estimated 150 to 200 people die each year from food allergy-related reactions (Food Allergy and Anaphylaxis Network, 2001).

People often minimize the severity of true food allergies. Food allergy, however, is the leading cause of anaphylaxis outside the hospital setting and accounts for an estimated 30,000 emergency room visits and 2000 hospitalizations each year (Food Allergy and Anaphylaxis Network, 2001). A minute amount, just a few grams, of the offending food can cause death (U.S. Food and Drug Administration [FDA], 1994). In the case of reaction to peanuts or tree nuts, an individual can have a severe reaction on the first exposure (Sicherer et al., 1998) and these reactions can become more severe over time (Sicherer et al., 2001).

A review of six pediatric deaths and seven near deaths attributed to food anaphylaxis revealed that the children were not only severely allergic to a specific food item such as peanuts, nuts, crab, milk, or eggs, but also had asthma and allergic rhinitis. All of the children ate the allergenic food accidentally in a prepared baked good such as a cookie or cake (40%), a candy (15%), or in a restaurant meal (30%). The difference between survival and death for these children seemed to be directly related to the time at which epinephrine was administered. In all of the children who died, more than 1 hour elapsed between the ingestion of the food and the administration of the epinephrine (Anderson, 1997).

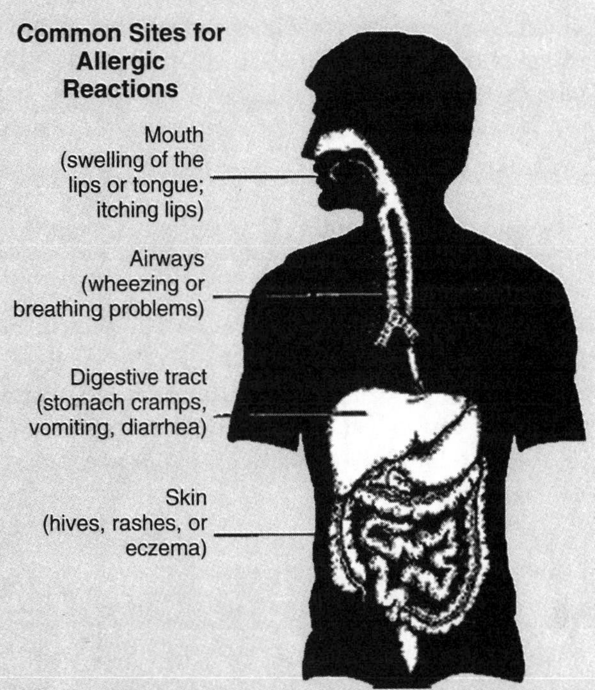

Figure 9-10 Common sites for allergic reactions. *(From FDA Consumer, 1994.)*

Adrenaline or epinephrine must be available at all times to someone who suffers from reactions to certain foods with severe, life-threatening anaphylaxis (Sicherer et al., 2001). Several drug delivery systems are available with a physician's prescription. As in the case of Tom, it is important to carry two, in case one malfunctions. Allergic individuals and their families must practice what to do in case of an accidental ingestion of a food and subsequent reaction. Caregivers, teachers, bus drivers, and anyone responsible for the care and supervision of children must be capable of giving an injection of epinephrine and calling for emergency healthcare (Nowak-Wegrzyn et al., 2001).

Oral Allergy Syndrome

Oral allergy syndrome is an allergic response triggered when a person consumes a fresh fruit or vegetable that is in the same botanic family as a plant that causes a pollen allergy. The response is characterized by tingling, itching, or swelling of the mouth. It can be differentiated from a true allergic reaction if the offending food is given in cooked form and the oral allergy syndrome reaction does not occur.

Diagnosis of Food Allergy

The diagnosis of a food allergy may be simple, as in the case of Marion's son Tom and his severe, systemic allergic reaction following the ingestion of a peanut butter cookie. However, given the variety of foods that people consume and the variability in the timing, presentation, and even severity of symptoms, pinpointing the food that caused the allergy is often difficult. A careful case history is essential. An allergist will complete a detailed medical history including a diet history. Questions may include the following:

- What was the timing of the reaction? Did the reaction come on quickly, within an hour of eating the food?
- Was allergy treatment successful? (Antihistamines should relieve hives, for example, if they stem from a food allergy.)
- Is the reaction always associated with a certain food?
- Did anyone else get sick? (If, for example, the person has eaten fish contaminated with histamine, everyone who ate the fish should be sick. In an allergic reaction, however, only the person allergic to the fish becomes ill.)
- How much did the patient eat before experiencing a reaction? (The severity of the individual's reaction is sometimes related to the amount of food ingested.)
- How was the food prepared? (Some people will have violent allergic reactions only to raw or undercooked fish. Complete cooking of the fish destroys those allergens in the fish to which they react. If the fish is cooked thoroughly, they can eat it with no allergic reactions.)
- Were other foods ingested at the same time of the allergic reactions? (Some foods may delay digestion and thus delay the onset of the allergic reaction.)

If it is suspected that the person had an allergic response to a food item, the physician or allergist may proceed with additional testing. These may include the following:

- Blood tests that measure the presence of food-specific IgE concentrations in the blood, such as Radioallergosorbent test (RAST); and serum immunoglobulin E concentration.
- Prick skin test: A dilute extract of the food is placed on the skin of the arm or back. The skin is then scratched with a needle and carefully observed for signs of an allergic reaction, such as a rash, swelling, or redness. If a reaction occurs, the patient has IgE on the skin's mast cells that are specific to the food being tested.
- Food challenges: A food item is placed in an opaque capsule and a patient is observed for allergic reaction after consuming the food-containing capsule. It is a "blind" test if the person does not know the food item being tested or "double-blind" if both the person consuming the food and the person administering the capsule and observing for symptoms do not know the content of the capsule.

Individuals can have a positive skin test or positive blood work and never have shown allergic symptoms in relation to that food. A food allergy is diagnosed when testing confirms the allergic history of an individual. Food challenges, however, are diagnostic for a food allergy. Caution must be taken with highly reactive individuals because severe, even life threatening, reactions may occur with food challenges or with any exposure to certain foods.

Treatment

The only effective treatment for a food allergy is to avoid the food in question. Once a food is identified as the culprit, a physician may prescribe an elimination diet. An elimination diet simply eliminates the suspected food from an individual's diet. A dietitian skilled in counseling for food allergies is an important resource to assist with planning a nutritionally adequate and acceptable diet. A person must learn how to read food labels to avoid the food as an ingredient in processed and prepared foods.

FOOD INTOLERANCE

A food intolerance is a generally localized, temporary, and rarely life-threatening reaction to a food. It involves the digestive system or a metabolic process and is not the result of an immune system response. Lactose intolerance is a common food intolerance. It is characterized by gastrointestinal symptoms such as cramping, bloating, flatulence, and diarrhea. These symptoms tend to occur 30 minutes to several hours after the ingestion of milk or a food containing lactose. The symptoms are directly attributable to the fermentation of the undigested lactose in the large intestine by naturally occurring bacteria. An estimated 30 million adults in the United States may have a low level of the intestinal enzyme lactase, although the prevalence of actual lactose intolerance is much lower (McBean, 1997).

Lactose intolerance should not, however, be confused with the actual allergic reaction to milk protein. Milk protein allergy occurs primarily in 1% to 3% of infants and young children. It is relatively rare in adults and it is thought that most children outgrow a milk protein allergy by age 3 years.

Food intolerances can also result from pharmacologic, metabolic, and toxic causes. Tyramine, found in some cheeses and red wine, can cause migraine headaches. Ingestion of monosodium glutamate (MSG), which is frequently added to processed or highly seasoned foods, can cause flushing, headache, and abdominal symptoms. It has been called the "Chinese restaurant syndrome" because many Asian foods include MSG (FDA, 1994). Any food item containing MSG must declare it on the label.

Bacterial or chemical contamination of foods can also cause adverse reactions. Brown oily fish, such as mackerel and tuna, that has spoiled can cause scombroid poisoning because of its high histamine level. Benzoic acid from citrus fruits can cause urticaria or hives.

Aspartame was found to be safe for use in foods by the FDA in 1981. Persons who have the genetic disease phenylketonuria (PKU) (see Chapter 5) are unable to metabolize the amino acid phenylalanine. High blood levels of this amino acid can cause brain damage. All food products that contain the artificial sweetener aspartame must be labeled so that those unable to metabolize this amino acid can avoid it.

Sulfites are a food additive used as an antioxidant to prevent the discoloration of light-colored fruits and vegetables such as apples and potatoes. They are also added to wine to inhibit the growth of microorganisms. Individuals, particularly asthmatics who are sulfite intolerant, can have what the FDA has termed an *allergic-type response*. Although it is not a true allergic reaction, the response to sulfites can range from mild to life threatening. All processed foods containing sulfites must be labeled and the FDA prohibits their use on fresh produce.

REFERENCES

Anderson JA: Milk, eggs and peanuts: food allergies in children, Am Fam Phys 56:1365, 1997.

Bindslev-Jensen C: Food allergy, BMJ 316:1299, 1998.

Dietitians face the challenge of food allergies, J Am Diet Assoc 100:13, 2000.

Food Allergy and Anaphylaxis Network: 10400 Eaton Place, Suite 107, Fairfax VA 22030, www.foodallergy.org, 2001.

Koerner CV and Munoz-Furlon A: Food allergies: tips from the nutrition experts, New York, 1998, Wiley.

McBean LD: Dairy food sensitivity: facts and fallacies, Dairy Council Digest 68:13, 1997.

Nowak-Wegrzyn A et al.: Food-allergic reactions in school and preschools, Arch Pediatr Adolesc Med 155:790, 2001.

Sampson HA and Burks AW: Mechanism of food allergy, Ann Rev Nutr 16:161, 1996.

Sicherer SH et al.: Clinical features of acute allergic reactions to peanut and tree nuts in children, Pediatrics 102:e6, 1998.

Sicherer SH et al.: A voluntary registry for peanut and tree nut allergy: characteristics of the first 5149 registrants, J Allergy Clin Immunol 109:128, 2001.

U.S. Food and Drug Administration: Food allergies rare but risky, FDA Consumer, Department of Health and Human Services, Food and Drug Administration Pub No (FDA) 94-2279, 1994.

CHAPTER 10

Nutrition for Children with Special Needs

Chapter Outline

Every weekday Scott climbs into a county van to ride from the home he shares with two other young men to his janitorial job downtown. In the year since he started his job, he has learned to clean, fluff, dust, and shine. "When you write me a list, I'll clean everything," Scott says. "I love cleaning. It feels good." The bus brings him home again in the evening.

He and his roommates share the cooking and cleaning chores. On Saturday a staff member from the county work/home program helps them shop and take care of their banking or other needs.

Scott, age 20, has Down syndrome, a genetic disorder that affects 350,000 Americans (i.e., 1 in 800 newborns). Down syndrome is characterized by mental slowness. Persons with Down syndrome have distinctive facial features, but the same ache for acceptance, independence, and love that motivates most people. Down syndrome makes achieving these things a bigger challenge.

Opportunities have soared for Scott and others like him in the quarter century since state institutions began releasing the mentally retarded into communities. They are beneficiaries of legislation and programs that have mainstreamed those with disabilities as much as possible. Special-education programs prepared them to care for themselves and for work, businesses are offering competitive wages in entry-level jobs, and not-for-profit agencies are making housing available.

INTRODUCTION/DEFINITIONS

- *Identify four criteria of a developmental disability, as specified in federal legislation.*
- *How do developmental delay and special needs or special health needs differ from developmental disability?*
- *What are five causes or risk factors for developmental disabilities or delays?*
- *What kinds of services are available for persons with developmental disabilities or delays?*

Developmental disabilities are a diverse group of physical, cognitive, psychologic, sensory, and speech impairments that begin anytime during development up to 18 years of age. In most instances the cause of the disability is unknown. That is why it is important to understand what

This chapter is a revision of a chapter contributed by Dr. Betty Kozlowski in the previous edition.

factors increase the chance that a child will have a developmental disability and what can be done to prevent the condition. The National Health Interview Survey estimated that approximately 12.6 million children suffered from chronic illness or conditions that create special developmental and health needs (Newacheck et al., 1998). Approximately 5% of the people in the United States have conditions that lead to the diagnosis of developmental disability (such as mental retardation or cerebral palsy [CP]) and require special education services or supportive care. But an estimated 17% of U.S. children under 18 years of age have developmental delays or disabilities.

Interrelated nutrition and feeding problems, such as those described for Peter in the Application at the end of this chapter, are common in many persons with developmental disabilities. Early identification of nutrition risk provides a basis for coordination of interdisciplinary support to minimize the adverse effects of the developmental problem and improve nutrition status. An important component of this process of promoting individual development is emphasis on increasing mealtime enjoyment for individuals with disabilities, their families, and other care providers. Therefore nutrition services are a central component of person- and family-centered, culturally competent, community-based, coordinated care. However, many more persons in this population could benefit from incorporation of nutrition services than those who currently receive them.

Developmental delays and disabilities vary widely with respect to their health and developmental characteristics, including those related to nutrition and feeding. Some persons have delays or deficits in cognitive development, but have physical development, feeding characteristics, and nutritional needs that are well within normal ranges. Other individuals, with widely varying levels of cognitive functioning, have complex medical problems in combination with physical, neuromotor, and behavioral disabilities. For many of these persons, health, growth, and development may be compromised or survival may be threatened by nutrition or feeding problems.

Nutrition intervention may be as basic as making adequate food available or as complicated as total parenteral nutrition, **enteral nutrition**, or a highly complex or severely restricted diet with a variety of supplements. Persons with developmental delays and disabilities are at increased nutrition risk because of a wide range of biologic, psychosocial, and environmental factors. Nutrition is one of the many variables that affect health, developmental potential, and the extent to which that potential is realized. It is critical for all people to have access to appropriate food and nutrition and, in many instances, nutrition services. People have many needs and nutrition and feeding must be viewed within the context of other needs and priorities.

ETIOLOGIES

- *Identify four factors that may contribute to developmental delays or disabilities.*
- *How does prematurity or low birth weight influence developmental delays and disabilities?*

Complex biologic and environmental factors have been identified as causes of developmental disabilities and delays, but for many disorders the causes are unknown. Some disorders are **inherited metabolic diseases,** such as **phenylketonuria,** Duchenne muscular dystrophy, and fragile X syndrome. Other disorders such as Down syndrome and myelomeningocele are the result of alterations that occur preconceptionally or early in embryonic development. Still other disorders are related to the result of harmful intrauterine factors, such as exposure to infections, alcohol (fetal alcohol syndrome is discussed on page 164), or drugs. Fetal undernutrition, complications associated with prematurity, and obstetric complications with full-term infants are substantial contributing factors for developmental disabilities. Other disorders are related to postnatal events such as physical trauma from accidents or child abuse, lead poisoning, or infections such as viral encephalitis and meningitis. But, for many infants and children, disabilities result from unknown causes.

In recent years advances in medicine and healthcare have reduced the prevalence of many risk factors for developmental disabilities and delays. Other risk factors have emerged, such as acquired immunodeficiency syndrome (AIDS), maternal alcohol or drug abuse, and child maltreatment. In particular the increase in the survival of preterm and very low-birth-weight (VLBW) infants is associated with a greater prevalence of long-term impairments than is seen in infants of higher birth weights. As survival rates of persons with many types of developmental disabilities or delays have improved, the number of adults and older persons with those disorders and the population of persons dependent because of developmental disabilities have expanded (American Dietetic Association, 1995).

Preterm, Growth-Compromised Birth

In recent years there has been an increase in the number of infants with disabilities associated with preterm birth. Although meticulous attention to fluid, electrolyte, nutrition, and temperature maintenance of preterm and low-birth-weight infants has reduced the risk of immediate mortality (Lee and Jain, 2000), the prevalence of developmental disabilities and delays among these tiny infants has increased.

A recent study of 283 30-month-old children, all of whom were born extremely preterm (less than 25 weeks of gestation), found that approximately one half had disability in the domain of mental and psychomotor development, neuromotor function, or sensory communication and approximately one quarter met the criteria for severe disability (Woods et al., 2000). Vohr et al. (2000) reported on the neurodevelopmental and function outcomes of extremely low-birth-weight infants in the National Institute of Child Health and Human Development Neonatal Research network during the first 3 years of life. The VLBW infants (born weighing less than 1500 g) were at significant risk of neurologic abnormalities, developmental delays, and functional delays at 18 months to 22 months and at 3 years of age. These infants had a greater incidence of large developmental delays and limitations in function. Among all infants, poverty, reliance on Medicaid and other government sources for health insurance, history of risky maternal behaviors, and inadequate prenatal care were associated with the occurrence of developmental disabilities (Vohr et al., 2000).

LEGISLATION, PROGRAMS, AND SERVICES

- *Describe major changes that have accrued in services for persons with developmental delays and disabilities.*
- *What are the implications of these changes for nutrition services?*

Federal legislation has promoted the development of services and support for improved health and developmental outcomes of individuals with developmental disabilities and delays. In 1935 Congress enacted Title V of the Social Security Act, authorizing Maternal and Child Health (MCH) Service Programs. The legislation provided foundations and structure for ensuring the health of mothers and children and a design for improving and measuring their health, including those with chronic illnesses and disabilities. Title V paid special attention to persons of low income or with limited availability of health services. Today Title V is administered by the MCH Bureau in the Health Resources and Service Administration of Department of Health and Human Services. The MCH programs stress prevention, early identification, intervention, and treatment of disabilities with the goal of maximizing function and preventing costly lifelong care.

In 1987 the U.S. Surgeon General made a national commitment to children with special health needs and their families through the promotion of family-centered, community-based, coordinated

KEY TERMS

enteral nutrition: feeding directly into the gastrointestinal tract through a tube

inherited metabolic disease: a hereditary condition from toxic accumulation, deficiency, or overproduction of a normally occurring substance and products that cause irreversible damage; in many of these diseases, modifications of dietary supply will alleviate manifestations

phenylketonuria: products of abnormal phenylalanine metabolism in the urine from the absence of an enzyme required for normal metabolism

care (U.S. Surgeon General, 1987). The Omnibus Budget Reconciliation Act of 1989 (Public Law 101-239) designated a minimum of 30% of the block grant funding under MCH Services Programs for children with special needs and their families. The purpose of Title V, to improve the health of all mothers and children, is guided by the *Healthy People* national health goals and objectives, which are revised each decade (see Chapter 1 for discussion of *Healthy People 2010*).

Public Law 101-496, the Developmental Disabilities Assistance and Bill of Rights Act of 1990, defined developmental disability as a severe chronic disability of a person 5 years of age or older that is attributable to a mental or physical impairment or combination of mental and physical impairments. By definition the disability is manifested before age 22 and is likely to continue indefinitely. The law also provided definitions for developmental delay, special needs, and special health needs (Box 10-1).

Another law affecting the lives of families of children with special health needs is the Individuals with Disabilities Education Act

Box 10-1 Definitions for Developmental Disabilities and Delays

DEVELOPMENTAL DISABILITY*

- A severe, chronic disability of a person 5 years of age or older, which is attributable to a mental or physical impairment or combination of mental and physical impairments
- Is manifested before the person attains age 22
- Is likely to continue indefinitely
- Results in substantial functional limitations in three or more of the following areas of major life activity:
    - i. Self-care
    - ii. Receptive and expressive language
    - iii. Learning
    - iv. Mobility
    - v. Self-direction
    - vi. Capacity for independent living
    - vii. Economic sufficiency
- Reflects the person's need for a combination and sequence of special, interdisciplinary, or generic care, treatment, or other services, which are of lifelong or extended duration and are individually planned and coordinated, except that such term, when applied to infants and young children, means individuals from birth to age 5, inclusive, who have substantial developmental delay or specific congenital or acquired conditions with a high probability of resulting in developmental disabilities if services are not provided

DEVELOPMENTAL DELAY†

- Development that is below accepted developmental norms
- Delays sometimes are overcome or remain so mild as to be of little consequence
- In other instances they are preliminary to the diagnosis of developmental disability

SPECIAL NEEDS OR SPECIAL HEALTH NEEDS‡

- These terms are used in relation to the pediatric population and include serious physical, cognitive, developmental, learning, or emotional problems or disabilities; social or socioeconomic disadvantage; or other conditions that may increase the vulnerability of particular children

*Developmental Disabilities Assistance and Bill of Rights Act of 1990, Public Law 101-496.
†States have developed definitions of developmental delay to use in conjunction with their respective early intervention programs and services, many of which serve children at biologic or environmental risk and those with identified delay or disability.
‡Aday LA: Health insurance and utilization of medical care for chronically ill children with special needs. Advance data from the Centers for Disease Control/National Center for Health Statistics, U.S. Department of Health and Human Services publication (PHS) 92-1250, 1992.

(Public Law 102-119), which amended the education law for children with developmental disabilities. As part of this legislation, states were required to develop agencies and interagency coordinating councils to develop and implement statewide systems to provide early intervention services for eligible infants and toddlers and their families. Family-centered, coordinated care (see the Application at the end of this chapter) is central in this legislation. Nutritionists are identified as qualified personnel who provide developmental services that include health services.

In addition strong political activity from parents, consumers, and healthcare professionals who work with persons with developmental disabilities provided support for legislative initiatives that have embodied principles of normalization, interdependence, and self-determination for persons with developmental disabilities. The overall result has been integration of large numbers of persons with developmental disabilities into the mainstream of public education, healthcare, employment, recreation, and community living. Services and supports have been provided as needed to promote quality of life in the least restrictive environment. The Developmental Disabilities Assistance and Bill of Rights Act of 1994 expresses a commitment for persons with developmental disabilities to achieve full integration into the community and society. Through the Americans with Disabilities Act (Public Law 101-336), civil rights protection was extended to people who are discriminated against because of their physical or mental handicaps.

With the integration of persons with developmental disabilities into community settings has come increasing involvement of communities in provision of services to this population. Improved basic healthcare and advances in health technology have altered morbidity and mortality rates and expanded the adolescent, adult, and elderly segments of this population.

Since the passage of Public Law 94-142, the Education for All Handicapped Children's Act of 1975, free public education in the least restrictive setting has been mandated for all children, ages 6 years to 21 years, despite disability. Child nutrition programs funded by the U.S. Department of Agriculture are required to provide special meals at no additional charge to children who have medical certification that disabilities restrict their diets. In addition the dining area must be accessible for children with disabilities and special feeding equipment must be provided if needed. State and federal education departments spend about $36 billion each year on special education programs for individuals with developmental disabilities who are 3 to 21 years old.

It is widely accepted that appropriate developmental support, including nutrition, reduces the occurrence of developmental delays and disabilities in infants and children who are at high biologic or environmental risk and minimizes the consequences of diagnosed disabilities. Part of the Individuals with Disabilities Education Act, or IDEA (Public Law 102-119), specifically addresses the development of services for very young children. Systems of service for early intervention have evolved around concepts of family-centered, community-based, culturally competent, coordinated, comprehensive care. Strong collaboration and coordination within and between disciplines involved in all aspects and levels of care are essential to promote the delivery of appropriate services to children and their families. Services are built on identified family needs and family perceptions of their needs. The roles of professionals are to collaborate and act in partnership with families and other service providers. The critical role of nutrition in preventive and rehabilitative services to children with disabilities and their families has been recognized for many years at the federal level in MCH programs (Egan and Oglesby, 1991).

EXAMPLES OF SELECTED DISORDERS WITH NUTRITION CONCERNS

- *What are the characteristics of several disorders associated with developmental disabilities and delay?*
- *How do these characteristics contribute to poor nutrition status?*
- *Identify major factors that contribute to the occurrence of feeding problems in persons with developmental delays and describe how diet and nutrition are likely to be affected.*
- *What are the implications of long-term tube feeding of individuals with developmental disabilities?*

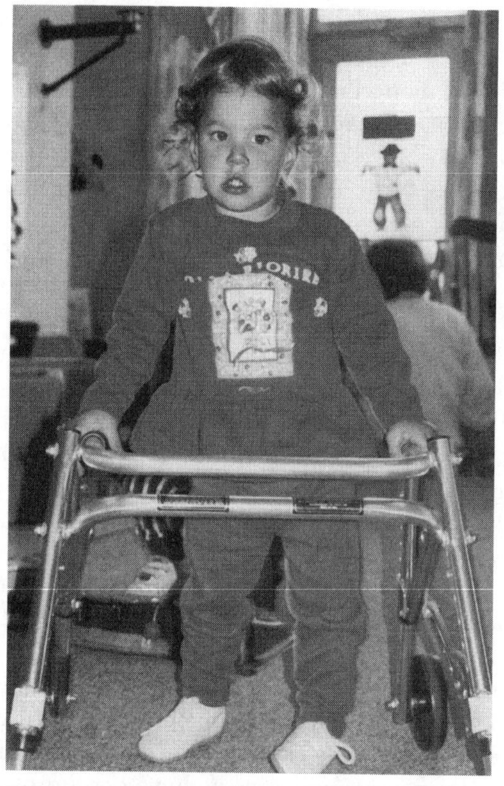

Figure 10-1 When movement disorders are present, mechanical efficiency, intensity, and/or duration of activity may be altered, thereby affecting energy needs. *(Photo credit: Betty Kozlowski.)*

Developmental disabilities comprise various disorders that have unique manifestations and require individualized diagnosis, treatment, and management. To illustrate the unique role of nutrition assessment and intervention in maximizing potential and reducing nutrition insult, several developmental disabilities—CP, autism spectrum disorders, Prader-Willi syndrome (PWS), Down syndrome, and myelomeningocele—are presented briefly before a general discussion of nutrition needs.

Cerebral Palsy

The progressive condition CP is characterized by disorganized movements, abnormal body postures, and poor muscle tone from damage of the brain (Bandini et al., 1993). Any cerebral disorder caused by genetic or developmental disorders, injury, or disease acquired before 5 years of age may produce CP. An estimated 5000 infants and approximately 1200 to 1500 preschool-age children are diagnosed with CP annually (Davis, 1997). The incidence of CP among infants has increased from improved survival rates for VLBW infants (Davis, 1997).

Children with CP possess varying degrees of physical and mental limitations, depending on the area of the brain affected (Bandini et al., 1993). Children may present variable muscle tone. The degree of neuromuscular dysfunction varies from child to child and influences the activity level of the child (Figure 10-1). The terms **spastic/hypertonic, athetoid,** or **ataxic** usually classify CP. Of all children with CP, approximately 60% have spasticity, 20% have athetosis, 1% have ataxia, and 25% to 30% have a mixture of symptoms. A given child is likely to have more than one. Depending on the area of brain injury, common problems may include cognitive delays; developmental delays; seizure disorders; orthopedic problems; oral-motor dysfunctions; impairment of sight, hearing, or speech; abnormal sensation and perception; and growth retardation (Bandini et al., 1993).

About one half of the people who have CP need to use devices such as braces, walkers, or wheelchairs to help them get around and almost 70% have other disabilities, primarily mental retardation. Depending on the severity of their disability, people with CP need specialized medical care, educational and social services, and other services throughout their lives from both their families and their communities.

Impact on Nutrition

Neuromuscular dysfunctions associated with medical problems, medications, perioral sensitivity, disturbance in hunger or satiety cues, and behavioral problems are risk factors for undernutrition or obesity in children with CP (Stevenson et al., 1995). Undernutrition may affect the alertness of children with CP and decrease their energy for emotional bonding, stimulation, and feeding. Undernutrition may also depress the immune system and increase the risk for recurrent illnesses. Obesity may further limit children's activity level and impair caregivers' ability to transport them.

Box 10-2 Factors That Contribute to Undernutrition in Children with Cerebral Palsy

Oral-motor dysfunction
- Limits ability to control and coordinate muscles for sucking, licking, chewing, and swallowing
- May involve perioral sensitivity
- May involve dental concerns such as poor dentition, dental caries, and poor oral hygiene

Limitations in motor abilities
- Impair self-feeding

Delayed language skills or auditory deficits decrease communication and stimulation
- Decrease ability to communicate related to eating

Disturbances in hunger and satiety cues
- May cause refusal to eat, discontinuation of eating too soon
- May keep normal hunger and satiety associations in infancy

Behavioral problems

Medications
- Anticonvulsants for seizure disorder
  - May decrease availability of vitamins D and K
  - Decrease serum calcium, magnesium, folate, and vitamins B_6, B_{12}, and C
- Antibiotics
  - May decrease absorption of some nutrients
  - May cause diarrhea

Medical problems
- Gastroesophageal reflux
- Chronic respiratory infections
- Constipation
- Decubitus ulcer

Because children with CP have multiple nutritional risk factors, early and frequent assessment and monitoring of nutrition status is recommended. Nutrition therapy may focus on maximizing growth potential, preventing undernutrition or obesity, providing rehabilitation, and improving the quality of life for these children. A multidisciplinary team can best address the medical, developmental, and nutrition concerns of children with CP (Chad et al., 2000).

Children with CP are at risk for undernutrition because of limitations in their motor abilities, medical problems associated with CP, medications, perioral sensitivity, disturbance in hunger or satiety cues, and behavioral problems (Box 10-2). Oral-motor dysfunctions are associated with undernutrition and growth retardation and are common among persons within this population (Davis, 1997). Compared with the general population of children, youngsters with CP require 2 to 12 times longer to eat a meal of pureed food and up to 15 times longer to eat one of solid food (Gisel and Patrick, 1988). Prolonged mealtimes, poor chewing and swallowing ability, and consumption of small portions of food have been observed (Dahl et al., 1996). Children with CP are at risk of aspiration (Mirrett et al., 1994). They require feeding assistance and adjustments in the consistency and textures of their diet, proper feeding position, supplemental tube feedings, or a combination of these options, depending on their chewing ability and swallowing ability (Mirrett et al., 1994).

Children with CP receive medications that may contribute to deterioration of their nutrition status. For the 35% to 60% of children with CP who have seizure disorders, anticonvulsant drugs may be prescribed for long periods. Anticonvulsant drugs, such as phenobarbital, may increase the metabolism of vitamins D and K and decrease serum levels of calcium, magnesium, vitamin B_6, vitamin B_{12}, vitamin C, and folate (Cloud, 1997). Laxatives prescribed for constipation may decrease the absorption of fat-soluble vitamins and deplete these nutrient stores in persons with CP. Antibiotics prescribed for infections may cause diarrhea and decrease nutrient absorption. Drowsiness from tranquilizers may interfere with food consumption and deter normal child-caregiver interactions, which are essential for communicating hunger or satiety.

KEY TERMS

spastic/hypertonic: characterized by stiffness and difficulty with movements

athetoid: characterized by involuntary and uncontrolled movements

ataxic: characterized by uncoordinated gait with disturbed sense of balance and depth perception

Delayed language skills or auditory deficits caused by brain injury can lead to decreased communication between the child and caregivers, decreased stimulation, and developmental delay. Approximately 70% to 80% of children with CP have moderate to profound vocal communication disorders and approximately 13% have hearing impairment. When children are unable to offer cues regarding their level of hunger, satiety, or thirst during feedings, it may be difficult for the caregiver to promote healthy feeding habits (Satter, 1990).

Behavioral Problems

Depending on the degree of neuromuscular development, children with CP may have low levels of physical activity and energy expenditure. This tendency to be sedentary increases their risk for obesity. Unfortunately obesity may further limit the activity level in children with CP and decrease caregivers' ability to transport them.

Autism Spectrum Disorder

Autism is a **spectrum** disorder classified as a pervasive developmental disorder (PDD) in the Diagnostic and Statistical Manual (DSM-IV) (American Psychiatric Association, 1998) (Box 10-3).

Autism affects the normal development of the brain in the areas of social interaction and communication skills. Children and adults with autism typically have difficulties in verbal and nonverbal communication, social interactions, and leisure or play activities. The disorder makes it hard for them to communicate with others and difficult to relate to the outside world. Persons with autism may exhibit repeated body movements (e.g., hand flapping or rocking), unusual response to people, attachments to objects, and resistance to changes in routines. Individuals may also experience sensitivities in the five senses of sight, hearing, touch, smell, and taste.

An estimated 1 in 500 children is diagnosed with autism (Dawson and Osterling, 1997). Autism is four times more prevalent in boys than in girls and knows no racial, ethnic, or social boundaries. Common behaviors among children with autism include difficulty with transitions, impaired communication skills, and difficulties with social interactions. Children with autism are often easily overwhelmed or overstimulated. There is no cure for autism; a behavioral approach to treatment seems to be the most effective. In some individuals with autism, the autistic mind has an odd capacity for genius and detachment.

Children with autism, in general, grow at rates typical for their age group with food patterns comparable to the intakes of typically developing children (Patterson, Ekvall, and Mayes, 1993; Raiten and Massaro, 1986). However, numerous case reports indicate feeding problems, especially food refusal and selectivity, that can lead to micronutrient deficiencies and can limit overall intake (Table 10-1). Behavior modification already in place in the educational setting can be extended to targeted food behaviors to increase the number of foods accepted and dietary variety (Ogata, 2000).

Box 10-3 Autism Spectrum Disorders

AUTISTIC DISORDER

- Characterized by impairments in social interaction, communication, and imaginative play prior to age 3 years
- Stereotyped behaviors, interests, and activities

ASPERGER'S DISEASE

- Characterized by impairments in social interactions and the presence of restricted interests and activities with no clinically significant general delay in language
- Testing in the range of average to above-average intelligence

RETT'S DISORDER

- A progressive disorder that to date has occurred only in girls
- Period of normal development and then loss of previously acquired skills
- Loss of purposeful use of the hands replaced with repetitive hand movements beginning at the age of 1 to 4 years

CHILDHOOD DISINTEGRATIVE DISORDER

- Characterized for at least the first 2 years by significant loss of previous skills

Table 10-1 FEEDING BEHAVIORS ASSOCIATED WITH AUTISM

Behavior Associated with Autism/ Pervasive Developmental Disorder	Possible Effects on Eating
Need for routine	Difficulty with changes in mealtime routines Refusal of food presented in an unfamiliar dish Restricted intake based on color, texture, and temperature Limited number of accepted foods and decreased acceptance of foods over time
Increased sensitivity to taste, temperature, and smell	Restricted intake from hypersensitivity Difficulty in making transitions to new textures
Short attention span	Loss of interest in eating after only a few minutes

The standard approach to treatment, known as applied behavioral analysis (ABA), involves conditioning children through constant reinforcement to behave appropriately. Tranquilizers and antidepressants can help ease the anxiety and compulsiveness that autism causes and stimulants such as Ritalin can help affected children focus their attention more easily. But no medication can correct the disorder itself and none is likely to take the place of intensive schooling. The side effects of the medications may be decreased food intake and potential deceleration of growth.

Prader-Willi Syndrome

The clinically diagnosed genetic disorder, PWS, results from a genetic alteration of chromosome 15 (Holm, 1994). **Hypotonia,** developmental delays, food-seeking behaviors, gorging behaviors, and other physical and behavioral factors that result in obesity are characteristic of the disorder, which occurs in 1 in 10,000 births to 1 in 25,000 births (Pipes and Glass, 1993). The effects of this disorder include **hypogonadism, hyperphagia** and obesity, **dysmorphic** appearance, mental retardation, behavioral problems, and other characteristics that are unique to PWS. Obesity is a major cause of morbidity and mortality among persons with PWS.

The major clinical criteria for diagnosis include neonatal and infantile hypotonia with feeding problems in infancy, hypogonadism, and global developmental delay resulting in mild to moderate mental retardation. Other concerns are short stature, altered temperature sensitivity, high pain threshold, and characteristic behavior problems (e.g., temper tantrums or obsessive-compulsive behavior).

Problems related to weight status characteristically change between infancy and early childhood in persons with PWS. Inadequate weight gain typically occurs during infancy, sometimes to the point that tube feeding is required. This is replaced by a very strong tendency toward development of obesity beginning in early childhood and continuing throughout the remainder of the life span. Both extremes of weight status can have life-threatening consequences and their prevention and treatment present the greatest management challenges associated with the disorder (Holm, 1994).

Recent studies have investigated the underlying physiologic mechanisms promoting obesity

KEY TERMS

spectrum: range; refers in this case to the fact that symptoms and characteristics of autism can present themselves in a wide variety of combinations, from mild to severe
hypotonia: reduced muscle tone
hypogonadism: underdevelopment of ovaries or testes
hyperphagia: increased hunger or appetite
dysmorphic: characterized by abnormal structure and features

in individuals with PWS. Although basal metabolic rate per unit of fat-free mass does not appear to be altered, research has demonstrated that fat-free mass is reduced (van Mil et al., 2000) and that energy expenditure at rest and during sleep is lower than in individuals without the disorder (Edgar et al., 2000). The finding that persons with PWS have a propensity to store fat may be supported by a recent report that the relationship between leptin and body fat was stronger for persons with PWS than it was for the control group in the study (Pietrobelli et al., 1998). Lindgren and colleagues (1999) found that the microstructure of eating behavior in subjects with PWS differs from that in obese and normal-weight control groups. Thus the eating behavior found in subjects with PWS might be from decreased satiation rather than increased hunger.

Most successful weight management has been described with early implementation of environmental controls and behavior management techniques to control food intake in combination with physical activity for energy expenditure and close professional monitoring and encouragement.

Myelomeningocele

Myelomeningocele, a form of spina bifida, occurs when the neural tube of the developing fetus fails to close. The defect involves the spinal cord and its coverings. Frequently a sac with the spinal cord and nerves protrudes from the infant's back. The level of lesions affects the degree of neurologic symptoms, which range from weakness in the lower extremities to complete paralysis, incontinence of the bladder and bowel, and loss of sensation (Ekvall, 1993).

Approximately 2500 infants are born in the United States each year with myelomeningocele or other forms of neural tube defects and an estimated 1500 additional fetuses with these disorders are aborted each year (Botto et al., 1999). Evidence has been presented in recent years that supplementation with folic acid during the periconceptional period is associated with reduced incidence of these birth defects, although the mechanisms involved are not yet known. This has led to recommendations for folic acid consumption by any woman who might become pregnant and extensive fortification of grains with folate (see Chapter 4).

Excessive weight gain and reduced stature are commonly associated with this disorder. Energy needs of persons with myelomeningocele vary widely because of wide variation in the extent of the muscle weakness and paralysis. The needs generally are lower, both absolutely and per centimeter of height, than for peers of the same age and sex in the general population (Dustrude and Price, 1990). Lean body mass and resting metabolic rate appear to be reduced. Increases in energy expenditure necessary to perform some tasks may be offset by decreased time spent in activity. Fat distribution is altered, with relatively greater amount of fat on the lower extremities (Bandini et al., 1991).

Deformities of the lower limbs, scoliosis, and an increased percentage of body fat present problems when standard growth charts are used to track growth of persons with myelomeningocele. Alternative ways of measuring are needed to assess nutritional status and growth accurately.

Atencio et al. (1995) have proposed growth charts for children with myelomeningocele based on measurements of 100 children between the ages of 5 years and 18 years who attended a myelomeningocele clinic.

Down Syndrome

Down syndrome is the most commonly recognized chromosomal disorder with which mental retardation is associated. It occurs in approximately 1 in 700 births worldwide (Hayes and Batshaw, 1993). Trisomy 21 (the presence of an extra chromosome 21) accounts for about 95% of the cases; mosaics (trisomy 21 in only some cells) and translocations involving chromosome 21 account for the remainder. The occurrence of all forms increases substantially with increasing maternal age. Some degree of mental retardation reduces muscle tone and short stature and distinctive facial features (Figure 10-2) are characteristic of the disorder (Blackman, 1990). Congenital cardiovascular malformations are

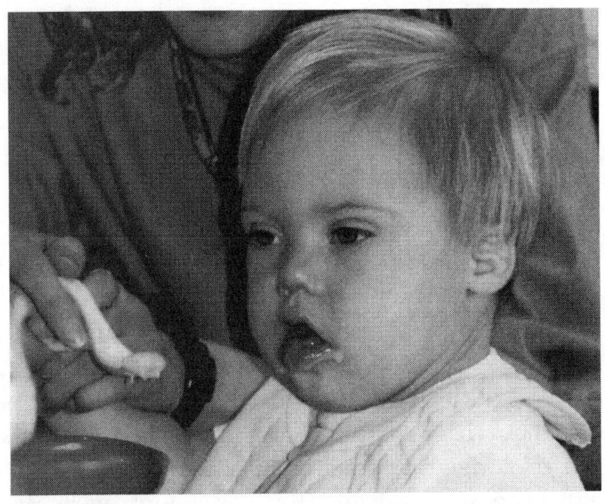

Figure 10-2 As illustrated by this child with Down syndrome, food may be lost from the mouth because of hyposensitivity, exaggerated tongue protrusion, or poor lip closure. *(Photo credit: Betty Kozlowski.)*

present about 50% of the time (Martin et al., 1989). In infancy these malformations, together with hypotonia and a weak suck, which also are common, may result in inadequate food intake. With developmental progression and treatment of heart disorders or other medical complications, caloric intake relative to need typically increases. Excessive weight-for-length is often present by age of 3 years and increased risk for obesity continues throughout life for many persons with Down syndrome (Cronk, 1978). Hypothyroidism and other forms of thyroid dysfunction are substantially more common than in the general populations and the prevalence apparently increases with age (Pueschel and Bier, 1992). Hypothyroidism can contribute to obesity and short stature.

Although a tendency toward obesity may be present in persons with Down syndrome, weight-for-stature is often maintained within general population normal limits through physical activity; careful monitoring of weight, growth, and diet; and implementation of dietary changes as the need is indicated. Energy needs vary in relation to activity and health characteristics. Because height is reduced, the total energy requirement is often lower than for other persons of comparable chronologic age, even if the need per centimeter is not reduced.

NUTRITION NEEDS, CONCERNS, AND RISK FACTORS

- *Cite three examples of alterations in physical size, body composition, or growth that occur in persons with developmental disabilities.*
- *Discuss major factors that alter energy needs of persons with developmental disabilities and factors that complicate assessment of those needs.*
- *Why are energy needs of persons with developmental disabilities often expressed in relation to height?*
- *What are the general nutrition concerns for persons with specific disorders (e.g., CP, PWS, or Down syndrome)?*
- *What are the major nutritional implications of anticonvulsant medications and psychotropic medications?*

Although many persons with developmental delays and disabilities have nutrition needs similar to those of the general population, other persons with disabilities have altered nutrition needs or increased difficulty of meeting their needs. Major factors affecting nutrition can be grouped in several broad categories (Box 10-4). These factors are often found in combination or in association with other problems related to a person's health or development.

Much of the difficulty in determining and meeting the nutrition needs of persons with developmental disabilities revolves around a triad of characteristics:

1. altered physical size, growth, or body composition
2. altered activity patterns, energy cost of activity, and energy needs
3. altered feeding characteristics

Deviations in any one of these areas complicate attempts to ensure that satisfactory nutrition can be achieved. When deviations in all three areas occur simultaneously, as is common in this population, the development of appropriate nutrition and feeding recommendations will hinge on evaluating the relationship of those deviations.

Altered Nutrition Needs

Alternations in nutrition needs result from many causes. Those most commonly observed in individuals with developmental disabilities include

Box 10-4 MAJOR FACTORS THAT ALTER NUTRITIONAL NEEDS, COMPLICATE ASSESSMENT OF NUTRITIONAL NEEDS, OR INCREASE NUTRITIONAL RISK OF PERSONS WITH DEVELOPMENTAL DELAYS OR DISABILITIES

A. Altered nutritional needs
   1. Altered physical size, growth, and energy needs
      a. Decreased linear growth
      b. Low weight-for-stature
      c. High weight-for-stature
      d. Altered energy needs
   2. Effects of medications
   3. Chronic constipation
   4. Other factors
      a. Stress of illness or surgery
      b. Metabolic or gastrointestinal disorders
      c. Other complex medical conditions
B. Food allergies or intolerances
C. Altered feeding characteristics
   1. Physical characteristics and health of mouth area
   2. Neuromotor factors
   3. Behaviors
   4. Tube feeding
D. Increased demands on time, energy, and financial and emotional resources
E. Inadequate information and support

altered physical size, growth, or energy needs; effects of medications; chronic constipation; stress of illness or surgery; metabolic or gastrointestinal disorders; or other complex medical conditions. Therefore the appropriateness of quantities of nutrients recommended for the general population must be evaluated on a person-by-person basis and adjusted for the individual's needs.

Alterations in Physical Size, Growth, and Energy Needs

Deviations in physical size and growth rate from those of the general population are common among persons with developmental delays and disabilities. Available research data, although limited, support clinical impressions that the body composition is altered with many disorders. For example an individual with PWS is likely to have a relatively lower lean body mass and higher body fat than another individual of the same age, height, and weight. The lower lean body mass will be reflected in lower levels of energy expended.

Physical growth and development are major components of nutrient and energy needs during infancy, childhood, and adolescence. Therefore they serve as key indicators of the adequacy of nutrition intakes. Low weight-for-stature, such as that described for Peter in the Application at the end of this chapter, is an early clinical sign of undernutrition in children. If nutrition deficits are prolonged or severe, gains in linear growth will be compromised. However, many variables influence size and growth and adequate nutrition does not ensure that physical development will occur in accordance with reference data for the general population (Garn and Weir, 1971; Roche, 1979).

Although particular patterns of physical size and growth are characteristic of certain disorders, variations occur among individuals within diagnostic groupings. Careful monitoring of growth, body weight, and nutrition is needed to ensure that nutrition is appropriate to support achievement of growth potential. Because body composition and stature often differ from those of the general population, energy and protein needs of persons with developmental disabilities are expressed in relation to the person's length or height rather than age or weight. Diet, biochemic, and other clinical parameters must be considered with diagnosis, physical size, and growth in evaluating the adequacy of the individual's intake. Assessing the relative contribution of nutrition to deviations in physical size and growth presents a major challenge.

Decreased Linear Growth

Decreased linear growth is common among persons with many disorders of known and unknown etiologies. Down syndrome, PWS, and fetal alcohol syndrome are examples of disorders for which reduced growth in length or height is characteristic, even when identified nutrition needs have been met (Holm, 1994). Reduced linear growth is also common among persons with myelomeningocele (Ekvall, 1993) and CP, although the variation in growth among persons with these diagnoses is greater than it is with the other syndromes. Ambulation and participation in other weight-bearing activity may influence linear growth and may be particularly significant in CP and myelomeningocele. All of the factors listed in Box 10-5 must be considered in determining whether inadequate nutrition is a contributing factor to short stature.

Low Weight-for-Stature

Low weight-for-stature is one of the primary reasons persons with developmental delays and disabilities are referred for nutrition assessment and intervention. It is very characteristic of individuals with CP to have low weight-for-stature, especially those with severe motor dysfunction and feeding problems (Stallings et al., 1993; Thommesson et al., 1991). Triceps fatfolds are generally more depleted than are subscapular fatfolds in persons with CP. Reduced body cell mass has been attributed to muscle atrophy from disease and low physical activity (Berg, 1970; Berg and Isaksson, 1970). Inadequate nutrient and energy intakes may also be contributing factors (Bandini et al., 1991; Pipes and Glass, 1993). Increases in weight-for-stature have been documented with initiation of tube feeding (Isaacs et al., 1994; Sanders et al., 1990).

For many individuals with developmental delays and disabilities, it is difficult to determine energy needs for activity and growth (including catch-up growth). Although it is hoped that research will yield guidelines for deriving estimates of energy needs of persons with CP and similar disorders, individual evaluation will continue to be a critical part of the process.

High Weight-for-Stature

For persons with developmental disabilities, the negative health and social implications associated with overweight status and obesity are superimposed on the health risks and social barriers related to disabling conditions. Excessive weight may compromise the ability of persons who have movement disorders to perform activities and may thereby decrease their activity levels, increase their risk for obesity, and potentially decrease the level of independence they are able to achieve. Excessive weight also makes it more difficult for caregivers to provide physical support to those who require it. The prevalence of obesity appears to be higher among adults with mental retardation, particularly women, than among the general population. The tendency toward excessive weight gain is particularly strong with Down syndrome, PWS, and myelomeningocele.

Although excess body fatness is visibly apparent, the degree may be difficult to assess. Variations in body segment ratios (e.g., proportion of height that is trunk length versus leg length), ratios of fat to lean body mass, and distributions of fat on the body are associated with some disorders. These differences may decrease the accuracy of body fat estimates that are derived by applying general population anthropometric criteria.

Box 10-5 MAJOR AREAS ADDRESSED IN NUTRITION ASSESSMENT OF PERSONS WITH DEVELOPMENTAL DELAYS OR DISABILITIES

Health, social, and developmental histories
Clinical/medical
Anthropometric
Biochemical
Dietary
Feeding

Altered Energy Needs

Resting energy expenditure and energy for activity are the major components of energy needs. Differences in growth account for some variation in energy needs in persons with developmental disabilities. Body composition influences the resting energy expenditure and also may be reflected in the amount of energy expended in activity, determining the burden and the efficiency of movement. When movement disorders are present, mechanical efficiency, intensity, or duration of activity may be altered, thereby affecting energy needs. Differences in intensity or duration of activity and the energy expended are related to behavioral characteristics. Medications; stresses of illness; surgery; cardiovascular, respiratory, and endocrine disorders; and other medical conditions influence energy needs.

Effect of Medications

Medication use is widespread among persons with developmental disabilities and may alter requirements for energy or specific nutrients. Medications may affect appetite, metabolism, elimination, or activity level, which then affect nutrient intakes or nutrition status (Table 10-2). Many persons receive multiple medications concurrently and for long periods, which generally increases the likelihood that nutrition-related effects will be clinically significant. The implications are even greater when nutrition status is already stressed by inadequate or excessive nutritional intakes or by effects of physical anomalies, disease, or surgery.

An estimated 20% to 40% of persons residing in institutions, intermediate care facilities for persons with mental retardation, and group homes and an estimated 6% to 18% of children with developmental disabilities who reside in the community receive anticonvulsant medications (Aman and Singh, 1988). Use is most prevalent among persons with the most severe handicapping conditions, many of whom are nonambulatory and among whom feeding problems also are most common. Increased requirements for folic acid, vitamin D, and calcium for persons receiving phenytoin, phenobarbital, and carbamazepine have been extensively described. Effects of other anticonvulsants on these nutrients and of these and other anticonvulsants on many other nutrients have been reported, but remain less well established. Persons receiving anticonvulsants should be considered at increased overall nutrition risk and at particular risk with respect to folate, vitamin D, and calcium. Anticipatory guidance and monitoring of diet and biochemical parameters should occur for persons receiving these medications. Prophylactic use of nutrient supplements is controversial because vitamin D intoxication can occur (Kozlowski, 1992).

Approximately 27% of 1000 adults included in a survey of disabled adults in community residential placements were receiving one or more psychotropic drugs, most commonly neuroleptic drugs (Reiss and Aman, 1997). Similar figures have been reported in previous years from several other studies (Aman and Singh, 1988). Use of medications for seizure control or treatment of behavioral disorders is prevalent among these same individuals. Many of the psychotropic drugs cause dry mouth, constipation, and changes in appetite. Stimulant medications such as methylphenidate and dextroamphetamine are used in combination with behavioral measures for treating attention deficit hyperactivity disorder in children. Loss of appetite, reduction in food intake, and a slowing of growth may accompany use of these drugs. Lucas (1993) has suggested timing food presentation to take advantage of peak appetite, which is within the first 30 minutes or 4 hours to 6 hours after administration of the stimulant drugs. The growth and weight status of children and nutrient and energy intakes of persons of any age who are receiving psychotropic drugs should be monitored.

Possible nutrition consequences should be considered with the use of any medication. Common medications that may affect the nutrition status of persons with developmental delays and disabilities include laxatives, antacids, medications to reduce acid toxicity of reflux, and antibiotics (American Dietetic Association, 1992; Brizee, 1992).

Persons with CP, myelomeningocele, Down syndrome, or one of many other disorders commonly experience chronic constipation. Hard, dry stools that are eliminated with difficulty may be the result of many factors, including inadequate intake of fluid and fiber, medication use, decreased physical activity, altered muscle tone, repeated failure to respond to physical signals of the need to defecate, and failure to establish a bowel routine.

Food Allergies and Intolerances

There is no evidence that **food allergies** and **food intolerances** are more common among persons with developmental disorders than among the general population. However, when disorders are present for which a cause or effective treatment has not been identified, individuals or their

Table 10-2 Nutritional Implications of Commonly Used Medications

Medication	General Effects	Generic Names	Nutritional Implications
Anticonvulsants	Control epilepsy and manage certain seizure disorders	General for most drugs in group	Constipation, diarrhea, nausea, vomiting, altered appetite
		Phenytoin, primodone, carbamazepine, phenobarbitol	Decreased folate in serum, red cells; may lead to megaloblastic anemia
		Phenytocin, phenobarbitol, carbamazepine	Depressed vitamin D status; may lead to rickets or osteomalacia; effect exacerbated by inability to ambulate
		Phenytoin	Gum atrophy may alter eating ability
		Valproic acid, valproate sodium, divalproex	Constipation, nausea, vomiting, altered appetite
Psychotropics Neuroleptics	Treat serious mental and emotional disorders; some are used to control agitation in certain individuals	Phenothiazine, thioridazine, chlorpromazine, fluphenazine, thiothixene, trifluoperazine	Dry mouth, constipation, weight gain
		Haloperidol	Dry mouth, loss of appetite, nausea, vomiting, constipation, diarrhea
Herterocyclic Antidepressants	Relieve certain types of mental depression	Amitriptyline, desipramine, doxepin, fluoxetine, imipramine, nortriptyline, trazadone	Dry mouth, constipation, weight gain
Monamine Oxidase Inhibitors	Relieve certain types of mental depression by blocking a chemical substance known as monamine oxidase	Phenelzine, tranylcypromine	Dry mouth, constipation, weight gain (with phenelzine), neurotoxicity may occur with tryptophan intake, acute hypertension with tryamine (most common in foods that are aged or fermented) intake, large amounts of caffeine-containing foods or beverages such as chocolate, cola, coffee, tea
Central Nervous System Stimulants	Used to treat attention-deficit hyperactivity disorder	Methylphenidate, dextroamphetamine, pemoline	Loss of appetite, weight loss, with long-term use slowing of growth
Atypical Antipsychotics	Treat symptoms of psychotic disorders such as schizophrenia, bipolar disorder, pervasive developmental disorders, autistic disorder	Resperidone, olanzapine	Significant weight gain in children and adolescents
Antacids	Relieve heartburn, sour stomach, or acid indigestion	Aluminum hydroxide, carbonate	Hypophosphotemia, bone demineralization with abuse of medication
		Sodium bicarbonate	High intake reduces folate absorption
		Magnesium hydroxide	Large doses have laxative effect
H-2 Receptor Antagonist	Reduce acid reflux	Cimetidine, famotidine	Reduce vitamin B_{12} absorption
Laxatives	Treat constipation		Chronic use may result in loss of fat-soluble vitamins (mineral oil), malabsorption, mineral depletion, gastrointestinal side effects, diarrhea

families sometimes hope that identification of an offending food substance may hold the key to the problem. Suspected allergy or intolerance should be called to the attention of a physician for evaluation according to techniques accepted by established medicine. Special attention is necessary to ensure that substances confirmed or highly suspected as offenders are eliminated from the diet, while also ensuring that nutrition needs are met and unnecessary restrictions are not placed on the individual. For many years adverse food reactions have been hypothesized to be a cause of negative behaviors.

NUTRITION SCREENING, ASSESSMENT, INTERVENTION, AND MONITORING

- *Describe the major areas addressed in nutrition assessment of the disabled or developmentally delayed population. How does it differ from that of the general population?*
- *Describe factors that complicate anthropometric assessment in this population.*
- *How may dietary assessment differ from that typically conducted with the general population?*
- *Identify three nutrition-related problems often addressed in dietary recommendations for individuals with developmental disabilities and delays.*
- *Why are nutrition monitoring and reassessment important aspects of nutrition service for this population?*

Screening

Screening for nutrition-related problems provides an opportunity for anticipatory guidance, which can prevent some potential problems. When the need is indicated, nutrition assessment can occur and intervention plans can be developed. Screening can be performed by trained members of the interdisciplinary team using criteria developed by the nutritionist or registered dietitian. Nutrition screening should begin in infants and occur throughout the person's life.

Assessment

Areas addressed in nutrition assessment of persons with developmental disabilities and delays are essentially those used in any assessment (see Box 10-5). The areas addressed and the manner in which assessment takes place are tailored to the characteristics of the individual and his or her support system. In the absence of feeding problems, complex medical problems, or diagnoses with specific nutrition or physical growth implications, nutrition assessment may differ little from that conducted with persons of similar age who do not have disabilities.

When more severe or more complex problems are present, a wide range of professionals may contribute, making the nutrition assessment interdisciplinary. Professionals whose expertise may be needed to complement that of the nutritionist include occupational and physical therapists, speech and language therapists, psychologists, special educators, early intervention specialists, nurses, dentists, dental hygienists, social workers, pediatricians, primary care physicians, and a variety of medical specialists. However, clients who have no complicating conditions have enhanced access to service if they use community-based primary nutrition services. An important goal in providing nutrition care to persons with developmental disabilities is to promote continuity of care and contribute to a coordinated system of comprehensive, community-based, culturally competent, person-centered and family-centered care (American Dietetic Association, 1995).

Health, Social, and Developmental Histories

Many individuals with developmental disabilities have very complex histories. Even at very young ages, they have received or are receiving a variety of services in many different locations. In addition to interviewing the individual or other significant family members and caregivers as part of the nutrition assessment process, review of extensive records and discussions with other service providers are very useful. Available background information may include diagnoses; medical or social complications; nutrition or feeding problems and interventions; physical growth patterns; weight patterns of adults; past and current services; strengths of the person's primary support system; and resources for accessing health, food, and nutrition services. Using this information helps to avoid unnecessary duplication of tests and enhances the assessment of the person's current physical size characteristics, feeding practices, nutrition status, and apparent nutritional needs. It also facilitates the development of recommendations and the delivery of integrated services that are person centered and family centered, culturally competent, coordinated, and comprehensive.

Clinical and Medical Assessment

Various medical specialists may contribute to the assessment of persons with complex medical conditions. They will evaluate the contribution of nutrition factors to the occurrence of health problems and the implications of various conditions with respect to diet and feeding recommendations. Examination should include subjective global assessment (see Chapter 2) for possible clinical signs of malnutrition. In persons who have communication difficulties or feeding problems, particular attention should be paid to possible signs of dehydration and deficiency of nutrients affected by medications the child is receiving.

The mouth area should be examined for structural characteristics and evidence of disease, including baby bottle tooth decay. Evaluation for **dysphagia**, aspiration, esophagitis, or gastroesophageal reflux may be indicated if the person is having feeding problems or shows signs of discomfort that could be related to eating. Review of elimination patterns often reveals needs for dietary change or medical treatment.

Radiographic techniques are used for evaluating characteristics of the skeleton, such as bone mineral density, bone age, or maturation pattern. Bone age, which is determined by radiographic assessment of either the wrist and hand area or the knee, is a better indicator of biologic maturity than chronologic age (Roche, 1979). Information about bone age or maturation patterns is sometimes used, for example, to elucidate physical growth deviation and may contribute to the nutritional assessment. Information about bone may be useful in evaluating nutritional status, effects of some anticonvulsant medications, and presence of disease such as osteoporosis.

Anthropometric Assessment

Frequently used anthropometric measurements and reference charts for interpretation were discussed in Chapters 2 and 7. In populations with developmental disabilities, measurements may need to be adjusted or adapted for the specific needs of the population served. Interpretation is difficult because individuals with developmental disabilities do not conform to values presented in the percentile on the CDC growth charts that are based on the National Health and Nutrition Examination Surveys (NHANES).

Anthropometric data are a key component of nutrition assessment of persons with developmental disabilities and are particularly useful when data are available from measurements repeated over time. Serial profiles of accurate anthropometric data provide an objective basis for evaluation of growth of children and are one of the best indicators of nutrition status. With adults and children, serial data for weight, length or stature, fatfolds, and various body circumferences provide objective means of quantifying changes in weight and are indirect indications of body composition and body fat distribution. Patterns of change in these variables often reveal the timing of significant events related to health or nutrition. When viewed in conjunction with information from other aspects of assessment, anthropometric data can serve as key indicators of the need for and response to nutrition intervention.

Interpretation of anthropometric measurements can be complicated by physical condition and neuromotor characteristics of some persons with developmental disorders. Sometimes it is impossible for measurement techniques used with the general population to be applied. In addition to more commonly used equipment

KEY TERMS

food allergies: immunologically mediated adverse food reactions

food intolerances: adverse reactions to food that are not proven to be immunologic; may be idiosyncratic, pharmacologic, metabolic, or toxic

dysphagia: difficulty in swallowing

described in Chapters 2 and 7, chair scales, bed scales, adult-sized length-measuring boards, and calipers for measuring knee height are useful with some subjects. Skilled personnel using accurately calibrated equipment and standardized techniques should perform measurements. Any difficulty encountered in performing a measurement and any deviation from standard measuring techniques should be documented.

Length or stature often presents the greatest measurement challenge with the developmentally disabled or delayed population. Measurement of length is recommended through age 2 years, and stature, which is 1 cm to 2 cm shorter than the recumbent measurement, is usually measured thereafter if the individual can be satisfactorily positioned. Many persons must continue to be measured in a recumbent position and even that is not feasible with persons who have physical deviations such as scoliosis or severe contractures.

Arm span is the distance between the tips of the longest fingers of each hand with both arms extended maximally to the level of the shoulders and the back pressed against a flat surface. It can be a very helpful measurement because it is highly correlated with stature and is sometimes used as a surrogate to approximate stature. Another surrogate, sitting height, is measured as the distance from the seating surface to superior point on the head of the subject in a sitting position.

Comparison of fatfold measurements with reference data for specific sites, such as triceps or subscapular fatfolds, and comparison of values over time can be useful in monitoring fat deposition at respective sites. Interpretation of anthropometric data may involve comparison with general population reference data, comparison of data collected for the individual over time, and, when available, comparison with disorder-specific reference data.

Biochemical Assessment

Like other aspects of nutrition assessment, biochemical assessment should be tailored to the characteristics of the individual. In addition to variables that are monitored in the general population, such as cholesterol in adults and hemoglobin or hematocrit in children and adults, tests may be ordered because of nutrient-drug interactions, overall low food intake, exclusion of particular food groups or nutrients from the diet, the presence of disease known to increase nutrition risk, or the presence of clinical signs of malnutrition. For example biochemical monitoring of calcium, vitamin D, and folate status is often recommended for persons receiving long-term treatment with certain anticonvulsant medications.

Dietary Assessment

Dietary information is collected in much the same manner as it is with the general population, with the exception that more persons may be needed as sources of information. The major source of information should be the person with the disability, with additional contributions from adults who are most knowledgeable of that person's food intake. In addition to family members and friends, this may include teachers, therapists, nurses, daycare providers, supported living providers, employers, and other personnel involved in programs that support work and independent living such as described in the case study about Scott.

Nutrient and energy intake information should be evaluated in relation to information obtained from other aspects of the nutrition assessment and to factors such as altered activity levels, altered physical growth potential, nutrient-drug interactions, and apparent nutrition deficiencies that may cause the person's needs to differ from those of the general population. Dietary standards, Recommended Dietary Allowances (RDAs), or Adequate Intakes (AIs) can be used as reference points in evaluating vitamin, mineral, and protein intakes, with the caveat that these standards are reported for a "reference size" that may be very different from that of the client.

Feeding Assessment

Dietary intake information needs to be augmented with an assessment of feeding skills of the person with developmental disabilities. When feeding development is delayed or performance is abnormal, it is highly desirable to use experts from other disciplines and a nutritionist. Occupational and physical therapists and language or speech therapists have expertise in assessing motor, sensory, and oral motor aspects; psychologists are most likely to have expertise in conducting in-depth assessment of behavioral aspects of feeding.

Observations of eating and feeding interactions and interactions surrounding this activity provide insights that are valuable for all team members in the assessment of an individual. Observations made in the client's usual environment, including home, school or work settings, have many advantages, but often are infeasible. In that case videotaping of feeding and eating sessions can be arranged. Alternatively, and probably most commonly, observations may be carried out in clinic settings. After team observation of the person eating independently or with feeding assistance, one or more team members often question or test various parameters related to feeding. If oral sensory motor feeding problems are present, dietary recommendations should be developed in accordance with consistencies, textures, temperatures, and volumes of intake determined by the therapist to be appropriate for the individual. Nutrient- and energy-dense foods are often indicated for a person with feeding problems. Examples of energy-dense foods often recommended for increasing energy intake are listed in Table 10-3. Care is necessary to maintain a reasonable distribution of calories from carbohydrate, protein, and fat in the diet within a feasible volume while also meeting fluid needs.

SUMMARY

Persons with developmental disabilities or delays are susceptible to the same factors that place other persons at nutrition risk and to additional factors less commonly seen in the general population. Growth patterns and physical size characteristics may differ from those of the general population and evaluating the nutrition implications of these differences is a major complicating factor in nutrition assessment and estimation of nutrition needs. Movement disorders and behavioral characteristics that affect efficiency, intensity, and duration of activity also have a major influence on dietary recommendations. Metabolic and gastrointestinal disorders

Table 10-3 Examples of Foods Used for Increasing Caloric Density of Diets

Food	Amount	Approximate Caloric Content*
Banana	½ medium	50
Peaches, pears, or fruit cocktail (canned, heavy syrup)	½ cup	45
Mashed potatoes	¼ cup	50
Sweet potato	¼ cup, mashed	85
Refried beans	¼ cup	70
Wheat germ	1 tbsp	25
Peanut butter	1 tbsp	95
Meat, commercial, infant or toddler	3.5 ounces	90-140
Evaporated milk, whole	2 tbsp	40
Nonfat dry milk	1 tbsp	25
Fluid milk, whole	2 ounces	40
Half and half	2 tbsp	40
Eggnog, commercial	¼ cup	80
Yogurt, whole milk	¼ cup	40
Cheese, cheddar	½ oz	55
Cream cheese	1 tbsp	50
Whipping cream, heavy	1 tbsp	50
Vegetable oil	1 tsp	40
Margarine or mayonnaise	1 tbsp	100
Jelly, jam, or fruit preserves	1 tbsp	50

*Values rounded to the nearest 5 kilocalories.

and other medical conditions or treatments may alter nutrition needs and may also affect food intake. Additional factors that increase nutrition risk include feeding problems; excessive demands on time, energy, and financial and emotional resources of caregivers; and inadequate knowledge and skills of individuals with developmental disabilities and their care providers.

Concepts to Remember

- Developmental disabilities and delays have a wide range of causes, manifestations, and consequences, which place individuals at nutrition risk.
- Early identification and intervention can improve the quality of life of persons with developmental disabilities and delays.
- A combination of general and specialized services from many agencies is often required, including healthcare, public education, employment, and recreation services and community-based support that is person centered and family centered.
- All persons with developmental delays and disabilities should have access to appropriate nutrition services and supports.
- Differences in physical size, growth patterns, diagnosis, physical abilities, and mental abilities influence the nutrition care modalities.

REFERENCES

Aman MG and Singh NN: Patterns of drug use, methodological considerations, measurements techniques, and future trends. In Aman MG and Singh NN, editors: Psychopharmacology of the developmental disabilities, New York, 1988, Springer-Verlag.

American Dietetic Association: Nutrition in comprehensive program planning for persons with developmental disabilities, J Am Diet Assoc 92:613, 1992.

American Dietetic Association: Position of the American Dietetic Association: nutrition services for children with special needs, J Am Diet Assoc 95:809, 1995.

American Psychiatric Association: Autism spectrum disorder. Diagnostic and statistical manual (DSM-IV). Washington, DC, 1998, American Psychiatric Association.

Atencio DJ et al.: Effect of level of lesion and quality of ambulation on growth chart measurements in children with myelomeningocele: a pilot study, J Am Diet Assoc 95:858, 1995.

Bandini L et al.: Body composition and energy expenditure in adolescents with cerebral palsy or myelodysplasia, Pediatr Res 29:70, 1991.

Bandini L et al.: Cerebral palsy. In Ekvall-Walberg S, editor: Pediatric nutrition in chronic disease and developmental disorders, New York, 1993, Oxford University Press.

Berg K: Effect of physical activation and of improved nutrition on the body composition of school children with cerebral palsy, Acta Paediatr Scand 204:S53, 1970.

Berg K and Isaksson B: Body composition and nutrition of school children with cerebral palsy, Acta Paediatr Scand 204:S41, 1970.

Blackman JA: Down syndrome. In Medical aspects of developmental disabilities in children birth to three, ed 2, Rockville, MD, 1990, Aspen Publishing.

Botto LD et al.: Neural tube defects, N Engl J Med 341:1509, 1999.

Brizee L: Drug-nutrient interactions: concerns for children with special health care needs, Nutr Focus Child Spec Health Care Needs 7:6, 1992.

Chad KE et al.: Body composition in nutritionally adequate ambulatory and non-ambulatory children with cerebral palsy and a healthy reference group, Dev Med Child Neurol 42:334-9, 2000.

Cloud HH: Expanding roles for dietitians working with persons with developmental disabilities, J Am Diet Assoc 97:129, 1997.

Cronk CE: Growth of children with Down's syndrome: birth to age 3 years, Pediatrics 61:564, 1978.

Dahl M et al.: Feeding and nutritional characteristics in children with moderate or severe cerebral palsy, Acta Paediatr 85:697, 1996.

Davis DW: Review of cerebral palsy, part I: description, incidence and etiology, Neonatal Network 12:7, 1997.

Dawson G and Osterling J: Early intervention in autism. In Guarlinck MD, editor: The effectiveness of early intervention, Baltimore, MD, 1997, Paul H. Brookes.

Dustrude A and Price A: Provision of optimal nutrition care in myelomeningocele, Top Clin Nutr 5:34, 1990.

Edgar A et al.: Energy expenditure at rest and during sleep in children with Prader-Willi syndrome is explained by body composition, Am J Clin Nutr 71:752, 2000.

Egan MC and Oglesby AC: Nutrition services in the maternal and child health program: a historical perspective. In Sharbaugh CO, editor: Call to action: better nutrition for mothers, children and families, Washington, DC, 1991, National Center for Education in Maternal and Child Health.

Ekvall SW: Myelomeningocele. In Ekvall SW, editor: Pediatric nutrition in chronic diseases and developmental disorders: prevention, assessment and treatment, New York, 1993, Oxford University Press.

Garn SM and Weir HF: Assessing the nutritional status of the mentally retarded, Am J Clin Nutr 24:853, 1971.

Gisel EG and Patrick J: Identification of children with cerebral palsy unable to maintain a normal nutritional state, Lancet 2:283, 1988.

Hayes A and Batshaw ML: Down syndrome, Pediatr Clin North Am 40:523, 1993.

Holm VA: Growth in children with developmental disabilities, Nutr Focus Child Spec Health Care Needs 9:2, 1994.

Isaacs JS et al.: Weight gain and triceps skinfold fat mass after gastrostomy placement in children with developmental disabilities, J Am Diet Assoc 94:849, 1994.

Kozlowski BW: Megavitamin treatment of mental retardation in children: a review of effects of behavior and cognition, J Child Adolesc Psychopharmacol 2:307, 1992.

Lee HL and Jain L: Physiology of infants with very low birth weight, Semin Pediatr Surg 9:50, 2000.

Lindgren AC et al.: Eating behavior in Prader-Willi Syndrome: normal weight and obese control groups, J Pediatr 137:50, 1999.

Lucas B: Stimulant medication. In Pipes PL and Trahms CM, editors: Nutrition in infancy and childhood, St. Louis, 1993, Mosby.

Martin GR et al.: Prevalence of heart disease in trisomy 21: an unbiased population, Pediatr Res 25:225A, 1989.

Mirrett PL et al.: Videofluoroscopic assessment of dysphagia in children with severe spastic cerebral palsy, Dysphagia 9:174, 1994.

Newacheck PW et al.: An epidemiologic profile of children with special health care needs, Pediatrics 102:117, 1998.

Ogata B: Autism, nutrition and the picky eater. Develop-Mental Issues: Dietitians in Developmental and Psychiatric Disorders Newsletter 18:4, 2000.

Patterson B, Ekvall SW, and Mayes SD: Autism. In Ekvall SW, editor: Pediatric nutrition in chronic diseases and developmental disorders, Oxford, 1993, Oxford University Press.

Pietrobelli A et al.: Prader-Willi syndrome: relationship of adiposity to plasma leptin levels, Obes Res 6:196, 1998.

Pipes PL and Glass RP: Developmental disabilities and other special health care needs. In Pipes PL and Trahms CM, editors: Nutrition in infancy and childhood, St. Louis, 1993, Mosby.

Pueschel SM and Bier JB: Endocrinologic aspects. In Pueschel SM and Pueschel J, editors: Biomedical concerns in persons with Down syndrome, Baltimore, 1992, Paul H. Brookes.

Raiten DJ and Massaro T: Perspectives on the nutritional ecology of autistic children, J Autism Dev Disord 16(2):133-42, 1986.

Reiss S and Aman MG: The international consensus process on psychopharmacology and intellectual disability, J Intellect Disabil Res 41:448, 1997.

Roche AF: Growth assessment in handicapped children, Diet Curr Ross Laboratories 6:5, 1979.

Sanders KD et al.: Growth response to enteral feeding by children with cerebral palsy, J Parenter Enteral Nutr 49:127, 1990.

Satter E: The feeding relationship: problems and interventions, J Pediatr 117:S181–189, 1990.

Stallings VA et al.: Nutritional status and growth of children with diplegic or hemiplegic cerebral palsy, Dev Med Child Neurol 35:997, 1993.

Stevenson RD et al.: The effects of nonnutritional factors on growth in cerebral palsy, Dev Med Child Neurol 37:124, 1995.

Thommesson M et al.: The impact of feeding problems on growth and energy intake in children with cerebral palsy, Eur J Clin Health 45:479, 1991.

U.S. Surgeon General: Children with special health care needs, Campaign '87: commitment to family centered, community based, coordinated care, DHHS Pub No (HRS) D/MC 87-2, Washington, DC, 1987, U.S. Department of Health and Human Services, Public Health Service.

van Mil et al.: Activity related energy expenditure in children with Prader-Willi syndrome, Int J Obes Relat Metab Disord 24:429, 2000.

Vohr BR et al.: Neurodevelopmental and functional outcomes of extremely low birth weight infants in the National Institute of Child Health and Human Development Neonatal Research Network, Pediatrics 105:1216, 2000.

Woods NS et al.: Neurologic and developmental disability after extremely preterm birth, N Engl J Med 343:378, 2000.

ADDITIONAL RESOURCES

Batshaw ML: Children with disabilities, ed 4, Baltimore, 1997, Paul H. Books.

Autism Society of America
National Office
7910 Woodmont Avenue, Suite 300
Bethesda, MD 20814-3015
(800) 3AUTISM
www.autism-society.org

APPLICATION

A Case of Nutrition Intervention in Cerebral Palsy

When Peter was born, his parents were in their early 20s. His father was employed full-time and his mother had decided to stay home with him. Pregnancy, labor, and delivery were uncomplicated and Peter was born at 39 weeks' gestation. His birth weight was 3.14 kg (6.9 lb) and he was 50.8 cm (20 in) in length (see Figures 10-3 and 10-4). Both measurements were near the fiftieth percentile on the National Center for Health Statistics (NCHS) growth charts. Breast-feeding was established without difficulty and Peter and his mother were discharged from the hospital when Peter was 2 days old. At 17 days of age, he became irritable, developed a fever, and began having seizures. Bacterial meningitis was the diagnosis and he was hospitalized for 3 weeks for treatment of the infection and associated complications.

During the hospitalization, Peter received **total parenteral nutrition** for 10 days and then received his mother's milk from a bottle for several days before returning to breast-feeding. At discharge he weighed 3.2 kg (7.1 lbs). He was receiving anticonvulsant medication for seizure control and showed muscle weakness, particularly on his right side. Peter and his parents were referred to the early intervention program in their home county. This provided Peter's parents the opportunity to learn about and gain access to developmental services and supports that were available.

total parenteral nutrition: feeding by infusion directly into the bloodstream

The central nervous system damage that Peter experienced as a result of the meningitis, although not progressive, became increasingly apparent in the weeks that followed and the diagnosis of CP was made. Peter showed little progress in developing head and trunk control and he exhibited abnormal muscle tone and abnormal reflex development. A therapist with the early intervention program began working with him and his parents and suggested activities for his parents to do with him at home. His developmental progress was slow, but he did turn his head toward noises and appeared to recognize the voices of people with whom he spent the most time. Peter's mother tried feeding cereal to him at 4 months, but he had trouble taking it. She wanted to begin weaning him at 6 months, but he had difficulty with all forms of nourishment except breast-feeding. After his hospitalization Peter's weight increased from 3.2 kg to 7.1 kg (15.8 lbs) by the time he was 6 months and his length was 65.1 cm (25.6 in), which is near the fifth percentile on the growth chart. At birth Peter's head circumference was reported to be within normal limits. At 7 months it was below the fifth percentile of reference data.

By the time Peter was 7 months old, his mother was pregnant. Although she wanted to wean Peter from breast-feeding, he refused to take a bottle, was unable to drink from a cup, and had difficulty taking food from a spoon. A great deal of effort was necessary to get even small quantities of food into him through spoon-feeding. Over the next several months Peter's growth pattern changed little. He was experiencing constipation, which provided evidence of neuromuscular involvement. His head circumference remained essentially the same between the age of 7 months and 15 months, reflecting the insult that had occurred to his brain. Peter was enrolled in the Women, Infants, and Children (WIC) Program and continued to receive developmental stimulation and therapy through an early intervention program. His WIC medical record noted when he was 12 months old that he had gained no weight in 5 months. By that time his weight had dropped from the fiftieth to below the fifth percentile.

When Peter was 14 months old, his family physician referred him for an interdisciplinary nutrition and feeding assessment in a clinic that specialized in services for children with developmental disabilities. Because Peter had poor pos-

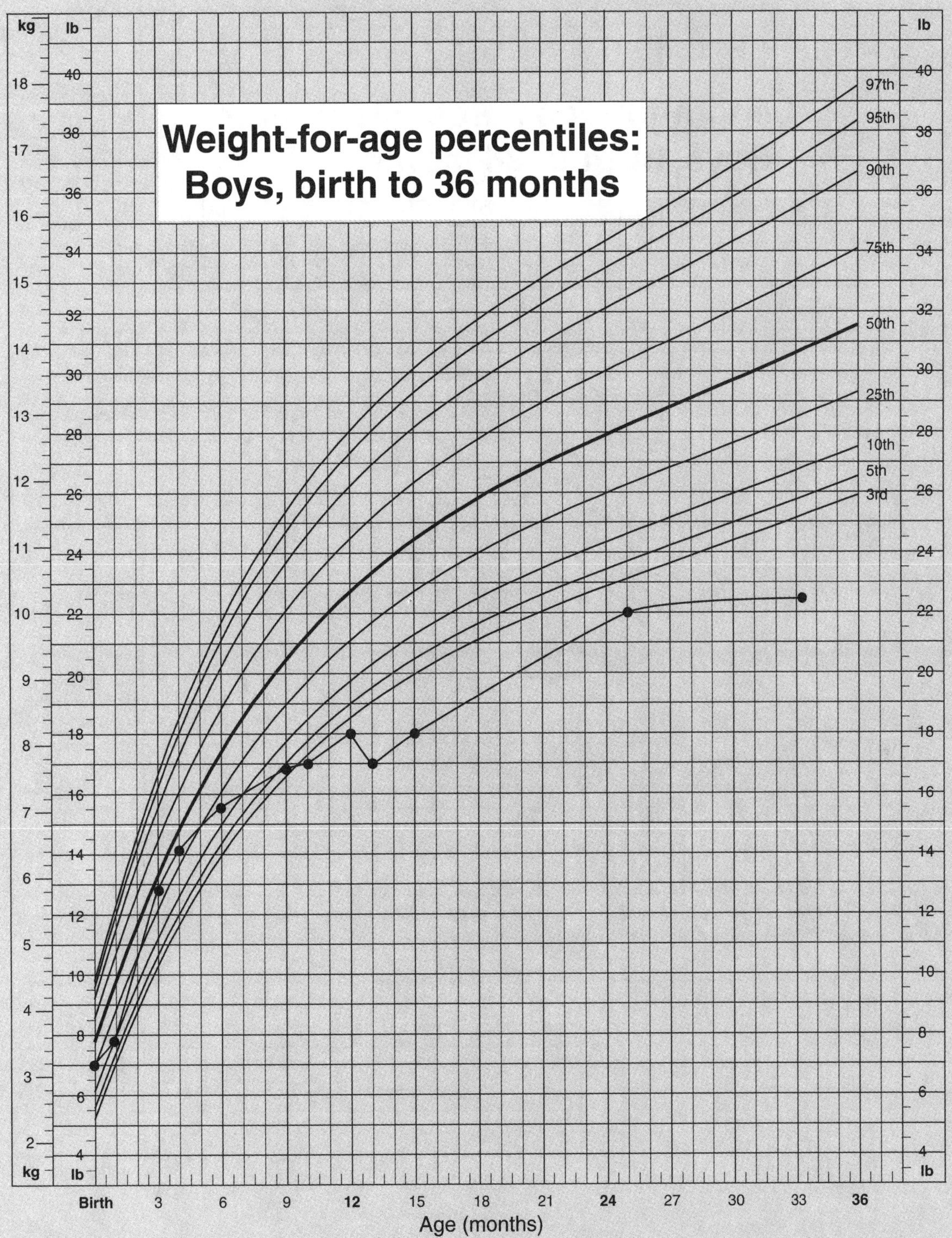

Figure 10-3 Weight data for Peter, plotted in relation to general population reference data on the weight-for-age percentiles for boys from birth to 36 months, CDC growth charts: United States. *(Growth chart only developed by the National Center for Health Statistics in collaboration with the National Center for Chronic Disease Prevention and Health Promotion, 2000.)*

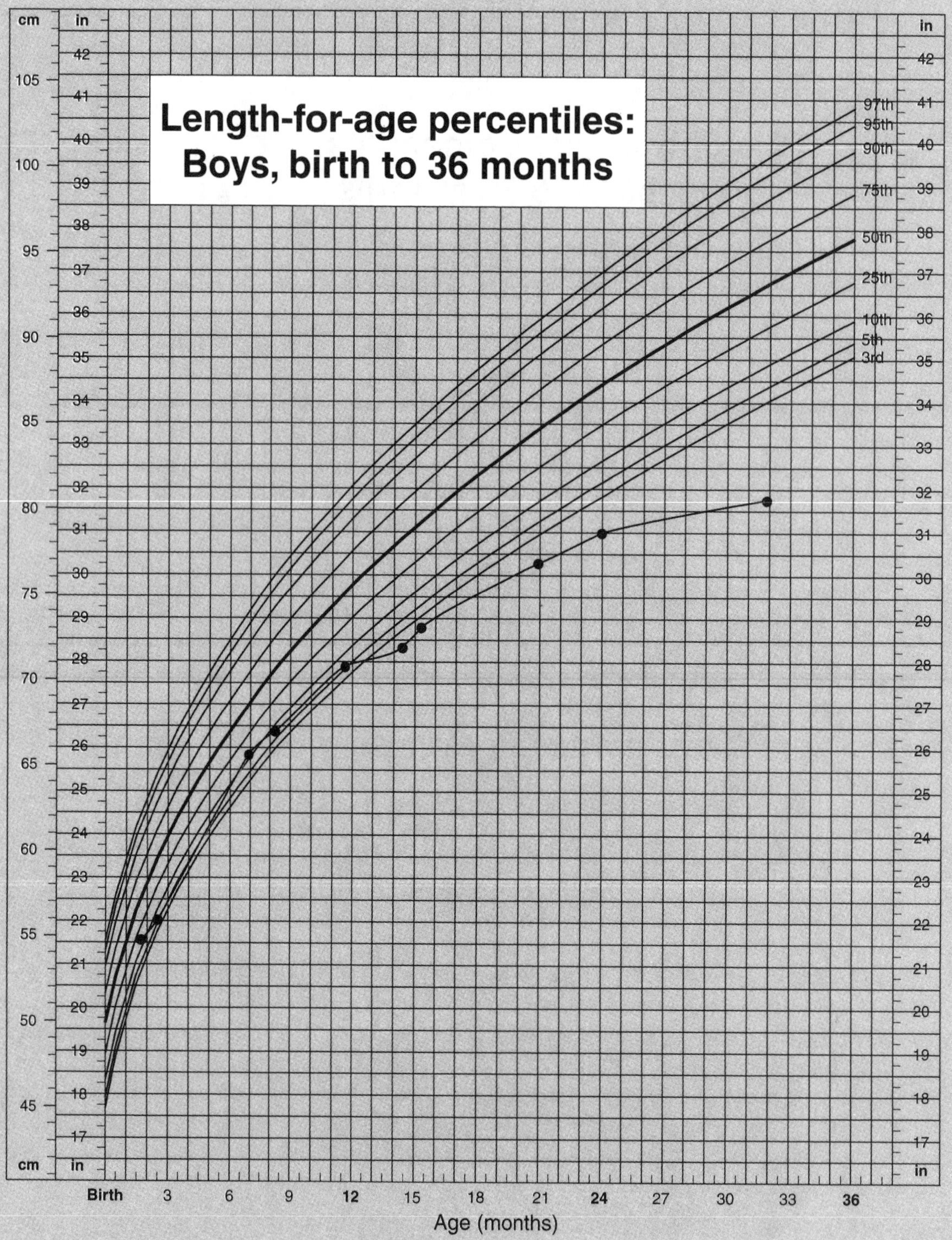

Figure 10-4 Length data for Peter, plotted in relation to general population reference data on the length-for-age percentiles for boys from birth to 36 months, CDC growth charts: United States. *(Growth chart only developed by the National Center for Health Statistics in collaboration with the National Center for Chronic Disease Prevention and Health Promotion, 2000.)*

ture control, which enhances oral motor problems in many persons with CP, the occupational therapist showed his mother how to position him to achieve stability. She also suggested equipment and techniques for placing the spoon in Peter's mouth to minimize his bite reflex. Getting more kilocalories and nutrients into Peter required finding ways to enhance his oral sensory motor functioning and increase his acceptance of a nursing bottle. The dietary recommendations were typical of those for feeding a developing infant.

His mother was anxious to receive assistance, but the new baby was born 3 weeks after Peter's assessment and circumstances were less than ideal for initiating intensive nutrition and feeding intervention. Progress often comes slowly and requires substantial input of time and energy of care providers, especially for patients with problems as severe as Peter's problems. As a result Peter's weight remained essentially the same for 3 months as his mother's attention was divided between him and the new baby. Gradually, when Peter was between 18 months and 20 months of age, his weight began to move upward toward the fifth percentile, but his length did not.

Feeding remained very difficult. The clinic that performed the interdisciplinary nutrition and feeding assessment was unable to follow Peter's progress for several months. Eventually his physician sent him for nutrition evaluation in another location, where the team recommended that Peter receive a concentrated formula, with margarine and glucose polymer added to further increase caloric density. Attention focused on caloric intake rather than overall nutritional value of his diet. At 25 months his mother returned with him to the interdisciplinary nutrition and feeding clinic. His weight of 22.5 lb, although still below the fifth percentile of reference data for boys his age, was at the twenty-fifth percentile in relation to his length. Recommendations for dietary change included some reduction in caloric density, with increased attention to overall nutrient intake and increased fluid intake. Extensive feeding evaluation was performed to assess his feeding status, identify appropriate forms of feeding him, and develop updated feeding recommendations. Drinking was more difficult for Peter than eating pureed foods, although neither was easy, and ensuring adequate fluid intake was a major challenge.

At age 3 Peter began attending a center-based development program. The teacher there agreed with Peter's parents that feeding and nutrition were major concerns and they included relevant goals and objectives in his individualized plan. Although Peter attended the developmental program only for half days, his parents and teachers devised a system in which he received breakfast at home, a second breakfast and lunch at school, and a second lunch, dinner, and one or two snacks at home. The fact that he was accepting food at all of those times, and actually showing some pleasure in it, illustrated a benefit often seen from small, frequent feedings. After attending the program for only a few months, Peter showed great improvement with respect to both his nutrition and his feeding. For the first time in over 2 years, Peter's weight reached the fifth percentile of reference data for boys his age.

Peter's nutrition and feeding problems are far from being resolved. Meals that appear to be generally pleasurable, although laborious for him and his care providers, have been established to provide nutritional intake that is much more adequate than it had been earlier in his life. The greatest progress may be the coordination and collaboration among home, school, and an evaluation center. Peter's nutrition and feeding needs will likely be an ongoing challenge.

CHAPTER 11

Nutrition during Adolescence

Chapter Outline

When David was 12 years old, he was an easy-going seventh grader who performed well in school and participated in several outside activities. His life centered on his family, especially his younger brother and sister. In the autumn, when David began eighth grade, he was 140 cm (55 in) tall and weighed 34 kg (75 lb). That year he began to "shoot up" in height and by Christmas he was an inch and a half taller. The jeans purchased for school in the fall were well above his shoe tops. He seemed to have more friends and was spending much of his time with them.

By the time David was 13 years old, he had grown 14 cm (5 in) and gained 11 kg (24 lb). Increased body hair and sexual development were becoming apparent, but he was concerned because he had "no muscles." He seemed to eat all the time. A usual breakfast consisted of two bowls of cereal, fruit juice, some kind of toast or pastry, and two large glasses of milk. He ate two or more portions of everything at dinner. For years David had been taking his lunch to school in a brown bag, but when high school began, he wanted to eat in the cafeteria or nearby fast food establishments. His first stop upon arriving home after school was at the refrigerator for a snack.

At the end of his freshman year, David was 168 cm (66 in) tall and weighed 55 kg (121 lb). That summer he worked at the local swimming pool and played baseball. It seemed he was never home except to eat and sleep. David's life became even busier when he returned to school. He tried out for and made the basketball team. This meant long hours of practice and now he was hungry all the time. He returned to taking his lunch to school because his lunch allowance did not buy enough "to fill him up." He would carry two lunches—one for noon and one for after school. Each included two sandwiches, fruit, and cookies. At noon he would add milk and potato chips from the cafeteria. After school he would have a soft drink from the vending machine. David ate dinner when he got home and then had a large dish of ice cream and a glass of milk before bedtime. Weekends found David either playing ball or hanging around with friends.

At the time of his physical examination in the fall of his junior year, David was 174 cm (68 in) tall and weighed 62 kg (136 lb). He was disappointed that he had not grown more and started lifting weights to "build himself up." He developed some problems with acne,

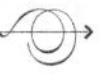

which made him very self-conscious. A friend suggested a product he had bought at the drug store to "dry up" the "zits," which seemed to help. Even though David was seldom home for family meals, he did consume large quantities of food there. When he was at home, he spent much of his time in his room with the door closed. He was impatient with his family and rejected many of the foods that had been his favorites.

By the time David entered his senior year, he was 177 cm (70 in) in height and 67 kg (147 lb) in weight. Although he was still not pleased with his body weight and shape, he had more muscle than a year ago. He believed lifting weights had helped. His acne was less bothersome than it had been. He still had a huge appetite, especially during basketball season, but he was not quite as ravenous as he had been the last couple of years. His relationships at home seemed more harmonious and he thought his parents were beginning to respect him as an individual.

As David approaches the close of his high school years, he is very different from that 12-year-old. He has grown another 2 inches and gained 8 pounds during his senior year and will continue to grow slowly after he leaves high school. His muscle mass and bone mass will continue to increase as he "fills out." David has a part-time job at a local restaurant. He is saving some of his earnings for a car. He is planning for his future after he leaves high school.

David's story is a rather benign example of the transitions of adolescence. In the United States teenagers constitute about 17% of the population (Committee on Nutrition, 2001). Adolescence, the period spanning the ages 10 years to 20 years, is the bridge from childhood to adulthood. It is a period of multiple transitions to physical maturity, a coherent sense of self, and emotional independence (Table 11-1). Because the time of onset of **puberty** varies among individuals and because the progression of puberty is uneven, chronologic age is a poor indicator of physiologic maturity. Adolescence is of longer duration than the defined stages of puberty. Except for increases in bone mass, the physical changes of puberty are usually completed around 17 years of age, but the overall transition from adolescence to young adulthood is generally reached between the ages of 17 years and 20 years. Understanding the growth and development patterns of adolescence is essential to the determination of nutritional needs and formulation of dietary recommendations for this age group.

GROWTH AND DEVELOPMENT

- *What are the characteristics of the growth and changes in body composition of puberty and how do boys and girls differ?*
- *What is the significance of the stage of sexual maturation in interpreting growth measurements?*
- *How do hormonal changes of puberty influence growth and development?*
- *Describe the cognitive and psychosocial changes of adolescence.*

Except for the first 2 years of life, there is no time when growth and development are as rapid as during the early teens. Puberty begins at different times for girls (8 to 13 years) than for boys (9.5 to 13.5 years) and at widely divergent times among age cohorts of boys and girls. The typical duration of puberty is 3 years to 4 years, but it can be much shorter or longer. Developmental stages of pubescence are considered the best guide of growth and maturation. The most frequently used sexual maturity ratings (SMR), developed by Tanner (1962), appear in Table 11-2. Once initiated, these changes follow a consistent pattern regardless of chronologic age. The stages of SMR, ranging from prepubertal (SMR 1) to adult (SMR 5), are defined by the development of primary and secondary sex characteristics in female adolescents (pubic hair and breasts) and male adolescents (pubic hair and mature genitalia).

Stage 1, characterized by rapid growth but no discernible physical changes, lasts 0.5 years to 2 years in boys and 0.2 years to 1.2 years in girls.

Table 11-1 Characteristics of Stages of Adolescent and Pubertal Development

Adolescence: General Characteristics	Puberty: Physical Development Characteristics
EARLY (10-13 y)	**EARLY (ONSET: BOYS, 10.5-14 y, GIRLS, 10-13 y)**
Onset of puberty; concern with developing body; expansion of social radius beyond family; concentration on relationship to peers; cognition usually concrete	Rapid growth; observable sexual maturation beginning—small amount of pubic hair, beginning of changes in genitalia
MIDDLE (14-16 y)	**MIDDLE ONSET: BOYS, 12.5-15 y, GIRLS, 12-14 y)**
Usually complete pubertal development; behavioral standards set by peer groups; persistence of family values; conflicts over independence; cognition beginning to be abstract	Increased pubic hair; larger penis and scrotum in boys; increased breast tissue, onset of menses in females; peak height and weight velocity in males
LATE (17-20 y)	**LATE ONSET: (BOYS, 14-16 y, GIRLS, 14-17 y)**
Physical maturation; complete established body image; more giving and sharing relationships; more individual than peer group; idealism; emancipation nearly secured; cognitive development complete; functional role beginning to be defined	Adult-type pubic hair distribution and genitalia

Adapted from Behrman RE et al., editors: Nelson textbook of pediatrics, ed 15, Philadelphia, 1996, WB Saunders.

Stage 2 is evidenced by breast budding in girls and appearance of pubic hair. The middle stage (SMRs 3 and 4) begins at 12 years to 14 years in girls and 12.5 years to 15 years in boys and lasts from less than 1 year to more than 2 years. Mean age of the onset of menarche is 12.8 years (SMR 3 or 4), but the normal range is from 10 years to 16.5 years. Late puberty (SMR 5) has its onset at 14 years to 16 years in girls and at 14 years to 17 years in boys. There is some evidence that, in North America, the onset of puberty is beginning earlier in girls, particularly African Americans.

Physiologic age, or **skeletal age,** can be assessed by comparing an X-ray of the wrist and hand with standard radiographs from a reference population (Cameron, 1993). The skeletal age of the individual adolescent is the chronologic age of the standard that his or her X-ray most closely resembles.

Growth

Height

Growth patterns change from a stable and linear pattern in childhood to a pattern of accelerated velocity in puberty (Denniston, 1994). The magnitude of growth during puberty is reflected in gains in height (Figure 11-1). At the onset of puberty (skeletal age of 10 years in girls and 12 years in boys), girls and boys have attained 84% of their ultimate height. They will acquire 95% of their ultimate height by a skeletal age of 13 years for girls and 15 years for boys (Roche and Davila, 1972).

Girls will add 23 cm to 28 cm (9 to 11 in) during pubertal development. Peak height velocity,

KEY TERMS

puberty: the dramatic changes in hormone concentrations, rapid somatic growth, changes in body composition, and sexual development that accompany reproductive maturation

skeletal age: a physiologic age determined from X-ray examination of the number and size of epiphyseal centers, the sharpness of outline of the ends of the bones, the distance separating the epiphyseal center and the bone shapes, and the degree of fusion between these two elements

Table 11-2 STAGES OF SEXUAL MATURATION (SEXUAL MATURITY RATINGS)

Male	Pubic Hair	Genital Development	Female	Pubic Hair	Genital Development
Stage 1	None	Prepubertal	Stage 1	None	Prepubertal
Stage 2	Small amount at outer edge of pubis; slight darkening	Enlargement of scrotum and testes Scrotum reddened and changed in texture Beginning of penile enlargement	Stage 2	Small amount; downy on labia majora	Elevation of breast as small bud Enlargement of areola diameter
Stage 3	Darker, coarser, and curled; sparsely covers pubis	Enlargement of penis Growth of testes and scrotum	Stage 3	Increase over junction of pubis; darker and curly	Further enlargement and elevation of breast and areola
Stage 4	Adult type; does not extend to thighs	Increased size of penis Testes and scrotum larger Scrotal skin darker	Stage 4	More abundant; coarse	Increased size of breast; areola and nipple form secondary mound
Stage 5	Adult type; now spread to thighs	Genitalia adult size and shape	Stage 5	Adult type; now spread to thighs	Adult distribution of breast tissue; continuous outline

Adapted from Tanner JM: Growth at adolescence, ed 2, Oxford, 1962, Blackwell.

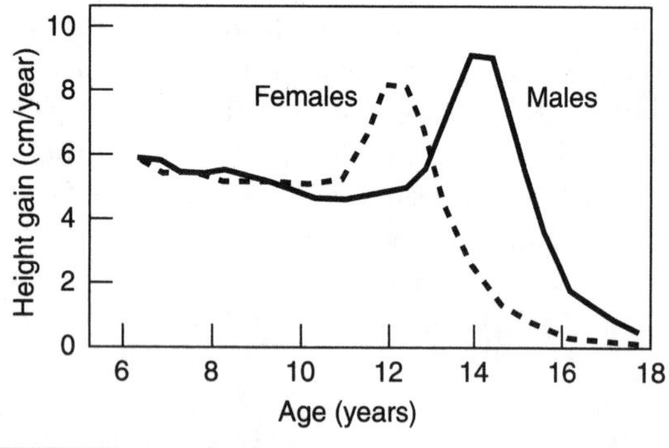

Figure 11-1 Maximum height gain (cm/y) for girls and boys from the peripubertal to pubertal period. *(From Tanner JM: Growth at adolescence, ed 2, Oxford, 1962, Blackwell.)*

the point at which the increase in height is at its greatest rate, occurs approximately 1 year after breast development begins and about 1 year before menarche, after which time gains range from 4.3 cm to 10.6 cm (1.7 to 4.2 in), as shown in Figure 11-2. An adolescent girl who has reached menarche is in the deceleration phase of growth. Girls who mature early will be taller sooner and attain their final height at a younger age, but final height is greater in girls who mature later because they have a longer preadolescent growth spurt (Biro et al., 2001). Early maturers also have greater ponderosity and adiposity.

Compared with girls, boys have a longer period of childhood growth before the adolescent spurt and achieve a higher peak height velocity at about 13.9 years (Figure 11-3). They accumulate an average of 28 cm (11 in) in the pubertal phase, resulting in an average final height that is 13 cm (5.2 in) taller than that of girls (Slap, 1986; Tanner, 1985).

With this rapid linear growth and increasing height comes lengthening of long bones and increased skeletal mineral mass. Adolescents gain about 40% of their eventual skeletal mass between SMR 3 and SMR 4 for boys and in SMR 2 for girls (Matkovik, 1993). The **epiphyses** are

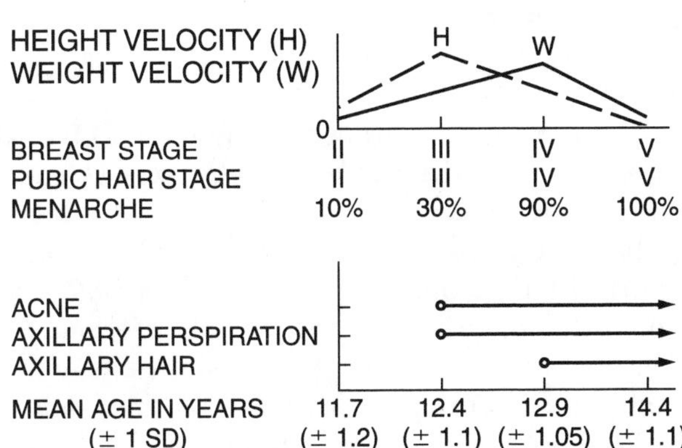

Figure 11-2 Sequence of maturation events in girls. *(From Marshall WA et al.: Variations in pattern of pubertal changes in girls and boys, Arch Dis Child 44:291, 1969.)*

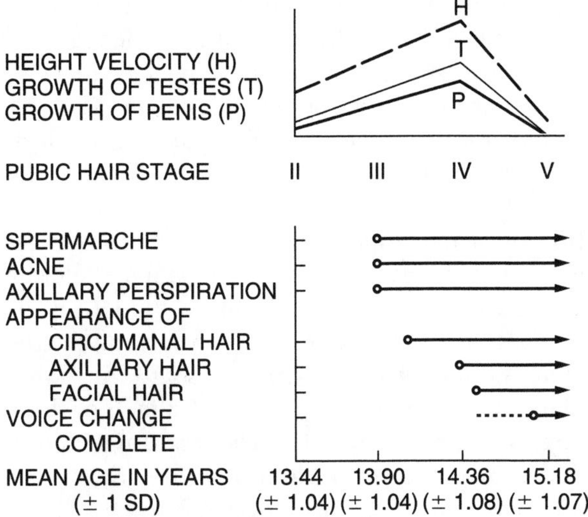

Figure 11-3 Sequence of maturation events in boys. *(From Marshall WA et al.: Variations in pattern of pubertal changes in girls and boys, Arch Dis Child 44:291, 1969.)*

found at the ends of long bones, on the margins of flat bones and at **tubercles.** During skeletal growth, the epiphyses are separated from the main portion of bone by a specialized fibrous connective tissue called **cartilage.** The final stage of skeletal maturation occurs at a median age of 17.3 years in girls and 21.2 years in males when, under the influence of the gonadal hormones of puberty, the epiphyses fuse with the main portion of the bones (Roche and Davila, 1972). When this process is complete, growth in stature ceases (Tanner, 1962), but increases in bone mass continue well into the mid20s.

Weight

The rate of weight gain during adolescence parallels the increase in stature. In girls, peak weight velocity occurs 6 months to 9 months before peak height velocity (Gong and Spear, 1988). From ages 10 years to 17 years, girls gain an average 24 kg (53 lb), approximately 42% of their young adult weight. The onset of menses is thought to occur with attainment of a critical body weight or body fatness (Merzenich et al., 1993). In boys, peak height velocity coincides with peak weight velocity. During the same period, ages 10 years to 17 years, boys accumulate an average of 32 kg (70 lb), which accounts for 51% of their adult body mass.

Development

Hormonal Changes That Influence Growth and Development

Sexual development is governed by hormones. Androgens are steroid sex hormones that promote development of masculine characteristics; estrogens are feminizing. Both types of hormones are normally secreted by both sexes. The testes secrete large amounts of androgens, principally testosterone, but they also secrete small amounts of estrogens. The ovaries secrete large amounts of estrogens and small amounts of

KEY TERMS

epiphyses: the end of the long bone, usually under the shaft and either entirely cartilaginous or separated from the shaft by a cartilaginous disk

tubercles: a nodule or rough, rounded prominence on a bone

cartilage: a specialized fibrous connective tissue

androgens. Androgens are also secreted by the adrenal gland in both sexes. The ovaries also secrete progesterone, which has special functions in preparing the uterus for pregnancy. The role of hormones in the normal menstrual cycle is discussed in Chapter 4.

In boys, androgens promote the accumulation of proportionately more muscle mass, less fat, greater linear growth, a heavier skeleton, and greater red blood cell mass than they do in girls. In addition to promoting growth and changes in body composition, testosterone stimulates development of the genitalia. For both boys and girls, elevated levels of androgens produced by the adrenal gland promote growth and are responsible for initiation of the growth of pubic and **axillary** hair. Another effect of androgens is increased size and secretions of the **sebaceous glands.** These effects are the forerunners of acne.

Estrogens and progesterone promote the deposition of proportionately more fat than lean body mass (LBM) in girls. Estrogens secreted in response to the follicle-stimulating hormone (FSH) from the pituitary gland stimulate growth of the ovaries and enlargement of the uterus and also influence breast development.

Physical Development

Puberty is characterized by accelerated muscular, skeletal, endocrine, and emotional development. During puberty the size of many of the abdominal organs increases. Skeletal changes other than those related to linear height become apparent. In boys the obvious changes are development of a more muscular torso and broader shoulders. Increases in shoulder width and leg length are more pronounced in boys than in girls. For boys the increases in LBM and testosterone during late puberty are associated with a marked increase in muscular strength. Girls experience an increase in the width of the hips, associated with a significantly broadened pelvic girth and increased fat deposition.

Alterations in craniofacial proportions entail mandibular (lower jaw) growth, with a more prominent chin and sharpening of the features. The well-recognized voice changes that occur in boys during puberty are the consequence of growth of the larynx and laryngeal muscles. By early adolescence the cuspids (canines) and first molars of the primary dentition are shed and permanent cuspids, first and second premolars, and molars erupt.

Body Composition

Lean body mass. Throughout childhood LBM is approximately the same in both sexes (Figure 11-4). Boys and girls accumulate LBM during puberty, but boys have a more rapid growth spurt of longer duration, so their final LBM exceeds that of girls by almost 50% (Bartlett et al., 1991). Shortly after the gain in stature is complete, muscle mass peaks. For girls this occurs at SMR 3 or SMR 4, usually by age 16 years to 18 years, and for boys it occurs at SMR 5, approximately 3 years later. As a percentage of body weight, LBM increases in boys from 80% to 90% of total body weight, whereas in girls, LBM decreases from 80% to 75% as girls accumulate proportionately greater amounts of body fat. The LBM is related to height and taller individuals have a larger LBM.

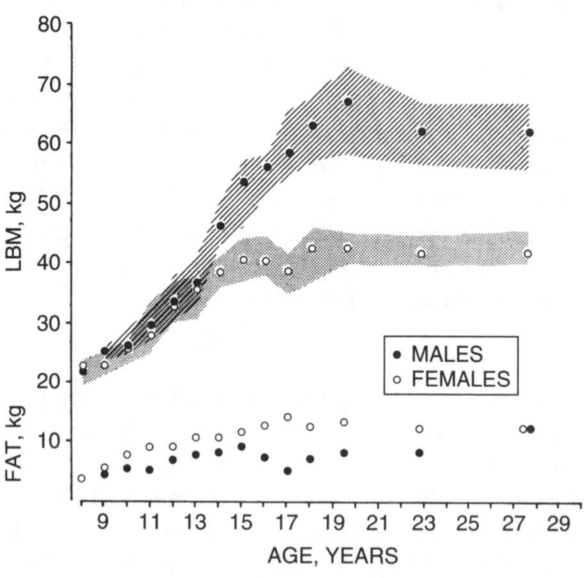

Figure 11-4 Plot of lean body mass (upper portion) and body fat (lower portion) for males and females, age 9 years to 29 years. Shaded areas include the 25th through 75th percentiles; dots mark the 50th percentile. *(From Forbes GB: Growth of lean body mass in man, Growth 36:325, 1972.)*

Body fat. There are great differences between males and females in body fat and LBM upon completion of the rapid body changes of puberty (see Figure 11-4). The percentage of body weight that is fat in females is about twice that in males. The mean body fat in boys increases from about 4% to 11% early in puberty (usually SMR 1-2) and remains relatively constant into adulthood. In girls each successive stage of pubertal development is associated with an increase in body fat content, which can range from 15% to 27% of weight. Girls characteristically have more subcutaneous adipose tissue in the pelvic, breast, upper back, and arm areas.

Bone mineral mass. From birth through about 16 years of age children have rapid bone growth and **modeling.** Puberty is a critical period for accumulation of bone mass; gains may be 7% to 8% per year (Figure 11-5) (Matkovik et al., 1990). **Peak bone mass** is achieved well into the third decade of life. After that period the skeleton is in a constant process of remodeling throughout life, but the accumulation of bone mass declines. Achievement of maximal bone mass at skeletal maturity is considered to be the best protection against age-related bone loss and subsequent fracture in later life (Weaver et al., 1999).

Body water. As a percentage of body weight, total body water decreases gradually across childhood and adolescence. Muscle tissue contains a relatively large amount of cellular water. As LBM increases, the proportion of water in the intracellular compartment increases and the proportion of extracellular water decreases. By approximately 16 years of age, body water is approximately 58% of total body weight and about 66% of that water is intracellular (Grande and Keys, 1980).

Neurodevelopment

Early adolescence is a period of continuing neurodevelopmental maturation. By 12 years of age most individuals manifest a mature response to all items of a standardized neurodevelopmental assessment, including the ability to distinguish left from right and to perform refined finger movements.

Cognitive Development

The rapid physical growth and maturation of early adolescence are associated with impulsive behavior. Adolescents have little ability to understand the etiology of that behavior, however. During this period logical thought development begins, integrating auditory, visual, and tactile signals. Individuals learn to organize (see Table 11-1). Middle adolescence is characterized by rapid growth in cognition as adolescents begin to understand complex abstract concepts and become capable of generating hypotheses to be tested before action is initiated. Self-control, judgment, and emotional regulation allow them to consider possible consequences of behavior and to modulate impulsive behavior. The final stage, in late adolescence, is characterized by

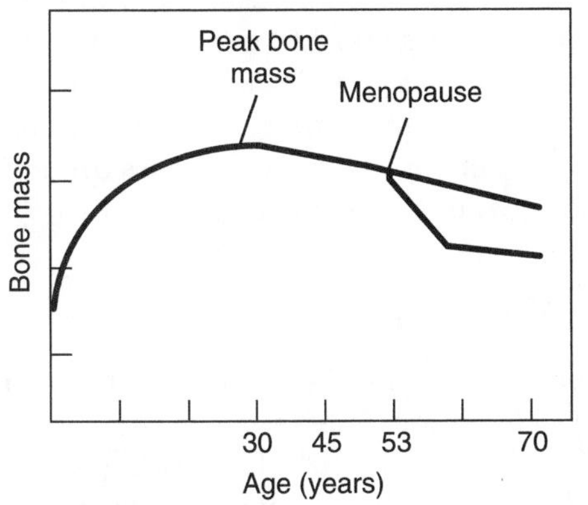

Figure 11-5 Bone mass rises in adolescent years and declines with aging.

KEY TERMS

axillary: upper chest, medial side of the arm, armpit

sebaceous glands: glands located at the base of the hair follicle that secrete sebum, a thick substance composed of fat and epithelial debris from cells

modeling: a continuing process of bone resorption and formation associated with general shaping of bones from adjustment to changes in body weight, stature, and proportion

peak bone mass: the maximum amount of bone an individual will accumulate

full maturity and establishment of personal identity and a functional role in society.

As adolescents become capable of understanding complex abstract concepts, they can consider options and make choices. Adolescence is an important time for development of positive health behaviors and sound nutritional practices because the individual is able to understand the potential consequences of behavior and make choices accordingly.

Psychosocial Development

Cognitive and psychosocial development are intertwined in adolescence. The developmental tasks of early, middle, and late adolescence change as the adolescent progresses toward independence. The psychologic changes of adolescence are often described as storm and stress. The adolescent must function in the arenas of family, peer group, and school; the criteria for success may be different in each arena.

The major psychosocial developmental change of early adolescence is initiating independence from the family. During this time rebellion may disrupt family homeostasis as an adolescent's need for limits comes in conflict with his or her need for autonomy.

In early adolescence the individual begins to expand his or her social radius beyond family and concentrate on relationships with peers (Figure 11-6). Middle adolescence is characterized by conflicts over independence. By late adolescence emancipation is complete and the budding young adult develops giving and sharing relationships. Conflict tends to subside after completion of puberty because of a general shift in family relations as the adolescent begins to assume adult responsibilities. As discussed later in this chapter, these sometimes turbulent changes affect the dietary intake of the adolescent as focus shifts from family food habits to peer group influence and, eventually, to the adolescent's own independent patterns. School provides structure to the learning and maturation experience and the completion of developmental tasks. Specifically the academic environment facilitates selecting a career, developing intellectual skills, learning to work with others, and following through with responsibilities.

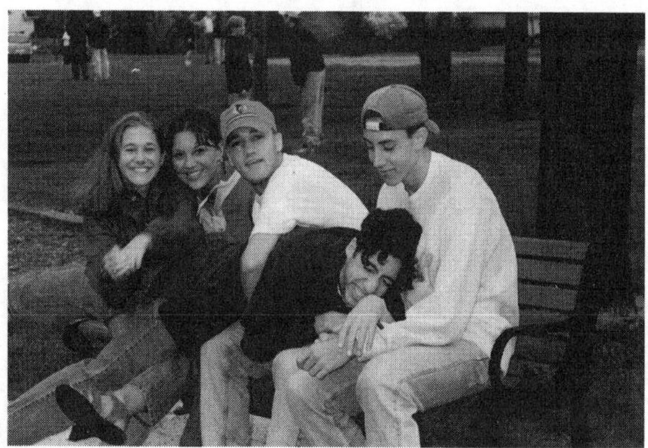

Figure 11-6 During adolescence, relationships with peers become very important.

ASSESSMENT OF NUTRITION STATUS

- *Describe the nutrition assessment techniques used for adolescents.*
- *How does the growth and development of puberty influence assessment?*

Nutrition assessment of adolescents involves anthropometric measurements, biochemical studies, clinical observations, and evaluation of dietary habits. Implementation and interpretation of these techniques are discussed in Chapter 2. The three important features of the adolescent growth spurt that must be considered in nutrition assessment are: (1) time of onset, (2) duration, and (3) magnitude. Although nutrition assessment is often considered in terms of evidence for risks associated with undernutrition, there is substantial evidence that risks of overnutrition and the attendant chronic diseases are apparent in adolescence and should be identified.

Anthropometry

Because adolescence is a period of rapid growth, much of nutrition assessment centers on changes in growth parameters. Monitoring growth or growth velocity is one of the most sensitive means for evaluation of the status of an adolescent because it reflects genetic makeup and adequacy of nutrition and the environment. Measurements of height, weight, and weight-for-height should be recorded and plotted on growth charts such as the Centers for Disease Control growth charts for boys and girls up to age 18 years (see Appendix E). David's gains in stature and weight are plotted in Figures 11-7 and 11-8, respectively. These charts are divided at the third, fifth, tenth, twenty-fifth, fiftieth, seventy-fifth, ninetieth, ninety-fifth and ninety-seventh percentiles. The area between any two percentiles on the growth chart is referred to as a growth channel. Crossing from one growth channel to another occurs frequently during the rapid growth of puberty. When two or more channels are crossed, further evaluation of nutrition status may be appropriate to identify factors contributing to changes in growth patterns.

During puberty girls accumulate substantial body fat, which is sustained into adulthood. Although boys also acquire some fat in early adolescence, overall their body fat stabilizes or even declines. Therefore neither body weight nor height suffices as an accurate indicator of nutrition status. Fatfolds at various body sites, most frequently triceps and subscapular fatfolds, are used to estimate body fat stores. The adolescent's measurement can be compared with age and sex percentiles from the National Health and Nutrition Examination Survey (NHANES) data, which appear in Appendix B. The midarm muscle circumference, or midarm muscle area, can be calculated using the midarm circumference and the triceps fatfold (see page 56). Comparison of these indicators with sex- and age-specific percentiles from the NHANES data (Appendix B) provides an estimator of somatic protein status.

Anthropometric assessment of nutrition status during puberty is complicated by the fact that the ratio of LBM and fat to height changes during normal growth and development. If the SMR of an adolescent is known, some assumption can be made about the composition of weight changes and the nutrition significance of growth deviations. For example for a girl at SMR 4, a weight and triceps fatfold at the eighty-fifth percentile may indicate she has excess body fat that may continue into adulthood, whereas for a girl of the same chronologic age who is at stage 1, the same values may be viewed as an indication of weight and fat accumulation preceding the pubertal growth spurt. The eighty-fifth percentile on NHANES charts for weight and fatfold measurements are typically considered criteria for overweight status or obesity in children and adolescents.

Biochemical Assessment

The biochemical measurements of nutritional status discussed in Chapter 2 are appropriate for assessment of visceral protein and hematologic status in adolescence. Certain risk factors for cardiovascular disease have their beginnings in childhood and adolescence, including elevations of total cholesterol (TC), low-density lipoprotein-cholesterol (LDL-C), insulin, and homocysteine (Washington, 1999). Increasingly adolescents are being screened for risk of cardiovascular disease or diabetes mellitus in the form of levels of TC, high-density lipoprotein-cholesterol (HDL-C), and LDL-C, and blood glucose and insulin levels.

Clinical Evaluation

Clinical evaluation is based on overt symptoms and signs of deficiency states. Table 2-7 in Chapter 2 outlines signs associated with various nutrient deficiencies. Because of their rapid growth, adolescents' nutrition deficiencies become apparent more quickly than do adults' nutrition deficiencies. Physical signs reflect advanced stages of undernutrition and accurate interpretation of clinical signs and symptoms requires an experienced clinician.

Dietary Intake

Dietary records, 24-hour dietary recalls, or food frequency questionnaires can be used to obtain dietary intake data from adolescents. A detailed nutrition history can yield information regarding typical dietary intakes. Each of these methods requires time and cooperation of the teenager. Because adolescents are likely to have irregular eating patterns, it may be difficult to get accu-

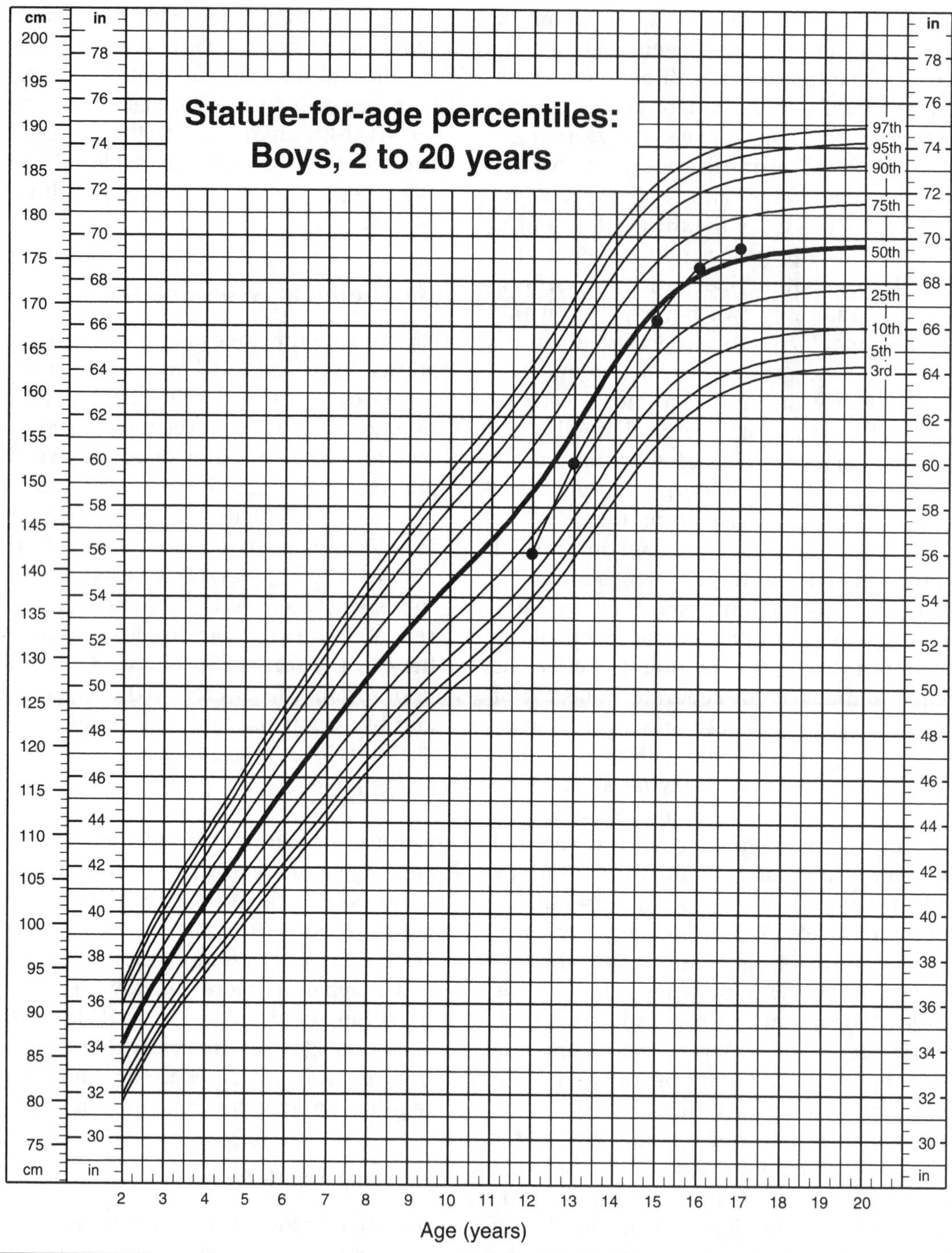

Figure 11-7 David's gains in stature plotted on the stature-for-age percentiles for boys age 2 years to 20 years. CDC growth charts: United States. (Growth chart only developed by the National Center for Health Statistics in collaboration with the National Center for Chronic Disease Prevention and Health Promotion, 2000).

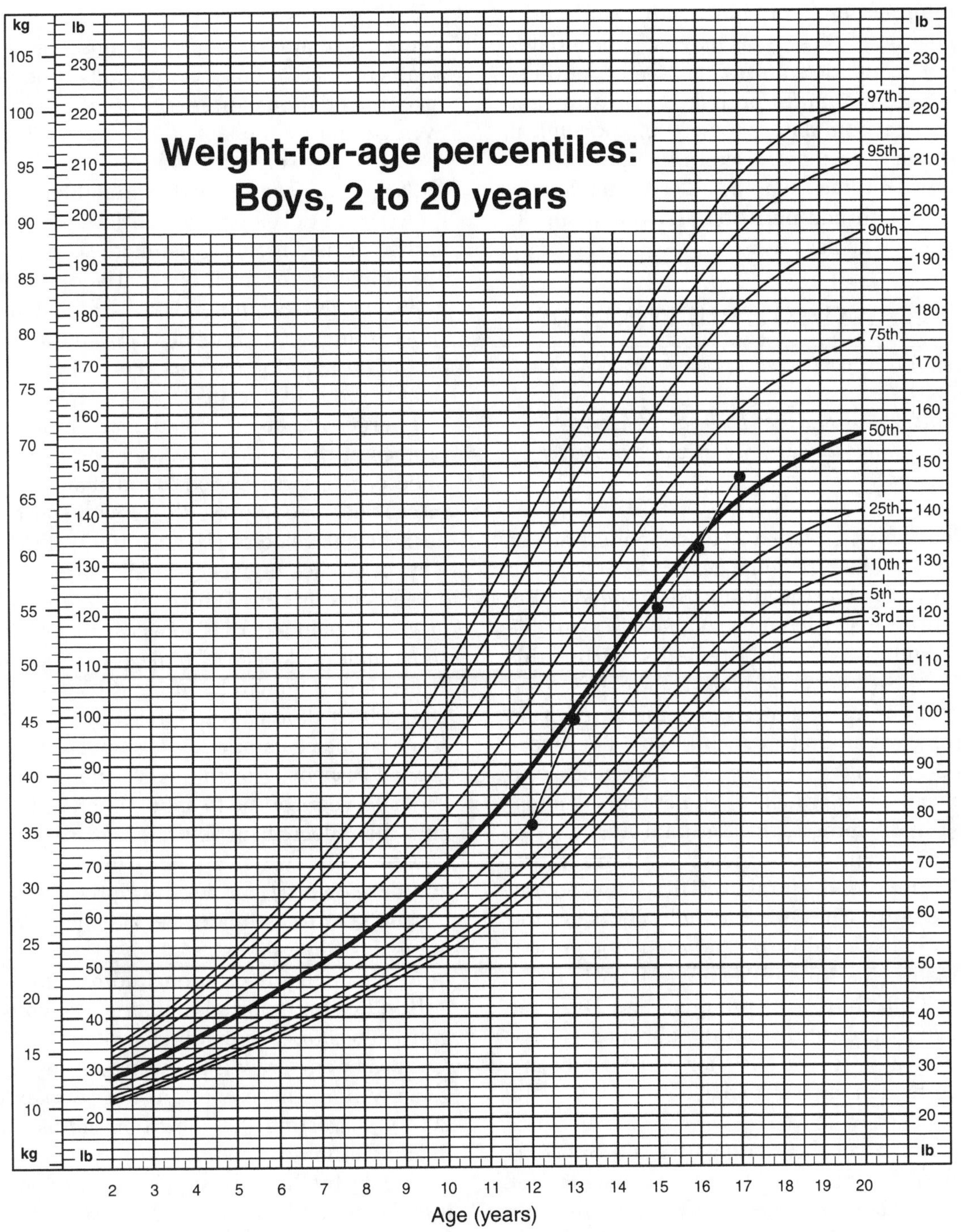

Figure 11-8 David's gains in weight plotted on the weight-for-age percentiles for boys age 2 years to 20 years. CDC growth charts: United States. (Growth chart only developed by the National Center for Health Statistics in collaboration with the National Center for Chronic Disease Prevention and Health Promotion, 2000).

rate information from some youngsters and a combination of these tools may be appropriate.

Overall nutrition assessment and identification of potential nutrition risk requires integration of data from anthropometric, biochemical, and dietary patterns. Determination of substance use or abuse may be an essential component of health and nutrition assessment in the population (see page 370).

ENERGY AND NUTRIENT NEEDS

- *What are the needs of adolescents for energy and nutrients?*
- *How well nourished are American adolescents?*
- *For which nutrients are there special concerns for adolescents?*

The section on growth and development makes it clear that the rapid changes of puberty result in markedly increased nutrition needs. Because little experimental evidence is available to determine exact requirements during this period, most recommendations are based on data from animal studies or extrapolated from research with adults or children. There are limited estimates of intakes associated with good health and growth of adolescents. As discussed in Chapter 1, the National Academy of Sciences is in the process of formulating Dietary Reference Intakes (DRIs) for energy and nutrients. The DRIs for adolescents are the intakes considered to be sufficient for growth and health (Institute of Medicine [IOM], 1997, 1998, 2000, 2001). In practice, the DRIs for adolescents are categorized by chronologic age rather than SMR. The DRIs for adolescence are divided by gender into two age groups: 9 to 13 years and 14 to 18 years.

At the time of this writing, the DRI Subcommittee on Energy and Macronutrients has not reported. Therefore the recommendations for energy and protein intakes reflect the 1989 Recommended Dietary Allowances (RDAs) (Food and Nutrition Board, 1989). For energy and protein the RDAs are presented by gender in three age groups: 11 to 14 years, 15 to 18 years, and 19 to 24 years.

Energy

Energy is required for growth, muscular activity, and synthesis of body compounds. The current recommendations for energy are estimated from average energy intakes of adolescents based on average body weights (Food and Nutrition Board, 1989). Because of the wide variability in rates of growth and development and levels of physical activity, it is difficult to estimate specific energy requirements for an individual adolescent. The 1989 energy recommendations for adolescents range from 2500 to 3000 kcal for males and 2100 and 2200 kcal for females (Food and Nutrition Board, 1989) (Table 11-3).

Energy intake is related to growth rate. Studies of the caloric intakes of girls across the pubescent growth period found that the highest intakes occurred during the growth spurt, or the peak height velocity (Daniel, 1982). From a review of studies of energy intake of children and adolescents in the United States, Heald et al. (1969) concluded that females appear to consume their peak caloric intakes, about 2550 kcal, at the time of menarche (around 12 years of age), after which time caloric intake levels slowly decline. In males caloric intakes appear to parallel the adolescent growth spurt, increasing until about 16 years of age to approximately 3400 kcal and then decreasing by the age of 19 years. Because of the wide variability in rates of growth and development and levels of physical activity, it is difficult to estimate specific energy requirements for adolescents.

A recent report of a longitudinal study of 67 girls in Boston reported that girls who consumed more kilocalories and animal protein 2 years before peak bone growth had a higher peak growth velocity than those who did not (Berkey et al., 2000), suggesting that nutrition status may influence ultimate growth.

Energy intake data support a relationship of total height and caloric needs in each age group. It appears that increments in height during adolescence are the most accurate representation of the anabolic effect of the growth period. Therefore the best index for determining energy needs is thought to be kilocalories per unit (centimeter) height (see Table 11-3).

Table 11-3 RECOMMENDATIONS FOR ENERGY AND PROTEIN INTAKE BASED ON HEIGHT

	Males				Females			
Age Group (y)	Reference Height (cm)	Total kcal/day	Energy (kcal/cm)	Protein (g/cm)	Reference Height (cm)	Total kcal/day	Energy (kcal/cm)	Protein (g/cm)
11-14	157	2500	15.9	0.29	157	2100	14.0	0.29
15-18	176	3000	17.0	0.34	163	2200	13.5	0.27
19-24	164	2700	16.4	0.33	164	2200	13.4	0.28

Adapted from Food and Nutrition Board: Recommended dietary allowances, ed 10, Washington, DC, 1989, National Academy Press.

The most accepted way to assess adequacy of energy intake is to evaluate growth and body composition. A common practice is to plot height on growth charts, which will reveal the position of the adolescent to the reference population. If multiple measures over time are available, changes in rates of linear growth of body mass can be detected (Gong and Spear, 1988).

Based on the first Health and Nutrition Examination Survey (U.S. Department of Health, Education and Welfare, 1974) and four U.S. Department of Agriculture (USDA) surveys of persons 11 to 18 years of age (Cavadini et al., 2001), overall total energy intakes of adolescents decreased indicating that poor dietary selections and physical inactivity contribute to excess body weight and potential health consequences. In contrast, among adolescents in North America, nutrition deficits associated with self-induced restriction of food or energy, sometimes accompanied by marked energy expenditure of training competition for some sports, make it difficult to assess the adequacy of growth (Rogol et al., 2000).

Macronutrients

Protein

The RDAs for protein are based on data for body composition and calculations of growth rate. As with kilocalories, the protein needs of the adolescent correlate more closely with the growth pattern than with chronologic age, making grams of protein per centimeter of height the most accurate method for estimating protein allowances. The daily protein recommendations for adolescents range from 0.29 g/cm to 0.34 g/cm height for males and 0.27 g/cm to 0.29 g/cm for females (see Table 11-3).

For most Americans, including adolescents, daily protein intakes exceed the RDA. Adolescents at risk of poor protein nutriture are those in low-income groups and those who severely restrict total food intake or exclude major food groups providing protein, such as strict vegetarians (see the Application at the end of this chapter).

Carbohydrate and Fat

The Food and Nutrition Board (1989) has not established recommended levels for dietary carbohydrate or fat, but levels sufficient to meet energy needs are necessary to spare dietary protein for protein synthesis rather than being utilized for energy. The Dietary Guidelines for adults are appropriate for adolescents—more than 55% of kilocalories consumed should be from carbohydrates and less than 30% of total kilocalories from fat.

A study of long-term trends of adolescent food consumption is based on data from four nationally representative USDA surveys of individuals age 11 years to 18 years (a total of 12,490 individuals) from 1965 to 1994 (Cavandini et al., 2001). The researchers found that during those years, the percentage of total energy from fat decreased from 39% to 32% and that from saturated fat fell from 15% to 12%. These changes were attributed to increased consumption of lower fat milk instead of whole milk. However, the total milk consumption decreased by 36%. The decrease was accompanied by an increase in consumption of soft drinks and noncitrus juices. Concurrent with the decrease in dairy fat intake was an increase in the intake of high-fat potatoes (French fries), pizza, and mixed dishes.

Data from NHANES III (1988 to 1994) indicated that one in four youths met recommendations for fat intakes (30%) and saturated fat (10%) (Troiano et al., 2000). Beverages contributed approximately 22% of energy and specifically soft drinks provided 8% of energy for adolescents.

Micronutrients

The 1977 to 1978 Nationwide Food Consumption Survey (USDA, 1984) and the NHANES I and II (National Center for Health Statistics [NCHS], 1979) have identified low dietary intakes and deficient or low biochemical measures of some vitamins (folate, riboflavin, and vitamins B_6, A, and C) and minerals (calcium, iron, and zinc). Female adolescents and those of low socioeconomic status were at particular risk. The DRIs for vitamins and minerals are based on the four reports from the IOM (IOM, 1997, 1998, 2000, 2001). The DRIs are discussed by nutrient groups of each report in the following section. The DRI values for adolescents appear in Table 11-4.

Calcium and Related Nutrients

The skeletal development of infancy and childhood accelerates during puberty and continues slowly into the third decade of life. The percentage of trabecular bone surface covered with **osteoids** is high during this period and declines in early adulthood, remaining low thereafter. Because of increased bone formation and accelerated muscular and endocrine development, calcium needs are greatest during puberty. A calcium deficiency during skeletal formation and maturation may be associated with a decrease in peak bone mass, which could contribute to increased risk of fracture later in life. Increasing dietary calcium during this growth period has been shown to enhance bone density (Cadogan et al., 1999).

If optimal peak bone mass is to be achieved, an adolescent must be in positive calcium balance. This means that both calcium intake and absorption have to be adequate to compensate for **obligatory losses** and to provide a surplus for skeletal growth. Accumulation of bone mass is optimal when the **threshold calcium balance** is met or exceeded. The DRI for calcium increases to 1300 mg during adolescence. Optimal utilization of dietary calcium requires adequate levels of vitamin D, a 1:1 calcium:phosphorus ratio, and adequate levels of other nutrients, including protein, magnesium, and vitamin C.

According to dietary surveys, calcium intakes of adolescent girls tend to be 400 mg to 700 mg below the Adequate Intake (AI) (Barr, 1994; Eck and Hackett-Renner, 1992). Higher intake levels have been reported by males. Limited use of calcium-rich dairy products, fewer total meals and snacks consumed each day, and increased consumption of soft drinks are largely responsible for inadequate calcium intakes in adolescents (Barr, 1994; Guenther, 1986). Substituting carbonated beverages for milk may substantially increase phosphorus intake, creating an unfavorable environment for bone formation. In African Americans, lactose intolerance may be a major contributing factor to low consumption of milk and other dairy products. A serving is considered to be one cup of milk or an equivalent that provided approximately 300 mg of calcium. Three servings would supply three fourths of the AI. The USDA Continuing Surveys of Food Intakes by Individuals found that only 30% of youth met the recommendations for dairy consumption (Munoz et al., 1997).

Vitamin D. Vitamin D is necessary for maintaining homeostasis of calcium and phosphorus in mineralization of bone. The RDA for vitamin D is 10 μg per day throughout adolescence. Because peak bone mass is not achieved before the third decade, this level is continued through 24 years of

KEY TERMS

osteoids: sites of new bone formation
obligatory losses: the amounts of nutrients lost through urine, feces, and skin in normal metabolic processes
threshold calcium balance: the level of calcium intake below which skeletal accumulation of calcium varies with intake and above which it remains constant

Table 11-4 Dietary Reference Intakes for Adolescence

	Females		Males	
Nutrient/Day	9-13 yr	14-18 yr	9-13 yr	14-18 yr
CALCIUM AND RELATED NUTRIENTS				
Calcium (mg)	*1300*	*1300*	*1300*	*1300*
Fluoride (mg)	*2*	*3*	*2*	*3*
Magnesium (mg)	**240**	**360**	**240**	**410**
Phosphorus (mg)	**1250**	**1250**	**1250**	**1250**
Vitamin D (μg)	*5*	*5*	*5*	*5*
B VITAMINS AND CHOLINE				
Thiamin (mg)	**0.9**	**1.0**	**0.9**	**1.2**
Riboflavin (mg)	**0.9**	**1.0**	**0.9**	**1.3**
Niacin (mg)	**12**	**14**	**12**	**16**
Vitamin B_6 (mg)	**1.0**	**1.2**	**1.0**	**1.3**
Folate (μg)	**300**	**400**	**300**	**400**
Vitamin B_{12} (μg)	**1.8**	**2.4**	**1.8**	**2.4**
Pantothenic acid (mg)	*4*	*5*	*4*	*5*
Biotin (μg)	*20*	*20*	*20*	*25*
Choline (mg/d)	*375*	*400*	*375*	*550*
ANTIOXIDANTS				
Vitamin C (mg)	**45**	**65**	**45**	**75**
Vitamin E (mg)	**11**	**15**	**11**	**15**
Selenium (μg)	**40**	**55**	**40**	**55**
OTHER VITAMINS AND MINERALS				
Vitamin A (μg)	**600**	**700**	**600**	**900**
Vitamin K (μg)	*60*	*75*	*60*	*75*
Chromium (mg)	*21*	*24*	*25*	*35*
Copper (μg)	**700**	**890**	**700**	**890**
Iodine (μg/d)	**120**	**150**	**120**	**150**
Iron (mg)	**8**	**15**	**8**	**11**
Manganese (mg)	*1.6*	*1.6*	*1.9*	*2.2*
Molybdenum (μg)	**34**	**43**	**34**	**43**
Zinc (μg)	**8**	**9**	**8**	**11**

Adapted with permission from the following Institute of Medicine publications: Dietary reference intakes for calcium, phosphorus, magnesium, vitamin D, and fluoride (1997); Dietary reference intakes for thiamin, riboflavin, niacin, vitamin B_6, folate, vitamin B_{12}, pantothenic acid, biotin, and choline (1998); Dietary reference intakes for vitamin C, vitamin E, selenium, and carotenoids (2000); and Dietary reference intakes for vitamin A, vitamin K, arsenic, boron, chromium, copper, iodine, iron, manganese, molybdenum, nickel, silicon, vanadium, and zinc (2001); Washington, DC, National Academy Press.
RDAs are printed in bold type; AIs are printed in italics.

age. The major source of dietary vitamin D is fortified milk, which may be consumed in decreasing amounts by adolescents, especially females.

B Complex Vitamins

Data on vitamin requirements for adolescents are even more limited than are those for minerals. The RDAs are extrapolated from data for other age groups, with estimates of increments for growth. Because of the increased energy demands of growth, the need for thiamin, riboflavin, and niacin is elevated. There are also heightened demands for vitamin B_6, folate, and vitamin B_{12}, which are required for normal deoxyribonucleic acid (DNA) and ribonucleic acid (RNA) synthesis and protein metabolism. The recent association of adequate folate intake during embryonic development with prevention of neural tube defects emphasizes the importance of adequate folate in the diets of teenage girls. Folate in the form of fortified foods or supplements has been recommended for any female who might become pregnant. This is particularly important for teens, for whom a high percentage of pregnancies are unplanned.

Antioxidant Nutrients: Vitamin C, Vitamin E, and Selenium

All three nutrients are important in maintaining the body's antioxidant pool. Vitamin C also participates in collagen synthesis in bone and other body tissues and a number of other biologic reactions. It is important in absorption and utilization of iron. Additional levels of vitamin C will be required for adolescents who smoke.

Vitamin E is well established as an antioxidant. In the body it protects polyunsaturated fatty acids, vitamin A, and ascorbic acid and cell membranes. Selenium is a component of enzymes that reduce the body's free radical pool.

Vitamin A and Other Nutrients

The major nutrients in this category are vitamin A, iron, and zinc. Information regarding the other nutrients can be found in Tables 1-2 and 1-3.

Vitamin A. Vitamin A is required for maintenance of epithelial cells and mucous membranes and formation of light-receptor pigments for vision. Vitamin A is essential for growth and reproduction. It is important that adolescents receive adequate amounts of vitamin A, preferably from dietary sources (dairy products, fortified cereals) for preformed vitamin A and particularly fruits and vegetables for carotenoid precursors of vitamin A. Pregnant teens should not take any supplements that contain vitamin A unless prescribed by their physician.

Iron. The increase in iron requirements during puberty is associated with the sharp increase in LBM, expanding blood volume, and red cell mass. More iron is needed for synthesis of myoglobin in muscle and hemoglobin in blood.

Dietary intake and absorption must be sufficient to compensate for losses through feces, urine, skin, and menstruation and to provide for tissue growth. In females the demands for growth are lower than those for boys, but the requirements for menstruation that starts after peak gains in height are estimated to require 1.3 mg/day. The DRIs for iron needed to reach adulthood with a storage level of 30 mg of iron are 12 mg for males and 15 mg for females. The iron content of the American diet is approximately 6 mg per 1000 kilocalories (Marino and King, 1980). For adolescent females, who typically have caloric intakes well below the RDA of 2100 to 2200 recommended and those who may lose iron associated with vigorous physical activity, inadequate iron intake is a problem.

Zinc. Zinc is essential for healthy growth and sexual maturation. Although there have been no controlled studies on the zinc requirements of adolescents, growth retardation and hypogonadism in adolescent boys with zinc deficiency have been reported in developing countries. Body zinc levels appear to decline during puberty (Thompson et al., 1986), which may reflect either an increased need for zinc during growth or a redistribution of plasma zinc from hormonal changes. Recommended levels for adolescents are the same as for adults.

Very little information is available on the requirements for other trace minerals during adolescence. Current recommendations have been extrapolated from adult values.

Until further research provides data for more precise nutrition recommendations for adolescents, the consumption of a varied diet remains the best assurance of adequate and safe intake levels of nutrients.

FACTORS THAT INFLUENCE FOOD HABITS

- *Describe the eating habits of teenagers.*
- *How does psychologic development influence dietary patterns?*
- *What social factors influence the food choices and nutrition status of teens?*
- *How does knowledge of nutrition science affect dietary intake?*

The eating patterns of adolescents are complex, influenced by an array of interwoven factors (Figure 11-9). These influences on food behavior are environmental (family, peers, models, and sociocultural factors) and personal (individual physiologic needs, development of self-concept, and food preferences). The food habits of adolescents are important not only in ensuring an adequate diet to support growth and development, but also in developing lifelong patterns for maintenance of health.

Eating Practices of Teenagers

The dietary habits of adolescents reflect those of the population in general. As adolescents make the transition to adulthood, their dietary intakes become less consistent because of busy schedules, the search for self-identity and peer group acceptance, and preoccupation with body weight, shape, appearance, or athletic prowess. Almost all schools' health education and science classes include some nutrition (Grunbaum et al., 1998) and most teenagers know what constitutes a good diet. For a teenager, eating the recommended number of servings from the groups in the Food Guide Pyramid may have low priority. Dieting, skipping meals, snacking, eating away from home, consuming fast foods, trying unconventional diets, and attempting to gain or lose weight are characteristic food behaviors among adolescents that relate to their physical, emotional, and social development. In many ways today's teens have many options for food choices and more responsibility for their own diets. Neumark-Sztainer and her coworkers (1999) have used focus groups with teenagers to study factors influencing food choices of adolescents and have identified general categories (Table 11-5).

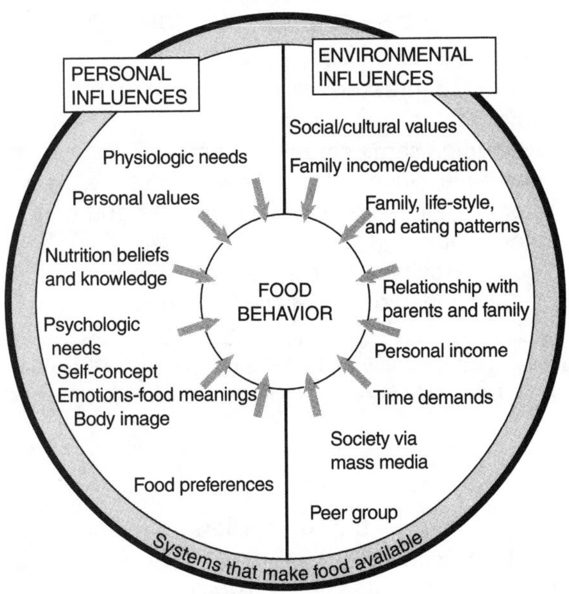

Figure 11-9 Illustration of factors that act in concert to influence the food behavior of adolescents.

Teenagers As Food Consumers

Traditionally mothers have been the gatekeepers of the family's diet, making shopping decisions and planning meals. With working mothers and single-parent families, many teens have become increasingly responsible for buying their own food and often that for the family as well. The Rand Youth Poll (1998), which surveys about 2700 teenagers semiannually, estimates that teenagers spent $48.8 billion in grocery stores in 1997, more than 10% of the total grocery industry sales. One half of the teenagers surveyed by Teen-Age Research Unlimited said they went to a grocery store at least once a week and 61% prepare a meal for themselves weekly and many prepare meals for younger siblings and whole families. Most buy their own breakfast and lunch plus snacks each day.

Responding to this transition in family food-buying patterns, many manufacturers and advertisers have targeted teenage food consumers with youth-focused advertising, web sites, and school promotions. Teenagers have food tastes ranging widely from pasta to pizza to sweet-and-sour chicken. They are becoming important buyers of "finished foods," one of the most rapidly growing sectors in North American supermarkets. Interviews with teenagers nationwide (Rand Youth Poll, 1998) depicted a generation of savvy shoppers who scoff at product hype and who are snack hungry, brand loyal, and drawn to familiar foods. Most buy on impulse, but are price conscious and want foods that they think taste good.

Table 11-5 FACTORS ADOLESCENTS VIEW AS INFLUENCING THEIR FOOD CHOICES

General Categories*	Subcategories and/or Description
LEVEL 1: FACTORS PERCEIVED AS MOST IMPORTANT	
Hunger/food cravings	Eating because of hunger or craving for a specific food
Appeal of food (primarily taste)	Taste/familiarity with food; appearance; smell; how food is prepared or served; temperature of food; if foods "go together"; variety
Time	Amount of time adolescent has or wants to spend on food; amount of time parents have (e.g., work schedules)
Convenience	Fast and easy to make (e.g., cereal) or get (e.g., fast food); easy to take with them on the bus or in a backpack; easy to obtain (home delivery or drive-through); don't have to wash dishes or clean up
LEVEL 2: FACTORS OF SECONDARY IMPORTANCE	
Availability	Food available and/or served in home (see "parent influence"), school (school lunch and vending machines), and region of country
Parent influence	Eating and cooking behaviors of parents: foods parents buy (or do not buy); rules surrounding eating/meals; parental concern about foods children eat; family meal patterns; overall parent-child relations; culture/religion of family
Perceived benefits	Get energy (to succeed in school or sports); influence body shape/condition (e.g., to look better or succeed at sports); feel full; be healthy; keep from feeling hungry or sick because of hunger
The situation	Who they are with (e.g., friends or family); what they are doing (e.g., teenage party or family event); when it is (e.g., time of day, season); where they are (e.g., nice restaurant or fast-food place)
LEVEL 3: FACTORS PERCEIVED AS LESS IMPORTANT (BUT COULD BE PRIMARY FACTORS FOR SOME STUDENTS)	
Mood	Eat differently when bored, depressed, stressed, or mad
Body image	Concerns about being too fat, skinny, or short
Habit	Eating as part of routine (e.g., same cereal in morning)
Cost	How much money they have; price of food; how much they want to spend (spend vs. save beliefs); parents' willingness and ability to spend money on food
Media	Discussed fast-food commercials and how good food looks
Vegetarian life-style	Some adolescents follow a vegetarian life-style for various reasons

Adapted from Neumark-Sztainer et al.: Factors influencing food choices of adolescents: findings from focus-group discussions with adolescents, J Am Diet Assoc 99:933, 1999.
*Listed in descending order by frequency discussed by youth.

According to students who participated in focus groups about nutrition, "junk food" tastes better than "health food" and is less expensive. In support of their claims, students reasoned they could purchase a popular combination meal at a fast food restaurant for less than they could purchase a healthful sandwich, salad, and milk (Neumark-Sztainer et al., 1999).

A study of 14 school stores of the San Diego County public middle schools with food merchandise stores reached similar conclusions regarding the importance of taste and price in food adolescent food choices (Wildey et al., 2000). All of these stores were open before and after schools and eight stores were open during lunch hours. Approximately 47% of the more than 1000 students returning questionnaires made food purchases from the store at least once every week. Analysis of food sold during the 1-week assessment period revealed 88.5% were snacks high in fat, sugar, or both. On average, students consumed 8.7 g fat and 23 g sugar per snack. Additionally 40% of all beverages sold were classified as soft drinks.

Eating Away from Home

Teenagers can obtain food from many places. Many earn their own money and can buy food they prefer to eat and discard foods they don't like. Adolescents often eat away from home. Sources of food include schools, fast food establishments, restaurants, vending machines, concessions at sporting events and movies, friends' houses, and ready-to-eat convenience foods and snacks from almost anywhere.

In the past three decades fast foods have become popular with most segments of the American population, but they have special appeal for teenagers. According to the Forecast Magazine Survey (1998), 75% of teens eat at fast food restaurants. Because it is relatively inexpensive, fast food fits into the budget of an adolescent. The menu items are well accepted and can be eaten with a minimum of utensils. In addition fast food restaurants provide a casual environment where teens feel comfortable.

A major criticism of fast food restaurants is the fact that their menu items tend to be calorically dense, high in fat and sodium, and low in fiber. In addition they may be low in several vitamins and minerals, including vitamins A and C, calcium, riboflavin, and folate.

Table 11-6 lists the nutrient, caloric, fat, saturated fat, cholesterol, and sodium content of menu items from several fast food restaurant chains. Some of these foods, such as Big Macs, chicken tenders, crispy chicken breasts, and tacos contain as much as 50% of kilocalories from fat. Fortunately many restaurants have begun to offer salads and sandwiches and yogurt sundaes with lower fat content. Although they are lower in fat, such items can still provide more than 30% of their kilocalories as fat. A salad can be low in kilocalories and fat, but adding dressings, croutons, bacon bits, cheese, ham, and eggs can increase the fat content greatly. For example a chef salad with many of these items provides 47% of its energy from fat. Given the prominent place of fast foods in the diet, it is important to encourage teens to make nutritious choices and to lobby the food industry to continue to offer more foods that are high in nutrient density and low in fat, sugar, and sodium.

Snacks and Meals

Only 21% of the adolescents interviewed in the Rand Youth Poll (1998) reported eating three meals a day. A study of breakfast consumption patterns of a national sample of adolescents aged 15 to 18 years defined breakfast as the consumption of food, beverage, or both (Seega-Riz et al., 1998). Based on that definition, 25% of boys and 35% of girls skipped breakfast. These researchers observed that although fewer teens are eating breakfast, the nutrition quality of foods consumed at breakfast has improved with the use of low-fat milk products. Of 711 ninth grade students in New Orleans, 14% of the boys and 23% of the girls skipped breakfast. Within ethnic groups 36% of nonwhite students and 20% of white girls skipped breakfast (Nicklas et al., 2000).

For many Americans and adolescents in particular, snacks have become the fourth daily meal. Snacking contributes significant amounts of energy and nutrients, particularly for adolescents (Jahns et al., 2001). Based on the USDA's nationally representative survey of adolescents, Zizza and colleagues (2001) reported a snacking prevalence of 84% among teens age 15 years to 18 years, and those snacks contributed 29% of total daily energy intake.

Over 90% of teenagers eat between meals (U.S. Department of Health and Human Services [USDHHS], 1991). Table 11-7 lists the nutrient content of some popular snack foods. Those low in fat are italicized. Snacking can be a liability, an asset, or a necessity, depending on the needs and choices of the adolescent. Many adolescents,

Table 11-6 ENERGY, FAT, SATURATED FAT, CHOLESTEROL, AND SODIUM OF SELECTED FAST FOOD ITEMS

Food Item	Serving Size	Energy (kcal)	Fat (g)	% kcal from Fat	Cholesterol (mg)	Sodium (mg)
Big Mac (McDonalds)		560	31	50	86	1070
French Fries (McDonalds)	medium	450	22	44	0	290
Onion Rings (Burger King)	medium	380	19	45	2	550
Chicken Tenders (Burger King)	8	350	22	57	65	940
Crispy Chicken Breast (KFC)	1	470	28	53	80	930
BBQ Chicken Sandwich (KFC)	1	256	8	29	57	782
6 inch Deep Dish Pizza (Domino's Pizza)	1 whole	595	27.5	41.5	23.5	1300
Taco (Taco Bell)	1	180	10	50	25	330
Burrito Supreme (Taco Bell)	1	440	19	39	35	1230
Veggie Fajita Wrap	1	420	19	40.5	20	980
Pita, Chicken Caeser (Wendy's)	1	490	18	34	65	1320
1 Baked Potato with Broccoli & Cheese (Wendy's)		470	14	28	5	470
Frosty Dairy Dessert (Wendy's)	small	330	8	24	35	200
Veggie Lover's Hand Tossed Pizza (Pizza Hut)	1 slice	240	7	25	20	650

Table 11-7 NUTRIENT CONTENT OF POPULAR SNACK FOODS

Item	Serving Size	Energy (kcal)	Protein (g)	Carbohydrate (g)	Fat (g)	Sodium (mg)
BREAKFAST DRINKS						
Instant Breakfast drink in skim milk	1 oz	130	7	23	1	136
CAKE						
Angel food	2 oz	142	4	32	0	142
Chocolate cupcake	1 oz	130	2	21	5	120
Yellow cake with icing	2 oz	268	3	40	11	191

Snacks low in fat are italicized.

Table 11-7 NUTRIENT CONTENT OF POPULAR SNACK FOODS—CONT'D

Item	Serving Size	Energy (kcal)	Protein (g)	Carbohydrate (g)	Fat (g)	Sodium (mg)
CANDY						
Caramels/chocolate	1 oz	115	1	22	3	74
Chocolate-coated peanuts	1 oz	160	5	11	12	19
Fudge	1 oz	115	1	21	3	54
M&Ms	1.5 oz	220	3	31	10	—
Jellybeans	10			17		1
Hard candy	1 oz	110		28		9
CEREALS						
Cheerios	1 c	88	3	16	1	246
Bran Chex	1 c	156	5	39	1	455
Corn Flakes	1 c	88	2	20		281
Trix	1 c	108	1.5	25		179
Product 19	1 c	126	3	27		378
Lucky Charms	1 c	125	2	26	1	227
COOKIES						
Chocolate chip	1	50	0.5	7	2	38
Oatmeal raisin	1	62	0.7	9	3	37
Chocolate cookie sandwich	1	50	0.5	7	2	63
CRACKERS						
Ritz	10	180		20	10	320
Cheddar snacks	10	70	1.5	11	2.5	140
Graham	4 (1 oz)	120	2	22	3.5	128
Wheat Thins	10	90	1	12	3.5	—
Saltines	5	63	1	10	1	185
ICE CREAM						
10% fat	1 c	269	4	32	14	116
2% fat	1 c	223	8	38	5	163
SHERBET						
2% fat	1 c	270	2	59	4	88
YOGURT						
Lowfat	1 c	144	13	16	2	159
Nonfat	1 c	127	13	17	0.5	174
POPCORN						
Light butter	6 c	150	0	25	7	310
Plain-air popped	5 c	125	5	25	0	
SOUP						
Cream of mushroom	1 c	203	6	15	14	1076
Vegetarian vegetable	1 c	72	2	12	2	823
Chicken noodle	1 c	75	4	9	2	1107
Tomato	1 c	86	2	16	2	872

especially those who are growing rapidly and are physically active, have high energy needs that require high-calorie snacks. For others with lower energy requirements, snacks can have a negative impact on the diet if they replace needed nutrient-dense foods. When chosen wisely and consumed in moderation, however, snacks can improve the adolescent's overall dietary intake and may, indeed, be essential for an adequate diet. Box 11-1 lists some nutritious snack food alternatives that are low in fat, sugar, and sodium.

Factors That Influence Food Behavior

Successful transition from childhood to adulthood is contingent on the interplay of physical, psychologic, and social forces. For example adolescents' characteristic repeated attempts to change their physical appearance and body shape to emulate a perceived desirable image is not simply a desire to conform to social and peer expectations, but the result of the struggle to integrate the physical changes of puberty into a stable body-image and self-image and to establish individuality and autonomy.

Box 11-1 Examples of Nutrient-Dense, Low-Fat Snack Foods

- 1%, 0.5% low-fat or skim milk
- Low-fat cheese, low-fat or nonfat yogurt
- Fresh or unsweetened fruits
- Raw vegetables
- Fruit juices or vegetable juices
- Pretzels, air-popped popcorn, bagels, baked tortilla chips
- Sandwiches: turkey, lean roast beef, lean ham, low-fat cold cuts, low-fat cheese, water-packed tuna with reduced-fat mayonnaise or salad dressing, peanut butter and jelly
- Hamburger/sloppy joes made with ground turkey
- Chicken tacos, enchiladas, bean burritos made with low-fat cheese
- Pizza with vegetables and low-fat cheese
- Frozen low-fat or nonfat yogurt, ice milk, sherbet, frozen fruit bars, fruit sorbets, pudding made with skim milk, commercial fat-free pudding

Psychologic Influences

Self-concept. Self-concept includes attributes an individual perceives he or she possesses and the perception of how others view him or her. Self-esteem, a facet of self-concept, involves perception of one's position in the social structure and how one sees himself or herself as a social object. Self-concept encompasses self-perceived attributes of physical appearance (including body image), personality features, and moral characteristics. Adolescents struggle to varying degrees to establish their own self-concept. Self-concept is one factor that can be a significant influence on eating patterns and, thus, on nutrient intakes (Pesa, 1999) (see Research Update box).

Body image. Approximately two thirds of adolescent girls report they are dissatisfied with their weight and slightly more than one half are dissatisfied with the shape of their bodies (Moore, 1993). These percentages increase as body weight increases. African-American girls are less likely to consider themselves overweight than are white or Hispanic girls (Serdula et al., 1993). Specific concerns of girls are perceived excess size of their thighs, hips, waist, and buttocks. Boys are more likely to be satisfied with their body weight, but approximately one third of boys expressed dissatisfaction with their body shape, desiring to appear strong and muscular, particularly in the upper body (Moore, 1993). Adolescents who attempt to lose weight or who struggle to maintain weight are not necessarily overweight by usual standards, but perceive themselves as overweight (Emmons, 1994). Such teens tend to have poorer body images and self-esteem than do those who are satisfied with their body weight and shape (Allen et al., 1993).

Emotional development. Eating habits have an emotional basis. Individuals eat not only because they are hungry, but also to fulfill myriad social and psychologic needs. Eating when lonely or bored or when treating oneself to special food as a reward are simple examples of the emotional use of food. More complex manifestations include denial of hunger or overeating associated with stress or anxiety, which can interfere with nutritional well-being. Adolescents become prone to

Research Update

*Self-Esteem, Body Image, and Food Habits of Adolescents**

Dietary intake during adolescence profoundly affects health, growth, and development of life-long eating behaviors. Relationships between nutrition and overall health are well recognized within the health and medical professions and yet nutrition principles have not been well received by adolescents.

A study by Custatis and Shannon (1996) found that, on average, students achieved a 46.6% adherence to Food Guide Pyramid recommendations. Both male and female students met recommendations for meat consumption and male students met recommendations for dairy food. Average intake of dairy products by female students was 80% of recommendations. Both groups fell short in terms of fruit, vegetable, and grain consumption. Sugar and fat consumption, however, were substantial among both male and female students (Custatis and Shannon, 1996).

Substantial data indicate that nutrition knowledge does not influence eating patterns of teenagers. Martin and colleagues (1999) reported that 43% of 630 adolescents surveyed exhibited anomalous eating behaviors, such as food restriction or bingeing accompanied by compensatory actions. Students with anomalous eating behaviors and those with normal eating behavior performed equally well on a questionnaire evaluating nutrition knowledge.

It does appear, however, that adolescent eating and general health behaviors are influenced by numerous personal and environmental factors (Custatis and Shannon, 1996). Personal factors include attitudes and beliefs toward nutrition, exercise, health, body image, and self-esteem. Environmental factors consist of factors forming the context in which behaviors take place. These include family structure, peer influences, school and community activities, and body size. Neumark-Sztainer and colleagues (1999) studied 141 male and female adolescents in 21 focus groups. Students were asked what they perceived as barriers to following recommended dietary guidelines. Students consistently expressed concern regarding time restraints. Eating healthy foods did not rank highly enough for it to gain their attention. Furthermore, many students felt they were too young to worry about their health, stating they will worry about nutrition issues when they are older and physically affected by declining health.

It is normal for adolescents to be self-conscious about or dissatisfied with their changing bodies. A society that emphasizes slimness and the bombardment of advertising that promises thinner thighs and slimmer waists or bigger muscles and a wonderful body creates a standard to which teenagers compare themselves, no matter how unrealistic the standard may be. An acute sense of how their bodies differ from the "ideal" may wreak havoc on adolescents' self-esteem. Girls are particularly prone to thinking obsessively about the shape of their bodies, but boys are not immune. In general girls desire thinner bodies, especially in the hips and thighs, and boys wish for larger, more muscular upper bodies.

Self-esteem is made up of two elements important to food behaviors and body satisfaction (Harter and Rosenberg, 1990). These include how a person believes others of importance view her or him and how a person performs a task viewed as personally important.

Self-esteem, body image, and eating behaviors are intertwined for female adolescents. Self-esteem was one of several components examined by the National Longitudinal Study of Adolescent Health, a study designed to collect data regarding social and physical factors affecting adolescents. Pesa's (1999) report on a subset of this data found a link between self-esteem and eating behaviors. Of the 2536 adolescent girls responding to questionnaires, 56% indicated unspecified eating disturbances. Within this group 43% were classified as having low self-esteem.

It is a concern that, in response to low self-esteem or low body image, many adolescents alter eating behaviors and develop unhealthy, disordered eating patterns. For example, in a questionnaire-centered study, Martin and colleagues (1999) examined body dissatisfaction; the use of a strict, slimming diet; and media and peer influence on disordered eating patterns. Among girls exhibiting altered eating patterns, only 17.7% were moderately or aesthetically obese, 26.8% were underweight, and

*This Research Update was contributed by Christine Kendle, MS.

Continued

Research Update

Self-Esteem, Body Image, and Food Habits of Adolescents—cont'd

55.4% were of an appropriate weight. The altered eating behavior was not justified by a real need to lose weight. Distorted body image was strongly related to eating patterns as evidenced by the increased number of times subjects with altered eating behaviors reported to view themselves in mirrors as opposed to individuals with normal eating behaviors. Custatis and Shannon (1996) found students' confidence in their abilities to be negatively correlated with their consumption of high-sugar snacks. These findings suggest that students who exhibit positive personal beliefs make healthier nutrition choices.

Adolescents' eating behaviors not only affect their current health status, but also result in future health implications. Therefore it becomes important to further investigate personal and societal factors influencing adolescents' food choices to implement educational programs to meet the needs of this vulnerable group.

these behaviors as they struggle to establish emotional independence.

Social Influences

Culture. Each individual requires the same nutrients to meet physiologic needs, yet the foods that are consumed to supply these nutrients are as different as the environments in which people live. It is very likely that each person cherishes a certain food, combination of foods, meal, or foods associated with a celebration from the past. Often these foods represent special occasions or memories of special events that relate to our personal culture. Often they are in the context of a larger culture. Culture represents the way in which people have adapted to their environment and reflects national, ethnic, and religious backgrounds and geographic, social, and economic environments. A composite of these factors provides the background against which adolescents eventually form their individual food habits. (See Appendix for summary of cultural influences on food habits.)

Family. Throughout childhood the family is the predominant influence on food habits and lifetime eating patterns. The family mediates a child's food behavior in two essential ways. The first, and most obvious, is the direct influence of the family as the main provider of food. The second, which shapes lifetime eating habits, is the influence exerted through the transmission of food attitudes, preferences, and patterns. Superimposed on this influence is the emotional component of food as a channel for interpersonal communication of love, approval, or even disapproval. These influences can have a positive or negative impact on food-related behavior.

The family can be an important unit for promoting healthy food habits and positive family relationships are associated with the acceptance of a wide variety of foods. Teens who eat with their families regularly usually have more nutritious diets than those who eat alone or with friends. During adolescence the child in each individual struggles to become an adult. This transition becomes evident in eating patterns, as the teen rejects (usually temporarily) family food traditions or preferences and seeks to assert his or her own autonomy. Difficulties during this transition are exaggerated by disordered family relationships. Adolescents whose parents are authoritarian and structured in relation to food patterns may use food to express rebellion against parental authority. Permissive parents and situations in which there is a breakdown in family relationships give teens little guidance with respect to eating and may consequently foster poor eating habits.

Peers. During adolescence the peer group defines what is socially acceptable and determines behavior standards. It is commonly assumed that adolescents are strongly influenced by the eating habits of their peers, but there is little research to support or contradict this assumption (Farthing, 1991). However, adolescents spend a lot of time with friends and eating is an important part of their recreation and socialization. In a group context, at least, it appears that foods may be selected to meet the approval of the peer group. For example many young adolescent girls who like and drink milk at home may choose to consume soft drinks when they are spending time with their friends.

Mass media. The extent to which adolescent food choices are influenced by the mass media is difficult to document. Today's adolescents have grown up in a time when mass media, through advertising and programming, have promoted the desirability of slim, trim, beautiful bodies and the fun and luxury of good eating. Prominent among foods promoted for good eating are soft drinks, fast foods, and other foods high in calories and fat and low in fiber. Although adolescents are better able to deal with the apparent contradictions between slimness and high-energy foods than are younger children, a lifetime of television viewing may have blunted their tendency to question the contradiction. In addition the physical, emotional, and social transitions of adolescence make adolescents especially susceptible to certain advertising, such as advertisements featuring weight control programs, diet aids, and bodybuilding products.

Financial Status

The increased nutrition needs of adolescents translate into a demand for a greater quantity of food. This can stress the family budget. Because today's adolescents eat at home less often than do adolescents in previous years, those with limited financial resources may find they are restricted in the amount of food they can afford or the food choices they can make when eating out. For example a teenager may be able to afford to buy lunch in the school cafeteria, but not to join friends at fast food establishments or restaurants.

The School Lunch Program provides free or reduced-cost lunches for youngsters from low-income families. It is important that such programs, if they are to be successful, provide not only nutritious meals, but also meals that are acceptable to the adolescent. Often families of children who receive free lunches are eligible to receive additional assistance through the use of food stamps. Dollar amounts allotted for food stamps are based on the USDA's food plans, which estimate the cost of food prepared at home. Although food stamps increase the availability of food to a family, the level of support is insufficient to afford "eating out."

Time pressures. In the hectic life of the typical teenager, the biggest obstacle to meeting nutrition needs may be making time to eat. A lunch period when both time and food are available is scheduled at school, but there are no guarantees that teens will use that opportunity to eat or, if they do eat, that they will make nutritious choices. After-school activities, sports, and employment create demands that interfere with regular eating patterns. Many teens may not eat until they arrive home hours after school is over. Possible solutions to this problem, such as packing an additional lunch at home to be eaten after school and planning ahead for nutritious snack alternatives, may be limited by time and financial resources.

NUTRITION-RELATED CONCERNS OF ADOLESCENCE

- *Beyond achieving a nutritionally adequate diet to support growth, what are the areas of concern related to nutrition for adolescents?*
- *How does nutrition relate to control of acne in teenagers?*
- *What role does nutrition play in the prevention of chronic disease in adolescence?*

Adolescence is a relatively healthy period of life, but because of the dramatic physical and lifestyle changes, teenagers often worry that something is wrong or will go wrong. Their concerns often relate to appearance, body image, and body weight. The increased physiologic demands of stresses, such as pregnancy and athletic performance, can place them at nutritional risk. It is important for their diets to provide a sound foundation to meet the demands during adolescence and to foster eating patterns and practices that will sustain them well into a healthy adulthood and even into old age.

Adolescent Pregnancy

In the United States, birth rates have consistently declined for all girls of reproductive age except those under 15 years of age, making adolescent pregnancy a major public health concern. Although pregnancy is a normal physiologic state, there are increased maternal, fetal, and neonatal risks for pregnant teens who are still growing. The nutrition status of the pregnant adolescent is influenced by the psychologic and social factors discussed in this chapter. In fact these factors may actually contribute to increased risk through poor dietary habits and inadequate weight gain. (Adolescent pregnancy is discussed in detail in Chapter 5.)

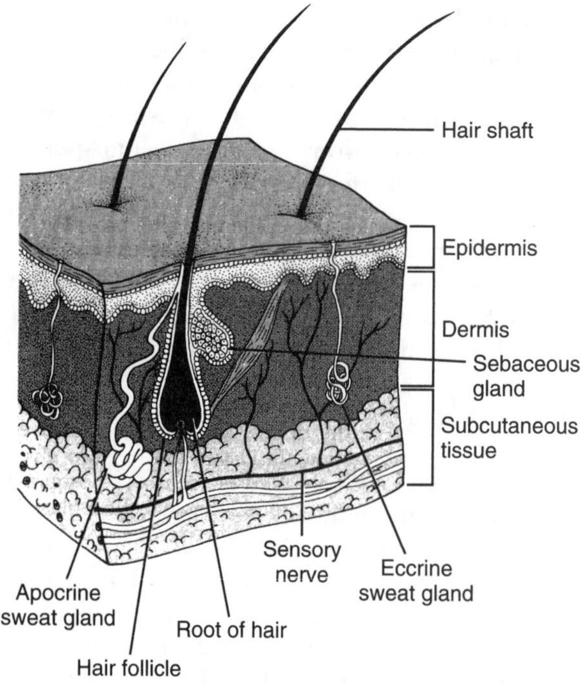

Figure 11-10 A pilosebaceous unit. *(From Betz CL et al.: Family-centered nursing care of children, ed 2, Philadelphia, 1994, WB Saunders.)*

Acne

Through the generations acne has been a scourge for teenagers. During no other time of life is appearance so important for self-esteem and peer acceptance. The face, the primary focus in determining attractiveness, is also a primary site of pilosebaceous follicles, the source of the blackheads and pimples known as acne vulgaris.

Acne is a disease of the pilosebaceous unit in the skin. This unit is made up of a hair follicle and a sebaceous gland, which are connected to the surface of the skin by a duct through which the hair passes (Figure 11-10). The sebaceous gland produces sebum, which helps keep the skin and the hair moist. Sebum also carries cells shed by the glands to the surface of the skin, a process called follicular keratinization. Pilosebaceous units are found all over the body, but they are more common on the face, upper chest, and back, which explains why acne usually occurs in these places.

Development

Acne develops when the sebaceous glands produce increased amounts of sebum, making the skin oilier. In the anaerobic depths of the sebaceous follicle, sebum provides a substrate for bacteria, resulting in the production of a wide variety of antigenic substances that induce an immune response such as inflammation. In response, cells stick together to form a thick layer that blocks the duct. As more cells and sebum pile up behind this layer, a compact plug called a comedo is formed.

If the sebum and accumulated cells remain below the skin surface, a "closed" comedo, or "white head," forms. If the orifice of a closed comedo dilates, the plug enlarges and pops out of the duct. This is called an "open" comedo, or "blackhead." The discoloration is from a buildup of melanin, the dark pigment in skin. If the wall of a closed comedo ruptures and releases its contents into the dermis, an inflammatory lesion results.

Approximately 80% of all teenagers develop some form of acne with the onset of puberty. The exact cause is unknown, but heredity and androgens that stimulate sebaceous glands are contributing factors. Boys are usually more severely affected than are girls. However, attractiveness has a greater impact on the social status of girls, so acne may be a greater concern for them. In girls, acne often worsens during the premenstrual period.

Most adolescents develop what is called noninflammatory acne, which usually involves the eruption of just a few blackheads or whiteheads every now and then. For some a more severe form, called inflammatory acne, causes a constant outbreak covering the face and sometimes the neck, back, chest, and groin. The pus-filled pimples and cysts can cause deep pitting and scarring.

For generations certain foods such as chocolate, nuts, cola drinks, potato chips, French fries, and other foods have been indicted in causing or exacerbating acne. No scientific evidence supports these claims, but some adolescents do notice that certain foods seem to increase their outbreaks. A nutritious, balanced diet is important for overall health of the adolescent, including the skin, to minimize the effects of acne.

Treatment

Mild acne can be controlled by washing the face once or twice daily. If these measures are ineffective, the next line of treatment is over-the-counter preparations that are applied directly to the skin. They may contain benzoyl peroxide, sulfur, resorcinol, or salicylic acid, all of which are approved by the Food and Drug Administration (FDA) for treating acne. Acne that does not respond to over-the-counter preparations requires medical consultation. Prescription drugs include both topical and oral antibiotics, such as tetracycline and erythromycin, and a derivative of vitamin A, tretinoin (Retin-A), that comes in cream, gel, or liquid form. Because tretinoin is applied externally, there appears to be no danger of toxicity.

A small percentage of adolescents and young adults develop deep **subcutaneous**, severe cystic acne, which can cause scarring. These individuals can be treated with another derivative of vitamin A. **Isotretinoin**, 13-cis-retinoic acid, known commercially as Accutane, is approved for the treatment of severe cystic acne (Committee on Drugs, 1992). Accutane is administered orally, usually over a period of 15 weeks to 20 weeks, until the total cyst count is decreased by 70%. Use of this drug is associated with a reduction in sebaceous gland size and a 75% to 90% decrease in sebum excretion. A course of treatment usually results in significant clearing of acne lesions and prolonged remission often follows.

However, isotretinoin is a potent human **teratogen.** If administered during pregnancy, it can result in serious congenital anomalies in the offspring (Lammer et al., 1985). Exposure to isotretinoin during embryosis produces defects in the central nervous system (e.g., hydrocephalus, microcephaly, microphthalmia), ears (e.g., microtia, anotia), and cardiovascular system and other abnormalities. Even exposed infants who have no external abnormalities show subnormal intelligence and other neuropsychologic impairments (Adams, 1990). Therefore Accutane is prescribed with caution for any female acne sufferer and is prescribed for any sexually active girl or woman only if dependable contraceptive protection is available.

Overweight Status and Obesity

Data on body mass index and triceps fatfold thicknesses obtained from national surveys indicate that between 15% and 25% of American adolescents are obese. The National Health Objectives, *Healthy People 2000* includes as one of its goals the reduction of overweight status to a prevalence of no more than 15% among adolescents age 12 years through 19 years, to be accomplished through sound dietary practices combined with regular physical activity. In addition there is evidence that anorexia nervosa, bulimia nervosa, and compulsive eating disorders are on the rise among adolescents. Eating disorders are discussed in Chapter 14 (Neumark-Sztainer, 1995).

KEY TERMS

subcutaneous: immediately beneath the skin
isotretinoin: 13-cis retinoic acid, a drug used to treat severe acne
teratogen: a substance that can cause physical defects in the developing embryo

This prevalence of eating disturbances is reflected in attitudes and eating behaviors of adolescents. Weight—too much or too little—is an actual or anticipated problem for many teenagers. For example the Youth Risk Behavior Survey, a national survey of health-risk behaviors of more than 11,000 students in grades 9 through 12, found that 44% of female students and 15% of male students were trying to lose weight (Serdula et al., 1993). An additional 26% of girls and 15% of boys reported they were trying to keep from gaining more weight. Preoccupation with body image, weight, or shape is apparent in adolescent behaviors, especially in weight control practices. Students in the Youth Risk Behavior Study reported using a variety of measures to control body weight, including exercising, skipping meals, taking diet pills, and inducing vomiting (Serdula et al., 1993). Chronic dieting is a risk factor for eating disorders (Neumark-Sztainer, 1995).

On the other hand many adolescents attempt to gain weight or increase muscle mass by using a variety of nutrient or food supplements, following highly restrictive diets, or engaging in rigorous physical training (aerobic or resistance exercise). To appear muscular and athletic, some teenagers may resort to taking **anabolic steroids** to stimulate muscle growth. Although these substances are controlled and require a prescription, 2.2% of high school students reported using steroids without a doctor's prescription (Kann et al., 1995). Although steroid pills are readily available on the black market to supply athletes, at least one fourth of high school boys are unaware of the health risks associated with anabolic steroid use (Wang et al., 1994). In the short term these drugs can cause problems such as fatigue, acne, **hirsutism**, and combative behavior (often referred to as " 'roid rages"). Long-term use increases the risk of early heart disease, osteoporosis, and liver tumors.

Physical Fitness

Despite the fact that more teenagers are participating in athletics, the overall fitness level of the entire adolescent population remains uncertain. Only 50% of adolescents regularly engage in vigorous physical activity (Centers for Disease Control, 2001). There is substantial evidence, however, that increased physical activity results in an improved level of fitness, lower body fat, and a more favorable lipid profile (Sutter and Hawes, 1993). The role of physical activity throughout the life span is discussed in Chapter 15.

Cardiovascular Disease

The prevalence of overweight adolescents in the United States and other developed countries has been rising over the past four decades (Troiano et al., 1995). Obesity at any age during childhood predicts obesity in adult life, but the predictive value of obesity in adolescence is higher than that in earlier childhood (Whitaker et al., 1997). Adolescent obesity is associated with cardiovascular risk factors, orthopedic conditions, lower self-esteem, and adverse social and economic outcomes in young adulthood (Gillman et al., 2001). Adolescent obesity predicts morbidity and mortality later in life. For these reasons, prevention is paramount.

Prevention

The adolescent years are often considered the healthiest in a person's life. Infectious childhood illnesses are in the past and it appears that chronic health problems of adulthood, particularly coronary heart disease (CHD), are in the distant future. Substantial evidence shows, however, that atherosclerosis or precursors of atherosclerosis have their origins in childhood and adolescence, progressing slowly into adulthood (Centers for Disease Control, 2001).

Fatty streaks are the earliest grossly visible lesions of the atherosclerotic process. Autopsy studies following untimely deaths of children, adolescents, and young adults (Strong, 1986) have revealed that fatty streaks appear in the coronary arteries and other blood vessels during early childhood and into the second decade of life. **Fibrous plaques**, the lesions that begin to narrow the arteries, appear in the coronary arteries of some young persons as early as the second decade. For youth and adults, blood levels of TC and LDL cholesterol are related to the development of early atherosclerotic lesions. There is evidence that identifying youngsters at risk of

CHD and preventing or reducing the effects of major risk factors (e.g., high blood lipid levels, hypertension, obesity, smoking, physical activity) can have long-term health benefits.

Atherosclerotic lesions are more prevalent in the arteries of adolescents who are obese or hypertensive or who smoke cigarettes (Newman et al., 1991) and loss of body weight is associated with a reduction of blood levels of the **atherogenic** factors (Wabitsch et al., 1994). Dietary intervention to reduce body weight and fat is more effective when exercise is included (Centers for Disease Control, 2001). In addition greater reductions in systolic and diastolic blood pressure occur in combined programs (Rocchini et al., 1993).

National Cholesterol Education Program

The Dietary Guidelines from the USDA and USDHHS, discussed in Chapter 1, are recommendations to promote healthy eating to decrease the long-term risk of disease. In addition the federally sponsored National Cholesterol Education Program (NCEP) has developed a two-phase approach to reduce the risk of CHD in children and adolescents. New NCEP guidelines for adults were released in 2000. These guidelines recommend more rigorous diagnostic criteria for recommending treatment and more aggressive treatment protocols. To date recommendations for children and adolescents are not available. However, it is reasonable to assume that detection and early treatment will be recommended for individuals with identified risk factors.

The guidelines can be implemented readily with moderation and common sense by selecting low-fat dairy products and protein alternatives that are low in total fat and saturated fat, such as poultry, fish, and legumes. Increasing the intake of fruits, vegetables, and whole-grain products can have the benefits of reducing fat in the diet and increasing fiber content. Introduction of low-fat nutrient-dense snack foods enhances nutritional adequacy (see Box 11-1). The more varied the diet, the more likely it is that a teenager's nutrient needs will be met. Analysis of diets of adolescents following these guidelines indicated that they do not compromise the level of micronutrients consumed (McPherson et al., 1990).

The American Heart Association recommends that children and adolescents who are identified as at increased risk for CHD make dietary changes to reduce total and saturated fat and increase physical activity (AHA, 2000).

PROMOTING POSITIVE FOOD HABITS

- *Why is it important to strive to improve the dietary intakes of adolescents?*
- *What are the long-term benefits of positive dietary habits in adolescents?*

Although many adolescents consume diets that approach nutritional adequacy, for a significant proportion, habitual intakes fall short of nutrient needs and dietary recommendations. Typical dietary patterns of adolescents are inconsistent with dietary guidelines. A national survey of dietary intakes of adolescents found that approximately 36% of calories came from fat and 13% from saturated fat (Kimm et al., 1990). Early results from NHANES III indicate that the percentages of energy from saturated fat were highest for those age 16 years to 19 years (Morbidity and Mortality Weekly Report, 1994). Because lifestyle habits observed in youth tend to persist over time, promotion of positive health and nutrition habits in adolescence seems to be warranted.

Creative approaches are needed to improve the overall health and nutrition status of adolescents. Effective nutrition education requires community-based support from parents, schools, healthcare professionals, and agencies to accomplish positive

KEY TERMS

anabolic steroids: synthetic versions of testosterone that stimulate muscle growth
hirsutism: abnormal or excessive body hair
fatty streaks: lipid accumulation on the intima (inside surface) of the artery
fibrous plaques: fatty streaks with an accumulation of connective tissue and various blood components
atherogenic: promote change that contributes to the development of atherosclerosis

changes in knowledge, attitudes, and behaviors. Late adolescence is a period when youngsters can consider possible consequences of their behaviors in making decisions about their dietary practices. The most effective changes occur when adolescents are armed with knowledge about nutrition and are in an environment in which standard or normative behaviors among their peers support sound health practices.

Some suggestions of how parents, teachers, and others who work with adolescents can deal with improving adolescent nutrition and fitness appear in Table 11-8. If changes are to be made, it is important to recognize the special emotional, physical, psychologic, and social needs of adolescents and to create programs that are sensitive and responsive to those needs.

Risk Behaviors in Adolescence

In the United States 73% of all deaths among school-age youth and young adults result from motor vehicle crashes, other unintentional injuries, homicide, and suicide. Results of the Youth Risk Behavior Surveillance System (YRBSS) suggest that many high school students practice behaviors that may increase the likelihood of death from these causes (Centers for Disease Control, 2000).

Adolescence is a critical period in initiation of risk behaviors, including substance use. Alcohol, tobacco, and marijuana are the most widely used substances among teenagers. The initiation of alcohol or tobacco use during adolescence often becomes the beginning of a lifetime pattern of substance use with negative consequences on health and longevity. Because the use of alcohol and tobacco usually precedes the use of illicit substances, the prevention of substance use and abuse is a primary public health concern.

A wide range of factors can influence risk behaviors by adolescents. For example Simons-Morton et al. (2001) found that smoking and drinking behaviors were associated with peer pressure and associating with friends who exhibit problem behaviors. Parent involvement, parent expectations, and parent regard had negative associations with smoking and drinking. On the other hand children from families that are too controlling or too lax and unsupportive tend to have more problems during adolescence. It is well documented that parental substance abuse predicts substance abuse in children (Biederman et al., 2000).

Tobacco

Cigarette smoking is the major preventable cause of premature disease and death in the United States. It has been causally linked to cancer, pulmonary disease, CHD, and a wide array of serious health consequences (Centers for Disease Control, 2000). Despite numerous anti-tobacco campaigns, smoking among adolescents continues to be a predominant public health issue (Hampl and Betts, 1999). Currently more than 3 million adolescents smoke cigarettes and more than 1 million, mostly boys, use smokeless tobacco (Centers for Disease Control, 2000). The good news is that a survey of 44,300 eighth, tenth, and twelfth grade students reports that there was a decline in prevalence of smoking among twelfth grade students from 36.5% in 1997 to 29.5% in 2001 (Institute for Social Research, 2001). Even greater decreases were found among eighth and tenth grade students.

Social factors, particularly having friends who smoke, are important in the early initiation of smoking by adolescents (Botvin et al., 1992). Other important determinants are perceived acceptability of smoking and intrapersonal factors such as self-efficacy and self-esteem (Bertrand and Abernathy, 1993). Compared with nonusers, students who use tobacco have lower self-image, are less independent and mature, are less involved with school and academic achievement, are of lower socioeconomic status, and have greater susceptibility to advertising and promotional activities (Lewis et al., 2001).

Active smoking during growth can reduce the rate of lung growth and the maximum level of lung function attained. Compared with nonsmokers, young smokers are more likely to experience shortness of breath, coughing spells, wheezing, and overall diminished physical health. Long-term health consequences of smoking are a function of the duration (years) and the intensity (amount) of use. Nicotine is highly addictive and initiating smoking at an early age increases the

Table 11-8 Nutrition Issues and Possible Alternatives for Adolescents

Current Issues	Personal Alternatives	Alternatives for Home	Supportive School/Community Activities
Improving overall diet quality	Encourage teens to seek food options that have greater nutrient density; especially low-fat dairy products, fruits and vegetables, and whole grains. Teach teen to use the food label in making food selections.	Have teen participate in food buying and food preparation.	Incorporate nutrition education throughout curriculum. Support group activities that promote positive life-style changes. Encourage student advocacy model for students related to promotion of more healthy food and physical activity options.
Consumption of high-fat snacks of low nutrient density	Teach teen how to make more healthful food choices in buying food and snacks in fast-food establishments, food markets and stores, and school cafeteria. Make teen aware of nutrient content information for fast-food items.	Make nutritious easy-to-prepare snack foods available. Make foods that are portable or of low caloric density available. Model family food habits. Discuss a role for fast-food choices in the diet.	Make nutritious food snacks available to students through school food service and snack bar/store. Assist teens in deciphering nutrition information in the media and on the web.
Limited time for food selection/preparation	Make more nutritious snack alternatives available. Develop a plan for serving-size foods or snacks that can be heated and eaten quickly. Select nutritious ready-to-eat products when shopping.	Have family members share in responsibility for meal and snack preparation. Plan simple meals that require little preparation.	Make nutritious food options available through school food service. Ensure that students eligible for free or reduced price meals can participate in the program.
Excess body weight, increasing body weight	Encourage increased physical activity via walking, climbing steps, social activities. Limit sedentary activities such as watching television, computer games, video games. Select foods of low caloric density.	Family members participate in activities with teen. Provide balanced diets that are moderate in fats and sugar. Make snacks and foods available that are of low caloric density, but increase nutrients such as fruits and vegetables, low fat dairy products, and whole grain products.	Provide opportunities for physical activity in class situations and in extracurricular activities. Encourage group activities. Provide the opportunity for students to purchase school meals/snacks of high nutrient density, but moderate calories.
Improving levels of physical fitness	Encourage participation in regular physical activity appropriate for fitness and skill level.	Provide physically active role models. Exercise with teen. Provide transportation and support for teen to participate in activities that will improve fitness. Emphasize the importance of physical activity to health.	Provide quality physical education classes with a physical education specialist to teach them. Provide physically active role models. Provide access to school buildings and community facilities that enhance safe participation in physical activity. Provide a range of extracurricular programs in schools and common recreation centers to meet needs and interests of specific adolescent populations.

probability of being an adult smoker. Adolescent use of tobacco increases the life years of exposure and possibly the intensity, thereby attenuating the risk of serious health consequences.

Cigarette smoke is a complex mixture of more than 4000 chemicals including free radicals and teratogenic and carcinogenic agents. Antioxidants may have a protective effect against oxidative damage in the plasma and tissues. Smokers are likely to have low levels of antioxidants, specifically vitamins C and E. Kallner and colleagues (1981) suggest that the vitamin C requirement for smokers should be 140 mg per day, but even this level may be inadequate to prevent the oxidative damage that results from cigarette smoke. A comparison of the nutrient content of diets of smokers and nonsmokers suggests that smokers have lower intakes of fiber, vitamins, and minerals. Both cigarette smokers and users of smokeless (chewing) tobacco have lower plasma levels of vitamins C and E (Giraud et al., 1995).

Tobacco is often considered a gateway drug because it is generally the first drug used by young people in a sequence that can include alcohol, marijuana, and other illicit drugs. It has been reported that 85% of adolescents admitted to substance treatment facilities were smokers (Myers and Brown, 1994). In fact there is a strong dose-dependent relationship between smoking and the use of alcohol and illicit drugs.

Smokeless (chewing) tobacco use has become popular with both school-age children and adolescents. Use of smokeless tobacco has been reported by more than 10% of high school students, most of whom were male (Centers for Disease Control, 1992). Health consequences of chewing tobacco range from halitosis to periodontal degeneration, soft tissue lesions, and various forms of oral cancer. Smokeless tobacco use is as addictive as cigarette smoking and users are likely to become cigarette smokers.

Because tobacco use by young people has substantial implications for long-term health, two of the national health-promotion and disease-prevention objectives for the year 2000 are related to tobacco use in young people.

Alcohol Use and Abuse

Although ethanol provides 7 kcal/g, it is not considered a nutrient. Beverages that contain alcohol provide few nutrients, if any, and displacement of food calories by alcohol calories reduces the total nutrient intake, even if caloric intake is the same or increased.

Ethanol is rapidly absorbed from the gastrointestinal tract. About 20% is absorbed through the lining of the stomach; the remainder enters the duodenum and, when absorbed, is carried via the portal vein to the liver. Alcohol dehydrogenase, the enzyme required for the oxidation of ethanol, converts ethanol to acetaldehyde. Acetaldehyde is metabolized to acetyl coenzyme A (CoA), which enters the tricarboxylic acid cycle to provide energy.

In the liver alcohol is metabolized preferentially (i.e., before carbohydrate and fat), but the rate of metabolism is limited by the availability of alcohol dehydrogenase. About 1 ounce of ethanol can be oxidized every 2 hours. When ethanol ingestion exceeds the amount that can be metabolized, ethanol enters the general circulation, reaching the brain, where it can influence the function of brain cells.

Small amounts of ethanol induce a sense of euphoria, the effect drinkers seek. The blood level of ethanol after two to three drinks increases to 0.05%, reducing inhibitions, restraint, and judgment. This level can double to 0.10% with four to five drinks and continue to rise to a level of 0.30, which is associated with stupor. Large amounts of ethanol depress the motor area of the brain, impairing muscle coordination, reflexes, speech, and auditory and visual discrimination.

The long-term consequences of alcohol abuse can affect nearly every organ. In the liver, the major site of alcohol metabolism, the influx of large amounts of ethanol over time changes glucose, fat, and protein metabolism. Prolonged abuse results in a "fatty liver" because of decreased fat oxidation, increased fatty acid synthesis, and mobilization of fat from body stores. In the early stages of alcohol abuse, fat accumulation can be reversed by abstinence from alcohol, but with prolonged abuse, liver cells become damaged and replaced by fibrous tissue, leading to cirrhosis.

Alcohol abuse is associated with reduced food intake, leading to malnutrition. Because of the central role of the liver in metabolism, alcohol-induced changes have far-reaching implications.

In addition to these changes, fat and glucose use is impaired and eventually defects occur in protein synthesis and transport and storage of vitamins and minerals. The undernutrition of alcoholism has many causes.

Alcohol consumption in the United States seems to be an accepted practice. Long before a child enters high school, he or she is likely to have had some experience with alcohol. Drinking that first beer or shot of whiskey often is one of the rebellious adolescent rites of passage. More than 90% of eleventh graders and 75% of eighth graders say that alcohol is easy to get (Johnston et al., 1996). The average age when alcohol is first used is around 13.1 years (Substance Abuse and Mental Health Services Administration, 1999). Unfortunately, many youngsters get hooked. In a national survey 31% of high school seniors reported heavy drinking (Substance Abuse and Mental Health Services Administration, 1999). In a 2001 survey 79.7% of twelfth grade students and 70.1% of tenth graders reported some alcohol use—a slight decrease from 2000 (Institute for Social Research, 2001). Today alcohol abuse ranks as the top drug problem among young people and is a major cause of morbidity and mortality.

Drinking during adolescence has biologic, social, psychologic, and economic consequences. Less alcohol is needed in teenagers than in adults to impair reflexes and bring about loss of control. Because of their smaller, lighter bodies, girls are less able to handle ethanol than are boys. Additionally girls have only about one half as much alcohol dehydrogenase as do boys (Frezza et al., 1990).

Alcohol abuse by adolescents is often concurrent with use of other drugs. Although little is known about the extent and pattern of polydrug use in adolescents, a recent study of 72 alcohol abusers admitted to an inpatient treatment center found that 96% of male and female alcohol abusers also used drugs other than alcohol (Martin et al., 1999).

There is no question that use of alcohol, tobacco, and other illegal substances can have a negative impact on nutrition status. An eating pattern that includes regular meals emphasizing complex carbohydrates, moderate amounts of protein, and conservative quantities of dietary fats with emphasis on balance, variety, and regularity will improve nutrition status.

Concepts to Remember

- Adolescence, the period spanning ages 11 years to 20 years, is a period of major physical, emotional, cognitive, and social transition.
- Puberty is a period of rapid physical growth, sexual maturation, and changes in body composition, which typically lasts 3 years to 4 years.
- Specific energy and nutrient needs, at their peak during puberty, are related more to the stage of physiologic development than to chronologic age.
- Because of the physical, social, and emotional changes of adolescence, eating habits become increasingly variable and can place some adolescents at nutritional risk.
- The food habits of adolescents are influenced by a multitude of personal and environmental factors.
- Nutrition-related concerns for adolescents include overweight status, eating disorders, low levels of physical fitness, poor dietary intake, acne, teenage pregnancy, and the future risk of chronic disease.
- Risky behaviors during adolescence, such as smoking and alcohol and drug use, compromise nutrition status and increase nutrition requirements.

REFERENCES

Adams J: High incidence of intellectual deficits in 5-year-old children exposed to isotretinoin "in utero," Teratology 41:614, 1990.

Allen KM et al.: Relationships between expectancies and adolescent dieting, J Sch Health 63:176, 1993.

American Academy of Pediatrics and Committee on Nutrition: Alcohol use and abuse: a pediatric concern, Pediatrics 108:32, 2000.

American Heart Association: AHA Dietary Guidelines. Revision 2000, Circulation 102:2284, 2000.

Barr SI: Association of social and demographic variables with calcium intakes of high school students, J Am Diet Assoc 94:260, 1994.

Bartlett HL et al.: Fat-free mass in relation to stature: ratios of fat-free mass to height in children, adults and elderly subjects, Am J Clin Nutr 53:1112, 1991.

Berkey CS et al.: Relation of childhood diet and body size to menarche and adolescent growth in girls, Am J Epidemiol 152:446, 2000.

Bertrand LD and Abernathy TJ: Predicting cigarette smoking among adolescents using cross-sectional and longitudinal approaches, J Sch Health 63:98, 1993.

Biederman J et al.: Patterns of alcohol and drug use in adolescents can be predicted by parental substance use disorders, Peditarics 106:792, 2000.

Biro FM et al.: Impact of timing of pubertal maturation on growth in black and white female adolescents: the National Heart, Lung, and Blood Institute Growth and Health Study, J Pediatr 138:617, 2001.

Botvin GJ et al.: Factors promoting cigarette smoking amount black youth: a causal modeling approach, Addict Behav 18:397, 1992.

Cadogan J et al.: Milk intake and bone mineral acquisition in adolescent girls: randomized controlled intervention trial, Brit J Med 315:1255, 1999.

Cameron N: Assessment of growth and maturation during adolescence, Horm Res 36(Suppl 3):9, 1993.

Cavadini C et al.: US adolescent food intake trends from 1965 to 1996, West J Med 175:235, 2001.

Centers for Disease Control: Physical activity and health. National Center for Chronic Disease Prevention and Health Promotion 2001. www.cdc.gov/nccdphp/sgr/adoles.htm

Centers for Disease Control: Recommendations to prevent and control iron deficiency in the United States, MMWR Morb Mortal Wkly Rep 47, 1998.

Centers for Disease Control: Selected tobacco-use among young people. A report of the Surgeon General, MMWR Morb Mortal Wkly Rep 43:2, 1994.

Centers for Disease Control: Results of the Youth Risk Behavior Surveillance System, MMWR Morb Mortal Wkly Rep 51:2, 2000.

Center for Disease Control: Selected tobacco-use behaviors, dietary patterns among high school students—United States, 1991. MMWR Morb Mortal Wkly Rep 41:417, 1992.

Committee on Drugs: Retinoid therapy for severe dermatological disorders. American Academy of Pediatrics, Pediatrics 90:119, 1992.

Committee on Nutrition, American Academy of Pediatrics: Pediatric nutrition handbook, Elk Grove Village, IL, 1998, The Academy.

Committee on Nutrition. American Academy of Pediatrics: Alcohol use and abuse: a pediatric concern, Pediatrics 108:32, 2001.

Custatis DC and Shannon BM: Influences on adolescent eating behavior, J Adolesc Health 18:27, 1996.

Daniel WA: Nutritional requirements of adolescents. In Winick M, editor: Adolescent nutrition, New York, 1982, Wiley.

Denniston CR: Assessing normal and abnormal growth, Primary Care 21:637, 1994.

Eck LH and Hackett-Renner C: Calcium intake in youth: sex, age, and racial differences in NHANES II, Prev Med 21:473, 1992.

Emmons L: Predisposing factors differentiating adolescent dieters and nondieters, J Am Diet Assoc 94:725, 1994.

Farthing MC: Current eating patterns of adolescents in the United States, Nutr Today 26:35, 1991.

Food and Nutrition Board. National Research Council: Recommended dietary allowances, ed 10, Washington, DC, 1989, National Academy of Sciences.

Forecast Magazine and Food Processing Magazine and Food & Beverage Marketing Magazine: Food and nutrition study. A national survey of teenagers. 14th annual study, Forecast Magazine, 1998.

Frezza M et al.: The role of decreased gastric alcohol dehydrogenase activity and first-pass metabolism, N Engl J Med 322:95, 1990.

Gillman MW et al.: Risk of overweight among adolescents who were breastfed as infants, JAMA 285:2461, 2001.

Giraud DW et al.: Plasma and dietary vitamin C and E levels of tobacco chewers, smokers and nonusers, J Am Diet Assoc 95:198, 1995.

Gong EJ and Spear BA: Adolescent growth and development: implication for nutritional needs, J Nutr Educ 20:273, 1988.

Grande F and Keys A: Body weight, body composition and calorie status. In Goodhart RS and Shils ME, editors: Modern nutrition in health and disease, ed 6, Philadelphia, 1980, Lea & Febiger.

Grunbaum JA et al.: Characteristics of health among secondary schools—School health education profiles, 1996, MMWR Morb Mortal Wkly Rep 47:1, 1998.

Guenther PM: Beverages in the diets of American teenagers, J Am Diet Assoc 86:493, 1986.

Hampl JS and Betts NM: Cigarette use during adolescence: effects on nutritional status, Nutr Rev 57:215, 1999.

Harter S and Rosenberg S: Self and identity development. In Feldman ST and Elliot G, editors: At the threshold: the developing adolescent, Cambridge, 1990, Harvard University Press.

Heald FP et al.: Caloric, protein and fat intake in children and adolescents. In Heald FP et al.: Adolescent nutrition and growth, New York, 1969, Appleton Century Crofts.

Institute of Medicine: Dietary reference intakes for calcium, phosphorus, magnesium, vitamin D and fluoride, Washington, DC, 1997, Institute of Medicine.

Institute of Medicine: Dietary reference intakes for thiamin, riboflavin, niacin, vitamin B_6, folate, vitamin B_{12}, pantothenic acid, biotin, and choline, Washington, DC, 1998, National Academy Press.

Institute of Medicine: Dietary reference intakes for vitamin C, vitamin E, selenium and carotenoids, Washington, DC, 2000, National Academy Press.

Institute of Medicine: Dietary reference intakes for vitamin A, vitamin K, arsenic, boron, chromium, copper, iodine, manganese, molybdenum, nickel, silicon, vanadium and zinc, Washington, DC, 2001, National Academy Press.

Institute for Social Research: Monitoring the future, University of Michigan, 2001, www.monitoringthefuture.org

Jacobson MS et al.: Adolescent obesity and cardiovascular risk: a rational approach to management, Ann NY Acad Sci 699:220, 1993.

Jahns L et al.: The increasing prevalence of snacking among US children from 1977 to 1996, J Pediatr 138:493, 2001.

Johnston LD et al.: National survey results on drug use from the monitoring the future study, 1975-1995, Vol I: secondary school students, Rockville, MD, 1996, NIH Publ No. 97-4139, National Institute on Drug Abuse.

Johnston CC Jr et al.: Calcium supplementation and increases in bone mineral density in children, N Engl J Med 327:82, 1992.

Kallner AB et al.: On the requirements of ascorbic acid in man: steady-state turnover and body pool in smokers, Am J Clin Nutr 34:22, 1981.

Kann L et al.: Youth risk behavior surveillance—United States, 1993, MMWR Morb Mortal Wkly Rep 44:1, 1995.

Kimm SYS et al.: Dietary patterns of U.S. children: implications for disease prevention, Prev Med 19:432, 1990.

Lammer E et al.: Retinoic acid embryopathy, N Engl J Med 313: 837, 1985.

Lewis PC et al.: Cigarette use in adolescents: the cardiovascular health in children and youth study, Res Nurs Health 24:27, 2001.

Marino DD and King JC: Nutritional concerns during adolescence, Pediatr Clin North Am 27:125, 1980.

Martin AR et al.: Unhealthy eating behavior in adolescents, Eur J Epidem 15:643, 1999.

Matkovik V: Calcium intake and peak bone mass, N Engl J Med 327:119, 1993.

Matkovik V et al.: Factors which influence peak bone mass formation: a study of calcium balance and the inheritance of bone mass in adolescent females, Am J Clin Nutr 52:88, 1990.

McPherson RS et al.: Intake and food sources of dietary fat among school children in the Woodlands, Texas, Pediatrics 86:520, 1990.

Merzenich H et al.: Dietary fat and sports activity as determinants for age at menarche, Am J Epidemiol 138: 217, 1993.

Moore DC: Body image and eating behavior in adolescents, J Am Coll Nutr 12:505, 1993.

Morbidity and Mortality Weekly Report: Preliminary findings from NHANES III, MMWR Morb Mortal Wkly Rep 43:116, 1994.

Munoz KA et al.: Food intakes of U.S. children and adolescents compared with recommendations, Pediatrics 100:323, 1997.

Myers MG: Smoking and health in substance-abusing adolescents: a two year follow-up, Pediatrics 93:561, 1994.

National Center for Health Statistics: Caloric and selected nutrient values for persons 1-74 years of age. First Health and Examination Survey, 1971-1974. DHEW Pub. No. (PHS) 79–1657, Series 11, No. 209, Hyattsville, MD, 1979, U.S. Dept of Health, Education and Welfare.

National Institutes of Health: Consensus Development Conference on Optimal Calcium Intake, Bethesda, MD, 1994, National Institutes of Health.

Neumark-Sztainer D: Excessive weight preoccupation, Nutr Today 30:68, 1995.

Neumark-Sztainer D et al.: Factors influencing food choices of adolescents. Findings from focus-group discussions with adolescents, J Am Diet Assoc 99:929, 1999.

Neumark-Sztainer D et al.: Weight-related behavior among adolescent girls and boys: results from a national survey, Arch Pediatr Adolesc Med 154:564, 2000.

Newman WP et al.: Autopsy studies in U.S. children and adolescents. Relationship of risk factors to atherosclerotic lesions, Ann NY Acad Sci 623:16, 1991.

Nicklas TA et al.: Breakfast consumption with and without mineral supplement use favorably impacts daily nutrient intake of ninth-grade students, J Adolesc Health 27:314, 2000.

Nieves JW et al.: Teenage and current calcium intake are related to bone mineral density of the hip and forearm in women aged 30-39 years, Am J Epidemiol 141:342, 1995.

Pesa J: Psychosocial factors associated with dieting behaviors among female adolescents, J Sch Health 69:196, 1999.

Rand Youth Poll: The marketing characteristics of American teenagers, New York, 1998, Rand Youth Poll.

Rocchini AP: Adolescent obesity and hypertension, Pediatr Clin North Am 40:81, 1993.

Roche AF and Davila GH: Late adolescent growth in stature, Pediatrics 50:874, 1972.

Rogol AD et al.: Growth and pubertal development in children and adolescents: effects of diet and physical activity, Am J Clin Nutr 72:521S, 2000.

Seega-Riz AM et al.: Trends in breakfast consumption for children in the United States from 1965-1991, Am J Clin Nutr 67:748S, 1998.

Serdula MK et al.: Weight control practices of U.S. adolescents and adults, Ann Int Med 119:667, 1993.

Simons-Morton B et al.: Peer and parent influences on smoking and drinking among early adolescents, Health Edu Behav 28:95, 2001.

Slap GB: Normal physiological and psychological growth in the adolescent, J Adolesc Health Care 7:13S, 1986.

Strong J: Coronary atherosclerosis in soldiers: a clue to the natural history of atherosclerosis in the young, JAMA 256:2863, 1986.

Substance Abuse and Mental Health Services Administration: National Household Survey on Drug Abuse: main findings 1997. Rockville, MD, 1999, Substance Abuse and Mental Health Services Administration.

Sutter E and Hawes MR: Relationship of physical activity, body fat, diet, and blood lipid profile in youths 10-15 yr, Med Sci Sports Exerc 25:748, 1993.

Tanner JM: Developmental age and the concept of physiological maturity. In Growth at adolescence, Oxford, 1962, Blackwell.

Tanner JM and Davies PSW: Clinical longitudinal standards for height and weight velocity for North American children, J Pediatr 107:317, 1985.

Thompson PR et al.: Zinc status and sexual development in adolescent girls, J Am Diet Assoc 86:892, 1986.

Troiano RP et al.: Overweight prevalence and trends for children and adolescents: the National Health and Nutrition Examination Surveys 1963-1991, Arch Pediatr Adolesc Med 149:1085, 1995.

Troiano RP et al.: Energy and fat intakes of children and adolescents in the United States: data from the national health and nutrition examination survey. Am J Clin Nutr 72:1343S, 2000.

U.S. Department of Agriculture: Nationwide Food Consumption Survey, nutrient intakes: individuals in 48 states, year 1977-78, Report No. 1-2, Hyattsville, MD, 1984, U.S. Department of Agriculture.

U.S. Department of Health and Human Services, Am Sch Health Assoc, Assoc Adol Health Educ, Soc Public Health Educ, Inc.: The National Adolescent Student Health Survey: a report of the health of America's youth 1989, Oakland, 1991, Third Party.

U.S. Department of Health, Education and Welfare: First health and nutrition examination survey, United States, 1971-1972: dietary intake and biochemical findings, Health Resources Administration (HRA) 74-219-1, Rockville, MD, 1974, National Center for Health Statistics.

Wabitsch M et al.: Body-fat distribution and changes in the atherogenic risk-factor profile in obese adolescent girls during weight reduction, Am J Clin Nutr 60:54, 1994.

Wang MQ et al.: Desire for weight gain and potential risks of adolescent males using anabolic steroids, Percept Motor Skills 78:267, 1994.

Washington RL: Intervention to reduce cardiovascular risk factors in children and adolescents, Am Fam Physician 59:2211, 1999.

Weaver CM et al.: Adolescent nutrition in the prevention of postmenopausal osteoporosis, J Clin Endocrinol Metab 84:1839, 1999.

Whitaker RC et al.: Predicting obesity in young adulthood from childhood and parental obesity, N Engl J Med 337:869, 1997.

Wildey MB et al.: Fat and sugar levels are high in snacks purchased from student stores in middle schools, J Am Diet Assoc 100:319, 2000.

Witte DJ, et al.: Relationship of self-concept to nutrient intake and eating patterns in young women, J Am Diet Assoc 91:1068, 1991.

Zizza AC et al.: Significant increase in young adults' snacking between 1977-1978 and 1994-1995 represents a cause for concern, Prev Med 32:303, 2001.

APPLICATION

Selecting Vegetarian Diets*

Kailey is a high school junior. Recently she and her family moved to a new community and Kailey settled into a new neighborhood and school. She says she is enjoying many new experiences in her school and has made several friends. Early in the year, a friend, Laura, invited Kailey to dinner with her family. To Kailey's surprise it turned out to be a vegetarian dinner with an entree and many foods she did not recognize. Her hosts encouraged her to try everything and explained the foods that were unfamiliar to her. Kailey was surprised at how good the food tasted and liked almost everything. As Kailey spent more time with Laura and some of her friends, she became more interested in vegetarianism. She learned that a vegetarian diet can be healthy and ecologically sound.

In Kailey's introductory biological science class, a guest speaker extolled the importance of conserving world resources and gave examples of the inefficiency of growing crops to feed to animals raised for human consumption. A few weeks later as part of her health class, Kailey read an article discussing the diet and heart disease link. Although she had been aware that her grandfather had reduced his intake of meat after his heart attack, it had not occurred to her why. Now she knew that saturated fats obtained mostly from animal sources can promote heart disease. She decided to learn more about vegetarianism.

A growing number of young people—college-age persons, teenagers, and even children—choose vegetarian diets although they live in nonvegetarian households. The prevalence of vegetarianism appears to be increasing, particularly among young women (Gilbody et al., 1999) and some researchers have suggested that vegetarianism may be related in a complex manner to weight-control efforts in some young women (Barr and Broughton, 2000).

Kailey considered becoming a vegetarian, but was unsure how to go about it. She talked to her mother, who was not opposed, but voiced a concern that someone who is still growing

*This section was contributed by Kelly Walsh.

might be unable to get an adequate diet without meat. Kailey mentioned her interest to one of her teachers, who suggested that she contact the registered dietitian (RD) who plans the school lunch menus and nutrition education programs for the school district.

When Kailey met with the dietitian, he assured her that a vegetarian diet could be nutritionally adequate with care in making food choices.

TYPICAL VEGETARIAN DIETS

lacto-ovovegetarian: consumes eggs and dairy products, but excludes meat, poultry, and seafood
lactovegetarian: consumes dairy products, but excludes eggs, meat, poultry, and seafood
vegan: refrains from eating animal products
pescovegetarian: consumes seafood, but excludes meat, poultry, eggs, and dairy products

Kailey mentioned that a friend says she follows a macrobiotic diet. The dietitian explained that the macrobiotic diet is very similar to vegan diets in that all animal products are excluded, but even nonmeat products are often highly restricted. A person on a macrobiotic diet may consume only a few grains and vegetables. The macrobiotic lifestyle generally involves spiritualism and harmony with an individual's environment obtained in part through diet (Mangles and Messina, 2001). Sometimes the diet may provide inadequate nutrition, depending on the practices of the individual. Regardless of the type of vegetarian diet, individuals who follow a vegetarian lifestyle must make wise selections to meet energy and nutrient needs.

HEALTH BENEFITS OF A VEGETARIAN DIET

There is ample evidence that a well-balanced vegetarian diet is associated with a decreased risk of hypertension, coronary artery disease, and cancer (Fraser, 1999). However, any comparison of the health consequences of a vegetarian diet and a typical American diet is complicated by the characteristics of a vegetarian lifestyle. It has been known for decades that individuals who follow a vegetarian diet tend to have lower body weights than average Americans (Appleby et al., 1999) and that, as a group, vegetarians tend to be physically active (Walter, 1997). Numerous studies have reported that vegetarians differ from control subjects in other respects. Vegetarians tend to have higher education and greater health consciousness as reflected in a lower prevalence of smoking and alcohol use (Fraser, 1999; Snowdon, 1988; Thorogood et al., 1994). Thus it is difficult to determine whether differences in body weight are associated with a vegetarian dietary pattern per se or are observed because of other differences in lifestyle practices or health consciousness.

Despite these limitations, a pervasive trend in research findings indicates that well-planned vegetarian diets foster improved health (American Dietetic Association [ADA], 1997). A diet rich in fruits and vegetables is likely to have a lower caloric density, higher levels of fiber and monounsaturated and polyunsaturated fatty acids, and lower levels of total and saturated fat and cholesterol than meat-based diets (Gilbody et al., 1999). All of these patterns are consistent with the 2000 Dietary Guidelines for Americans. Thus vegetarians would be expected to have lower rates of heart disease (Mann et al., 1997; Ornish, 1990), hypertension (McDougall et al., 1995), and cancer (Fraser, 1999; Key et al., 1996) than their nonvegetarian counterparts. In addition the antioxidants present in fruits and vegetables may have some chemoprotective effects on the disease process.

In plant-based diets the monounsaturated fats of seeds and nuts and the polyunsaturated fats of vegetable oils are **inversely associated** with heart disease (Coulston, 1999). Vegetarian diets are generally higher in dietary fiber, another factor that is negatively associated with higher levels of blood lipids.

inversely associated: as one variable goes up (vegetable oils in the diet), the other variable declines (incidence of heart disease)

A vegetarian diet does not ensure that an individual will have a diet low in fat. If a vegetarian chooses to consume whole milk and whole milk products, such as cheese and sour cream, and salad dressings, deep-fried vegetables, pastries, or desserts, the increased fat consumption will increase health risks to levels similar to those of the omnivores. Both vegetarian and omnivore diets require careful planning, particularly in today's environment of extra large portion sizes and unlimited buffet choices. If diets are not properly planned, they can provide inappropriate energy intakes and a lack of essential nutrients.

NUTRITIONAL ADEQUACY

Adolescents like Kailey may need assistance in adopting a vegetarian diet. Taste and convenience are key factors in adolescent food choices. However, for the vegetarian, particularly the vegan, meal planning for adequacy and balance are important. It is important to develop appropriate, available, and healthful food choices.

The lower caloric density of the foods in a vegetarian diet is usually an asset for adults. It is possible for children to be well nourished following a vegetarian diet, but the volume of food consumed may become a limiting factor, particularly if dairy products are excluded. For adolescent vegetarians looking for healthful menu choices, a number of issues arise, involving principles of good nutrition, availability of foods, and cost.

The Food Guide Pyramid has been adapted for vegetarian diets. Planning optimal menus for replacing meat with plant sources is more complex than simply replacing meat with a plant source, such as soy protein. A diet that excludes all animal products demands particular attention to nutrients that animal products typically contain, such as protein, calcium, vitamin B_{12}, iron, zinc, and vitamin D.

Protein

Protein is the nutrient that most individuals assume is lacking in a vegetarian diet. The dietitian tells Kailey that this generally is not the case. Adequate protein intakes can be achieved with vegetarian diets (Young et al., 1994). Lacto-ovovegetarians who use animal-derived foods such as milk and eggs receive high-quality proteins and can easily meet their protein needs. Those who adopt a plant-based diet will require greater planning to ensure adequate protein intake. They can increase their protein consumption by using a variety of vegetable protein sources based on whole grains, legumes, seeds, nuts, and vegetables combined to provide all the essential amino acids. Adequate energy intakes are important to ensure that dietary protein is used for protein synthesis.

Additional sources of plant proteins are soy products and meal analogs. Soy products include foods such as **tofu, tempeh,** soy nuts, and soy milk. Meat analogs are food products designed to resemble the taste and texture of meat. In many instances these products are made from textured vegetable protein (TVP) and may contain egg and wheat gluten. Commercial meat analogs are becoming more popular and may be found in almost any grocery store. Meatless versions of hot dogs, burgers, chicken nuggets, chicken patties, sausage, bacon, bologna, ham, and pepperoni are just some of the meat analogs currently being manufactured. These foods are produced to meet the nutritional needs of vegetarians. Therefore many manufacturers fortify these products with nutrients such as iron, calcium, zinc, and vitamin B_{12}. As an added benefit, meat analogs are precooked, which makes them more convenient than their meat counterparts.

tofu: a curd made from soybeans that is rich in protein and often fortified with calcium; used in a variety of vegetarian dishes
tempeh: a fermented soybean food that is rich in protein and fiber

The dietitian recommends that Kailey consume meat alternatives, nuts, legumes, dairy products, or eggs to meet her daily protein needs. He also points out that meat analog products may be fortified with important vitamins and minerals and encourages her to read the labels carefully.

MEAT ALTERNATIVES

veggie burgers: soy protein based or vegetable based and textured vegetable protein
meat analogs: imitation meat products including vegetarian sausage, chicken patties, fried chicken products, bacon, and lunch meat
dairy analogs: cheese and milk-like products made from vegetable proteins

Calcium

Adequate calcium is essential for bone development. For a teenage girl it is even more critical to have sufficient calcium to achieve peak bone mass, reducing the risk of osteoporosis later in life. Studies of spinal bone mineral density in premenopausal women revealed that women who had followed vegetarian diets for a long period had lower bone densities than omnivores (Barr et al., 1998). The dietitian explains to Kailey that her calcium intake can be compromised depending on which type of vegetarianism she chooses. Calcium intake is generally not a problem for lacto-ovovegetarians and lactovegetarians because they consume calcium-rich dairy products (Weaver and Plawecki, 1994). Individuals who follow vegan or macrobiotic diets do not consume dairy foods and must obtain their dietary calcium from other sources. Calcium-fortified foods, such as juices, soymilk, tofu, and vegan meat analogs are alternative sources of calcium. Vegetables can be a good source of calcium; however, not all of the calcium is bioavailable. For example, spinach has a significant amount of calcium, but it also contains large quantities of oxalic acid. Oxalic acid can bind with calcium, thereby decreasing the amount of calcium that is absorbed (Weaver, 1992). Another potential problem is caused by phytates. Phytates are compounds found in foods, such as whole grains, that can also interfere with calcium absorption.

Table 11-9 CALCIUM CONTENT OF SELECTED FOODS

Food	Amount	Calcium (mg)
Soy milk	8 oz	150-300 mg
Collard greens, cooked	1 cup	350 mg
Broccoli, cooked	1 cup	102 mg
Kale, cooked	1 cup	175 mg
Blackstrap molasses	2 tbsp	340 mg
Tofu, processed with calcium sulfate	4 oz	200-300 mg
Calcium-fortified orange juice	8 oz	300 mg
Tofu, processed with nigari	4 oz	100-200 mg
Tahini	2 tbsp	120 mg
Almonds	¼ cup	90 mg

A calcium supplement may be needed if the particular vegetarian diet provides inadequate amounts of calcium (Table 11-9).

Vitamin B_{12}

Conversely, vitamin B_{12} is found only in foods of animal origin and some yeasts grown in a vitamin B_{12}-enriched environment. Microorganisms produce vitamin B_{12} in the intestines of animals. Vitamin B_{12} is present in meats, eggs, and dairy products. Ovovegetarians and lactovegetarians are able to obtain sufficient dietary sources of vitamin B_{12}. Individuals excluding all animal products from their diets will need a supplemental source of vitamin B_{12}. Many commercial vegan foods are currently fortified with this vitamin. Once again, it is essential to read the product labels to ascertain the vitamin B_{12} content.

Iron

Potentially, iron can pose a problem for vegetarians, especially girls and women, because of their greater iron requirements and lower total food intake. Dietary iron is categorized as heme iron or non-heme iron. Heme iron is the form that comes from animals. Non-heme iron constitutes the majority of iron consumed by vegetarians. Unfortunately non-heme iron is absorbed less effectively than heme iron. To avoid iron deficiency, it is important to enhance the absorption of non-heme iron.

To some extent, iron absorption from plant sources increases as the body adapts to a plant-based diet (Hunt and Roughead, 1999). From a dietary standpoint, however, increasing non-heme iron consumption is best accomplished by consuming a source of ascorbic acid (vitamin C) with a meal that contains a substantial source of non-heme iron. Research indicates that ascorbic acid can greatly increase the amount of non-heme iron that is absorbed (Hallberg et al., 1986). Whole grains and enriched breads, fortified cereals, and legumes are good sources of non-heme iron. Cooking foods (especially acidic foods such as spaghetti sauce) in cast iron cookware can also increase the amount of non-heme iron in food. Consuming these iron-rich foods with fruits and vegetables can compensate for

Table 11-10 IRON CONTENT OF SELECTED FOODS

Food	Amount	Iron (mg)
Soybeans, cooked	1 cup	8.8
Blackstrap molasses	2 tbsp	7.0
Lentils, cooked	1 cup	6.6
Kidney beans, cooked	1 cup	5.2
Chickpeas, cooked	1 cup	4.7
Lima beans, cooked	1 cup	4.5
Swiss chard, cooked	1 cup	4.0

the lower amount of heme iron in a vegetarian diet (Table 11-10).

Zinc

Zinc, like iron, is highest in meat although it is present in both animal and vegetable foods. Zinc from plant sources is less well absorbed (Gibson, 1994). An individual following a vegetarian diet should also be concerned about zinc. Consuming foods such as whole grains and legumes can effectively meet a vegetarian's zinc requirement (Hunt et al., 1998).

Vitamin D

Vitamin D is a nutrient we often take for granted. If we get sufficient exposure to sunlight, the precursor to vitamin D in the skin will be activated. For those who spend less time in the sun, we have come to depend on vitamin D-fortified milk. For vegans or ovovegetarians (who consume no milk products), a supplement of vitamin D may be necessary. This is particularly true of individuals in northern climates during the winter months.

GUIDELINES FOR VEGETARIAN DIETS

Vegetarians should keep in mind the following guidelines for achieving a nutritionally balanced diet:

- Base diets on whole grains, vegetables, and fruits.
- Include moderate amounts of legumes and nuts or seeds daily.
- Choose vegetable fats such as olive oil or canola oil, and use them in moderation.
- Identify foods that are rich in calcium and consume enough of them to provide 1000 mg of calcium per day. Use a supplement to achieve recommended intakes if necessary.
- Consume a good source of vitamin B_{12} and of vitamin D daily. For vegans these will be fortified foods or supplements. In the case of vitamin D, sun exposure may negate the need for dietary sources.
- Consume enough food to maintain appropriate weight.

In general, adults who eat vegetarian diets can reduce their risks of mortality and several chronic diseases, including obesity, high blood pressure, heart disease, and cancer (Fraser, 1999). There is nothing mysterious or magical about the vegetarian diet and its apparent benefits for reducing disease risk. It simply includes ample fruits, vegetables, whole grains, and legumes—foods that are higher in fiber, richer in antioxidants (vitamins and other compounds), and lower in fat than meat-based diets.

Kailey received a significant amount of information in her meeting with the dietitian. At the end of the session the dietitian reassured Kailey that a well-planned vegetarian diet can be quite healthy and gave her a copy of the Vegetarian Food Guide Pyramid and some detailed information on sources of various nutrients. With this information, Kailey decided to pursue a vegetarian lifestyle. She has a number of health benefits and a world of discovery waiting for her.

REFERENCES

American Dietetic Association. Vegetarian diets (position statement), J Am Diet Assoc 97:1317, 1997.

Appleby PN et al.: The Oxford Vegetarian Study: an overview, Am J Clin Nutr 70:S255, 1999.

Barr SI and Broughton TM: Relative weight, weight loss efforts, and nutrient intakes among health-conscious vegetarian, past vegetarian and nonvegetarian women ages 18 to 50, J Am Coll Nutr 19:781, 2000.

Barr SE et al.: Spinal bone mineral density in premenopausal vegetarians and nonvegetarian women: cross-sectional and prospective comparisons, J Am Diet Assoc 98:760, 1998.

Coulston AM: The role of dietary fats in plant-based diets, Am J Clin Nutr 70:S512, 1999.

Fraser GE: Associations between diet and cancer, ischemic heart disease, and all-cause mortality in non Hispanic white California Seventh Day Adventists, Am J Clin Nutr 70:S538, 1999.

Gibson RJ: Content and bioavailability of trace elements in vegetarian diets, Am J Clin Nutr 59:1223, 1994.

Gilbody SM et al.: Vegetarianism in young women: another misuse of weight control? Int J Eat Disord 26:87, 1999.

Hallberg L et al.: Effect of ascorbic acid on iron absorption from different types of meals. Studies with ascorbic acid-rich foods and synthetic ascorbic acid given in different amounts with different meals, Hum Nutr Appl Nutr 40:97, 1986.

Hunt JR and Roughead ZK: Non-heme-iron absorption, fecal ferritin excretion, and blood indexes of iron status in women consuming controlled lacto-ovo-vegetarian diets for 8 weeks, Am J Clin Nutr 69:944, 1999.

Hunt JR et al.: Zinc absorption, mineral balance, and blood lipids in women consuming controlled lactovegetarian and omnivorous diets for 8 weeks, Am J Clin Nutr 67:421, 1998.

Key TJA et al.: Dietary habits and mortality in 11,000 vegetarians and health conscious people: results of a 17 year follow up, BMJ 313:775, 1996.

McDougall J et al.: Rapid reduction of serum cholesterol and blood pressure by a twelve-day, very low fat, strictly vegetarian diet, J Am Coll Nutr 14:491, 1995.

Mangels AR and Messina V: Consideration in planning vegan diets, Infants J Am Diet Assoc 101:670, 2001.

Mann JI et al.: Dietary determinants of ischaemic heart disease in health conscious individuals, Heart 78:450, 1997.

Ornish DM et al.: Can lifestyle changes reverse coronary heart disease? The Lifestyle Heart Trial, Lancet 336: 129, 1990.

Snowdon DA: Animal product consumption and mortality because of all causes combined, coronary heart disease, stroke, diabetes, and cancer in Seventh-day Adventists, Am J Clin Nutr 48:S739, 1988.

Thorogood M et al.: Risk of death from cancer and ischaemic heart disease in meat and non-meat eaters, BMJ 308:1667, 1994.

Walter P: Effects of vegetarian diets on aging and longevity, Nutr Rev 55:561, 1997.

Weaver CM: Calcium bioavailability and its relation to osteoporosis, Proc Soc Exp Biol Med 200:157, 1992.

Weaver CM and Plawecki KL: Dietary calcium: adequacy of vegetarian diet, Am J Clin Nutr 59:1238S, 1994.

Young VR et al.: Plant proteins in relation to human protein and amino acid nutrition, Am J Clin Nutr 59:1203S, 1994.

VEGETARIAN WEB SITES

Vegetarian Resource Group: http://www.vrg.org/nutshell.htm

Vegetarian Resource Center: http://www.tiac.net/users/vrc/wdex.ntm

World Guide to Vegetarianism: http://www.veg.org/veg/guide

The Vegetarian Page: http://www.veg.org/veg/

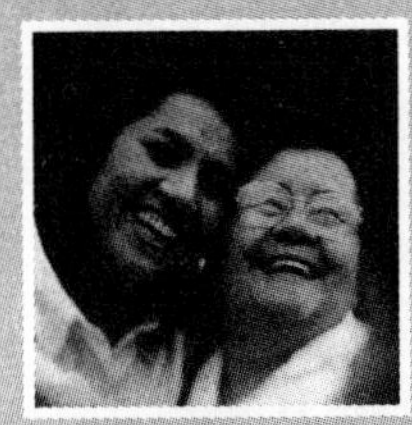

PART **FOUR**

THE ADULT YEARS

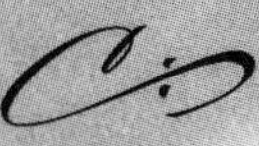

CHAPTER 12 ADULTHOOD

Chapter Outline

- Physiologic Changes
- Psychosocial Development
- Nutrition Assessment
- Energy and Nutrient Needs
- Chronic Health Concerns of Adults: Cardiovascular Disease
- Cancer
- Promoting Health and Well-Being

Andrew, a 42-year-old office manager, lives in a suburb of a large New England city with his wife Sara, his daughter, and two sons. The boys are in elementary school and the daughter has just begun high school. To make ends meet and to plan for college expenses, Sara has taken a job at a nearby school district and Andrew has started selling real estate part time. The children are busy with sports, church, and school activities. Andrew and Sara try to attend as many of the children's activities as they can, but their busy schedules mean they are on the go all the time.

Sara is a good cook and Andrew helps out in the kitchen sometimes, too. The family tries to have dinner together each evening, but it is often at odd hours. In the morning everyone makes his or her own breakfast—usually fruit or fruit juice and cereal with milk. There is always toast and sometimes muffins and donuts. The children buy a school lunch most days, but sometimes pack a lunch from home. Sara always packs a sandwich and fruit for lunch. Andrew eats in the cafeteria in his building or at a fast-food restaurant down the street.

Andrew is 188 cm (74 in) tall and weighs 105 kg (230 pounds). He has a bit of a "gut" and could afford to lose some weight. He knows that he should exercise consistently, but he has difficulty finding time. Sara gave him an exercise bicycle the previous Christmas, which he uses once or twice a week. Andrew doesn't like feeling fat especially around his midsection. He wants to eat better to live longer and healthier, but doesn't know where to begin.

Andrew does most of the family grocery shopping. He is interested in nutrition and checks the Nutrition Facts label, particularly for calories and fat content. He tries to control his weight by avoiding snacks, especially cakes, cookies, and chips and dip. He tends to categorize these foods as "bad" and many of the foods he likes less he considers "good" because they are more nutritious. When Andrew gets the urge for something sweet, he'll eat as many as a dozen cookies at one sitting, then will avoid them for weeks.

Andrew really wants to improve his diet, but he gets confused about what to do and frustrated at his apparent lack of progress. He reports eating more good foods, fruits, and vegetables than he used to eat. Despite these efforts, in the last three days the only good foods he has had were two 4-oz glasses of orange juice, a half cup of stir-fried broccoli and

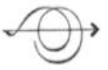

mushrooms, two lettuce leaves, and half a tomato. Andrew wonders if he should take a supplement of some kind to improve his diet.

Last month Andrew wasn't feeling very well and went to see his family physician. The doctor treated him for a throat infection, but insisted that he come back in 2 weeks for a complete physical examination and some blood work. When the laboratory results came back, the physician told Andrew that his total blood cholesterol and low-density lipoprotein cholesterol (LDL-C) were too high and that his high-density lipoprotein cholesterol (HDL-C) levels were a little low. He recommended that Andrew make some changes in his diet and get more exercise and also suggested he lose a few pounds. He said this was particularly important because of Andrew's family history of diabetes mellitus and heart disease.

Andrew's situation is representative of the many nutrition-related issues facing adults as they approach middle age. With maturation and the first discernible stages of aging, adulthood focuses on nutrition for promoting lifelong health. This focus includes physical fitness and optimum dietary intakes to promote well-being and minimize the progression of chronic diseases and their impact on quality of life.

Physiologically, adulthood begins with the attainment of sexual maturity and the completion of growth; the former occurs in the late teen years, the latter occurs well into the third decade of life. Emotionally, it is often associated with significant life events such as completing education, getting a first job, getting a credit card, or reaching the age of eligibility to vote or legally buy alcoholic beverages. Typically, young adulthood begins at 18 years and encompasses at least the next 2 decades. Middle age remains one of the least studied phases of life. It is uncharted territory in human development without set stages or transition points. By conventional definition, middle age starts at age 40 years. However, as the human life span increases, it becomes more difficult to define middle life. Individuals who are called middle age today are very different from those of a generation ago. The baby boomers (those born between 1946 and 1964) have not been referred to as middle age until they turned 50 or older. In fact this group seems to be programmed to never get old and many baby boomers will not confront old age until well into their 70s (Chernoff, 1995). As in the growth years, a great diversity exists in individual responses to maturation and aging. Although the rate of change is determined by genetics, it is influenced by growth during early life and by adult life-styles (McGill et al., 1996).

PHYSIOLOGIC CHANGES

- *What physiologic changes occur across adulthood?*
- *How do body weight and composition change as an individual moves from adolescence through adulthood?*
- *What is menopause and what are its long-term health implications? What are the advantages and disadvantages of hormone replacement therapy (HRT)?*

There are no dramatic markers in physical development in the adult. Physiologic maturity is defined as the completion of skeletal growth, as characterized by the achievement of maximum height and the formation of peak bone mass. Most body systems reach their peak efficiency and optimum functioning before age 30 years. The human body is a dynamic organism and stability is the major physiologic characteristic of adulthood. In general, the cells of most tissues are catabolized and replaced at approximately the same rate. With time, catabolism slightly exceeds anabolism, resulting in small changes in function or performance. Most of these changes accelerate after middle age and are discussed in greater detail in Chapter 13.

Musculoskeletal Changes

Approximately 5 years after maximum height is attained, an adult reaches maximum strength, endurance, and agility. From this point there is a gradual, but steady, decline. Bone mass increases well into the third decade. In young adult women, this increase is positively influenced by physical activity, dietary calcium, and use of oral contraceptives (Recker et al., 1992). Data from cross-sectional studies indicate that beginning in the third decade, both men and women experience a continuous loss of trabecular bone mineral density (BMD). For females the marked decrease in estrogen and progesterone production of menopause is associated with an acceleration in loss of cortical bone.

Muscle mass increases into the third decade and then declines. Because the decrease is gradual, these changes may not become apparent for more than a decade. Physical activity, especially resistance training, may attenuate or prevent the bone and muscle mass loss associated with aging (Vuori, 1996).

Oral Health

Although the process of tooth decay can continue beyond childhood, tooth loss during the adult years most frequently is from **periodontal disease.** Periodontal disease is promoted by the same factors that contribute to dental caries. Accumulation of bacteria-containing plaque can cause the gums around the teeth to become inflamed and bleed easily, a condition called gingivitis. If the symptoms are ignored, the gingiva become scarred, and bacteria work their way below the gum line and into the jawbone. The ensuing infection results in destruction of the bone that holds in the teeth, resulting in tooth loss.

Perimenopause

During a woman's childbearing years, the ovaries produce estrogen and progesterone that signal the **endometrium** to grow and thicken. One of the ovaries releases an ovum each month. If the ovum is not fertilized, it moves to the uterus and is absorbed. Consequently hormone levels decline and the endometrial tissue breaks up and is discharged during menstruation. The normal menstrual cycle is discussed in Chapter 4.

Perimenopause occurs toward the end of a woman's reproductive period, when estrogen and progesterone levels fluctuate wildly and progressively decline. Menstrual cycles may become irregular and menstrual flow is usually lighter and of shorter duration. Eventually ovulation ceases and menstruation ends. Menopause, the point at which a year has passed since the last menstrual period, is a marker between perimenopause and postmenopause. A woman is not completely without estrogen even after menopause, but levels are severely diminished. Postmenopause is an open-ended era that begins after menopause and is characterized by increased vulnerability to heart disease, osteoporosis, breast cancer, and other conditions. Drug and supplement manufacturers, healthcare professionals, and other concerned groups have been attempting to provide approaches to symptom relief and risk reduction for the perimenopausal woman.

Hormone Replacement Therapy

For many women a variety of symptoms are associated with perimenopause, ranging from mild discomfort to hot flashes with extreme flushing of the skin, vaginal dryness, fatigue, anxiety, sleep disturbances, memory and concentration problems, and many other symptoms (Kuller et al., 2001a). For more than 30 years, estrogen in all its myriad forms has been used to mitigate the acute symptoms of menopause. *Estrogen* is a blanket term for several chemically related compounds, the most active of which is 17 beta estradiol. Estrogen works indirectly, stimulating receptor molecules in the cell nucleus, stimulating cell growth and proliferation. The receptors

KEY TERMS

periodontal disease: a disease of tissues supporting the teeth—gingiva, ligaments, and bone
endometrium: lining of the uterus
perimenopause: the time around menopause that, for some women, may be characterized by a variety of symptoms including hot flashes and insomnia

can pair up with other molecules that bear a chemical similarity to estrogen, including plant compounds called **phytoestrogens** or "designer drugs" (selective estrogen receptor modulators [SERMs]) made to imitate estrogen. In reality, the form of estrogen will determine its overall effects by stimulating or blocking receptors. That may explain the wide variation in effects that have been observed in different studies. For example the first SERM, tamoxifen, was developed in the 1970s to act as a treatment for breast cancer by blocking estrogen receptors in breast-cancer cells. One of the newest SERMs is raloxifene (Evista). Raloxifene performs as an estrogen mimic in some tissues and as an estrogen block in others. It reduces fractures, lowers serum LDL-C levels, and may reduce the risk of breast cancer.

Estrogen replacement therapy (ERT) decreases the average lifetime risk of osteoporosis and reduces the risk of hip fracture. There have been some reports that estrogen helps alleviate wrinkling by stimulating the production of collagen, a major protein of the skin. In addition some observational studies have indicated that estrogen may reduce the risk of colon cancer. It is theorized that estrogen may work by suppressing bile acid production in the liver, producing a less-favorable climate for tumors in the colon. Estrogen reduces the risk of Alzheimer's disease, protects LDL cholesterol from being oxidized (a first step on the formation of atherosclerotic plaque), and relieves many of the symptoms of perimenopause. However, estrogen also stimulates the growth of the endometrium and increases the risk of endometrial cancer and breast cancer. Estrogen therapies that include a natural or synthetic progesterone, known as HRT, may reduce the excess uterine cancer risk. Use of progestin counters estrogen's effect on endometrial growth, but does not appear to negate the other positive effects of estrogen (Writing Group for the PEPI Trial, 1996). However, adding progestin may increase such side effects as breast tenderness, bloating, irritability, depression, monthly vaginal bleeding, and irregular bleeding, which usually subside within the first year of treatment.

KEY TERMS

phytoestrogens: products of plant origin that have some estrogen-like effects on the body

A dietary approach, which has been described as efficacious among women who consume diets high in phytoestrogens, involves consumption of generous amounts of soy protein, flax, and some herbs. These foods may alleviate symptoms, but there are few data on the preventive effects of phytoestrogens at this time.

It has been suggested that postmenopausal women who received HRT tended to gain less weight or develop less abdominal fat than do women who received a placebo, but other studies have provided inconsistent results. A 5-year prospective and cross-sectional cohort study of 6871 postmenopausal women found that intermittent or continuous HRT was not associated with any differences in the central obesity commonly observed in postmenopausal women (Kirtz-Silverstein and Barrett-Connor, 1996).

Basic laboratory research has shown that estradiol is a neuroprotective factor involved in the growth and protection of neurons and their connections (Wise et al., 2001). Estrogen and SERMs such as raloxifene act on the hippocampus, an area of the brain associated with memory. Research on how estrogen and SERMs affect the brain may become a new frontier in HRT. Recent studies have associated estrogen treatment (Yaffe et al., 1998) and serum concentrations of oestradial (Yaffe et al., 2000) with improvements in memory and cognition in healthy postmenopausal women and women with Alzheimer's disease (Asthana et al., 1999). However, studies have varied in size, length, and design, and the results have been inconsistent (Shaywitz and Shaywitz, 2000). There have been questions regarding the effect of progesterone in the beneficial effects of estrogen. LeBlanc et al. (2001) completed a meta-analysis of 29 randomized, controlled trials and cohort studies of the effect of HRT on cognitive decline and dementia in healthy postmenopausal women. The conclusions were that women symptomatic from menopause had improvements in memory, viligance, reasoning, and motor speed, but generally no benefits in asymptomatic women. However, the authors emphasized that possible biases, lack of control of potential confounders, made generalizations difficult without additional research.

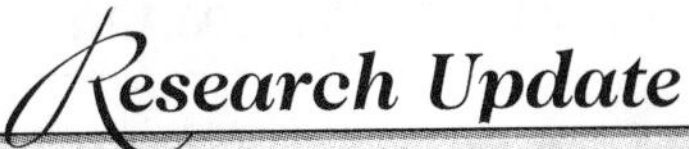

Can Hormone Replacement Therapy Prevent Heart Disease in Healthy Postmenopausal Women?

Many observational studies have found that estrogen lowers rates of coronary heart disease (CHD) (Col et al., 1997; Wegner, 1998). In fact reduction of CHD risk was well documented in epidemiologic studies, making it an additional benefit of estrogen therapy. Early studies indicated that taking estrogen may have an effect in reducing a woman's risk of developing coronary artery disease (CAD) by lowering LDL-C, the form most readily incorporated into arterial deposits and by raising HDL-C levels. However, such effects were not observed in a study of more than 2500 postmenopausal women with established coronary disease studied for 4.1 years at 20 U.S. clinical centers (Hulley et al., 1998). The blinded, randomized, placebo-controlled trial found no significant differences between women taking estrogen and nonestrogen control groups in myocardial infarction or CHD deaths contradicting earlier results suggesting that estrogen decreases heart disease. However, the researchers did note a favorable pattern of CHD events for women who had been taking estrogen for several years. They suggest that for women already receiving estrogen, continuation of estrogen treatment may be appropriate.

The Estrogen Replacement and Atherosclerosis (ERA) study came to the same conclusion, that postmenopausal women with heart disease did not do better on HRT than they did on placebo (Herrington et al., 2000). The ERA was a 3-year intervention trial that measured CAD progression with **angiograms.**

A third study, the Heart and Estrogen/Progestin Replacement Study (HERS), was the first randomized clinical trial of combined hormone therapy and secondary prevention of coronary events in postmenopausal women with previous heart disease (Grodstein et al., 2001). Initially the researchers found no significant effects of estrogen/progestin on coronary events, but did report an unexpected increased risk for recurrent events in the initial year (relative risk 1.25 compared to nonusers), followed by a decrease during the final years. A more long-term analysis of data for 2489 postmenopausal women found a significant trend of decreasing risk for recurrent major CHD events with increasing duration of hormone use (a relative risk of 0.38 compared with nonusers).

Some studies have investigated the effects of 17 beta estadiol on the thickness of the carotid artery via ultrasound in postmenopausal women taking HRT compared with those taking no hormones and found that HRT seemed to encourage thickening of the layers with the highest connective tissue component and delay the atheromatous imtima layer (Baron et al., 1998; Sator et al., 1998), supporting a cardioprotective effect. If this effect is verified, the impact of HRT may be similar to that of **statins,** the most widely prescribed cholesterol-lowering drugs. The investigators also found that HDL-C increased more and LDL-C levels decreased more in the women taking estradiol than in the placebo group (Davidson et al., 2000).

The issue of HRT is being addressed in a trial of 27,000 women in the Women's Health Initiative, a 15-year project sponsored by the National Heart, Lung and Blood Institute. Most of the data collected have been in short-term studies (2 to 5 years).

In this situation the research results can be both encouraging and confusing. The results of some studies are encouraging for healthy postmenopausal women. They are consistent with biologic and some observational studies that have suggested that estrogen improves lipid profiles and arterial elasticity. However, there are important issues. One obviously centers around short- and long-term effects of HRT. Another is the differences in the form of estrogen used. The most positive results seem to be associated with 17 beta estradiol (a pure form of estrogen that occurs naturally in women). The other studies used Premarin, which is derived from pregnant mares' urine and consists of several types of estrogen and other substances, the effects of which are not completely known. Also, there may be differences between women who were healthy at the start of the trial. It could be that the effects of estrogen are inconsistent between women with no cardiovascular disease (CVD) and those with some degree of involvement.

KEY TERMS

angiograms: radiographic images obtained when a dye is injected into the arteries of the heart via cardiac catheterization

statins: a group of drugs, HMG-Co-A reductase inhibitors, that block the enzyme that catalyzes the early step in cholesterol synthesis, thereby lowering blood levels of cholesterol

Metabolism

During adulthood the resting energy expenditure (REE) decreases, gradually at first and then at an accelerating rate as muscle mass declines. Diminished REE translates into reduced caloric requirements. Failure to adjust levels of dietary intake and physical activity to compensate for this decline in energy expenditure has the potential to promote excess gains of body weight and fat.

Body Weight

In the United States, average body weight increases throughout the seventh decade in both sexes. Not all adult Americans gain weight—by the age of 50 years, those who lose weight are as prevalent as those who gain weight, but gainers gain more than losers lose and averages climb (Garn, 1996). However, body weight has a relationship to mortality, which is manifested in a "J curve" with increased mortality at either end of the range of body mass index (BMI), with a greater mortality with excess body weight because of the higher degree (Figure 12-1).

"Middle-age spread" is not a myth. Weight gain begins as early as a person's 20s and 30s and accelerates with age. A 10-year follow-up of 5115 African-American and white men and women age 18 years to 30 years from the Coronary Artery Risk Development in Young Adults (CARDIA) study reported that the prevalence of being overweight (BMI >25.0 kg/m^2) increased markedly and prevalence of severe obesity (BMI >40.0 kg/m^2) doubled in all race and sex categories (Lewis et al., 2000). For example African-American women gained 0.96 kg per year and white women gained 0.55 kg per year. On the longer term, the Atherosclerosis Risk in Communities study found that for individuals first measured at age 25 years and followed for an average of 29 years, weight gains for white men and African-American men were 9.7 kg and 10.1 kg, respectively. Over the same period, gains for white women were 12.0 kg and gains for African-American women were 20.8 kg (Stevens et al., 1998). The First National Health and Nutrition Examination Survey (NHANES) Follow-Up Study included 10,000 adults age 25 years to 74 years (Williamson et al., 1990). During the decade

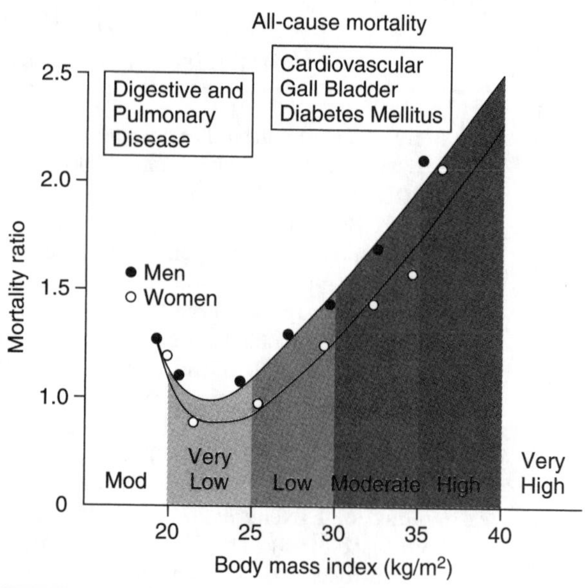

Figure 12-1 Mortality curve associated with BMI. *(Reprinted from Bray GA: Handbook of obesity, New York, 1998, Marcel Dekker, Inc., p. 846, by courtesy of Marcel Dekker, Inc.)*

following the initial measurements, weight gains in individuals between 25 years and 44 years of age were 3.4% of baseline weight for men and 5.2% for women.

Extra pounds often tend to settle around the midsection. As waistlines increase, so do health risks. Figure 12-1 illustrates the mortality curve associated with BMI. A 3-year prospective study among 29,122 men age 40 years to 75 years found that weight gain was associated with increased risk of CHD (Rimm et al., 1995). Similarly, the Nurses Health Study, a prospective study that followed more than 100,000 registered nurses over 14 years, found that among women of normal weight, gains of 5 kg or more after 18 years of age increased the risk of both fatal CHD and nonfatal **myocardial infarction** (Willett et al., 1995). In addition women who gained 5 kg or more experienced increased risk of diabetes mellitus (Colditz et al., 1995). Women who lost 5 kg or more, however, had a decreased risk of diabetes. These researchers suggest that the long-held assumption that it is normal for body weight to increase with age is erroneous and that maintenance of the weight

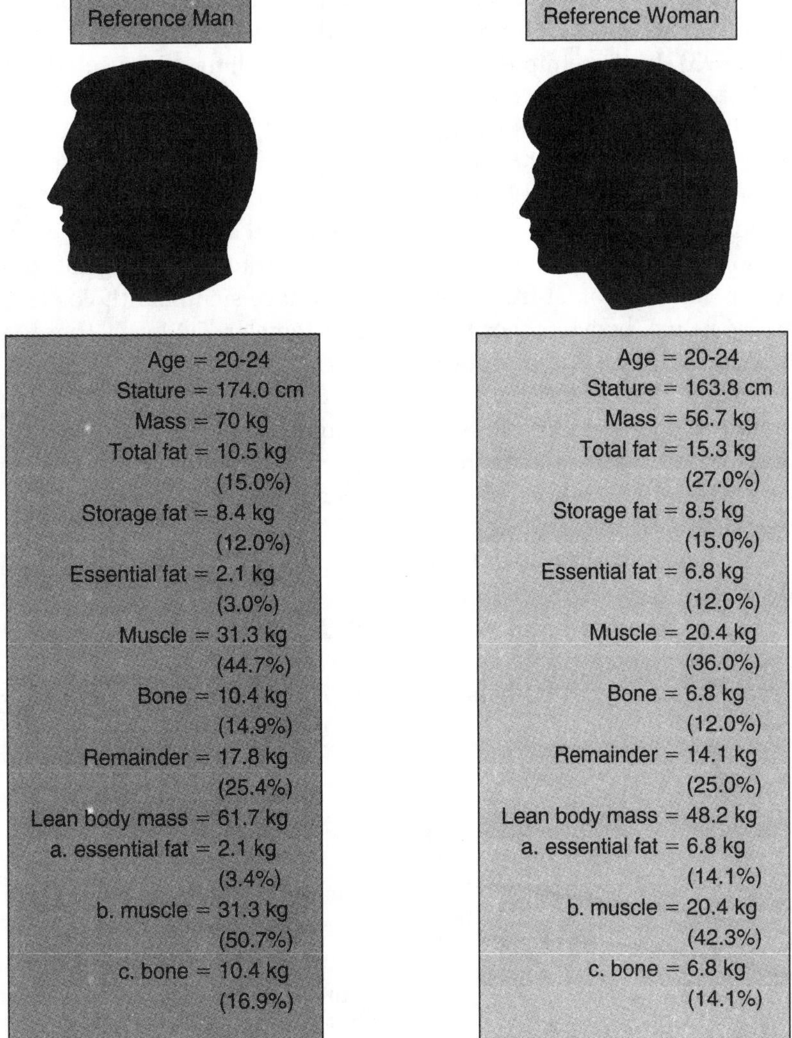

Figure 12-2 Body composition of reference man and reference woman. *(From Katch FI and McArdle WD: Introduction to nutrition, exercise and health, ed 4, Philadelphia, 1993, Lea & Febiger.)*

of early adulthood is an appropriate lifetime goal. A review of available research on the impact of age on associations between weight and mortality led Stevens (2000) to conclude that the lowest mortality falls at the weight within the age range of 18.5 years to 24.9 years for both men and women.

Body Composition

At a genetically determined point, overall growth is achieved and an adult pattern of body composition is established. The major structural components of the human body are muscle, fat, and bone. Figure 12-2 summarizes body composition for a reference man and reference woman 20 years to 24 years of age. These standards are not

KEY TERMS

myocardial infarction: an area of tissue necrosis in the heart muscle from obstruction of circulation

considered ideal or average, but are a frame of reference to which individuals may be compared (Katch and McArdle, 1993). In these models, essential fat refers to that stored in the marrow of bones; in the heart, liver, spleen, kidneys, intestines, and muscles; and in the central nervous system. The storage fat is the most variable component of body composition.

At entry to adulthood, women have a larger body fat mass and lower lean body or fat-free mass (FFM) than do men. Over time, body composition changes. As illustrated in Figure 12-3, the average percentage of body weight that is fat mass increases. This is accompanied by a decline in lean mass in both men and women. Based on data from more than 2 decades, Forbes (1999) estimated that adults who maintained their weight lost 1.5 kg FFM per decade, those who gained weight lost FFM more slowly, and those who lost weight lost even more FFM. During the middle adult years, these changes are reflected in increased fatfold thicknesses for both males and females, but body fat is greater and fluctuates more in females. Increased body fatness is associated with increased risk of diabetes mellitus, CHD, and hypertension.

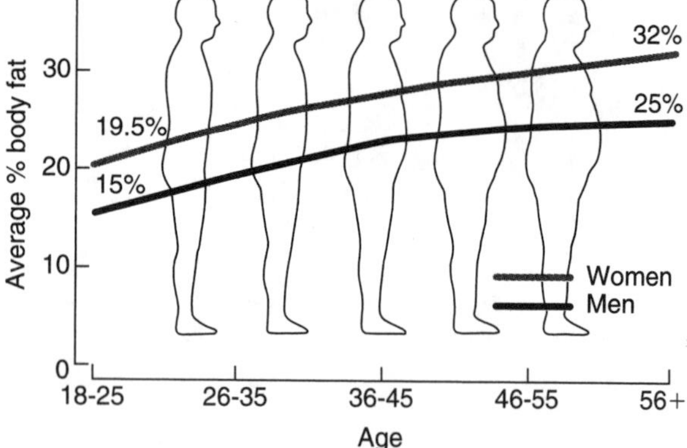

Figure 12-3 Average body fat increases with age. Average body fat for young men is about 15%. For young women, the average range is 18 to 23%. With age, the amount of muscle tends to drop and fat accounts for a greater percentage of weight. By age 60, body fat gradually increases to about 25% in men and 32% in women. *(From Medical Essay: Supplement to Mayo Clinic health letter, Rochester, MN, 1994, Mayo Foundation for Medical Education and Research. © 2001 Mayo Foundation for Medical Education and Research, Rochester, MN. 55905. Reprinted with permission.)*

Blood Lipid Levels

Serum total cholesterol (TC) levels increase in men until about 50 years of age. This pattern differs markedly from that observed in women, who have significantly lower levels than do men. For females TC levels increase after menopause from 50 years to 65 years of age, reaching the levels of males about 10 years later. Throughout adulthood males have a much greater ratio of TC to HDL-C, but after age 50 years this ratio is similar in males and females.

PSYCHOSOCIAL DEVELOPMENT

- *What psychosocial changes are associated with the adult years?*
- *How do stress and social and psychological issues influence dietary patterns?*

Psychosocial development of adulthood is characterized by changing patterns as societal roles develop and evolve. The early adult years are characterized by the formation of personal relationships, career development, establishment of home, rearing of young children, and assumption of a role within the community.

Gradual changes to middle adulthood are accompanied by adaptation to growing families, greater economic responsibilities, stable careers, and greater self-identity. Many of today's middle-age individuals find themselves sandwiched between generations, caring for aging parents and, because of delayed childbearing, raising young children.

There are approximately 76.8 million baby boomers born between 1946 and 1964, making up 28% of the U.S. population. This generation is very different from previous generations in numbers and characteristics. They have delayed childbirth and had fewer babies; they are better educated than previous generations and more women work (Chernoff, 1995). As their children mature and leave home, transitions of middle-age adults are accompanied by less-demanding family responsibilities, preparation for retirement, and renewed opportunities for personal development. Overall they spend 15% of their income on food, of which 23% is spent on food away from home (Dinkins, 1995). They also reported spending 4% on healthcare and 64% report worrying about healthcare in the future. Sixty-two percent are concerned about healthcare for an aging parent.

Physiologic needs form the foundation for health and nutrition status, but overall dietary patterns probably are more influenced by social and psychologic factors. Psychologic well-being is a multifaceted phenomenon that comprises both emotional functioning and satisfaction with life (Stewart and Ware, 1992). Psychologic well-being has been equated with the absence of anxiety and depression, the presence of positive affect, high levels of self-esteem, the capacity to deal with daily stresses, and positive ratings of satisfaction with personal life circumstances (Gauvin and Spence, 1996).

A combination of psychologic stress, social pressures, and sedentary life-style can contribute to poor dietary and activity patterns with negative health implications. As discussed in Chapter 3, the challenge is to motivate adults to make modest changes, primarily in food habits and exercise patterns, to improve their well-being and reduce the risk of disease. An understanding of the individual's life-style and psychosocial behaviors is central to monitoring and improving nutrition status.

NUTRITION ASSESSMENT

- *What tools are used for assessment of nutrition status of adults?*
- *Why is it appropriate to include identifiers of chronic disease in nutrition assessment?*
- *How are risks of chronic disease measured and monitored?*

The anthropometric, biochemical, clinical, and dietary techniques of nutrition screening and assessment are discussed in Chapter 2. Particular attention is given to identification of individuals at risk of undernutrition. This chapter presents additional measurements used for assessment of risk for nutrition-related chronic diseases. Such measurements are essential for early identification and intervention and for monitoring the effectiveness of nutrition care. Of particular importance is monitoring of those parameters related to major causes of death and disability: obesity, diabetes mellitus, hypertension, and CVD.

Excess Body Weight

Traditionally overweight and obesity are defined by comparison of an individual's weight-for-height to a reference standard such as the Metropolitan Relative Weight (MRW) or BMI. In the past the reference weight has been designated as "ideal" or "desirable." Such terms are misleading because there is no single appropriate weight for all individuals. Reference weights can be useful when they are associated with decreased health risks.

In 1996 the American Health Foundation (a nonprofit organization dedicated to finding preventive strategies to reduce chronic diseases) convened an expert panel that identified a healthy weight as one associated with the lowest morbidity (Meisler and St. Jeor, 1996). A BMI of less than 25 was considered the upper limit, beyond which morbidities of obesity are identifiable and weight-related disease risks become a concern (Table 12-1). These data, converted to weight-for-height, regardless of sex, are illustrated in Table 12-2.

Fatfold measurements increase and decrease with body fat. Values can be compared with the percentiles of reference data from NHANES (Appendixes B2 and B3). Deposition of increased body weight as abdominal fat during adulthood is a risk factor for hypertension and diabetes mellitus, and thus CHD, beyond that of excess weight alone (Croft et al., 1995). To identify increased risk associated with an accumulation of abdominal fat, routine measurement of waist circumferences is recommended. Table 12-1 indicates disease risk associated with weight and waist circumference. A waist circumference of 40 inches in males or 35 inches in females is associated with a significant increase in the incidence of disease.

Table 12-1 CLASSIFICATION AS OVERWEIGHT OR OBESE BY BMI, WAIST CIRCUMFERENCE, AND ASSOCIATED DISEASE RISKS

			Disease Risk[a] Relative to Normal Weight and Waist Circumference[b]	
	BMI (kg/m2)	Obesity Class	Men ≤102 cm (≤40 in) Women ≤88 cm (≤35 in)	>102 cm (>40 in) >88 cm (>35 in)
Underweight	<18.5		—	—
Normal	18.5-24.9		—	—
Overweight	25.0-29.9		Increased	High
Obesity	30.0-34.9	I	High	Very High
	35.0-39.9	II	Very High	Very High
Extreme Obesity	≥40	III	Extremely High	Extremely High

From National Heart, Lung, and Blood Institute: The practical guide. Identification, evaluation, and treatment of overweight and obesity in adults, NIH Pub # 00-4084, 2000. The evidence report, Bethesda, Md, preprint June 1998:228pp. This is Table ES-4 in the original report.

[a]Disease risk for type 2 diabetes, hypertension, and CVD.

[b]Increased waist circumference can also be a marker for increased risk, even in persons of normal weight.

Table 12-2 HEALTHY-WEIGHT TARGET FOR ADULTS REGARDLESS OF SEX, AS DERIVED FROM A BODY MASS INDEX OF 25

Height		Maximum Weight	
cm	in	kg	lb
147	58	54	119
150	59	56	124
152	60	58	128
155	61	60	132
157	62	62	136
160	63	64	141
163	64	66	145
165	65	68	150
168	66	70	155
170	67	72	159
173	68	75	164
175	69	77	169
178	70	79	174
180	71	81	179
183	72	84	184
185	73	86	189
188	74	88	194
190	75	91	200
193	76	93	205

From Meisler JG and St Jeor S: Summary and recommendations for the American Health Foundation Panel on Healthy Weight, Am J Clin Nutr 63(Suppl):476S, 1996. © Am J Clin Nutr. American Society for Clinical Nutrition.

Screening for Diabetes Mellitus

Diabetes mellitus is characterized by an abnormal metabolism of glucose that results from an absolute or relative lack of the hormone insulin. Type 2, or non–insulin-dependent diabetes mellitus (NIDDM), is more common in individuals with obesity. Screening and diagnostic testing are particularly important when an individual is obese, has a family history of diabetes mellitus, or has symptoms that suggest the presence of the disease. Screening for diabetes mellitus is based on plasma glucose levels.

When urine is tested as part of a routine physical examination, diabetes may be detected by the presence of glucose. A random plasma glucose level above 200 mg/dL is suggestive of the presence of diabetes. Although neither glucose in the urine nor a single elevated blood glucose is diagnostic for diabetes mellitus, an elevated level in the presence of symptoms or a family history of diabetes mellitus is an indicator for a glucose tolerance test (GTT) for diagnosis. A GTT involves the measurement of fasting blood glucose levels, administration of a glucose "load" (a solution containing 75 to 100 g glucose), and measurement of plasma glucose levels up to 3 to 5 hours later to determine **glucose tolerance.** There are several variations of the GTT. The values in Table 12-3 represent normal plasma glu-

Table 12-3 BLOOD GLUCOSE VALUES ASSOCIATED WITH DIABETES MELLITUS

Blood Glucose	Normal Value (mg/dL)	Diagnostic for Diabetes Mellitus (mg/dL)
Random glucose	<200	≥200 with signs and symptoms of diabetes mellitus
Fasting glucose	115	≥140 on at least two occasions
GLUCOSE TOLERANCE TEST		
Glucose load		
After 60 minutes	200	>200
After 120 minutes	140	200

cose levels in response to a glucose load and those that would be considered to confirm the diagnosis of diabetes mellitus. However, specific values may vary somewhat based on the measurement used and the laboratory completing the analysis.

It is estimated that as many as one third of individuals with type 2 diabetes are undiagnosed and up to 20% of those have evidence of vascular disease. Therefore early diagnosis becomes a goal. Inflammation is hypothesized to play a role in development of type 2 diabetes mellitus. It has been postulated that markers for inflammation, C-reactive protein, and Interleukin 6 (IL-6) may be useful for diabetes. Data from the Women's Health Study of a cohort of more than 27,000 women free of diagnosed diabetes mellitus, CVD, and cancer at baseline found that for women diagnosed 4 years later, elevated levels of C-reactive protein and IL-6 predicted the development of type 2 diabetes mellitus. Further confirmation of this observation may provide a diagnostic tool to identify diabetes so early treatment may be initiated.

Hypertension

Chronic hypertension is a major risk factor for CHD, cerebrovascular disease, and renal insufficiency. Blood pressure is measured in millimeters of mercury (mm Hg), a standard unit for the measurement of pressure.

Hypertension, a major public health problem, is defined as blood pressure exceeding the upper limit of normality; the upper limit is generally accepted as **systolic pressure** greater than 140 mm mercury (Hg) and **diastolic pressure** greater than 90 mm mercury (Hg) (Joint National Committee on the Detection, Evaluation and Treatment of High Blood Pressure, 1997).

Serum Lipids and Lipoproteins

Elevated levels of serum TC and LDL-C and low levels of HDL-C have been correlated with increased rates of CHD. They are used routinely for assessment of risk and monitoring of intervention. Approximately 7% of the body's cholesterol circulates in the blood. Because lipids such as cholesterol and triglycerides are fat soluble, they must be transported in the bloodstream from sites of absorption or synthesis to sites of storage or metabolism on lipoproteins. Lipoproteins are spheric macromolecular complexes of lipids (triglycerides, cholesterol, cholesterol ester, and phospholipids) and special proteins known as apoproteins. The apoprotein portion controls the interaction and metabolic fate of a given lipoprotein. Apoproteins activate enzymes that modify the composition and structure of lipoproteins, are involved in the binding and uptake of lipoproteins by cells, and participate in the exchange of lipids between lipoproteins of different classes. Major transport lipoproteins are chylomicrons, high-density lipoproteins (HDLs),

KEY TERMS

glucose tolerance: efficiency with which the body can clear a bolus of glucose from the blood

systolic pressure: pressure that occurs with contraction of the heart muscle

diastolic pressure: pressure during relaxation of the ventricles

low-density proteins (LDLs), and very-low-density lipoproteins (VLDLs).

Chylomicrons, synthesized in the small intestine, transport dietary triglyceride from the small intestine to adipose tissue, muscle, and the liver. They are 90% triglyceride. The dietary cholesterol they carry is taken up by the liver for production of bile acids or later incorporated in VLDLs. Chylomicrons are found in the serum in the postprandial state.

The VLDLs are 60% triglyceride by weight and contain 10% to 15% of the serum's TC. Synthesized in the liver, VLDLs carry triglycerides to the cells for storage and metabolism. When triglycerides are removed from VLDL, the remaining smaller and denser lipoprotein particles are known as intermediate density lipoprotein (IDL) because the density of IDL falls between that of VLDL and LDL. Approximately one half the IDLs are catabolized by the liver and the remaining IDLs undergo changes that transform them into LDLs.

The LDL contains approximately 70% of the serum TC. Its primary role is to transport cholesterol to various cells of the body. The LDL is considered the most atherogenic lipoprotein. About 70% to 80% of LDL-C is removed from the serum by LDL receptors located on the plasma membranes of hepatic and peripheral cells. The remaining 20% to 30% are degraded by **macrophages.**

Most clinical laboratories do not measure LDL-C directly. Instead, it is calculated based on measurements of TC, HDL-C, and triglycerides. In this procedure, VLDL-cholesterol is estimated by dividing the triglyceride measurement by 5. The following equation for calculating LDL-C is recommended by the National Cholesterol Education Program (NCEP):

$$\text{LDL-C} = \text{TC} - \text{HDL-C} - (\text{Triglyceride}/5)$$

This formula cannot be used when the triglyceride level is greater than 400 mg/dL.

HDL is the smallest and most dense of the lipoproteins. Secreted by the liver and small intestine in a disk-shaped form, HDL eventually assumes a spheric shape as it takes up phospholipids and cholesterol from other lipoproteins and body cells. It appears that HDL picks up cholesterol from the bloodstream, other lipoproteins, and various cells of the body and transports it to the liver where it is excreted in the bile, converted to bile acids, or reprocessed into VLDL. This reverse transport process is thought to be at least part of the explanation for the strong **inverse relationship** between serum HDL-C and CHD risk.

The National Institutes of Health's National Cholesterol Education Program (2001) encourages Americans to modify their diets to reduce the risk of CHD. The NCEP Guidelines define risk status according to levels of TC, HDL-C, and LDL-C (Table 12-4). These measurements are used in conjunction with other major risk factors (Box 12-1) to evaluate risk and formulate guidelines for intervention.

Table 12-4 RISK STATUS ACCORDING TO TOTAL SERUM CHOLESTEROL AND LDL AND HDL CHOLESTEROL

LDL CHOLESTEROL	
<100	Optimal
100-129	Near or above optimal
130-159	Borderline high
160-189	High
≥190	Very high
TOTAL CHOLESTEROL	
<200	Desirable
200-239	Borderline high
≥240	High
HDL CHOLESTEROL	
<40	Low
≥60	High

From Third Report of the National Cholesterol Education Program (NCEP) Panel on Detection, Evaluation and Treatment of High Blood Cholesterol in Adults (Adult Treatment Panel II), Bethesda, Md, 2001, National Heart and Blood Institute. National Institutes of Health.
LDL, low-density lipoprotein; HDL, high-density lipoprotein.

ENERGY AND NUTRIENT NEEDS

- *What are the Recommended Dietary Allowances (RDAs)?*
- *How do energy and nutrient needs change across adulthood?*
- *For which nutrients are there concerns about adequate intakes (AIs)?*

Box 12-1 Major Risk Factors for Coronary Heart Disease*

- LDL-cholesterol >130 mg/dL
- Cigarette smoking
- Hypertension (blood pressure ≥140/90 mm Hg or on antihypertensive medication)
- Low HDL cholesterol (<40 mg/dL)†
- Family history of premature CHD (CHD in male first-degree relative <55 years; CHD in female first-degree relative <65 years)
- Age (men ≥45 years; women ≥55 years)

From Third Report of the National Cholesterol Education Program (NCEP) Panel on Detection, Evaluation and Treatment of High Blood Cholesterol in Adults (Adult Treatment Panel II), Bethesda, Md, 2001, National Heart and Blood Institute. National Institutes of Health.

*Diabetes is regarded as a coronary heart disease (CHD) risk equivalent. LDL indicates low-density lipoprotein; HDL, high-density lipoprotein.

†HDL cholesterol ≥60 mg/dL counts as a "negative" risk factor; its presence removes 1 risk factor from the total count.

At the time of this writing, a panel of experts of the Institute of Medicine is preparing the Dietary Reference Intake (DRI) report for energy and macronutrients (protein, amino acids, fats and fatty acids, carbohydrates, and fiber). In the following discussion of energy and macronutrients, recommended intakes for energy and protein are based on the 1989 RDAs (Food and Nutrition Board, 1989). Remember that the term *RDA* is used to describe nutrients for which levels have been established based on the criterion for a RDA—namely, that a requirement can be established as the basis for the recommendation. For other nutrients, AI levels are given when an RDA cannot be established. Upper limits for all nutrients for which they have been established can be found inside the front cover of this text. Be sure to ask your instructor about progress on the DRI changes for energy and macronutrients.

During the adult years, excluding pregnancy and lactation, nutrients are used for body repair and maintenance. The 1989 RDAs are levels recommended. For adults the 1989 RDA levels for energy and protein intakes were divided into the age groups—19 years to 24 years, 25 years to 50 years, and older than 50 years—which are different from the age groups established for the DRI. The heights and weights of the reference males and females for these age groups are designated to quantify daily levels. Actual levels needed or consumed by healthy adults vary with individual age, body size, and activity level.

Energy and Macronutrients

The energy need of an individual is the level required to balance that used for REE, physical activity, and the thermic effect of food. For most adults the REE represents the largest component of total energy used each day, and as mentioned previously, it is highly correlated with lean body mass. Therefore males have higher REEs than females and lean individuals have higher levels than do those with greater proportions of body fat. Except in individuals who engage in vigorous physical activity, daily energy expenditure for physical activity is less than that for REE.

Energy needs vary widely. They are determined, to some extent, by age, sex, body size and composition, genetic factors, energy intake, activity level, and ambient temperature. The RDA for energy assumes that an individual's body size and composition and level of physical activity are consistent with long-term good health. The RDA for adults, expressed as kilocalories per kilogram of body weight, appear in Table 12-5. Energy recommendations range from 40 kcal/kg for the reference 72-kg male, age 19 years to 24 years, to 37 kcal/kg at age 25 years to 50 years, to 30 kcal/kg for those older than 50 years. Energy levels for the reference female in these three age categories are 38 kcal/kg, 35 kcal/kg, and 30 kcal/kg body weight, respectively.

Mean daily total food energy intakes of adults age 20 years to 59 years participating in the third NHANES (NHANES III) appear in Table 12-6. It is

KEY TERMS

macrophages: large phagocytic cells located within connective tissue

inverse relationship: a decrease in one variable (e.g., CHD risk) as another variable (e.g., HDL-C level) increases; also called *negative relationship*

apparent that energy intakes decline with age for both men and women. It is important to note that for women of all ages and men age 40 years to 49 years, mean food energy intakes are consistently below the RDA. Despite this fact, the prevalence of overweight among Americans has increased dramatically in the last decade (Kuczmarski et al., 1998). Such observations have led to concerns about the nutrient adequacy of American diets with kilocalorie levels below recommended amounts and potentially reduced energy output from physical activity. Any nutrient or dietary recommendations to support health must be based on this consideration.

Table 12-5 RECOMMENDED ENERGY INTAKES FOR ADULTS

Age (y)	Weight (kg)	kcal/day	kcal/kg
MALES			
19-24	72	2900	40
25-50	79	2900	37
51+	77	2300	30
FEMALES			
19-24	58	2200	38
25-50	63	2200	35
51+	65	1900	30

From National Academy of Sciences, Food and Nutrition Board, National Research Council: Recommended dietary allowances, ed 10, Washington, DC, 1989, National Academy Press.

Protein

The 1989 recommended protein intakes of 0.8 g/kg body weight per day for adult men and women assume that a diet of mixed sources of protein is consumed. Mean protein intakes in NHANES III were 15% of kilocalories, a level adequate for most individuals (McDowell et al., 1994). If an individual restricts his or her total food intake or restricts intake of some protein foods, careful dietary planning is required to achieve the RDA. Equally important, the recommendations for protein are based on the assumption that the individual consumes an adequate amount of energy to spare dietary protein for protein synthesis. If energy intake is below maintenance levels, additional protein is required to compensate for that catabolized to meet energy needs.

Fats and Fatty Acids

Total fat consumption among Americans has decreased from approximately 41% of energy intake in the late 1970s to 36% in the mid-1980s to 33% in 1994 (Agricultural Research Service, 1996). However, only one third of adults met the

Table 12-6 MEAN DAILY TOTAL FOOD-ENERGY INTAKE (TFEI) AND PERCENTAGES OF TFEI FROM TOTAL DIETARY FAT AND FROM SATURATED FAT, BY AGE GROUP AND SEX

Age Group	Sample Size	Daily TFEI	TFEI from Total Dietary Fat (%)	TFEI from Saturated Fat (%)
MALES				
20-29	844	3025	34.0	12.0
30-39	735	2872	34.6	11.9
40-49	626	2545	33.9	11.4
50-59	473	2341	35.7	11.8
FEMALES				
20-29	838	1957	34.0	11.9
30-39	791	1883	34.2	11.9
40-49	602	1764	34.9	11.8
50-59	456	1629	33.8	11.4

From Third National Health and Nutrition Examination Survey, Phase I, 1988-91, Morb Mortal Wkly Rep 116, 1994.

recommendation of getting 30% or fewer kilocalories from fat. Data from NHANES III indicate that saturated fat constitutes a mean of 12% of kilocalories in the diets of Americans (McDowell et al., 1994). The NHANES I Epidemiologic Follow-Up Survey (NHEFS) found that from the survey in 1971 to 1974 to a decade later, the percentage of energy intake from fat and weight change were inversely related in women, but positively associated in men (Kant et al., 1995).

A review of the U.S. Dietary Association's National Food Consumption Survey (FCS) and the Continuing Survey of Food Intake by Individuals (CSFII) evaluated intake from fat over time (1965 to 1995) and found that use of low-fat food products were more likely to meet the Dietary Guidelines for fat and saturated fat (Kennedy et al., 1999).

Vitamins and Minerals

As indicated in the discussion of DRIs in Chapter 1, four reports have been completed and reference intakes have been established for vitamins and minerals, thus completing the vitamins and most elements (Table 12-7). A review of electrolytes (such as sodium, potassium, chloride) and water is yet to be initiated. (Estimated minimum requirements for sodium, chloride, and potassium appear in Appendix A.)

Table 12-7 Dietary Reference Intakes for Vitamins and Minerals for Adults

Nutrient	Females 19-30 y	Females 31-50 y	Males 19-30 y	Males 31-50 y
Calcium, mg	*1000*	*1000*	*1000*	*1000*
Phosphorus, mg	**700**	**700**	**700**	**700**
Magnesium, mg	**310**	**320**	**400**	**420**
Fluoride, mg	*3*	*3*	*4*	*4*
Vitamin D, µg	*5*	*5*	*5*	*5*
Thiamin, mg	**1.1**	**1.1**	**1.2**	**1.2**
Riboflavin, mg	**1.1**	**1.1**	**1.3**	**1.3**
Niacin, mg	**14**	**14**	**16**	**16**
Vitamin B_6, mg	**1.5**	**1.5**	**1.7**	**1.7**
Folate, µg	**400**	**400**	**400**	**400**
Vitamin B_{12}	**2.4**	**2.4**	**2.4**	**2.4**
Pantothenic Acid, mg	*5*	*5*	*5*	*5*
Biotin, µg	*30*	*30*	*30*	*30*
Choline, mg	*550*	*550*	*425*	*425*
Vitamin C, mg	**75**	**75**	**90**	**90**
Vitamin E, mg	**15**	**15**	**15**	**15**
Selenium, µg	**55**	**55**	**55**	**55**
Vitamin A, µg	**700**	**700**	**900**	**900**
Vitamin K, µg	*90*	*90*	*120*	*120*
Chromium, µg	*25*	*25*	*35*	*35*
Copper, µg	**900**	**900**	**900**	**900**
Iodine, µg	**150**	**150**	**150**	**150**
Iron, mg	*18*	*18*	*8*	*8*
Manganese, mg	*1.8*	*1.8*	*2.3*	*2.3*
Molybdenum, µg	**45**	**45**	**45**	**45**
Zinc, mg	**8**	**8**	**11**	**11**

Adapted with permission from the following Institute of Medicine publications: Dietary reference intakes for calcium, phosphorus, magnesium, vitamin D, and fluoride (1997); Dietary reference intakes for thiamin, riboflavin, niacin, vitamin B_6, folate, vitamin $B_{12,}$ pantothenic acid, biotin, and choline (1998); Dietary reference intakes for vitamin C, vitamin E, selenium, and carotenoids (2000); and Dietary reference intakes for vitamin A, vitamin K, arsenic, boron, chromium, copper, iodine, iron, manganese, molybdenum, nickel, silicon, vanadium and zinc (2001). Washington, DC, National Academy Press.
RDAs are printed in bold type; AIs are printed in italics.

For adults the DRIs are reported for the age group 19 to 50 years.

Calcium and Related Nutrients

Calcium

The AI level for calcium is 1000 mg per day for men and women from 19 years to 50 years to promote development and maintenance of maximum peak bone mass and, potentially, to reduce the risk of osteoporosis in later life. As discussed in Chapter 13, the link between calcium intake and reduced risk of progressive osteoporosis is well documented. In fact supplements of 600 mg of calcium are frequently recommended for postmenopausal women to reduce the risk of progressive osteoporosis. In addition there is evidence that intakes of calcium and/or dairy products are inversely related to colon cancer (Holt, 1999) and breast cancer (Lipkin and Newmark, 1999).

Vitamin D

The AI levels for vitamin D in this age group are 5 μg; however, most adults are likely to get sufficient exposure to sunlight to meet their needs. As discussed in Chapter 13, to minimize the effects of osteoporosis, sufficient vitamin D must be available to facilitate calcium absorption and bone formation. If an individual has little exposure to sunlight and does not consume vitamin D-fortified milk, a supplemental source should be considered. Most calcium supplements include vitamin D.

Fluoride

An AI level of fluoride is 3 μg and 4 μg for women and men, respectively. Over one half of the U.S. population has access to water with optimal fluoride concentration—about 1 mg per day per person.

B Complex Vitamins

Vitamin B_6

Vitamin B_6 is required for a variety of metabolic reactions, particularly those in protein metabolism as the coenzyme pyridoxal phosphate (PLP) that participates in the transfer of amino groups. Vitamin B_6 is involved in conversion of tryptophan to serotonin and the synthesis of heme. There is evidence that B_6 influences cognitive performance and immune function. Because of its central role in protein metabolism, the allowance for vitamin B_6 has been set at a level that appears to maintain adequate blood values for most indices of vitamin B_6 status. The recommended levels are higher than those in many countries around the world because they reflect the fact that protein intake levels in the United States may be as much as 50% to 100% greater than recommended levels.

Folate

Current dietary allowances for folate reflect levels that maintain adequate folate status and liver stores. The allowance, 3 μg per kg body weight, is an amount within the range of typical consumption levels by healthy adults in the United States and Canada. Folate is critical in early embryonic development for the formation of the neural tube. Evidence from clinical intervention studies indicates that intakes of folate above the RDA (400 μg) during the period before conception and during early pregnancy can reduce the recurrence of neural tube defects in newborns significantly (see Chapter 4, page 106). The U.S. Public Health Service (Centers for Disease Control and Prevention, 1992) recommended that women of childbearing age consume at least 400 μg of folic acid daily to reduce their risk of having a pregnancy in which the child is affected with spina bifida or other neural tube defect. To significantly increase the daily folate intake, the Food and Drug Administration (FDA) mandated that effective January 1, 1998, folate must be added to most enriched flour, breads, corn meals, rice, noodles, macaroni, and other grain products (Federal Register, 1996). Fortification of grains to improve folate intake will improve intake levels for the whole population, which has the potential of having a positive impact on CVD by reducing elevated blood levels of homocysteine, a recognized independent risk factor for CHD.

Vitamin B_{12}

The AI levels for Vitamin B_{12} for adult males and females are based on levels that will sustain metabolic functions, maintain normal serum concentrations, and promote accumulation or maintenance of substantial body stores. Vitamin B_{12} and folate are closely related. Each depends on the other for activation. Regeneration of the amino acid methionine and synthesis of deoxyribonucleic acid (DNA) and ribonucleic acid (RNA) depend on folate and Vitamin B_{12}. Also, B_{12} maintains the sheath that surrounds and protects nerve fibers and promotes their normal growth. It is unique among vitamins in that it is found almost exclusively in foods derived from animals. For vegans who opt not to consume animal products, B_{12} supplements or B_{12}-fortified foods are recommended.

Antioxidants

Vitamin C

Vitamin C functions as a water-soluble antioxidant, which means it neutralizes oxidizing agents before they can damage cells in the body. It is required for the synthesis of collagen, carnitine, and neurotransmitters. The recommended allowance for vitamin C for adults is 75 mg for females and 90 for males, levels considered sufficient to provide an average body pool of 1500 mg and a margin of sufficiency because vitamin C is poorly retained in the body. It is well recognized that cigarette smoking increases the destruction of vitamin C and higher levels of intake are recommended for smokers.

Vitamin E

A specific role for vitamin E in a required function has not been established. Its major function is as a chain-breaking antioxidant that is soluble in fatty substances. The vitamin E recommendations are based on alpha tocopherol only. The RDA levels are set at 15 mg. Persons who consume large amounts of polyunsaturated fatty acids (PUFAs) need more vitamin E.

Other Vitamins and Minerals

Vitamin A

Vitamin A plays many roles in the body. In particular, it is required for normal vision, gene expression, reproduction, embryonic development, and immune function. In addition to its established biologic roles, there has been substantial interest in the use of creams containing retinoic acid (traditionally a medication to treat acne) to prevent wrinkling or diminish the brown age spots that begin to appear on the skin of some individuals in middle age. Recommendations are expressed as **retinal activity equivalents** (RAEs).

Vitamin K

Vitamin K is required for normal blood coagulation. Adequacy of status is assessed by maintenance of plasma prothrombin concentrations. Anticoagulant drugs function by interfering with the use of vitamin K in the process of blood coagulation. Individuals who are treated with these drugs should have their vitamin K status monitored carefully. Treatment of individuals with broad-spectrum antibiotics may reduce gastrointestinal absorption of vitamin K and make them susceptible to deficiency.

Iron

Iron is a component of hemoglobin and numerous enzymes. The recommendations for iron are based on amounts required to replace daily iron losses, which are estimated to be 8 mg for men and postmenopausal women and 1.8 mg in menstruating women. Assuming an overall absorption of 10% for dietary iron, the RDA for iron is 8 mg for men and postmenopausal women and 18 mg for premenopausal women.

Adult men have an iron store of about 1 g; menstruating women have a store of about 300 mg. When total body iron is increased 5-fold to 10-fold, clinical manifestations of damaging effects of iron occur (Lynch, 1995).

Iron can mediate the production of free radicals that lead to tissue damage. Evidence suggests that oxidation of LDL within the arterial wall may depend on the presence of iron or copper. Salonen and coworkers (1992) found a strong association between high serum ferritin concentrations and the risk for acute myocardial infarction in men, particularly in those with

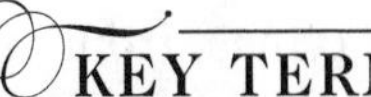

KEY TERMS

retinal activity equivalents (RAEs): one μg of retinal and 12 μg of beta carotene

elevated serum LDL-C concentrations, but results of other studies have been inconsistent.

A major difficulty with current epidemiologic surveys is dependence on a single measure of iron status (Sempos et al., 1994). A second limitation is the absence of reports of vascular damage in patients with hereditary disorders of severe iron overload. An association between increased iron stores and the prevalence of cancer has also been postulated on the basis of epidemiologic studies (Knekt et al., 1994), but iron storage status has not been adequately characterized in these studies.

Iodine

Iodine is required as a component of the thyroid hormones, thyroxine and triiodothyronine. In the 1900s iodine deficiency goiter was widespread in the United States. Iodine supplementation of salt and other foods reduced the risk of goiter and by the 1960s, iodine-related problems were more likely to be associated with too much rather than too little of this essential nutrient (Lee, 1999). Recent data suggest a sharp decline in iodine intake during the last 20 years, especially in women of reproductive age (Hollowell et al., 1998). It appears that at the start of the twenty-first century, iodine deficiency may create health concerns for some, especially in women, and for excess iodine in certain individuals who are at risk because of preexisting thyroid pathology.

Zinc

Zinc supports numerous proteins functioning in many metabolic processes. Zinc stabilizes cell membranes by strengthening their defense against free radical attacks. It supports immune function and growth and development. It is required for utilization of vitamin A. The RDA levels for females and males of all ages are 8 and 11 mg per day, respectively.

The recommended levels of nutrients are based on the assumption that the diet contains adequate energy to maintain a healthy weight and includes recommended servings from all food groups. The potential benefits of eating a variety of foods include preventing excesses or deficiencies of micronutrients, promoting balance among nutrients, and limiting exposure to any one type of food and thereby to any associated contaminants. Less-tangible advantages are increased personal choices and enjoyment of eating. However, a single value or group of values must be considered in the context of the overall diet, which contains foods from all food groups. As will become apparent in the following section, the potential role of specific nutrients in prevention or treatment of chronic disease is an area of great interest. If future research does support such a benefit, the DRIs will be revised to support dietary intake levels for that purpose.

CHRONIC HEALTH CONCERNS OF ADULTS: CARDIOVASCULAR DISEASE

- *How does atherosclerosis develop and progress?*
- *What are the major risk factors for CHD?*
- *What effect does excess body fatness and its distribution have on risk of chronic disease?*
- *How do dietary factors influence levels of blood lipids, lipoproteins, and platelet aggregation?*
- *What dietary recommendations are appropriate to prevent CHD for all Americans? For individuals at risk?*
- *Why are diabetes mellitus and hypertension risk factors for CHD?*
- *Can nutrition intervention for diabetes mellitus influence the development of CHD?*
- *What are the roles of excess body weight and dietary intake in development and control of hypertension?*

Despite a decline of more than 50% in the death rate from CHD since 1950, CVD is the most common cause of death in the United States, accounting for more than 260.6 deaths per 100,000 population. In 1999 it was estimated that 58 million Americans live with some form of CVD, with an estimated cost of $287 billion (Centers for Disease Control and Prevention, 2000).

When the coronary arteries supplying the heart with oxygen and nutrients become narrowed and inelastic because of atherosclerosis, CHD results. Atherosclerosis begins with the deposition of fatty streaks in macrophages and smooth muscle cells within the inner lining of large elastic and muscular arteries. High levels of LDL-C are atherogenic. Evidence supports the hypothesis that LDL undergoes oxidative modification that targets it for uptake by macrophages. Lipoprotein-loaded macrophages (foam cells) accumulate in fatty streaks, which are the earliest identifiable lesions in atherogenesis. Foam cells may become nonfunctional and die, releasing cytotoxic contents that damage the overlying endothelium. These early lesions do not substantially diminish blood flow in the affected artery. Eventually, however, more lipid accumulates and a **fibrous plaque** develops that projects into the channel or lumen of the artery, resulting in ischemia, or impaired blood flow. Ischemia within the myocardium can result in **angina pectoris.** If the impairment of blood flow is severe, the tissues nourished by the obstructed artery may die. When this process affects the coronary arteries, a myocardial infarction occurs; in cerebral arteries, a stroke results. Atherosclerotic changes within other arteries can result in peripheral vascular disease.

An individual's risk of developing CHD and the rate at which atherosclerosis progresses are influenced by many factors. They include some that cannot be modified, such as age, sex, and family history of premature CHD. Others, such as body weight, cigarette smoking, blood pressure, blood lipid levels, and diabetes mellitus, may be modified to reduce the risk of myocardial infarction or death.

Risk Factors for Cardiovascular Disease

The good news about CVD is the remarkable decline in mortality from heart disease and stroke. The bad news is that young people in the United States today are smoking more, weigh more, and are less physically active than in the past (Hennekens, 1997). Numerous risk factors for CVD have been identified. Prominent factors include excess body weight, elevated TC and LDL-C, and hypertension. Life-style factors include exercise, diet, use of alcohol and cigarettes, and stress. For example a 16-year NHEFS review (Gartside et al., 1998) of coronary events revealed a positive association with age, serum cholesterol, BMI, and cigarette use. There was an inverse relationship with female gender, fish intake, alcohol use, moderate exercise, and moderate and heavy habitual physical activity.

Gender

Epidemiologic studies show that women do not develop heart disease and other complications of atherosclerosis until 10 years after their male counterparts. By menopause, however, estrogen levels have started to decline and body weight and cholesterol levels tend to rise, as does the risk of suffering a heart attack or stroke. Nonetheless, when women are stricken, they are more likely to die and survivors are more likely than are male survivors to have another heart attack or stroke.

The Women's Healthy Lifestyle Project was designed to determine if changes in life-style could help women fend off the increases in cholesterol (and body weight) that so often accompany menopause in women 44 years to 50 years of age. The project evaluated the effects of reducing intake of calories (1300 kcal), fat (30% of kcal), saturated fat (7% of kcal), and cholesterol (300 mg) and increasing physical activity in 535 women who were just about to enter menopause and had average risk of heart disease (Kuller et al., 2001b). The 5-year intervention program began with an intensive group component during the first 6 months and individual and group follow-up sessions for the remainder of the study. All of the women were given a modest weight-loss goal of 5 pounds to 15 pounds, depending on how overweight they were at the beginning of the program. Researchers recommended burning 1000 kcal to 1500 kcal per week through physical activity. At 54 months, compared with the control group, the women who followed the intervention had a smaller increase in LDL-C, a weight gain of only 0.2 lb versus 5.2 lbs, and a slight decrease in waist circumference. These findings are quite encouraging because it demonstrates that life-style changes can blunt the rise in LDL-C that typically

KEY TERMS

fibrous plaque: the lesion of atherosclerosis that bulges into the lumen. It is composed of lipid, cell debris, smooth muscle cells, and collagen

angina pectoris: chest pain caused by insufficient blood flow to the heart

occurs around menopause. In addition women in the intervention group were able to avoid adding pounds, at least for the duration of the study. Because they maintained their premenopausal body weight, these women can expect significant health benefits including a lower risk for heart disease, diabetes, high blood pressure, and arthritis. However, a separate paper from this research group reported that women in the intervention group who modified their life-style to lose weight had a significantly higher rate of decline in BMD at the hip and lumbar spine (Salamone et al., 1999).

Overweight and Regional Adiposity

Overweight constitutes a substantial burden because it leads to a worsening of all the elements of the cardiovascular risk profile (Must et al., 1999). Systolic and diastolic blood pressures are higher, serum TC and LDL-C are increased, and concentrations of glucose in the blood are moderately greater. Furthermore, there is a graded relation so that risk is proportional to the degree of adiposity (Hubert et al., 1983). Reduction of weight has the potential to reduce the incidence of many risk factors. For example a follow-up of data from the Framingham Study showed improvement in blood pressure and plasma cholesterol with weight loss (Kannel et al., 1996). Weight gain can offset other heart-positive changes. In the more than 85,000 women in the Nurses' Health Study, reduction in smoking, improvement in diet, and an increase in postmenopausal hormone accounted for a decline in the incidence of coronary disease, but the decline appeared to have been slowed by the prevalence of obesity (Hu, 2000).

The Expert Panel of the American Health Foundation has defined healthier weight goals as a reasonable upper limit for body weight that would offer a reduction in disease risk for most overweight adults (Table 12-8). It has been postulated that these goals of 10 to 16 pounds, if achieved, will reduce health risks for chronic diseases and that the goal weights are attainable for most overweight adults (Meisler and St. Jeor, 1996).

Regional obesity appears to be an independent contributor to CVD. For men under the age of 65 years, obesity, regardless of fat distribution, is a risk factor for CHD (Rimm et al., 1995). For older men, the waist circumference is the best predictor of risk of death from CVD (Baik et al., 2000). Central obesity is associated with a greater risk of developing diabetes than is adiposity (Haffner et al., 1991). Reduction of body fat has the potential to reduce risk for each of these diseases.

Table 12-8 HEALTHIER-WEIGHT GOALS FOR ADULTS WHO ARE ABOVE THE HEALTHY-WEIGHT TARGET FOR A GIVEN HEIGHT, REGARDLESS OF SEX, AS DERIVED FROM TWO-UNIT EQUIVALENTS OF THE BODY MASS INDEX

Height		Weight Loss	
cm	in	kg	lb
147	58	4.5	10
150	59	4.5	10
152	60	4.5	10
155	61	5	11
157	62	5	11
160	63	5	11
163	64	5.5	12
165	65	5.5	12
168	66	5.5	12
170	67	6	13
173	68	6	13
175	69	6.5	14
178	70	6.5	14
180	71	6.5	14
183	72	7	15
185	73	7	15
188	74	7.5	16
190	75	7.5	16
193	76	7.5	16

From Meisler JG and St Jeor S: Summary and recommendations from the American Health Foundation Panel on Healthy Weight, Am J Clin Nutr 63:(suppl):476S, 1996. © Am J Clin Nutr. American Society for Clinical Nutrition.

Blood Lipid Levels

The risk factors most directly associated with CHD are elevated serum TC and LDL-C and reduced HDL-C. Guidelines for classifying TC,

LDL-C, and HDL-C levels in adults appear in Table 12-4. Figure 12-4 shows the distribution of high LDL-C and low HDL-C in the U.S. population as reported in data from NHANES III. It has been demonstrated in controlled prospective studies that lowering TC and LDL-C with diet (Schaefer et al., 1995) or drug therapy (Gotto, 1995) halts the progression of atherosclerotic lesions and may stabilize the rupture-prone lesions that are present, thereby reducing the subsequent risk of CHD morbidity and mortality (Stamler et al., 2000).

In 2001, the Expert Panel on Detection, Evaluation, and Treatment of High Blood Cholesterol Adult Treatment Panel III (ATP III) issued new guidelines for prevention, diagnosis, and treatment of CAD. Characteristics of the ATP III guidelines are focused on primary prevention, identification of multiple risk factors, complete lipoprotein profile for screening, new lower levels for lipids and lipoprotein levels as thresholds for intervention and more aggressive life-style changes and medical interventions to lower cholesterol levels.

Primary prevention. The primary concern for CVD is to decrease risk by modifying individual risk factors when possible. The *Dietary Guidelines for Americans,* presented in Chapter 1, are general guidance for heart healthy life-styles. The American Heart Association recently released its *AHA Scientific Statement: AHA Dietary Guidelines* (Kraus et al., 2000), which are outlined in Box 12-2.

Risk assessment. The first step in risk assessment is a complete lipoprotein profile obtained after a 9- to 12-hour fast, measures TC, LDL-C and HDL-C, cholesterol and triglycerides. Knowing the LDL-C is the target of therapy. The ATP III recommends that all adults aged 20 years and older obtain a fasting lipoprotein profile at least every 5 years.

In the second step of risk assessment, the presence of clinical atherosclerotic disease (clinical CHD, symptomatic carotid artery disease, peripheral artery disease, or abdominal aortic aneurysm) is determined. Clinical atherosclerotic

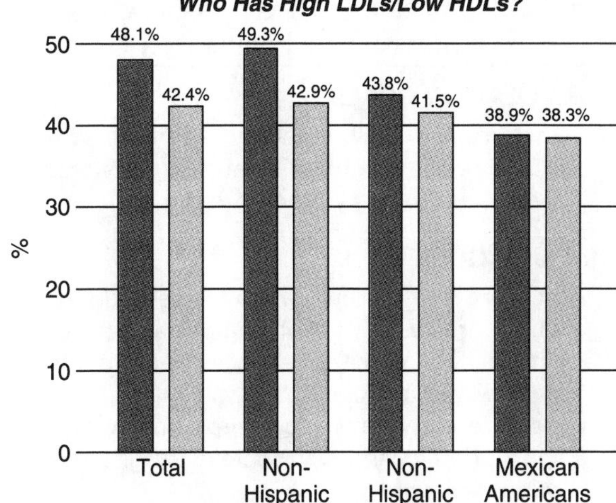

LDL: Percentage of Americans age 20 years and older with LDL cholesterol greater than 130 mg/dL (borderline high).

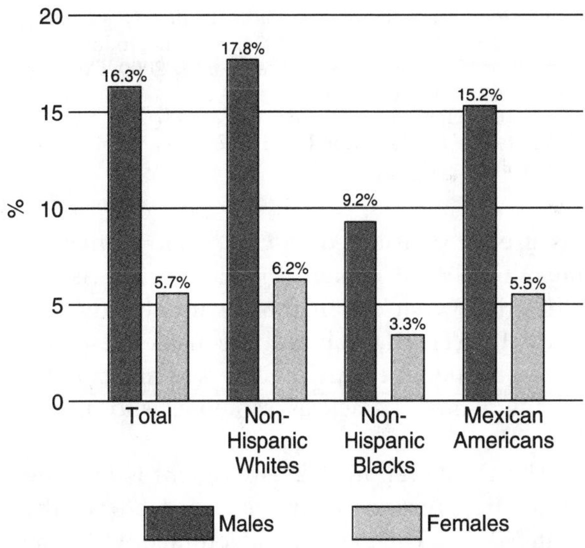

HDL: Percentage of Americans age 20 years and older with HDL cholesterol of 35 mg/dL or lower (increased risk or coronary heart disease).

National Health and Nutrition Examination Survey III (NHANES III)

Figure 12-4 Distribution of high LDL and low HDL cholesterol levels from the National Nutrition Examination Survey (NHANES III).

Box 12-2 American Heart Association Summary of Population Goals

POPULATION GOALS

- Encourage a healthy eating pattern, appropriate body weight, desirable cholesterol profile, and healthy blood pressure.

MAJOR GUIDELINES

- Increase the variety of fruits, vegetables, whole grains, low-fat or nonfat dairy products, fish, legumes, poultry, and lean meats in the American diet.
- Match energy intake to energy needs with appropriate changes to achieve weight loss when necessary.
- Limit foods high in saturated fat and cholesterol, substituting unsaturated or monounsaturated fats found in vegetables, fish, legumes, or nuts.
- Limit salt and alcohol.
- Maintain a healthy body weight.

From American Heart Association: AHA dietary guidelines: revision 2000, Circulation 102:2284, 2000. Reproduced with permission. Dietary Guidelines Revision.
The "AHA Scientific Statement" prepared by the Nutrition Committee of the American Heart Association details the revised guidelines.

disease is considered a CHD risk equivalent, meaning that it confers the same high risk for CHD risk events as in those who already have CHD. In ATP III, diabetes is considered a CHD risk equivalent because it confers as high a risk of having a heart attack as someone who already has CHD.

The third step in risk assessment is to determine the presence of major risk factors other than LDL-C. The major risk factors for CHD that modify the LDL goal are listed in Table 12-4.

If two or more risk factors are present without CHD or a CHD risk equivalent, a scoring system (Framingham Risk Assessment) is used to estimate short-term (10-year) risk. The system uses age, TC, smoking status, HDL-C level, and systolic blood pressure to estimate 10-year risk for heart disease. The ATP III divides those with multiple (2 or more) risk factors into three categories based on the 10-year risk for CHD >20%, 10 to 20% and <10%. The LDL goal of therapy is based on which of the three categories of CHD the individual falls into:

- Persons with clinical atherosclerotic disease or a 10-year risk >20% are placed in the highest risk group. The LDL goal for this highest risk group is <100 mg/dL.
- Persons with two or more risk factors and a 10-year risk <20% have an LDL goal of 130 mg/dL.
- Individuals who have a zero to one major risk factor usually have a 10-year risk of less than 10%. The LDL goal for persons with zero to one risk factor is 160 mg/dL.

Lowering Coronary Heart Disease Risk. To lower CHD risk, a multifaceted life-style approach termed therapeutic life-style changes (TLCs) are appropriate. The TLC is for anyone whose LDL is above his or her goal level. The components of this intervention are diet, weight management, and increased regular physical activity. Principles for weight management and increasing physical activity are discussed in Chapters 14 and 15, respectively. Specific dietary recommendations outlined in Box 12-3 are based on the Dietary Guidelines with greater restriction of fat and cholesterol and suggested use of foods or food products that can reduce cholesterol absorption in the gut (plant stanols and soluble fiber). Nutrient composition of the TLC appear in Table 12-10.

Drug treatment to lower cholesterol. The total life changes indicated may lower the LDL-C to the goal in many persons, but for others, especially those with multiple risk factors and those with CHD or CHD risk equivalent, may need drug therapy. Table 12-10 outlines drugs used to reduce LDL-C.

The metabolic syndrome. Some individuals have a constellation of metabolic risk factors (see Box 12-1) that dramatically increases the risk of coronary events. The metabolic syndrome is a strong contributor to early heart disease as is cigarette smoking. In addition insulin resistance that goes with the syndrome is one of

Table 12-9 DRUGS AFFECTING LIPOPROTEIN METABOLISM

Drug Class, Agents	Lipid/Lipoprotein Effects	Clinical Trial Results
HMG-CoA reductase inhibitors	Decrease LDL 18-55% Increase HDL 5-15% Decrease TG 7-30%	Reduced major coronary events, CHD deaths, stroke, and total mortality
Bile acid sequestrants	Decrease LDL 15-30% Increase HDL 3-5% No change in TG	Reduced major coronary events and CHD deaths
Nicotinic acid	Decrease LDL 5-25% Increase HDL 15-35% Decrease TG 20-50%	Reduced major coronary events and possibly total mortality
Fibric acids	Decrease LDL 5-20% Increase HDL 10-20% Decrease TG 20-50%	Reduced major coronary events

Adapted from Third Report of the National Cholesterol Education Program (NCEP) Panel on Detection, Evaluation and Treatment of High Blood Cholesterol in Adults (Adult Treatment Panel II), Bethesda, Md, 2001, National Heart and Blood Institute. National Institutes of Health.
LDL, low-density lipoprotein; HDL, high-density lipoprotein.

Box 12-3 THERAPEUTIC LIFE-STYLE CHANGES (TLC) IN CHOLESTEROL LOWERING

Dietary Modifications

Saturated fat <7 percent of total calories
Cholesterol <200 mg
Consideration of plant stanols/sterols (2 g/day) and viscous (soluble) fiber (10-20 g/day)

Weight Management

Increased Physical Activity

From Third Report of the National Cholesterol Education Program (NCEP) Panel on Detection, Evaluation and Treatment of High Blood Cholesterol in Adults (Adult Treatment Panel II), Bethesda, Md, 2001, National Heart and Blood Institute. National Institutes of Health.

the underlying causes of type 2 diabetes. The metabolic syndrome should be addressed after the LDL goal is achieved.

Medications for lowering cholesterol include *bile acid sequestering agents,* which reduce body cholesterol by binding bile acids in the gut, thereby increasing fecal excretion, and *fibric acid derivatives,* which increase the breakdown of lipoproteins and excretion of sterols, including cholesterol (see Table 12-9). *Reductase inhibitors* (statins) inhibit the enzyme 3-hydroxy-3 methylglutaryl coenzyme A (HMG-CoA) reductase, thereby reducing hepatic cholesterol synthesis, thereby stimulating the synthesis of LDL receptors and the uptake of LDLs, decreasing blood cholesterol. Niacin (1.5 to 3.0 g/d nicotinic acid), in doses many times the RDA, lowers TC, lowering LDL-C and raising HDL-C levels.

Fatty Acids

In 1994 Americans consumed approximately 33% of kilocalories from fat, an amount higher than the 30% recommended in the Dietary Guidelines and by the American Heart Association. Although total dietary fat has been linked to several chronic diseases, the effects of individual fatty acids are just beginning to be explored. Evidence is accumulating that individual fatty acids can affect TC and LDL-C levels and that the fatty acid composition of the LDL particle can influence lipoprotein oxidation, the key factor in the atherogenic effects of the LDL particle (Jonnalagadda et al., 1996). Overall, it has been recognized that satu-

Table 12-10 NUTRIENT COMPOSITION OF THE THERAPEUTIC LIFE-STYLE CHANGES (TLC) DIET

Nutrient	Recommended Intake
Saturated fat*	<7% of total calories
Polyunsaturated fat	Up to 10% of total calories
Monounsaturated fat	Up to 20% of total calories
Total fat	25%-35% of total calories
Carbohydrate†	50%-60% of total calories
Fiber	20-30 g per day
Protein	Approximately 15% of total calories
Cholesterol	<200 mg per day
Total calories‡	Balance energy intake and expenditure to maintain desirable body weight/prevent weight gain

From Third Report of the National Cholesterol Education Program (NCEP) Panel on Detection, Evaluation and Treatment of High Blood Cholesterol in Adults (Adult Treatment Panel II), Bethesda, Md, 2001, National Heart and Blood Institute. National Institutes of Health.
LDL, low-density lipoprotein; HDL, high-density lipoprotein.
**Trans* fatty acids are another LDL-raising fat that should be kept at a low intake.
†Carbohydrates should be derived predominantly from foods rich in complex carbohydrates including grains, especially whole grains, fruits, and vegetables.
‡Daily energy expenditure should include at least moderate physical activity (contributing approximately 200 kcal per day).

rated fatty acids (SFAs) tend to increase TC and are significantly correlated with carotid artery wall thickness (Folsom et al., 1993) and 5-year incidence of CHD (Keys, 1970). Myristic, palmitic, and lauric acids increase serum TC and stearic acid appears to be neutral (Yu et al., 1995). It has been suggested, however, that palmitic acid may play a role in improving the LDL/HDL ratio. Monounsaturated fatty acids (MUFAs), which can be obtained from both plant and animal sources, appear to lower TC and LDL-C levels when substituted for saturated fatty acids.

Among the PUFAs, it is well established that the omega-6 fatty acids (linoleic acids) lower TC and LDL-C levels. The MUFAs elicit a neutral effect or are hypocholesterolemic, but less potent than PUFAs. Omega-3 fatty acids lower blood triglyceride levels. A statistically significant inverse relationship between omega-3 fatty acids and both death from CHD and all-cause mortality has been observed (Nordoy and Goodnight, 1990).

Studies have demonstrated the antithrombotic effects of omega-3 PUFA, or fish oil. In general, subjects given omega-3 PUFAs consistently show a mild prolongation of bleeding time and decreased reactivity to platelet aggregation (Nordoy and Goodnight, 1990). By substituting for arachidonic acid and reducing the precursor available for **thromboxane** synthesis, these fatty acids also reduce blood platelet aggregation and decrease interactions of the platelets within the vessel wall, thereby reducing the tendency for blood to clot.

Trans fatty acids have been the topic of much debate among nutrition scientists. They are byproducts of hydrogenation of liquid vegetable oils in the manufacture of margarines and hydrogenated fats to formulate commercially prepared baked goods and fried foods (Lichtenstein, 1995). The average per capita consumption in the United States is estimated to be approximately 12.5 g per day, approximately 8% of total fat intake (Hunter and Applewhite, 1991).

The concern regarding *trans* fatty acids has centered around feeding studies that have demonstrated decreases in HDL-C and increases in LDL-C concentrations (Judd et al., 1994; Katan et al., 1995). However, elevations of the LDL-C concentrations shown with *trans* fatty acids are less than those that would occur with consumption of highly saturated fats such as butter or palm oil. In 1995 the Expert Panel on *Trans* Fatty Acids and Coronary Heart Disease (Kris-Etherton

Research Update

Plant Stanols to Lower Serum Cholesterol

Do you put plant stanols in your cart at the supermarket? What are plant stanols? You don't know? Perhaps you will recognize the name Benecol—that expensive "light" spread some folks buy regularly at the supermarket.

Plant stanols are found in small quantities in foods such as corn, wheat, rye, oats, and olive oil. In the amounts they are consumed in the typical Western diet, they have no discernable effect on serum cholesterol. Plant stanol esters, which are plant stanol derivatives, were developed in Finland, where they have been marketed since 1995 as Benecol, a margarine-like spread.

As long ago as the 1950s, plant sterols were studied for lowering cholesterol. However, the effect was small and eventually plant stanols, the saturated derivatives of plant sterols, were found to be more effective than plant sterols (Levine and Cooper, 2000). When sufficient quantities of plant stanols are present in the digestive tract, they can reduce the amount of cholesterol transported from the intestinal tract to the liver by mimicking the cholesterol molecule's action. The net effect is the reduction of the amount of cholesterol in the liver, which in turn stimulates the liver to increase LDL receptor activity that pulls cholesterol out of the blood, leading to a reduction in serum cholesterol and LDL-C levels.

Plant sterols (sitosterol, campesterol, and stigmasterol) and stanols are minimally absorbed in the intestines of humans (Heinemann et al., 1993). It appears that sitostanol, a saturated sitosterol derivative, reduced cholesterol absorption more effectively than sitosterol. In the early 1990s, Finnish researchers developed a process that solubilized the plant stanol sitostanol into fat, allowing it to be easily and effectively incorporated into the diet in the form of a margarine-like spread.

Extensive and rigorous placebo-controlled intervention trials have documented the cholesterol-lowering abilities of plant stanol esters. A direct comparison of sitostanol and sitosterol found that the former reduced cholesterol absorption by 85% and the latter by 50% (Heinemann et al., 1993). The clinical trials with stanols have consistently demonstrated a lowering of total and LDL cholesterol by an average of 10% and 14%, respectively (Denke et al., 1994; Miettinen et al., 1995). This reduction is greater than that achieved in free-living participants who followed diets from the American Heart Association (Walden et al., 1997).

Consumers are driving the demand for early, nonpharmacologic health solutions. The Dietary Supplement Act of 1994 and new product developments such as plant stanols are welcomed by those who seek out health claims and products with nutrition information in making dietary choices.

and Nicolosi, 1995) concluded that evidence for a link between *trans* fatty acids in the diet and CHD risk is weak and inconsistent.

Alcohol

Alcohol appears to play several roles in relation to CVD. A 10-year follow-up of subjects in NHANES I and II reported that moderate drinkers had a life span 3% to 4% longer than that of nondrinkers or light drinkers (Coate, 1993). There is evidence that drinking in moderation (1 to 2 drinks a day) can be beneficial in reducing the risk of heart attack. However, three or more drinks a day increase blood pressure. The most significant benefit of moderate alcohol intake appears to be raising HDL-C, which clears cholesterol from the

KEY TERMS

thromboxane: a compound of released endothelial cells and platelets following activation of thrombin; interacts with a variety of molecules to induce platelet aggregation (clotting)

blood, thus avoiding the build-up of deposits along the artery walls (Linn et al., 1993).

Alcohol appears to help render **platelets** less sticky and therefore less likely to aggregate and form a clot that could result in a myocardial infarction. This may occur because endothelial cells exposed to alcohol increase the production of endogenous **tissue plasminogen activator (t-PA).** In participants in the Physicians' Health Study, a direct association was observed between moderate alcohol intake and plasma levels of endogenous t-PA that was independent of HDL-C levels (Ricker et al., 1994).

Diabetes Mellitus

Type 2 NIDDM is estimated to affect 15 million Americans and the incidence is increasing and is associated with an augmented risk for CVD, especially in women (Harris et al., 1998). Diabetes is a major cause of morbidity and premature mortality. Individuals with NIDDM have blood lipid profiles that are consistent with high risk of CHD and are usually associated with poor control of blood glucose levels. Obesity increases insulin resistance (Pi-Sunyer, 1996). In data from NHANES II, the relative risk of developing diabetes was 2.9 times greater for obese persons than for persons of normal weight (van Itallie, 1985).

Weight reduction improves blood glucose control in diabetics. The effect of energy restriction from reduced energy intake improves glucose control very quickly, even before much weight loss occurs (Pi-Sunyer, 1996). As weight is lost, the concentration of **glycohemoglobin** drops. Some individuals are able to cease or reduce taking insulin and can even manage their disease without hypoglycemic agents. Even a 5% loss of weight can decrease blood glucose concentration by improving insulin sensitivity and glucose uptake into muscle and adipose tissue. Nutrition therapy consisting of foods that are low in fat and high in complex carbohydrate accompanied by daily aerobic exercise can improve glycemic control and reduce serum lipid levels.

Hypertension

Hypertension is the most prevalent chronic condition in the United States. Because hypertension is generally asymptomatic, its progression is often insidious. Its implications are significant, however. Hypertension accelerates aging of the circulatory system and is a major risk factor for CHD, cerebrovascular disease, renal insufficiency, and vascular disease. The atherosclerotic process, in which the arteries lose their elasticity, increases hypertension.

Data from NHANES III concluded that 24% of the U.S. population had hypertension (Burt et al., 1995.) The incidence increases with age, occurring in 50% or more of those older than 55 years and in 63% of those age 65 years to 74 years. The prevalence is highest in African-Americans (32%) (Joint National Committee on the Prevention, Detection, Evaluation, and Treatment of High Blood Pressure, 1997).

Most causes of hypertension are unknown and it is probable that causes are multiple and interrelated. In epidemiologic studies elevated systolic and diastolic pressures have been associated with diets high in calories, sodium, simple sugars, and saturated fat and diets low in calcium, iron, potassium, fiber, and complex carbohydrates (Preuss et al., 1996).

Weight loss is effective in lowering blood pressure and in decreasing the risks of other chronic diseases (Hunt et al., 1998). Mechanisms that contribute to the relation between body weight and blood pressure include elevated cardiac output with expanded intravascular and cardiopulmonary volume in the presence of a normal peripheral resistance. A positive correlation between peripheral insulin concentrations and arterial pressure in overweight hypertensive individuals suggests that the metabolic disturbances of obesity are related to the blood pressure elevation (McCarron and Reusser, 1996).

Numerous clinical intervention trials have documented the effectiveness of weight loss in lowering blood pressure. One national multicenter program of nonpharmacologic interventions on blood pressure involving more than 2000 men and women with high to normal blood pressure measurements found that weight loss was the single most effective means of lowering blood pressure (Joint National Committee on the Prevention, Detection, Evaluation, and Treatment of High Blood Pressure, 1997). Modest reductions in weight (3 to 5 kg) can improve blood pressure in both those who are hypertensive and those who are normotensive, regardless of sodium intake (McCarron and Reusser, 1996). Changes in blood pressure were found to be proportional to weight loss among overweight men and women who had mild hypertension for 5 years (Davis et al., 1993). For almost 25% of the participants, weight loss lowered blood pressure to the normal range and kept it there. For others, weight loss significantly reduced the requirement for antihypertensive medication.

The 2000 Dietary Guidelines recommend moderation of salt consumption (see Chapter 1). The American Heart Association (2000) maintains that available evidence indicates that a high intake of salt adversely affects blood pressure and recommends that salt intake be limited to 6 g per day (2400 mg sodium). A meta-analysis of 32 clinical trials testing the effects of sodium intake on blood pressure concluded that there is no evidence that moderate sodium reduction presents any safety hazards. As an overview of the study, Cutler et al. (1997) project that blood pressure reduction from a substantial lowering of dietary sodium in the U.S. population could reduce the cardiovascular morbidity and mortality (see Box 12-3).

Reducing blood pressure involves a variety of life-style changes including physical activity and diet. Hypertension may be an insulin-resistant; changes that improve glucose tolerance also improve blood pressure measurements.

The Dietary Approaches to Stop Hypertension (DASH) clinical trial of dietary patterns was designed to test the effectiveness of diet modification, particularly by increasing intake of foods rich in potassium, calcium, and magnesium rather than single nutrient modifications. The 459 adults enrolled were randomly assigned to receive one of three provided diets. The first was rich in fruits and vegetables; the second, a combination diet, was also rich in fruits and vegetables with added low-fat dairy products; and the third was a control diet, similar to the typical American diet. The main results of the study showed that subjects provided with the combination diet, with 8 to 10 servings of fruits and vegetables and 2 to 3 servings of low-fat or nonfat dairy foods, experienced significant lowering of blood pressure compared with subjects on the control diet. The declines in blood pressure were greater proportionally for individuals with hypertension.

The effectiveness of the DASH diet (Table 12-11) under optimal conditions for compliance was only the beginning. Translating the diet into general practice such as when people are counseled to make dietary changes, but the foods are not provided, and sustaining such changes is a challenge being addressed in new studies and demonstration projects.

Epidemiologic studies have documented an inverse relationship between calcium intake and systolic and diastolic pressure (McCarron et al., 1990; Pryer et al., 1995). However, the range of values is large, and substantial differences exist among population subgroups (sex, age, and ethnicity). It appears that a portion of individuals with hypertension respond to increased calcium intake, supporting calcium insufficiency as one of the contributors to this multifactorial disorder (Morris and Reusser, 1995). Because many adults consume calcium at levels well below those recommended, encouraging adequate calcium intake has important benefits for hypertension. A meta-analysis of pooled data from 2412 subjects in 33 randomized controlled trials of calcium supplementation showed a reduction in systolic blood pressure (but not diastolic blood pressure) with calcium supplementation (Bucher et al., 1996).

KEY TERMS

platelets: disk-shaped structures found in blood that lack a nucleus and DNA; known chiefly for their role in coagulation

tissue plasminogen activator (t-PA): an enzyme secreted by endothelial cells that plays a central role in the regulation of intravascular fibrinolysis

glycohemoglobin: hemoglobin with glucose attached to the terminal of the amino acid chain; the amount of glucose increases in hyperglycemia (uncontrolled diabetes mellitus)

Table 12-11 The DASH Diet

Food Group	Daily Servings	One Serving Equals	Examples and Notes	Significance of Each Food Group to the DASH Diet Pattern
Grains and grain products	7-8	1 slice bread ½ c dry cereal ½ c cooked rice, pasta, or cereal	Whole-wheat breads, English muffin, pita bread, bagel, cereals, grits, oatmeal	Major sources of energy and fiber
Vegetables	4-5	1 c raw leafy vegetable ½ c cooked vegetable 6 oz vegetable juice	Tomatoes, potatoes, carrots, peas, squash, broccoli, turnip greens, collards, kale, spinach, artichokes, beans, sweet potatoes	Rich sources of potassium, magnesium, and fiber
Fruits	4-5	6 oz fruit juice 1 medium fruit ¼ c dried fruit ½ c fresh, frozen, or canned fruit	Apricots, bananas, dates, grapes, oranges, orange juice, grapefruit, grapefruit juice, mangoes, melons, peaches, pineapples, prunes, raisins, strawberries, tangerines	Important sources of potassium, magnesium, and fiber
Low-fat or nonfat dairy foods	2-3	8 oz milk 1 c yogurt 1.5 oz cheese	Skim or 1% milk, skim or low-fat buttermilk, nonfat or low-fat yogurt, part-skim mozzarella cheese, nonfat cheese	Major sources of calcium and protein
Meats, poultry, fish	2 or less	3 oz cooked meats, poultry, or fish	Select only lean; trim away visible fats; broil, roast, or boil instead of frying; remove skin from poultry	Rich sources of protein and magnesium
Nuts	1-2	1.5 oz or ⅓ c or 2 tbsp seeds ½ c cooked legumes	Almonds, fiberts, mixed nuts, peanuts, walnuts, sunflower seeds, kidney beans, lentils	Rich sources of energy, magnesium, potassium, protein, and fiber

From U.S. Department of Health and Human Services, National Institutes of Health, National Heart, Lung, and Blood Institute: Facts about the DASH diet, NIH Pub #01-4082, Revised May 2001.

CANCER

- *Why is it difficult to identify nutrition or dietary components that may promote or prevent cancer?*
- *For which cancers might nutrition be a contributing factor?*
- *What dietary recommendations are appropriate for cancer prevention?*

Cancer is the second leading cause of death in the United States. During the 1970s large-scale **epidemiologic** studies observed substantial international differences in the prevalence of cancer rates, suggesting correlations with environmental factors, including diet (Armstrong and Doll, 1975). Evidence for environmental influences, including diet, in cancer causation is supported by observations that migrating populations adopted, sooner or later, the cancer rates of their new host population.

In the most general terms, **carcinogenesis** can be thought of as requiring one or more **genotoxic** events, resulting in a **mutation** and the proliferation of mutated cells. Early research focused on possible mutagens, such as those occurring naturally in many foods or produced by cooking food at high temperatures. Current research also focuses on the likelihood that protective factors may alter the metabolism of potential mutagens or act as antioxidants or cofactors for antioxidant enzymes.

Nutrition could contribute to the causation and prevention of cancer in many ways. Dietary factors influence the rate at which cells multiply through the availability of energy and essential nutrients. Some dietary components have hormonal effects or act indirectly by influencing the endogenous synthesis or metabolism of hormones. Some nutrients have physiologic roles in regulating gene expression (e.g., vitamin A) or in the normal regulation of cell differentiation and proliferation (e.g., folate) and thus may also affect the likelihood that a mutation is reproduced.

Although evidence of a diet-cancer connection does not establish a cause and effect relationship, substantial epidemiologic (Block et al., 1992) and experimental evidence in animal models suggests that some dietary components may increase or decrease the risk of particular cancers. A variety of approaches are being used to explore the significance of dietary factors. Case control and **cohort** epidemiologic studies provide the opportunity to study the effects of specific dietary factors with much greater capacity to control for confounding variables than in the early general comparisons of populations. However, the effects of specific dietary factors may be difficult to disentangle when they exist together in foods such as vitamin A and carotene. Table 12-12 summarizes current evidence in the relationship between various cancers and major food groups, energy-generating nutrients, salt, alcohol, and indicators of energy balance. The following discussion summarizes some of the most pronounced relationships between dietary factors and cancer.

Dietary Factors and Types of Cancer

Oral and Laryngeal Cancer

Oral and laryngeal cancer are marked by two risk factors that appear far more powerful than nutrition—tobacco use and alcohol consumption. Case control evidence indicates that a diet emphasizing fruits and vegetables may protect against oral cancer even after statistical adjustment for alcohol and tobacco use (Marshall and Boyle, 1996). For laryngeal cancer, available studies provide no estimate of risk of the role of diet in subjects not exposed to tobacco and alcohol (Riboli et al., 1996).

Esophageal Cancer

A protective effect of fruit and vegetable consumption is supported by a large body of evidence, especially from case control studies. Intervention studies in areas of China with a high incidence of esophageal cancer suggest that micronutrient supplements may have a modest effect in reducing risk (Cheng and Day, 1996), but the implication of these results is uncertain.

Stomach Cancer

Substantial ecologic evidence supports a role of dietary factors in determining the risk of stomach cancer. High salt intake has been associated with an increased risk in many case control studies and limited cohort studies. There has been a consistent **negative association** with consumption of fresh vegetables and fruits in numerous case control studies in different populations (Kono and Hirohata, 1996). Both epidemiologic and experimental data suggest that vitamin C intake is inversely related to stomach cancer mortality

KEY TERMS

ecologic: studies across populations, usually international
carcinogenesis: production of a malignant new growth made up of epithelial cells tending to infiltrate surrounding tissue
genotoxic: damaging to DNA
mutation: permanent transmissible change in genetic material, usually of a single gene
cohort: group of individuals sharing a characteristic (such as date of birth or exposure to asbestos) who are used in epidemiologic studies
negative association: as one variable increases (fruit and vegetable consumption), the other decreases (cancer risk); also called *inverse association*

Table 12-12 RISK IMPLICATIONS FOR MAJOR FORMS OF CANCER BY CONSUMPTION OF FOODS IN MAJOR GROUPS; INTAKE OF ENERGY-GENERATING NUTRIENTS, ALCOHOL, AND SALT; AND NUTRITION-RELATED INDICATORS

	Oral Cavity	Nasopharynx	Esophagus	Stomach	Large Bowel	Liver	Larynx	Lung	Breast	Endometrium	Ovary	Prostate	Urinary Bladder
MAJOR FOOD GROUPS													
Cereals				Increase?									
Vegetables	Reduce		Reduce	Reduce	Reduce	Reduce?	Reduce	Reduce	Reduce?	Reduce?	Reduce?	Reduce?	Reduce
Fruits	Reduce		Reduce	Reduce	Reduce	Reduce?	Reduce	Reduce	Reduce?	Reduce?	Reduce?		Reduce
Red meat					Increase								
Fish													
Milk and milk products													
Eggs and egg products				Increase?									
Sugars					Increase?								
MACRONUTRIENTS													
Animal proteins					Increase?					Increase?			
Carbohydrates (total)				Increase?									
Fiber					Reduce?								
Saturated fat (as animal)					Increase?			Increase?	Neutral	Increase?		Increase	
Monounsaturated fat									Reduce?				
Polyunsaturated fat					Neutral?				Neutral?				
NONNUTRIENTS													
Alcohol	Increase		Increase		Increase				Increase				
Salt (NaCl)		Increase		Increase									
NUTRITIONAL COVARIATES													
Height					Increase?				Increase			Increase?	
Obesity					Increase				Both	Increase			
Physical activity					Reduce				Reduce	Reduce?		Reduce?	
Hot drinks			Increase										

From Willett WC and Trichopoulos D: Nutrition and cancer: a summary of the evidence, Cancer Causes Control 7:178, 1996 (Table 1).

(Ocke et al., 1995). However, evidence is sparse and inconsistent with reference to protective effects of carotene, vitamin E, or selenium.

Lung Cancer

Lung cancer is the leading cause of cancer death in men and women. Cigarette smoking has been established as the dominant risk factor in lung cancer deaths in men and women. Diet may be of particular importance, because prevention is considered the only viable strategy for reducing lung cancer mortality. Early detection of lung cancer has not been successful because symptoms often do not appear until the disease is advanced, thereby reducing the effectiveness of treatment.

Prospective and retrospective studies suggest strongly that increased vegetable and fruit intake is associated with reduced risk in men and women—in smokers, former smokers, and those who have never smoked—for all types of lung cancer (Ziegler et al., 1996). Some prospective studies have observed that blood levels of beta carotene (a biomarker of vegetable and fruit intake) are consistently related to lower risk of cancer (van Poppel and Goldbohm, 1995). In a 25-year follow-up of the participants in the Seven Countries Study, average intake of vitamin C, alpha or beta carotene, or alpha tocopherol showed no relationship to mortality from lung cancer (Ocke et al., 1995).

Colorectal Cancer

Inheritance and numerous environmental and life-style factors such as diet, low levels of physical activity (Glynn et al., 1996), and obesity (Lee et al., 1991) have been implicated in carcinogenesis of the colon (Shike, 1996).

There is strong evidence from epidemiologic studies and experimental studies in animals that a diet high in fat and energy and low in fruits, vegetables, and dietary fiber strongly predisposes humans and animals to the development of colon cancer (Wynder et al., 1996; Ziegler, 1991). As meat consumption rises, so does risk, but this is not explained solely by the fat content of meat (Potter, 1996). Mutagenic compounds, particularly heterocyclic amines, which are produced when protein is cooked, plausibly explain the meat association.

Many **phytochemicals** in vegetables and fruits prevent cancer in experiments with animals. The results of clinical trials to test the ability of antioxidant vitamins to prevent colorectal adenomas have been inconsistent. High dietary fiber intake is associated with lower risk, but fiber alone does not account for this association.

Data from epidemiologic studies suggest that dietary calcium may have a protective role for colon and rectal cancer (Garland et al., 1991). Recent clinical trials in individuals at high risk for development of **adenomas** have reported a reduction in hyperproliferation of epithelial cells in the **colonic crypts** when calcium is added to the diet (Alberts et al., 1996; Bostick et al., 1995) and no improvement in mucosal cell proliferation in similar patients given 1200 mg of calcium per day for 6 months to 9 months (Baron et al., 1995). A recent double-blind, placebo-controlled study of calcium in families with hereditary colorectal cancer did not find any increase in epithelial cell proliferation with calcium supplementation (Cate et al., 1995).

Breast Cancer

Breast cancer is the second leading cause of cancer mortality in women. The incidence of breast cancer increases with age and adiposity. However, factors that predict risk of breast cancer in premenopausal women are different from those for postmenopausal women. For example obese women appear to be at decreased risk for developing premenopausal breast cancer, but increased risk of developing and dying from postmenopausal breast cancer (Ballard-Barbash and Swanson, 1996).

The role for dietary fat and individual fatty acids to the risk of breast cancer have been a source of

KEY TERMS

phytochemicals: substances derived from naturally occurring ingredients that may have health-promoting potential
adenomas: benign epithelial tumors
colonic crypts: deep indentations or pits in the lining of the colon

controversy in recent years. Epidemiologic evidence shows a positive correlation between total dietary fat and breast cancer rates (Whittemore and Henderson, 1993). Nonetheless these observations are not supported by a large cohort study of 88,975 U.S. women followed for 14 years (Holmes et al., 1999). It may be the case that if fat intake is relevant to breast cancer, the relationship is to intakes during early life. This explanation is consistent with an emerging hypothesis that higher energy intake and growth rate in childhood and adolescence increases risk (Hunter and Willett, 1996).

Considerable evidence suggests that low intakes of vegetables modestly increase the risk of breast cancer; however, the responsible dietary components remain elusive (Fredudenheim et al., 1996). In a 3-year prospective study of 2569 women, Negri and colleagues (1996) found an inverse relationship between risk of breast cancer and dietary levels of beta carotene, vitamin E, and calcium, but not dietary levels of vitamin C. Such observations raise important questions regarding components of fruits, vegetables, grains, and other food components that may affect cancer risk.

Phytoestrogens, a group of phytochemicals that are weaker versions of human estrogen, are of particular interest in the areas of breast and prostate cancer. Phytoestrogens of dietary origin, lignins and isoflavinoids, occur in more than 300 plants, but major amounts are found in soybean and whole-grain products and various seeds. Evidence for positive effects of phytoestrogens relates to observations that in areas where large amounts of soy products are consumed, such as Japan, China, and Korea, symptoms of menopause, breast cancer rates, and death from prostate cancer are much lower than in the West.

The effects of phytoestrogens may vary with menopausal status. It is speculated that before menopause, phytoestrogens act as antiestrogens, staving off breast cancer by blocking the action of some of the body's naturally occurring estrogens. After menopause, when production of endogenous estrogen dramatically declines, phytoestrogens may provide some hormone activity without raising breast cancer risk. In men phytoestrogens appear to act as a blocker of testosterone, the male hormone that can spur the growth of prostate tumors (Adlecreutz, 1995).

Exploring Nutrient Relationships

On the basis of epidemiologic observations and studies in laboratory animals, antioxidants, particularly beta carotene and vitamin A, have attracted wide interest as agents to prevent cancer. It is difficult to determine from observational studies whether the apparent benefits of fruit and vegetable consumption are from beta carotene, other substances in those foods, other dietary habits, or other nondietary life-style characteristics (Hennekens and Buring, 1993).

In principle, **randomized clinical trials** are the most powerful tool in determining the effects of dietary factors on cancer risk. Three large, randomized, placebo-controlled trials in well-nourished populations were designed to validate the protective effects of beta carotene. The first, a study by the ATBC Cancer Prevention Study Group (1994) on the effects of alpha tocopherol and beta carotene (ATBC), assigned 29,000 Finnish male smokers to receive beta carotene, vitamin E, both active agents, or neither for an average of 6 years. There were no benefits of supplementation in terms of the incidence of cancer or cardiovascular death; indeed, rates of lung cancer were somewhat higher among the subjects given beta carotene. The second clinical trial, the Beta Carotene and Retinol Efficacy Trial (CARET), was designed to assess the chemopreventive efficacy and safety of beta carotene and retinyl palmitate in 18,314 smokers, former smokers, and workers exposed to asbestos (Omenn et al., 1996). For heavy smokers receiving beta carotene, the risk of lung cancer was higher than the placebo group. These two studies raised the possibility that beta carotene is not only ineffective in preventing cancer, but also potentially harmful to smokers.

The Physicians' Health Study, a randomized, double-blind, placebo-controlled trial, tested aspirin and beta carotene in primary prevention of CVD and cancer in 22,071 male physicians (40 to 84 years of age at enrollment) in the United States (Hennekens et al., 1996). Average duration of treatment was 12 years. In this largely nonsmoking population, supplementation with beta carotene neither increased nor reduced the incidence of cancer, CVD, or death from all causes.

None of the studies showed a benefit from supplementation with beta carotene and the estimated excess risks in smokers were small. It remains unclear whether beta carotene is truly harmful or whether it might prove to be beneficial over a longer period. The **induction period** for cancers is often unknown and may be decades (Willett and Trichopoulos, 1996). Because the duration of these studies was relatively short, they leave open the possibility that benefit, especially in terms of cancer risk reduction, would become evident with longer treatment and follow-up. In addition the nutrition factors that influence cancer development may interrelate with one another and may differ with the type of cancer.

Regardless of the results of these studies related to beta carotene, there is substantial evidence that diets that include moderate energy and fat; abundant vegetables, fruits, and grains; and adequate calcium can provide important practical assistance in cancer prevention.

PROMOTING HEALTH AND WELL-BEING

Health has traditionally been defined as the absence of disease or illness. Major strides in medicine (particularly the control of infection), food safety, and public health have resulted in increased life span and life expectancy. As individuals live longer, the advances that prolong life should be employed to ensure that the additional years are healthy years.

Because of these changes, today health is viewed as a complex concept that encompasses physical, mental, emotional, social, and spiritual well-being. This broad definition of health focuses on the individual and his or her needs and abilities to attain optimum health. Obviously, nutrition is an integral part of each of the components of health.

Health Promotion

Health promotion is an exciting area offering the opportunity to improve and maintain the health status of individuals, families, and communities. It is integrated into healthcare, but emphasis is on prevention of disease in community or work settings. The purpose of health promotion is to improve the health status of individuals by facilitating permanent changes in life-style that will promote **wellness** behaviors. Wellness encompasses day-to-day habits, including food eaten, exercise taken, sleep patterns, and management of stress. As described in Chapter 3, wellness depends on the individual's knowledge of what constitutes good health behaviors and on development of techniques to apply that knowledge in modifying current behaviors and developing new behaviors and life-styles. In addition health promotion is most effective in a family, work, or community environment that supports wellness behaviors.

Promoting Nutrition Health

Nutrition is a critical part of all aspects of health. The role of nutrition is complex and is integrated with other health behaviors. *Healthy People 2010* outlines national health-promotion and disease-prevention objectives for Americans with a goal for achievement by the year 2010 (see Box 1-1 in Chapter 1). One of the three broad goals is to increase the span of healthy life for Americans. Obviously nutrition is a component of this goal.

Promotion of nutrition health begins with the Food Guide Pyramid (see Figure 1-6 in Chapter 1). This foundation will allow individuals to develop basic understanding and practice in positive eating behaviors to meet nutrition needs. An important component of wellness is the prevention of disease. The 2000 Dietary Guidelines for Americans from the U.S. Departments of Agriculture and Health and Human Services (see Figure 1-4 in Chapter 1) can provide guidance for food choices that will minimize nutrition health risks as they are currently perceived. The most recent edition of the Dietary Guidelines

KEY TERMS

randomized clinical trials: a research technique in which subjects are assigned randomly to experimental (treatment) groups or to control groups
induction period: the period it takes for specific cellular changes to occur
health promotion: a set of strategies to increase the level of health of individuals
wellness: a focus on enhancing the level of health

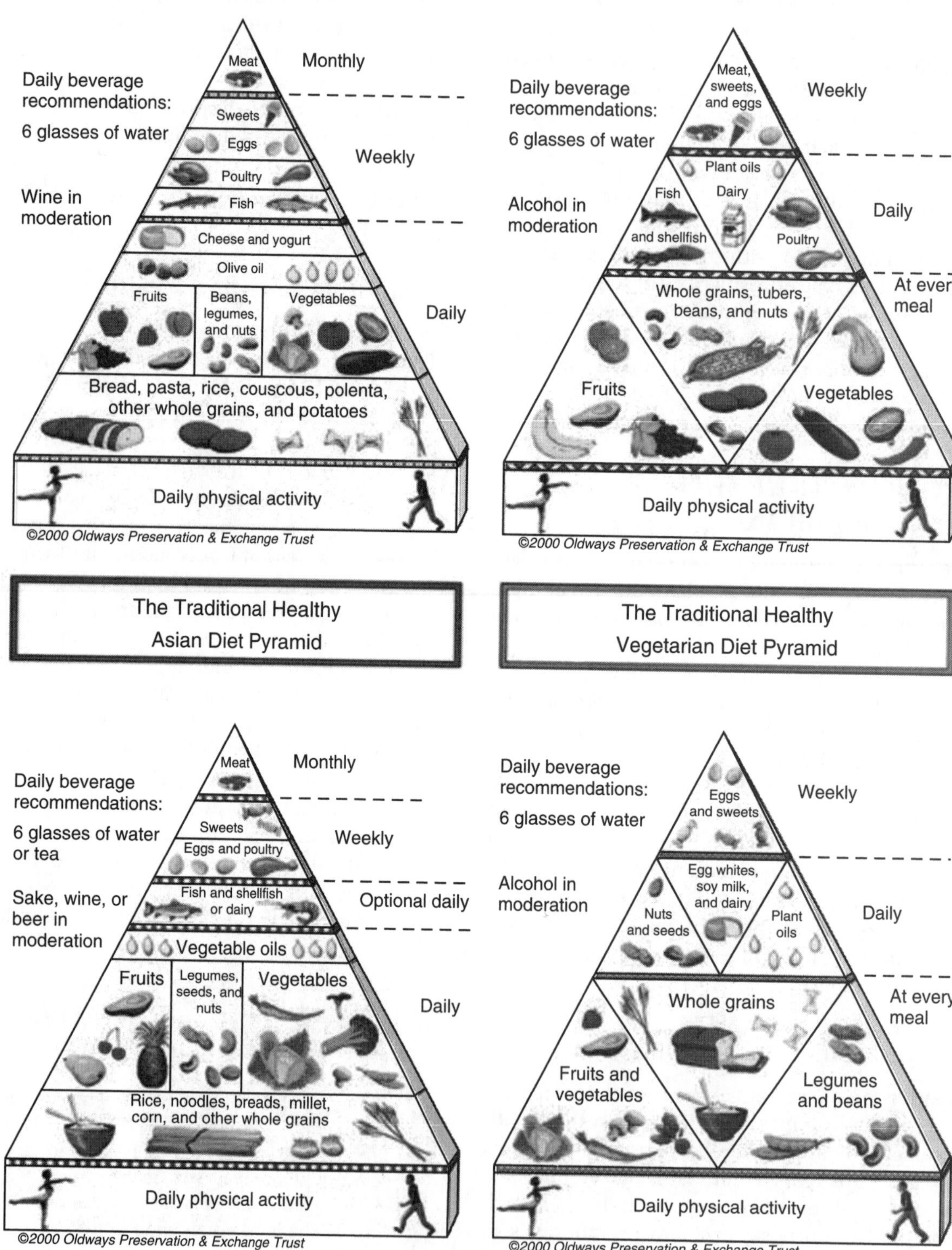

Figure 12-5 Four Traditional Healthy Food Guide Pyramids. © 2000, Oldways Preservation and Exchange Trust.

emphasizes the importance of diet and exercise in the maintenance of body weight. This emphasis reflects a trend toward using the synergy between diet and physical activity to create the greatest health benefit (Blair, 1995; Eaton et al., 1993; Paffenbarger et al., 1993).

It has been known for decades that, compared with North America, populations living in other regions of the world have low rates of chronic disease, especially CHD, and increased life expectancies (Willett et al., 1995). The Mediterranean Food Pyramid; other ethnic food pyramids including the Asian Food Guide Pyramid and the Latin American Food Guide Pyramid; and the Vegetarian Food Guide Pyramid (Figure 12-5) characterize the diet of populations. At the base of these pyramids are a variety of grains (including many that are unknown or are just becoming popular in the United States, such as couscous, polenta, bulgur, and others), fruits, and vegetables. Other foodways that may represent diets that promote health and reduction in the risk of chronic disease. The guides include emphasis on beans, other legumes, and nuts and fruit and vegetable subsection. In these pyramids, animal protein foods and dairy products appear toward the top with recommended servings being much fewer. Fish, poultry, and eggs are consumed only a few times a week rather than daily and red meat is typically consumed only a few times a month. The guides also encourage regular physical activity.

Many Americans use these models for healthy eating because the models reflect their cultural backgrounds or because they are willing to explore and enjoy consuming healthy diet alternatives. They are examples of acceptable and health-promoting dietary patterns.

Concepts to Remember

- Adulthood begins with the completion of growth and is a period of physiologic homeostasis characterized by gradual changes of aging.
- For women menopause and declining estrogen levels have implications for increased risk of CHD, osteoporosis, and cerebrovascular disease.
- Hormone replacement therapy can be used during menopause and to reduce risk of osteoporosis and heart disease.
- The REE decreases with age and may contribute to a gradual increase in body weight
- Nutrition assessment for adults includes screening body weight and risk factors for chronic disease.
- Energy and nutrient needs are relatively stable during adulthood, but caloric intakes tend to vary widely.
- Homocysteine is a nutrition-related risk factor for CAD.
- Nutrition plays a role in the development or progression of chronic diseases.
- Dietary changes, particularly of energy and fat intake, may have health benefits for CVD, diabetes mellitus, hypertension, and cancer.
- Exercise is an important adjunct to dietary interventions for disease.
- Reductions in dietary fat and changes in the type of fat can reduce blood TC and LDL-C.
- There is substantial evidence linking consumption of certain food groups with the occurrence of some chronic diseases.
- There is much speculation, but little evidence, linking specific nutrients to the occurrence or progression of chronic disease.
- The unique health concerns of women may require specific nutrition modifications.

REFERENCES

Adlercreutz H: Phytoestrogens: epidemiology and a possible role in cancer protection, Environ Health Perspect 103:103, 1995.

Agricultural Research Service: Continuing survey of food intakes by individuals, Riverdale, Md, 1996, U.S. Department of Agriculture.

Alberts DS et al.: Randomized, double-blinded, placebo-controlled study of effect of wheat bran fiber and calcium on fecal bile acids in patients with resected adenomatous colon polyps, J Natl Cancer Inst 88:81, 1996.

American Heart Association: AHA dietary guidelines revision 2000, Circulation 102:2284, 2000.

Anger P et al.: Effect of oral postmenopausal hormone replacement on progression of athersclerosis: a randomized controlled trial, Arterioscler Thromb Vasc Biol 21:262, 2001.

Armstrong B and Doll R: Environmental factors and cancer incidence and mortality in different countries, with special reference to dietary practices, Int J Cancer 15:617, 1975.

Asthana S et al.: Cognitive and neuroendocrine response to transdermal estrogen in postmenopausal women with Alzheimer's disease: results of a placebo-controlled, double-blind, pilot study, Psychoendocrinology 24:657, 1999.

The ATBC Cancer Prevention Study Group: The effect of vitamin E and beta carotene on the incidence of lung cancer and other cancers in male smokers, N Engl J Med 330:1029, 1994.

Baik I et al.: Adiposity and mortality in men, Am J Clin Nutr 152:264, 2000.

Ballard-Barbash R and Swanson CA: Body weight: estimation of risk for breast and endometrial cancers, Am J Clin Nutr 63:437S, 1996.

Baron JA et al.: Calcium supplementation and rectal mucosal proliferation: a randomized controlled trial, J Natl Cancer Inst 87:1303, 1995.

Baron YM et al.: Carotid artery changes in estrogen treated and untreated postmenopausal women, Obstet Gynecol 91:982, 1998.

Blair SN: Diet and activity: the synergistic merger, Nutr Today 30:108, 1995.

Block G et al.: Fruit, vegetables, and cancer prevention: a review of the epidemiological evidence, Nutr Cancer 18:1, 1992.

Bostick RM et al.: Calcium and colorectal epithelial cell proliferation in sporadic adenoma patients: a randomized, double-blinded, placebo-controlled clinical trial, J Natl Cancer Inst 87:1307, 1995.

Bucher H et al.: Effects of dietary calcium supplementation on blood pressure: a meta-analysis of randomized controlled trials, JAMA 275:1016, 1996.

Burt VL et al.: Prevalence of hypertension in the U.S. population: results from the Third National Health and Nutrition Examination Survey 1988-1991, Hypertension 25:308, 1995.

Cate A et al.: Randomized, double-blinded, placebo-controlled intervention study with supplemental calcium in families with hereditary nonpolyposis colorectal cancer, J Natl Cancer Inst 87:598, 1995.

Centers for Disease Control and Prevention: Recommendations for the use of folic acid to reduce the number of cases of spina bifida and other neural tube defects, MMWR Morb Mortal Wkly Rep 44:1, 1992.

Centers for Disease Control and Prevention: Preventing cardiovascular disease: addressing the nation's leading killer, Atlanta, Ga, 2000, U.S. Department of Health and Human Services, Centers for Disease Control.

Cheng KK and Day NE: Nutrition and esophageal cancer, Cancer Causes Control 7:33, 1996.

Chernoff R: Baby boomers come of age: nutrition in the 21st century, J Am Diet Assoc 95:650, 1995.

Coate D: Moderate drinking and coronary heart disease mortality: evidence from NHANES I and the NHANES II follow-up, Am J Public Health 83:888, 1993.

Col NR et al.: Patient-specific decisions about hormone replacement therapy in postmenopausal women, JAMA 277:1140, 1997.

Colditz GA et al.: Weight gain as a risk factor for clinical diabetes in women, Ann Intern Med 122:481, 1995.

Croft JB et al.: Waist-to-hip ratio in a biracial population: measurement, implications, and cautions for using guidelines to define high risk for cardiovascular disease, J Am Diet Assoc 95:60, 1995.

Cutler JA et al.: Meta analysis of the effects of reducing sodium intake on blood pressure, Am J Clin Nutr 65:643S, 1997.

Davidson MH et al.: Effects of continuous estrogen and estrogen-progest in replacement regimens on cardiovascular risk markers in postmenopausal women, Arch Intern Med 21:3315, 2000.

Davis BR et al.: Reduction in long-term antihypertensive medication requirements: effects of weight reduction by dietary intervention in overweight persons with mild hypertension, Arch Intern Med 153:1773, 1993.

Denke MA et al.: Individual responses to a cholesterol-lowering diet in 50 men with moderate hypercholesterolemenia, Arch Intern Med 154:317, 1994.

Dinkins JM: Per capita income and expenditures of baby-boomer households, Fam Nutr Rev 8:27, 1995.

Dyer AR and Elliott P: The Intersalt study: relations of body mass index on blood pressure, J Hum Hypertens 3:299, 1989.

Eaton CB et al.: Self-reported physical activity predicts long-term coronary heart disease and all-cause mortalities, Arch Fam Med 4:323, 1993.

Expert Panel on Detection, Evaluation, and Treatment of High Blood Cholesterol in Adults: executive summary of the third report of the National Cholesterol Education Program (NCEP), Adult Treatment Panel II, JAMA 285:2486, 2001.

Federal Register: Folic acid fortification, Federal Register 61:8781, March 5, 1996.

Folsom AR et al.: Association of hemostatic variables with prevalent cardiovascular disease and asymptomatic carotid artery atherosclerosis: the Atherosclerosis Risk in Communities (ARIC) study, Arterioscler Thromb 13:1829, 1993.

Food and Nutrition Board, National Research Council: Recommended dietary allowances, ed 10, Washington, DC, 1989, National Academy of Sciences.

Forbes GB: Longitudinal changes in adult fat-free mass: influence of body weight, Am J Clin Nutr 70:1025, 1999.

Fredudenheim JL et al.: Premenopausal breast cancer risk and intake of vegetables, fruits and related nutrients, J Natl Cancer Inst 88:340, 1996.

Garland CG et al.: Can colon cancer incidence and death rates be reduced with calcium and vitamin D?, Am J Clin Nutr 54:193S, 1991.

Garn SM: Fractionating healthy weight, Am J Clin Nutr 63:412S, 1996.

Gartside PS et al.: Prospective assessment of coronary heart disease risk factors: the NHANES Epidemiologic Follow-up Study (NHEFS) 16-year follow-up, J Am Coll Nutr 17:263, 1998.

Gauvin L and Spence JC: Physical activity and psychological well-being: knowledge base, current issues and caveats, Nutr Rev 54:S53, 1996.

Glynn SA et al.: Alcohol consumption and risk of colorectal cancer in cohort of Finnish men, Cancer Causes Control 7:214, 1996.

Gotto AM: Lipid risk factors and the regression of atherosclerosis, Am J Cardiol 76:3A, 1995.

Grodstein F et al.: Postmenopausal hormone use and secondary prevention of coronary events in the nurses' health study: a prospective observational study, Ann Int Med 135:1, 2001.

Haffner S et al.: Greater influence of central distribution of adipose tissue in incidence of non-insulin dependent diabetes in women than men, Am J Clin Nutr 53:1312, 1991.

Harris MI et al.: Prevalence of diabetes, impaired fasting glucose and impaired glucose intolerance in U.S. adults: the Third National Health and Nutrition Examination Survey 1988-1994, Diabetes Care 21:518, 1998.

Heinemann T et al.: Comparison of intestinal absorption of cholesterol with different plant sterols in man, Eur J Clin Invest 23:827, 1993.

Hennekens CH: Antioxidant vitamins: current and future directions, Lydia J Roberts Lecture, Chicago, December 1997.

Hennekens CH and Buring JE: Observational evidence, Ann N Y Acad Sci 703:18, 1993.

Hennekens CH et al.: Lack of effect of long-term supplementation with beta carotene on the incidence of malignant neoplasms and cardiovascular disease, N Engl J Med 334:1145, 1996.

Herrington DM et al.: The estrogen replacement and atherosclerosis (ERA) study: study design and baseline characteristics of the cohort, Control Clin Trials 21:257, 2000.

Hollowell JG et al.: Trends and public health implications: iodine excretion data from National Health and Nutrition Examination Surveys I and III (1971-1974 and 1988-1994), J Clin Endocrinol Metab 83:3401, 1998.

Holt PR: Dairy foods and prevention of colon cancer: human studies, J Am Coll Nutr 18:379S, 1999.

Hu FB: Trends in the incidence of coronary heart disease and changes in diet and lifestyle in women, N Engl J Med 343:530, 2000.

Hubert HB et al.: Obesity as an independent risk factor for cardiovascular disease: a 26-year follow-up of participants in the Framingham Heart Study, Circulation 61:968, 1983.

Hulley S et al.: Randomized trial of estrogen plus progestin for secondary prevention of coronary heart disease in postmenopausal women, JAMA 280:605, 1998.

Hunt SC et al.: Angiotensinogen genotype, sodium reduction, weight loss, and prevention of hypertension: trials of hypertension prevention phase II, Hypertension 32:393, 1998.

Hunter DJ and Willett WC: Nutrition and breast cancer, Cancer Causes Control 7:56, 1996.

Hunter JE and Applewhite TH: Reassessment of trans fatty acid availability in the U.S. diet, Am J Clin Nutr 54:363, 1991.

Joint National Committee on the Detection, Evaluation and Treatment of High Blood Pressure: sixth report (JNC VI), Arch Intern Med 151:2413, 1997.

Jones DY et al.: Dietary fat and breast cancer in the National Health and Nutrition Examination Survey I: epidemiologic follow-up study, J Natl Cancer Inst 79:465, 1987.

Jonnalagadda S et al.: Effects of individual fatty acids on chronic diseases, Nutr Today 31:90, 1996.

Judd JF et al.: Dietary trans fatty acids: effects on plasma lipids and lipoproteins of healthy men and women, Am J Clin Nutr 59:861, 1994.

Kannel WB et al.: Effect of weight on cardiovascular disease, Am J Clin Nutr 63:419S, 1996.

Kant AK et al.: Proportion of energy intake from fat and subsequent weight change in the NHANES I epidemiologic follow-up study, Am J Clin Nutr 61:11, 1995.

Katan MB et al.: Trans fatty acids and their effects on lipoproteins in humans, Annu Rev Nutr 15:473, 1995.

Katch FI and McArdle WD: Introduction to nutrition, exercise, and health, ed 4, Philadelphia, 1993, Lea & Febiger.

Kennedy ET et al.: Dietary-fat intake in the U.S. population, J Am Coll Nutr 18:207, 1999.

Keys A: Coronary heart disease in seven countries, Circulation 41:1S, 1970.

Kirtz-Silverstein D and Barrett-Connor E: Long-term postmenopausal hormone use, obesity, and fat distribution in older women, JAMA 275:46, 1996.

Knekt P et al.: Body iron stores and risk of cancer, Int J Cancer 56:379, 1994.

Kono S and Hirohata T: Nutrition and stomach cancer, Cancer Causes Control 7:41, 1996.

Kraus RM et al.: AHA scientific statement: AHA dietary guidelines, revision 2002: a statement for healthcare professionals from the Nutrition Committee of the American Heart Association, Circulation 102:2284, 2000.

Kris-Etherton PM and Nicolosi RJ: Trans fatty acids and coronary heart disease risk, International Life Sciences Institute, Technical Committee on Fatty Acids, Washington, DC, 1995, ILSI Press.

Kuczmarski RJ et al.: Increasing prevalence of overweight among U.S. adults: the National Health and Nutrition Examination Surveys 1960 to 1991, JAMA 272:205, 1998.

Kuller LH et al.: Estrogen and women's health: interrelationship of coronary heart disease, breast cancer and osteoporosis, J Steroid Biochem Mol Biol 74:297, 2001a.

Kuller LH et al.: Healthy lifestyle project: a randomized clinical trial: results at 54 months, Circulation 130:32, 2001b.

Lee I-M et al.: Physical activity and risk of developing colorectal cancer among college alumni, J Natl Cancer Inst 83:1324, 1991.

Lee K: Too much versus too little: the implications of current iodine intake in the United States, Nutr Rev 57:1977, 1999.

Levine BS and Cooper C: Plant stanol esters: a new tool in the dietary management of cholesterol, Nutr Today 35:61, 2000.

Lewis CE et al.: Weight gain continues in the 1990s: 10-year trends in weight and overweight from the CARDIA study, Coronary Artery Risk Development in Young Adults, Am J Epidemiol 151:1172, 2000.

Lichtenstein AH: Trans fatty acids and hydrogenated fat: what do we know?, Nutr Today 30:102, 1995.

Linn S et al.: High-density lipoprotein cholesterol and alcohol consumption in U.S. white and black adults: date from NHANES II, Am J Public Health 83:811, 1993.

Lipkin M and Newmark HL: Vitamin D, calcium and prevention of breast cancer: a review, J Am Coll Nutr 18:392S, 1999.

Lynch SR: Iron overload: prevalence and impact on health, Nutr Rev 53:255, 1995.

McCarron DA and Reusser ME: Body weight and blood pressure regulation, Am J Clin Nutr 63:423S, 1996.

McCarron DA et al.: Dietary calcium and chronic diseases, Med Hypotheses 31:265, 1990.

McDowell M et al.: Energy and macronutrient intakes of persons ages 2 months and over in the United States: Third National Health and Nutrition Examination Survey, Phase I, 1989-1991, Advance Data No. 225, page 1, October 24, 1994.

McGill HC et al.: Early determinants of adult metabolic regulation: effects of infant nutrition on adult lipid and lipoprotein metabolism, Nutr Rev 54:S31, 1996.

Marshall JR and Boyle P: Nutrition and oral cancer, Cancer Causes Control 7:101, 1996.

Meisler JG and St. Jeor S: Summary and recommendations from the American Health Foundation's expert panel on healthy weight, Am J Clin Nutr 63:474S, 1996.

Miettinen TA et al.: Reduction of serum cholesterol with sitostanol ester margarine in mildly hypercholesterolemia population, N Engl J Med 333:1308, 1995.

Morris CD and Reusser ME: Calcium intake and blood pressure: epidemiology revisited, Semin Nephrol 15: 490, 1995.

Must A et al.: The disease burden associated with overweight and obesity, JAMA 282:1523, 1999.

National Heart, Lung, and Blood Institute: Clinical guidelines on the identification, evaluation, and treatment of overweight and obesity in adults: the evidence report, Obes Res 6:515, 1998.

National Heart, Lung, and Blood Institute: The practical guide. Identification, evaluation, and treatment of overweight and obesity in adults, NIH #00-4084, 2000.

National Institutes of Health Consensus Development Panel on Physical Activity and Cardiovascular Health: Physical activity and cardiovascular health, JAMA 276:241, 1996.

Negri E et al.: Intake of selected micronutrients and the risk of breast cancer, Int J Cancer 65:140, 1996.

Nordoy A and Goodnight SH: Dietary lipids and thrombosis: relationships to atherosclerosis, Atherosclerosis 10:149, 1990.

Ocke MC et al.: Average intake of anti-oxidant (pro) vitamins and subsequent cancer mortality in the 16 cohorts of the Seven Countries Study, Int J Cancer 61:480, 1995.

Omenn GS et al.: Effects of a combination of beta carotene and vitamin A on lung cancer and cardiovascular disease, N Engl J Med 334:1150, 1996.

Paffenbarger RS et al.: The association of changes in physical activity and other lifestyle characteristics with mortality among men, N Engl J Med 328:538, 1993.

Pi-Sunyer FX: Weight and non-insulin-dependent diabetes mellitus, Am J Clin Nutr 63:426S, 1996.

Potter JD: Nutrition and colorectal cancer, Cancer Causes Control 7:127, 1996.

Pradhan AD et al.: C-reactive protein, interleukin and risk of developing type 2 diabetes mellitus, JAMA 286:327, 2001.

Preuss HG et al.: Association of macronutrients and energy intake with hypertension, J Am Coll Nutr 15:21, 1996.

Pryer J et al.: Dietary calcium and blood pressure: a review of the observational studies, J Hum Hypertens 9:597, 1995.

Recker RR et al.: Bone gain in young adult women, JAMA 268:2403, 1992.

Riboli E et al.: Nutrition and laryngeal cancer, Cancer Causes Control 7:147, 1996.

Ricker PM et al.: Association of moderate alcohol consumption and plasma concentration of endogenous tissue-type plasminogen activator, JAMA 272:929, 1994.

Rimm EB et al.: Body size and fat distribution as predictors of coronary heart disease among middle-aged and older U.S. men, Am J Epidemiol 14:1117, 1995.

Salamone LM et al.: Effect of a lifestyle intervention on bone mineral density in premenopausal women: a randomized trial, Am J Clin Nutr 70:97, 1999.

Salonen JT et al.: High stored iron levels are associated with excess risk of myocardial infarction in Eastern Finnish men, Circulation 86:803, 1992.

Sator MO et al.: The effect of hormone replacement therapy on carotid arteries: measurement with a high frequency ultrasound system, Maturitas 30:63, 1998.

Schaefer EJ et al.: Body weight and low-density lipoprotein cholesterol changes after consumption of ad libitum diet, JAMA 274:1450, 1995.

Selhub J et al.: Association between plasma homocysteine concentrations and extracranial carotid-artery disease, N Engl J Med 332:286, 1995.

Selhub J et al.: Vitamin status and intake a primary determinant of homocysteinemia in an elderly population, JAMA 270:2693, 1993.

Sempos CT et al.: Body iron stores and the risk of coronary heart disease, N Engl J Med 330:1119, 1994.

Shaywitz BA and Shaywitz SE: Estrogen and Alzheimer's disease. Plausible theory, negative clinical trial, JAMA 283:1055, 2000.

Shike M: Body weight and colon cancer, Am J Clin Nutr 63:442S, 1996.

Stamler J et al.: The relationship of baseline serum cholesterol levels in 3 large cohorts of younger men to long-term coronary, cardiovascular, and all-cause mortality and to longevity, JAMA 284:3118, 2000.

Stevens J et al.: Body weight change and carotid artery wall thickness: the Atherosclerosis Risk in Communities (ARIC) study, Am J Epidemiol 147:563, 1998.

Stevens J: Obesity and mortality in African-Americans, Nutr Rev 58:346, 2000.

Stewart AL and Ware JE, editors: Measuring functioning and well-being: the medical outcomes study approach, Durham, NC, 1992, Duke University Press.

Trials of Hypertension Prevention Collaborative Research Group: The effects of nonpharmacologic interventions on blood pressure of persons with high normal levels: results of the trials of hypertension prevention, phase I, JAMA 267:1213, 1992.

U.S. Department of Health and Human Services, National Institutes of Health, National Heart, Lung, and Blood Institute: Clinical guidelines on the identification, evaluation, and treatment of overweight and obesity in adults: the evidence report, Bethesda, Md, June 1998, Table ES4.

U.S. Public Health Service: National Center for Health Statistics data 2010: Healthy People 2010 database, 1999. http://www.cdc.gov/nchs/aboutactupdate.2010/about.hp.htm

van Itallie T: Health implications of overweight and obesity in the United States, Ann Intern Med 103:983, 1985.

van Poppel G and Goldbohm RA: Epidemiologic evidence for beta carotene and cancer prevention, Am J Clin Nutr 62:1393S, 1995.

Vaziri SM: The impact of female hormone usage on the lipid profile: the Framingham offspring study, Arch Intern Med 153:2200, 1993.

Vuori I: Peak bone mass and physical activity: a short review, Nutr Rev 54:S11, 1996.

Walden CE et al: Lipoprotein response to the National Cholesterol Education Program Step II diet by hypercholestolemic and combined hyperlipidemia women and men, Arterioscler Thromb Vasc Biol 17:375, 1997.

Wegner NK: Postmenopausal hormone therapy: is it useful for coronary prevention? Cardiol Clin 161:1725, 1998.

Whittemore AS and Henderson BE: Dietary fat and breast cancer: where are we?, J Natl Cancer Inst 85:762, 1993.

Willett WC and Trichopoulos D: Nutrition and cancer: a summary of the evidence, Cancer Causes Control 7: 178, 1996.

Willett WC et al.: Dietary fat and fiber in relation to risk of breast cancer, JAMA 268:2034, 1992.

Willett WC et al.: Weight, weight change, and coronary heart disease in women, JAMA 273:461, 1995.

Williamson D et al.: The 10-year incidence of overweight and major weight gain in U.S. adults, Arch Intern Med 150:655, 1990.

Williamson DF et al.: Intentional weight loss and mortality among overweight individuals with diabetes, Diabetes Care 23:1499, 2000.

Wise PM et al.: Minireview and neuroprotective effects of estrogen: new insights into mechanisms of action, Endocrinology 142:969, 2001.

Working Group on Hypertension in the Elderly: Statement on hypertension in the elderly, JAMA 256:70, 1986.

Writing Group for the PEPI Trial: Effects of hormone replacement therapy on endometrial histology in postmenopausal women, JAMA 275:370, 1996.

Wynder EL et al.: High fiber intake: indicator of a healthy lifestyle, JAMA 275:488, 1996.

Yaffe K et al.: Serum estrogen levels, cognitive performance, and risk of cognitive decline in older community women, J Am Geriatr Soc 46:816, 1998.

Yaffe K et al.: Cognitive decline in women in relation to non-protein-bound oestradiol concentrations, Lancet 356:708, 2000.

Yu S et al.: Plasma cholesterol-predictive equations demonstrate that stearic acid is neutral and monounsaturated fatty acids are hypocholesterolemic, Am J Clin Nutr 61:1129, 1995.

Ziegler RG: Vegetables, fruits and carotenoids and the risk of cancer, Am J Clin Nutr 53:251S, 1991.

Ziegler RG et al.: Nutrition and lung cancer, Cancer Causes Control 7:157, 1996.

APPLICATION

Foods, Supplements, Herbs?

Abby is a 36-year-old wife and mother of two sons who are 2 years and 3 years of age. Her husband is a salesperson. She contributes to the family income by teaching aerobic dance classes two evenings a week, but she says they always have difficulty making ends meet.

Abby is very concerned about her health and appearance. She is 165 cm (65 in) and she weighs 60 kg (132 lb). In addition to teaching aerobic dance classes, she walks 2 miles with a neighbor three to four times a week and works out at least twice a week using a set of weights she purchased at a garage sale. Abby says she doesn't want to "get old" like her mother did.

Abby is convinced that nutrition is an important component of her campaign to stay young. She tries to eat a balanced diet, but feels she needs supplements to help her feel and look better. Abby drinks ***ginseng*** *tea with every meal and takes the following supplements, which she buys at the health food store or by mail from a catalogue:*

- *1 multivitamin supplement with trace minerals and* ***lutein***
- *1 vitamin supplement of* ***antioxidants*** *(vitamins A, E, C, and beta carotene)*
- *2 soft gel capsules for mental enhancement, each of which contains the following:*

Vitamin B_6	*2 mg*
Vitamin B_{12}	*6 μg*
Lecithin	*120 mg*

- *3 capsules for joint health, each of which contains the following:*

Carbohydrate	*2g*
Vitamin C	*180 mg*
Vitamin E	*69 IU*
Iron	*0.78 mg*

- *3* ***Glucosamine chondroitin*** *sulfate tablets*
- *2* ***melatonin*** *capsules*
- *3* ***garlic*** *tablets, 220 mg garlic powder each*

ginseng: the root of the Chinese shrub *Panax schinseng,* which contains compounds called saponins that interact with neurotransmitters in the body
lutein: a carotenoid with antioxidant activity
antioxidants: substances that prevent tissue damage by trapping organic free radicals or deactivating excited oxygen molecules, which occur as a byproduct of many metabolic reactions
glucosamine: a natural compound present in most human tissue, including joints; has an important role in protein metabolism in cartilage
chondroitin: larger substance composed of many glucosamine molecules; clinical trials suggest that glucosamine chondroitin sulfate may be mildly effective in releiving the pain of osteoarthritis
melatonin: a hormone that is secreted mostly at night by the pineal gland, which regulates many cyclical body functions, such as sleep and fertility; natural levels in the body decrease with age
garlic: an herb that has been promoted to lower blood cholesterol; however, the effect appears to be very small

As illustrated by Abby's story, dietary supplements can be varied. Figures from national surveys reveal that 30% to 60% of adults take one supplement product or another on a regular basis (American Dietetic Association, 2001; Hensrud et al., 1999). Supplement users tend to be healthy people and often their diets are more likely to provide recommended nutrient intake levels than those nonsupplement users. Although the most commonly used supplements are multivitamins, supplements of single nutrients and small groups of nutrients are gaining in popularity. In 1992 the nutritional supplement market in the United States amounted to approximately $4 billion. Of that amount, $123 million was spent for vitamin E alone and $22 million for beta carotene.

Traditionally, nutrient supplements, defined as single or multiple vitamins or minerals, were used to replace nutrient deficits from poor dietary intake. Over time the concept of supplements has evolved from insurance against nutrient inadequacy to protection and improvement of health and prevention of disease. It is the position of the American Dietetic Association (2001) that the best nutritional strategy for promoting optimal health and reducing the risk of chronic disease is to choose wisely from a wide variety of foods. Although no dietary supplement can replace a healthful diet, experts agree that providing the body with adequate nutrient intake is especially important in light of the increasing prevalence of degenerative diseases, particularly heart disease, stroke, cancer, and osteoporosis (Yates et al., 1998).

The characteristics of individuals who choose to use supplements have been profiled in numerous studies. In general, a typical supplement user has been described as female, healthy, with a higher income and educational level, and a tendency to consume diets that provide recommended nutrient intake levels greater than have those of nonsupplement users. However, there is great diversity among users and studies based on consumer characteristics of a group generally can predict only about one third of the individuals' diet-related behaviors (Baranowski et al., 1999).

Data from national surveys suggest that 30% to 60% of adults take one or more supplements regularly (Greger, 2001). Although the most commonly used supplements are multivitamins, supplements of single nutrients and small groups of nutrients and food components are gaining in popularity. Usage of supplements is changing. Increasingly, consumers are taking charge of their health and seeking alternative forms of medicine, including **dietary supplements** (Eisenberg et al., 1998). In 1999 consumers spent $47 billion on dietary supplements, an almost sixfold increase in just 5 years (Global Nutrition Industry, 2000).

> **dietary supplements:** a new category of foods that includes vitamins and minerals and herbal or other botanical ingredients (often referred to as phytochemicals), amino acids, and dietary substances used to increase total dietary intake

Scientific research has begun to identify specific components in foods that have health benefits beyond meeting nutrient needs. Confusion exists about how to describe this newly evolving area of food and food components. Numerous interchangeable names have been used, such as **herbals**, medicinals in food, **phytochemicals**, phytomedicinals, **nutraceuticals**, and **functional food.** Common to all these terms is the assumption that the food or components have a potentially beneficial role in prevention and treatment of disease (American Dietetic Association, 1996). The Dietary Supplement Health and Education Act (DSHEA) of 1994 includes these substances as dietary supplements. By definition this includes the ginseng tea, garlic tablets, and melatonin taken by Abby, and her vitamin and mineral supplements.

> **herbals:** plants used to produce a desired effect on the body
> **phytochemicals:** botanical ingredients that may have beneficial properties
> **nutraceuticals:** any substance (food or part of food) that provides medical or health benefit
> **functional food:** any modified food or ingredient that may provide a health benefit beyond the traditional nutrients it contains

For purposes of clarity, studies of dietary supplements may separate vitamin and mineral supplements from other supplements, often referring to them as nonvitamin, nonmineral supplements. Although there has been some controversy about use of vitamin and mineral supplements above the levels of the DRI, supplements have been shown to be beneficial in certain circumstances. There is evidence that supplements of vitamin B_6 may prevent the onset of **carpal tunnel syndrome,** that nicotinic acid lowers blood total plasma cholesterol, that folate before and during early pregnancy helps reduce the occurrence of neural tube defects, and that calcium and vitamin D aid in the prevention of osteoporosis.

> **carpal tunnel syndrome:** a complex of symptoms resulting from compression of the nerves in the wrist, which causes pain, burning, or tingling in the fingers and hand

Many argue that dietary supplements are necessary because they extend beyond the prevention of deficiency diseases to the prevention or delay of aging and of chronic diseases such as cancer (Nayga and Reed, 1999). Over the last decade evidence has been accumulating that a variety of dietary components may have a protective effect in relation to changes associated with aging and some chronic diseases. Many epidemiologic studies have observed a relationship between foods containing antioxidants (vitamins C and E and carotenoids) and risk of chronic disease, particularly cancer, CVD, and cerebrovascular disease, the three major causes of mortality in adults (Radimer et al., 2000). A chief limitation of observational studies is their inability to control for all factors that might independently affect health risk.

For example it is recognized that oxidation of the lens proteins plays a central role in the formation of age-related cataracts, and dietary antioxidants may play an important role in preventing or delaying the progression of the cataract forming process. Persons consuming low amounts of fruits and vegetables have been observed to be at increased risk of cataract (Jacques and Chylack, 1991). Dietary manipulation may change blood carotenoids, but that may or may not reflect the amount present in the human lens (Bowen et al., 1993). In fact carotenoids such as beta carotene, lypopene, and beta cryptoxanthin have not been found in the human lens, whereas lutein and zeaxanthin have been measured in small amounts and vary widely between individuals (Bates et al., 1996). Intakes of lutein and zeaxanthin in the form of supplements or foods high in lutein and zeaxanthin have been shown to increase the amount of macular pigment (Hammond et al., 1997; Landrum et al., 1996), suggesting a potential protective role. In the Nurses' Health Study, a 12-year follow-up found that an increase in the frequency of intakes of spinach and kale, which are foods rich in lutein, was associated with a moderate decrease in risk of cataract (Chasan-Taber et al., 1999). From a practical standpoint, this research is intriguing and provides the impetus for further investigation of the health-promoting role of lutein. As a result of these preliminary, but promising, observations the marketing of lutein has skyrocketed as a dietary supplement and as an addition to other supplements including daily multiple vitamin and mineral products.

An important effect of the DSHEA of 1994 is the fact that, in contrast to foods and drugs, for dietary supplements it places the legal burden on the FDA to prove that a supplement product is unsafe rather than requiring the manufacturer to prove it is safe. Products may be marketed if there is a history of use or other evidence of safety establishing that the product is reasonably expected to be safe when used under the conditions recommended or suggested in its labeling.

In 2000 the FDA issued a final rule for claims on dietary supplements under DSHEA. Dietary supplements may bear "structure/function" claims—claims that the products affect the structure or function of the body—without prior FDA review. They may not, without prior FDA review, bear a claim that they can prevent, treat, cure, mitigate, or diagnose disease (a disease claim).

ALLOWABLE CLAIMS ON LABELS OF DIETARY SUPPLEMENTS

- The statement claims a benefit to a classic nutrient deficiency disease and discloses the prevalence of such disease in the United States.
- It describes the role of a nutrient or dietary ingredient intended to affect the structure or function in humans.
- It characterizes the documented mechanism by which a nutrient or dietary ingredient acts to maintain such structure or function.
- It describes general well-being from consumption of a nutrient or dietary ingredient.

The FDA final rule precludes express disease claims ("prevents osteoporosis") and implied disease claims ("prevents bone fragility in postmenopausal women") without prior FDA review. The final rule clarifies that such express and implied disease claims can be made through the name of a product, through a statement about the formulation of a product ("contains aspirin"), or through the use of pictures, vignettes, or symbols (e.g., electrocardiogram tracings). The rule permits claims that do not relate to disease. These include health maintenance claims ("maintains a healthy circulatory system"), other nondisease claim ("for muscle enhancement," "helps you relax"), and claims for common, minor symptoms associated with life stages ("for common symptoms of PMS," "for hot flashes").

Under DSHEA and existing regulations, dietary supplement manufacturers are already required to have, in their files, substantiation of any structure or function claims they make. They must also include a disclaimer on their labels that the dietary supplements are not drugs and receive no FDA premarket approval. Finally, they must notify FDA of the claims they are making within 30 days of marketing a given dietary supplement.

Manufacturers are now required to provide a nutrition facts label for all supplements. Products labeled "high potency" must provide at least 100% of the nutrients' Daily Value. Products described as antioxidants must have the ability to neutralize free radicals. None of these statements indicates that a supplement will actually enhance health or that is safe. Similarly the presence of an FDA-approved label does not mean that the product has been evaluated or supported by the FDA.

The Office of Dietary Supplements Research (ODSR), a division of the NIH, has been established and is responsible for regulating herbs and other dietary supplements and for deciding whether to allow manufacturers' claims for the products. The FDA is called in if the ODSR decides that a product presents a danger to public health.

Experts in traditional medicine lack information of supplements and herbals. More research is needed on the efficacy, toxicity, and bioavailability of supplements and herbal medicines.

Studies of the efficacy of dietary supplements such as lutein illustrate the complexity of identifying compounds from other dietary components that may have protective effects. It may be that the positive effects of fruits and vegetables on cancer are from other substances in the foods and interactions among food components.

The origin of these observations between nutrition and aging or disease is the diet. Obviously food is more than the sum of its nutrients. Some supplements in large doses may have beneficial effects on nutrition status and health; others may have detrimental effects from direct toxicity of the supplement or interference with other nutrients (Thomas, 1996). Therefore it is appropriate to emphasize the importance of food as the best source of essential nutrients and disease prevention factors by recommending eating a wide variety of foods and exercising caution in using supplements.

An estimated 29,000 different dietary supplements are available to consumers and an average of 1000 new products are added each year (Sarubin, 2000). Sometimes supplements are promoted by commercial and other forces on the basis of incomplete or preliminary evidence. As the number of these dietary supplements appearing on the shelves increases, it becomes essential that consumers be assisted in making careful selections (McNutt, 1995). Because dietary supplements are not sold in standardized doses and do not come with a list of possible adverse responses, as the FDA requires for all pharmaceuticals, consumers may be unaware of the side effects that could result from taking the products.

Therefore recommendations to use dietary supplements should be based on well-accepted scientific evidence (American Dietetic Association, 1996). Although few are likely to be harmful, *natural* is not a synonym for *safe*. Nutrients and other dietary substances relevant to health are already available in familiar and attractive packages called fruits, vegetables, legumes, grains, and animal products. They come in concentrations and in combinations with which humans have long had cultural familiarity (Thomas, 1996).

REFERENCES

American Dietetic Association: Position of the American Dietetic Association: phytochemicals and functional food, J Am Diet Assoc 95:493, 1995.

American Dietetic Association: Position of the American Dietetic Association: vitamin and mineral supplementation, J Am Diet Assoc 96:73, 1996.

American Dietetic Association: Position of the American Dietetic Association: food fortification and dietary supplements, J Am Diet Assoc 100:115, 2001.

Bates CJ et al.: Quantitation of vitamin E and carotenoid pigment in cataractous human lenses, and the effect of a dietary supplement, Int J Vitam Nutr Res 66:316, 1996.

Baranowski T et al.: Psychological correlates of dietary intake: advancing dietary intervention, Annu Rev Nutr 19:17, 1999.

Bowen PE et al.: Variability of serum carotenoids in response to controlled diets containing six servings of fruits and vegetables, Ann N Y Acad Sci 691:241, 1993.

Chasan-Taber et al.: A prospective study of vitamin supplement intake and cataract extraction among U.S. women, Epidemiology 10:679, 1999.

Eisenberg DM et al.: Trends in alternative medicine use in the United States, 1990-1997: results of a follow-up national survey, JAMA 280:1569, 1998.

Global Nutrition Industry 2000, Nutr Bus J 5:10, 2000.

Greger JL: Dietary supplement use: consumer characteristics and interests, J Nutr 131:1339S, 2001.

Hammond BR et al.: Density of the human crystalline lens is related to the mocular pigment carotenoids, lutein and zeaxanthin, Optom Vis Sci 74:499, 1997.

Hensrud DD et al.: Underreporting the use of dietary supplements and nonprescription medications among patients undergoing periodic health examination, Mayo Clin Proc 74:443, 1999.

Jacques PF and Chylack LT Jr: Epidemiologic evidence of a role for the antioxidant vitamins and carotenoids in cataract prevention, Am J Clin Nutr 52:352S, 1991.

Landrum JT et al.: The macular pigment: a possible role in protection from age-related macular degeneration, Adv Pharmacol 38:537, 1996.

McNutt K: Medicinals in food. Part II: what's new and what's not, Nutr Today 30:261, 1995.

Nayga RM and Reed DB: Factors associated with the intake of dietary supplements, Fam Econ Nutr Rev 12:43, 1999.

Radimer KL et al.: Nonvitamin, nonmineral dietary supplements: issues and findings from the NHANES III, J Am Diet Assoc 100:447, 2000.

Sarubin A: The health professional's guide to popular dietary supplements, Chicago, 2000, American Dietetic Association.

Thomas PR: Food for thought about dietary supplements, Nutr Today 31:46, 1996.

Yates AA et al.: Dietary reference intakes: the new basis for recommendations for calcium and related nutrients, B vitamins and choline, J Am Diet Assoc 98:699, 1998.

ADDITIONAL RESOURCES

DeBusk R and Treadwell P: Herbs as medicine: what you should know, Tallahassee, Fl, 1998, Debusk Communications.

INTERNET-BASED RESOURCES

Natural medicines comprehensive database: http/www.naturaldatabase.com.

CHAPTER 13

Aging and Older Adults

Chapter Outline

Martha is a 75-year-old widow. She married in her late thirties and had no children, but she does have a niece and nephew close by. She worked intermittently during her life, but has not been employed for the last 2 decades. Her husband owned extensive property and had a moderate pension, so she has few financial concerns. She had smoked two or more packs of cigarettes each day since her early twenties, but she stopped about 2 years ago because she began to have difficulty breathing. Approximately 1 year ago, Martha was hospitalized for emphysema and returned home on oxygen and medication. Several weeks later she was moved to an extended-care facility. Her activities consist of bathing, dressing, and watching television. She dresses each day, but refuses to go to the dining room for meals and has to be coaxed to walk occasionally in the halls. Martha is frequently curt with the staff and refuses to interact with the other patients. She complains little and does not indicate that she wants to be anywhere else, but she doesn't seem very happy and isn't responsive to the staff or visitors.

Ethel is 80 years of age. She and her husband Bob live in a suburb of a western city. Ethel has a degree in Home Economics, but was employed for only a short time before her marriage. Ethel and Bob have sufficient income to maintain their current life-style. They have one son and one daughter and five grandchildren—most in college or working—and they own a spacious ranch-style home. Ethel is active as a volunteer, plays bridge several days a week, and participates in church activities. Ethel no longer drives, but Bob takes her wherever she wants to go. In the summer she plays golf 2 or 3 days a week, playing nine holes and pulling her clubs on a small cart. She got a new set of clubs last year that improved her game dramatically. She would play golf more frequently, but her other activities keep her too busy.

The process of aging converts healthy adults into frail ones with diminished physiologic reserves and increased vulnerability to disease. Yet, as seen in these two women, there is marked variety among older adults and the ways in which they age. Ethel might be considered an example of what has been termed "successful" aging with a gradual progressive functional decline. Increased morbidity with aging is usually associated with progressive illness and rapid functional decline or a catastrophic event, such as a stroke or a hip fracture with some degree of improvement after rehabilitation (Vellas et al., 1992). In Martha's case quality of life is compromised by health problems associated with a lifetime of poor health habits (Gray-Donald, 1995). Because of such factors, she is frail and requires assistance with the basic activities of living. What makes the difference in their lives? Genetics, environment, health, lifestyle, nutrition? All of the above.

The physiologic and psychologic changes of aging influence an individual's ability to function independently and determine his or her quality of life. Researchers in **gerontology** have identified some characteristics common to individuals who are able to function actively at an advanced age (Box 13-1).

Box 13-1 FACTORS ASSOCIATED WITH THE ABILITY TO FUNCTION AT AN ADVANCED AGE

Genetic potential for longevity
Intelligence, motivation, curiosity
Well-developed sense of humor
Pursuit of active challenges
Stimulating, highly organized, complex daily life
Social contacts maintained
Capacity to adapt to changing events
Religious conviction
Financial independence
Living arrangements—independence, convenience, safety, contact with younger people, preferably family
Responsibility
Family integrity—strong family bonds
Intimacy—marriage, intimate friendships, love and mutual understanding
Moderate body size—improves agility and decreases risk of systemic disease
Life habits of moderation—avoidance of substance abuse (alcohol, smoking, drugs); prudent diet (i.e., avoidance of excess)
Availability of community health care
Relative freedom from accidents

AGING

- *How old is old?*
- *What are the characteristics of the older adult population?*
- *What are some of the theories of why we age?*

The most apparent consequences of aging are gray hair, wrinkles, age spots on the skin, changes in physique, decreased strength and endurance, and declines in the acuity of taste and smell. The overall process is more complex, however, encompassing molecular, cellular, physiologic, and psychologic changes that are influenced by genetics and socioeconomic environment.

Being old is less a chronologic age than a state of mind and physical status. No two people age in exactly the same way and older adults are a remarkably diverse group. Older adulthood is often defined as beginning at age 65 years because that is the age at which eligibility for Medicare and Social Security benefits begins. However, many people choose to retire while still in their fifties, whereas others continue to work and lead active lives into their seventies and eighties and beyond.

The Aging Population

Since 1900 life expectancy in the United States has increased by approximately 29 years. A baby girl born in 2000 can expect to live 79 years and a male about 4 years less (U.S. Census Bureau, 2001). Increased life expectancy from control of infections, reduced death rates for children and young adults, and improved treatment of chronic diseases has contributed to the "graying of America." If an individual lives to 65 years, the life expectancy from that point is 19 years for a woman and 15.8 years for a man.

At the beginning of the twentieth century, only 4% of the population of the United States was over 65 years of age. In 2000 12.7% of

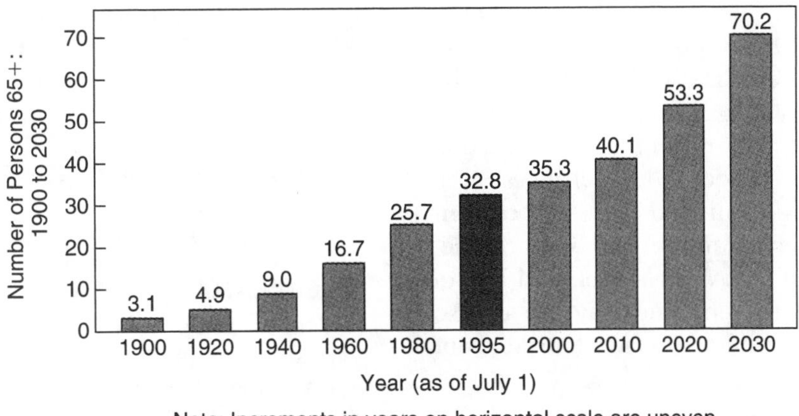

Figure 13-1 Predicted increases in the number of persons 65 years and older by the year 2030.

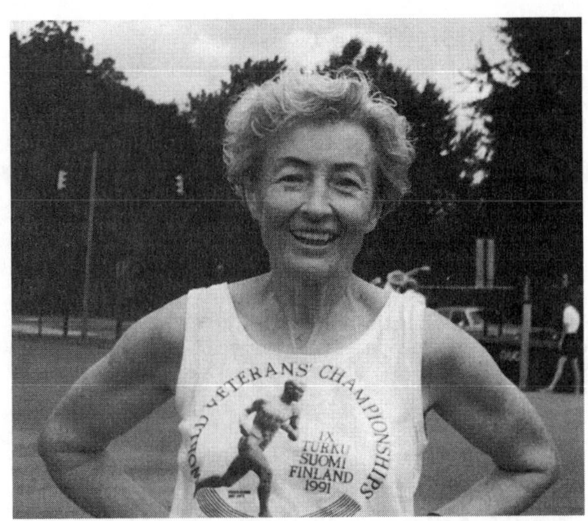

Figure 13-2 Most older adults are active, involved individuals. This 67-year-old woman competes in track events all over the world. *(Photographer: Mary Kay Mitchell.)*

Americans, or 34.6 million (20.3 million women and 14.3 million men), were 65 or older. The number increases at the rate of 5422 per day (U.S. Census Bureau, 2001). Of persons age 65 or older, almost one third (12 million) are between 75 years and 84 years and 4 million are the "oldest old," those 85 and over. Analysis of 1990 census data estimates that nearly 70,000 people are age 100 years or older and four of five of these are women. It is estimated that by the year 2030, about 70 million individuals will be over 65 and 17% of that group will be over 85 (Figure 13-1). In 1999 16.1% of persons over 65 were minorities. By 2030 minorities will represent 25% of the population of older adults, with the largest increases in Hispanics and Asians.

The majority of older adults are free-living, active individuals (Figure 13-2). In 1998 67% of community-dwelling persons 65 years and older lived in a family setting. Overall only 4.3% of older adults are in long-term care facilities and less than 17% require assistance with the day-to-day activities of living. With increasing age, however, chronic illnesses and health conditions result in greater dependency on others for performing daily activities of living (U.S. Census Bureau, 2001).

Theories of Aging

Gerontologists have documented many changes of the gradual process of aging, but the fundamental processes that control the rate at which people age and how **senescence** leads to the diseases of

KEY TERMS

gerontology: the scientific study of all aspects of aging

senescence: the process or condition of growing old

aging are essentially unknown (Hollozy, 2000). The factors that are known to affect longevity do so by their influence on disease development. The majority of theories of aging suggest that an intracellular molecule, cell, or organ that loses function over time triggers age-dependent changes in a whole range of body organs and cells. Most current theories relate to some form of impairment of deoxyribonucleic acid (DNA) replication and loss of viability of the cell and hence the body's organs. No single theory explains all of the facts known about aging.

PHYSIOLOGIC CHANGES OF AGING

- *How does body composition change with aging?*
- *Describe the major age-related changes that occur in the senses and body systems.*
- *What is the impact of the physiologic changes of aging on function and quality of life?*

Changes in body and organ function occur throughout adult life, making old age the culmination of diverse processes that began at earlier ages. Overall, in the absence of disease, older adults maintain physical function, but their **reserve capacity** diminishes with time. With aging, there are declines in the number of active cells and in organ size and function. In Table 13-1 there are percentages of the age-related changes in major physiologic systems and functions that occur between ages 30 years and 70 years. Aging is associated with a loss of strength, flexibility, and cardiovascular fitness, which leads to a further decrease in activity. Table 13-2 presents a brief summary of the age-related changes in physiologic systems.

Table 13-1 Age-Related Changes in Physiologic Function at 70 Years as a Percentage of That Function at Age 30

CARDIOVASCULAR SYSTEM	
Cardiac output	70
Maximum heart rate	75
RESPIRATORY SYSTEM	
Vital capacity	60
Residual volume	130-150
Maximum O_2 uptake	40
MUSCULOSKELETAL	
Muscle mass	70
Hand grip, flexibility	70
Bone mineralization	70-80
Renal function	60
NERVOUS SYSTEM	
Conduction velocity	85
Resting glucose uptake	100
Taste and smell	10
METABOLISM	
Fasting blood glucose	100
Basal metabolic rate	85

From Berry EM: Undernutrition in the elderly: a physiological and pathological process? In Munro H and Schlierf A, editors: Nutrition of the elderly, Nestle Workshop Series vol 29. Nestle Ltd. New York, 1992, Vervey/Raven Press.

Body Composition

Age is associated with slow declines in weight and modifications in body composition, or **sarcopenia,** declines in bone mass, and gradual accretion of adipose tissue (Rubenoff and Hughes, 2000; Tessari, 2000). In addition to having less muscle and bone mass, elderly people have expanded extracellular fluid volumes and reduced body cell mass compared with younger adults (Baumgartner, 2000). In general adults gain weight until the sixth decade, after which there is a gradual decline, typically 10% between 70 years and 80 years. Extremes in body weight are associated with a greater risk of functional impairment in older adults (Galanos et al., 1994).

The decline in muscle mass is almost linear, at approximately 2% to 3% per decade (Fontera et al., 1991) (Figure 13-3). As lean body mass decreases, the percentage of body fat increases. In

KEY TERMS

reserve capacity: the ability to respond to stress
sarcopenia: loss of skeletal muscle and strength

Table 13-2 PHYSIOLOGIC CHANGES ASSOCIATED WITH AGING

System/Function	Physiologic Change
Basal metabolic rate	Decrease of 20% between 20 years and 90 years that accelerates with age
Senses	General decline
Taste	Decreased taste buds and papillae on tongue; loss of ability to detect salt and sweet
Smell	Decrease in olfactory nerve endings
Hearing	Bilateral symmetric hearing loss
Sight	Decreases in dark adaptation, distance vision, visual acuity; thickening and loss of elasticity of crystalline lens; cataracts
Gastrointestinal oral cavity	Reduced saliva flow; thinning of gum tissue, shrinking of connective tissue; periodontal disease causing loss of teeth
Esophageal function and swallowing	Minor changes, including disordered contractions
Gastric function	Decreased secretion of hydrochloric acid, intrinsic factor, and pepsin (atrophic gastritis); increased pH in small intestine may contribute to bacterial overgrowth; decreased bioavailability of some minerals and vitamins
Liver and biliary function	Decreased liver size, reduced blood flow to liver; decreased rate of albumin synthesis; reduced activity of drug metabolizing enzymes
Pancreatic secretion	Slightly reduced output of bicarbonate and enzymes
Small intestine	Decreased absorption of calcium and vitamin B_{12}
Laxation	Decreased motility; delayed transit; retention of feces within rectum, constipation common
Respiratory function	Linear decline from ages of 20 years to 80 years; decreased vital capacity
Cardiovascular	Decreased heart size; increased rigidity of arterial walls causes a decrease of blood flow to tissue; decreased contractibility; general loss of tolerance for physical stress
Skin	Dryness, wrinkling, mottled pigmentation, loss of elasticity; changes accelerated by exposure to sunlight; increased water loss from surface; decrease in sebaceous gland activity
Hair	Graying, hair loss
Nails	Slow growth, thickening
Neuromuscular	Progressive loss of cells, neuromuscular loss (decline in number of nerve fibers and contractile process), motor function and muscle strength decline; 15% decrease in nerve conduction velocity; decrease in muscle mass
Skeletal system	Decrease in bone mass
Kidneys	Fewer nephrons after age 40 years; glomerular filtration rate declines about 50% at age 80, decreased ability to concentrate or dilute urine
Endocrine	Decreased response of beta cells of pancreas to glucose; reduced glucose tolerance and production of insulin, slight changes in other endocrine secretions; large decreases in estrogen, some decrease in activity of testosterone
Immune system	Decline in size and function of immune system, especially cell-mediated

addition there is a shift from subcutaneous to central or truncal body fat, with fat deposited in the abdomen and on the thighs and buttocks.

Resistance training exercise can preserve fat-free mass and increase muscle strength in the aged. In a study of 100 elderly male nursing home residents who completed a program of resistance training, Fiatarone and colleagues (1994) demonstrated that the men improved muscle strength and gait velocity and enhanced thigh muscle area,

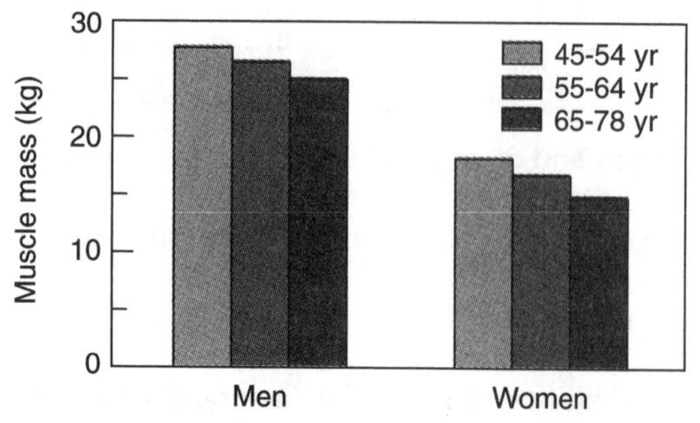

Figure 13-3 Declining muscle mass with age.

stair climbing power, and levels of spontaneous activity. Other studies have shown that combined exercise and dietary intervention with a hypocaloric diet can augment lean mass while further reducing fat mass (Singh, 1998). Guo and coworkers (1999) found that physical activity can improve lean body mass in men and women. In fact they reported that the effects were more profound in women after menopause and that the effects were augmented by hormone (estrogen) replacement.

Basal Metabolic Rate

As lean body mass declines after age 30 years, there is a gradual, but accelerating, decrease in the basal metabolic rate (BMR). Early in the process the decrease in energy output may contribute to weight gain and obesity. However, over time dietary intakes appear to diminish and being underweight becomes more common. The decrease in weight further reduces lean body mass; therefore the BMR declines even more. With lower energy intakes, it becomes difficult for older persons to satisfy all of their nutrient needs.

The Senses

Vision

Age-related reductions in visual acuity vary widely from person to person. The central area of the **retina** is the most sensitive site of visual perception and it tends to degenerate with age. There is a loss of ability to focus on near objects (presbyopia) because of the inability of the aging lens to change in curvature in response to needs of near vision. An increase in lens size and a narrowing of the angle between the **cornea** and the **iris** may impair drainage of fluid present in the anterior chamber of the eye, leading to a buildup of interior or intraocular pressure and impaired vision, referred to as glaucoma.

In natural aging changes in chemical composition of the lens contribute to **cataracts,** which can reduce visual acuity. The lens becomes less resilient and less transparent. Fibers in the lens become compressed and the lens turns more rigid. Clarity fades as proteins coagulate. In the early stages, night vision is reduced. Later there is progressive loss of vision, which can be relieved by surgical extraction of the lens. A growing body of evidence suggests that development of cataracts can be retarded by avoidance of smoking and long-term exposure to ultraviolet-B (UVB) rays from the sun. In addition adequate levels of antioxidant nutrients in and around the lens of the eye may have a protective effect. This protection has been reported with increasing levels of the antioxidant vitamins C and E and beta carotene in the diet and in the circulation (Vitale et al., 1993). Brown and coworkers (1999) reported that in a study of U.S. men, carotinoids and zeaxanthin intake in fruits and vegetables was associated with a decreased risk of cataract and cataract extraction.

Age-related macular degeneration (AMD) is a slow, insidious atrophy of the photoreceptors in the **macula** on the retinal pigment epithelium. It is the most common irreversible cause of blindness in older adults. Macular degeneration affects almost 30% of Americans over the age of 65 and the proportion increases with age. People with AMD experience blurred vision and the inability to clearly see things in front of them. It is the foremost cause of legal blindness in people over 55. Smoking can accelerate AMD damage; quitting smoking and using sunglasses that block blue UVB wavelengths may provide some protection. Evidence is accumulating for a protective effect of antioxidant nutrients to prevent the progression of AMD, but a definitive effect will await the results of ongoing trials (Seddon et al., 1994).

Hearing

Age-related hearing loss disorders result from impaired function of the inner ear (cochlea) or the connections of the auditory nerve close to or within the brain. These changes may result from several factors, but are most commonly related to genetics, occupational noise exposure, chronic middle ear disease, or atherosclerosis.

Taste and Smell

The diminished senses of taste (hypogeusia) and smell (hyposemia) common with advancing age can contribute to inadequate food intake and to compromised nutrition status. The losses reach statistical significance at approximately 60 years of age and become increasingly severe after 70.

The receptor cells for taste are arranged in buds located on the surface of the tongue, the roof of the mouth, the passage between the mouth and the windpipe, and the upper third of the esophagus. Signals from taste buds are transmitted via the cranial nerves. The cells in taste buds have an average turnover time of about 10 days. Some age-related losses in taste are caused by interruption of turnover of taste cells.

The receptor or olfactory cells of the sense of smell are located in the upper part of the nasal cavity. Like taste cells, they are in a constant state of flux, turning over about every 30 days. Olfactory cells project to the olfactory bulbs, which contain groups of cells called glomeruli. During the aging process the number of glomeruli decreases. Olfactory information is processed by the limbic system of the brain, which is the emotional seat of the brain. Therefore stimulation of olfactory bulbs can affect emotions and the ability to perceive odor.

The Gastrointestinal Tract

Oral Cavity

Age-related changes in teeth include abrasion or wearing down of crowns. On the other hand, there is an increased resistance to tooth decay because of maturation of enamel and dentin. However, the gums deteriorate with age, causing loss of teeth and **periodontal** disease, which afflicts up to 90% of adults over the age of 65 years. Older adults often have missing teeth or poor-fitting dentures that impair mastication, resulting in reduced food intake. Masticatory efficiency is also compromised by loss of mobility of the mandibular (lower jaw) joint, often caused by osteoarthritis (a noninflammatory joint disease occurring chiefly in older persons).

In a healthy mouth copious amounts of saliva containing essential electrolytes, glycoproteins, and antimicrobial enzymes continually lubricate and protect the teeth and oral mucosa. Aging is associated with decreased salivary flow, which can cause the healthy mouth to become susceptible to painful deterioration. **Xerostomia** is particularly prevalent among the aged. Inadequate lubrication and moisture within the mouth, lack of ability to taste, food sticking to the tongue, and difficulty swallowing are among the most devastating manifestations of xerostomia in older adults; xerostomia is a major contributor to **geriatric** malnutrition in the United States (Rhodus and Brown, 1990).

Xerostomia is a potential side effect of many drugs widely used in geriatrics. Treatment is aimed at increasing the flow of saliva when possible or providing oral moisture by other means.

Esophagus, Stomach, and Small Intestine

Older people report gastrointestinal complaints more frequently than do younger adults and some disorders, such as diverticulosis, occur primarily in the elderly. Older adults also take more medications, which may affect gastrointestinal

KEY TERMS

retina: innermost layers of the eyeball
cornea: transparent structure forming the anterior portion of the eye
iris: the circular pigmented membrane behind the cornea
cataracts: opacities of the crystalline lens of the eye
macula: retinal area responsible for sharp central vision
periodontal: around the teeth; related to structures that support the tooth including bony socket and collagenous ligament that connects the root to the gum tissue
xerostomia: the feeling of dry mouth caused by a severe reduction in the flow of saliva
geriatric: branch of medicine that treats problems particular to old age and the aging process

function and food intake. Age-related changes in the anatomy and physiology of the digestive tract are small overall.

There is a slight decline in gastrointestinal motility and a general reduction in secretory ability of digestive glands, resulting in lower levels of enzymes, especially amylase, pepsin, and trypsin. In the stomach, gastric **atrophy** and **atrophic gastritis** increase significantly with age. Reduced hydrochloric acid secretion may result in decreased bioavailabilty of calcium, iron, folate, and vitamins B_6 and B_{12}, and increased risk of bacterial overgrowth of the small intestine. At typical intake levels, absorption of carbohydrate, lipid, and protein appears unaffected by age in healthy elderly persons. However, high-fat diets (greater than 100 g per day) are less tolerated (Holt and Balint, 1993).

Colon

Age-related alterations in motility of the colon may contribute to the retention of feces and constipation. Constipation is more common in older adults, partially from decreased activity, limited fluid intake, low-fiber diets, and, possibly, medications used. With low fiber intakes, increased intraluminal pressure and greater muscle contraction is required to move the digestive contents through the colon. The resulting weakening of the muscle wall may result in "outpouching," or the formation of small pouches in the wall of the colon, a condition known as diverticulosis.

Pancreas and Liver

Although morphologic changes occur in the liver and pancreas, digestive function appears to be adequate on usual intakes. The liver is the major site of drug metabolism in the body. The rate at which drugs are metabolized and detoxified is slower in older persons than in younger persons, causing drugs to remain in the body longer and to exert their effects over a longer time.

Anorexia of Aging

Anorexia of aging is a term used to describe the decline in appetite and loss of weight that are common with advancing age. Many factors contribute to anorexia and weight loss (Box 13-2). Depression and side effects of medication are the two most common treatable causes of weight loss in older persons (Birrer, 1998). In addition restricted diets with limited taste appeal, such as those low in cholesterol or salt, often precipitate weight loss.

Box 13-2 Factors That May Contribute to Anorexia of Aging

Hypothalamic control: decreased opioid feeding drive
Senses: decreased sense of taste and smell
Food ingestion: chewing difficulties from endentulous problems, xerostemia
Gastrointestinal: delayed gastric emptying—early satiety, difficulties in swallowing, increased cholecystokinin—increased satiety, abdominal angina (pain)
Chronic constipation
Psychosocial: poverty, depression, dementia, social isolation
Physical: impaired mobility
Disease states: cancer, chronic obstructive pulmonary disease
Medications: digoxin, psychotropic and analgesic/antiinflammatory drugs, other medications

Respiratory System

With aging comes a reduction in surface area of the alveoli (air sacs), which is accompanied by deterioration of the elastic properties of lung tissue. These decreases are almost linear between the ages of 20 years and 80 years and by age 80 years the level is approximately 30% of maximal young adult values. Because of these changes, the lungs become stiffer and alveolar tissue less distensible and less permeable to respiratory gases; therefore gas exchange is lowered. **Vital capacity** decreases with age and the ability to exercise is reduced.

Cardiovascular System

Cardiac output may decline with aging by as much as 30%. This change is from increased rigidity of arterial walls, decreased blood flow to tissues, and decreased oxygen uptake, all of which contribute to age-related changes in other tissues such as the kidney. There is an overall decrease in the size of the heart muscle and the size of the cavity of the ventricle (lower chamber of the heart) and an increase in the size of the left atrium (chamber). The heart valves become more rigid because of thickening from increased collagen and there is calcification in aortic valve. Hypertrophy (enlargement) of individual muscle fibers of myocardium occurs to compensate for other muscle fibers that are lost. The aging heart tolerates physical stress less well; there is reduced tolerance of strenuous exercise and, possibly, increased systolic blood pressure.

Skin, Hair, and Nails

The **collagen** content of the body is altered with age, and cross-linkages between molecules can result in many changes in skin and the loss of elasticity. The many age-related changes in the skin include dryness, wrinkling, enlarged sebaceous glands (but decreased sebaceous gland activity), mottled pigmentation, loss of elasticity, dilation of capillaries, and senile purpura (bleeding into skin in response to minor trauma). Chronic exposure to sunlight causes premature aging of these tissues. Solar effects on the skin are not limited to wrinkling and changes in pigmentation. Ultraviolet (UV) light accelerates the loss of elasticity in the walls of the tiny vessels that feed the skin, contributing to their permanent dilation. There are also the changes of graying of hair and more hair loss. The nails grow more slowly and may be thicker.

Neuromuscular System

Generalized age-related muscle weakness is related to a decline in the number of functioning muscle fibers, a general loss of muscle mass, and a decrease in the contractile process itself (Carmeli and Reznich, 1994). Because there is some loss of peripheral motor neurons, muscle response to nerve stimulation declines. The extent of these age-related changes varies from muscle to muscle.

Aging brings progressive loss of brain cells, particularly in the cortex, the area responsible for higher mental function, movement perception, and behavioral reactions. Therefore memory may decline, but the degree varies greatly. Although there may be some loss of memory that affects ability to learn and retain information, it is not an inevitable consequence of aging. There is evidence that consistent engagement with intellectually stimulating activities such as reading, working puzzles, playing a musical instrument, or painting reduce these effects.

It is possible that subclinical vitamin deficiencies play a role in the pathogenesis of declining neurocognitive function with aging. Attention has focused on vitamins C, B_6, B_{12}, E, and folate. Administration of vitamin B_{12} has been shown to reverse both cognitive and peripheral nervous system deficits in older adults who have no evidence of the hematologic abnormalities of vitamin B_{12} deficiency (Lindenbaum et al., 1994).

Skeletal Tissue

From infancy through young adulthood, bone mass increases rapidly during growth, especially at sites composed largely of **cortical bone.** Gains continue into the third decade of life, when peak bone mass is achieved, and then plateau. After peak bone mass is achieved, bone loss begins in the fourth or fifth decades and persists until the end of life. Bone loss is proportionately less for men than for women. A woman can lose 20% to 30% of **cancellous bone.** Among women the decline in estrogen secretion after menopause contributes to

KEY TERMS

atrophy: diminution of cell tissue or organ
atrophic gastritis: chronic inflammation of the stomach with decreased thickness of the mucosa and disappearance of gastric pyloric glands
vital capacity: the volume of gas that can be expelled from the lungs after full inspiration
collagen: protein substance of white fibers of the skin, tendon, bone, cartilage, and other connective tissue
cortical bone: compact bone, found primarily in long bones
cancellous bone: trabecular or spongy bone

accelerated bone loss; then, after a time, the rate of loss slows. The clinical importance of low bone mass is the increased risk of subsequent fractures. Osteoporosis, or accelerated bone loss, is discussed on page 457.

Kidney Function

Kidney function deteriorates with age. There is a net loss of **nephrons** and decreased blood flow through the kidney. As a result the rate at which blood is filtered through the kidney (the glomerular filtration rate) declines so that the rate of blood filtration at age 80 years is approximately 50% of that at age 25 years. The ability to concentrate or dilute urine is also decreased. This reduces the ability of the kidneys to deal with large fluctuations in the workload so that, for instance, it takes longer to excrete a large amount of dietary sodium from a food or meal high in salt.

Endocrine System

Aging is associated with myriad changes in the endocrine system. The most prominent may be a decline in glucose tolerance and in the production of insulin in response to an oral load of glucose. Reduced insulin levels are thought to contribute to adiposity, especially abdominal obesity (Tessari, 2000), and are associated with an increased incidence of non–insulin-dependent diabetes mellitus (NIDDM) with age. For women the dramatic decline in estrogen production at menopause has substantial implications for bone mass and osteoporosis.

Immune System

Throughout adult life the mass of immune tissue declines, with loss of immune function and an increased incidence of infections, cancer, and autoimmune disorders (Yung, 2000). Some immune cell functions decrease rapidly; others resist change or are even disproportionately elevated.

Nutrition can influence both immune function and the aging process. In fact most age-related changes of the immune system parallel those observed in protein energy undernutrition (PEU) (Chandra, 1995). Krause et al. (1999) examined immune function in older (62 to 88 years) versus younger (20 to 40 years) women. They found the most immune parameters were not compromised with aging in well-nourished women. Specific nutrient deficiencies have been shown to produce some impairments of immune function in older people. These include vitamin E (Meydani et al., 1995), zinc, and vitamins A, B_6, and C (Bogden et al., 1994; Rosenberg and Miller, 1992), which have been responsive to supplementation. However, oversupplementation, or "megadoses," of some nutrients may also suppress the immune system. More studies are needed before specific recommendations can be made.

PHYSICAL, ECONOMIC, PSYCHOSOCIAL, AND HEALTH FACTORS ASSOCIATED WITH AGING

- *Describe the kinds of nonphysiologic factors that influence health and nutrition status in older adults.*
- *How do economic factors influence dietary intake?*
- *What are activities of daily living (ADL) and instrumental activities of daily living (IADL) and what is their significance in determining quality of life and nutrition health?*
- *How is social isolation related to health and nutrition status in older adults?*
- *What are the effects of cigarette smoking and alcohol consumption on the health of older adults?*

Although age-related physiologic changes reduce the ability of the older person to respond to stress, many other factors influence the health, well-being, and quality of life of older adults. For example being poor, being a member of a minority, and living alone and in poor health are factors that reduce social integration and can lead to social alienation, isolation, and powerlessness. Box 13-3 summarizes physical, economic, psychosocial, health, and dietary factors that may occur with aging and that interact to influence the process of aging and nutrition status.

Physical

Physical mobility determines the level of independence and, therefore, the quality of life for all in-

Box 13-3 Physical, Economic, Psychosocial, and Health Factors Associated with Aging

PHYSICAL

Functional status
Activities of daily living
Instrumental activities of daily living
Disabling conditions
- Immobility
- Inactivity

Inability to obtain and prepare food

ECONOMIC

Limited income
Inadequate housing
Limited access to medical care
Access to economic assistance programs
Access to food
Medical expenses

SOCIAL STATUS

Social isolation
Support systems—family, friends
Living arrangements
Access to community services/transportation

PSYCHOLOGICAL

Depression
Dementia
Alzheimer's disease
Cognitive impairment
Emotional impairment

FOOD INTAKE

Frequency of food consumption
Quantity
Quality
Dietary modifications
Use of supplements
Use of alcohol/tobacco
Food quackery

HEALTH CONDITIONS

Underweight or overweight
Alcohol or tobacco abuse
Oral health

CHRONIC DISEASES

Cardiovascular
Cerebrovascular
Diabetes mellitus
Rheumatoid arthritis
Cancer

CHRONIC MEDICATION USE

Control
Polypharmacy

dividuals, but particularly for the older generation. Increasing infirmity, **osteoarthritis,** and failing eyesight are common with aging and all can reduce mobility. Simple things, such as inability to read labels or prices while shopping or the inability to stand or move about for cooking and cleaning up, can compromise quality of life and reduce food intake. Older persons may have to depend on family members, friends, or public transportation to shop, seek healthcare, and socialize.

An individual's ability to perform the customary ADL is often referred to as functional status. Functional status is measured by the degree of assistance required with basic self-management activities called ADLs or with home management activities referred to as IADLs. Box 13-4 outlines the components of these two groups of activities. In 1999 about 14% of older people living in the community had difficulty with one or more ADLs and 21% had difficulty with one or more IADLs (U.S. Census Bureau, 2001). The percentages needing help were greater in women than in men and increased sharply with age for both sexes, especially after 80 years, at which point

KEY TERMS

nephrons: functional units in the kidney for filtering blood
osteoarthritis: a noninflammatory degenerative joint disease accompanied by pain and stiffness

Box 13-4 Functional Activities Associated with Mobility and Independence in Older Adults

ACTIVITIES OF DAILY LIVING (ADL)

Bathing
Continence
Dressing
Eating
Toileting
Transferring from bed or chair
Walking
Getting outside

INSTRUMENTAL ACTIVITIES OF DAILY LIVING (IADL)

Food preparation
Use of the telephone
Housekeeping
Laundry
Use of transportation
Responsibility for medication
Money management
Shopping

27.5% of the elderly had difficulty with ADLs and 40.4% with IADLs.

Physically impaired older adults are likely to have poor dietary intakes because of the inability to perform one or more daily activities related to eating, food procurement, or food preparation. This inability serves as a warning sign of increased nutrition risk. Preventable factors that have been associated with functional decline include smoking, frequent alcohol use, lack of regular physical activity, and use of sedatives or tranquilizers.

A minimal level of aerobic fitness appears necessary for independent living. For older adults without functional impairments, regular physical activity may improve cerebral function and sleep patterns, provide opportunities for social contact, and increase energy intake and expenditure.

Economic Factors

As the number and percentage of older people in the United States continue to increase, financial and economic status is an increasingly important public health issue. The overall well-being of older individuals is inextricably linked to their economic well-being. It is a determinant of lifestyle, including standards of housing, levels of healthcare, availability of economic assistance programs, and dietary adequacy. In 1999 9.7% (3.2 million) of elderly persons were classified as poor (income below the poverty level) and 6.1% (20 million) were near poor (income between the poverty level and 125% of this level) (U.S. Bureau of the Census, 2000).

Approximately 8.3% of elderly whites, compared with 22.7% of elderly African Americans and 20.4% of elderly Hispanics, were poor or near poor. Women were more likely than men to be poor, as were older adults living alone or with nonrelatives (U.S. Bureau of the Census, 2000).

Low-income elderly persons often have limited access to food and fewer food choices, particularly when needs perceived as more pressing take precedence. Housing costs may consume as much as one-third of their incomes and, for many, medical care (even with Medicare) may consume a large portion of the budget, limiting the availability of dollars to purchase adequate food. It is estimated that 2.5 million community-dwelling older adults are likely to suffer from **food insecurity** in any 6-month period (Older Americans Report, 1994).

The nutritional consequences of food insecurity are largely undocumented. Lee and Frongillo (2001) analyzed data from the Third National Health and Nutrition Examination Survey (NHANES III) (1988 to 1994) and the Survey of the Elderly in New York State (1994) for nutrient intakes, nutrition status (fatfold thickness), and self-reported health status and nutrition risk. Food-insecure elderly persons had poor nutrition status (e.g., lower fatfolds) and significantly lower intakes of energy, protein, carbohydrate, saturated fat, niacin, riboflavin, vitamins B_6 and B_{12}, magnesium, iron, and zinc than food-secure older adults. Even food-secure older persons consumed less than the dietary recommendations for eight nutrients.

Psychosocial

As illustrated in the case study at the beginning of this chapter, there is great diversity among

Table 13-3 TEN MOST COMMON CHRONIC CONDITIONS IN NONINSTITUTIONALIZED OLDER PERSONS

Condition	Percent of Adults Over 65 Years Affected
Arthritis	48
Hypertension	36
Hearing impairment	32
Heart disease	32
Deformity or orthopedic impairment	19
Cataracts	17
Chronic sinusitis	16
Diabetes	11
Visual impairment	9
Tinnitus	9

From U.S. Department of Health and Human Services Vital and Health Statistics: Current estimates from the National Health Interview Survey: United States, 1992. Washington, DC, 1994, National Center for Health Statistics.

people who have exceeded age 65. Most are healthy and independent, leading active, productive lives. With time mental processes may slow, but the typical individual remains in touch with reality and is well oriented, consuming a variety of foods for a balanced diet. People with positive health habits, who maintain a healthy weight and exercise regularly, live longer and have fewer disabilities (Vita et al., 1998).

Important contributors to poor food intake of older adults include psychologic factors such as bereavement, confusion, depression, and **dementia.** A small percentage of people over age 65 suffer from some type of dementia, with the prevalence increasing to approximately 20% or more by age 80 (Wolf-Klein and Silverstone, 1994). Manifestations of dementia are memory loss, disorientation, indifference, impaired judgment, and coexistent anxiety and restlessness. These symptoms often lead to reduced food intake and alteration in physical activity. Dehydration, often unrecognized in older adults, may exacerbate the dementia.

Depression is more common with increasing age. Depression disorders have a significant impact on level of function, productivity, and perceived physical and mental health. Frequent components of depression are loss of enthusiasm and appetite and declining body weight and nutrition status. Distorted attitudes toward food and body image may occur in some older adults, particularly women, but the pattern of abnormalities may not be consistent with classic anorexia nervosa (Stevens et al., 1994).

The longer individuals live, the more likely they are to lose spouse, family, neighbors, and vital social and occupational roles in the community. The older individual lives in an increasingly isolated world. Because eating is generally a social activity, social isolation may result in reduced food intake and compromised nutrition status. Older adults who live alone and who, for whatever reason, are unable to go out regularly and have few friends or relatives to visit them may lose the incentive to prepare and consume regular nutritious meals.

Health Status

Degenerative diseases that first appear in middle life persist and become more severe in old age. Most older persons have at least one chronic condition and many have multiple conditions (Table 13-3). Treatment of chronic health problems increases the demand for economic and social services and healthcare resources.

In 1997 49% of all days of care in hospitals involved older people (U.S. Bureau of the Census, 2000). Compared with younger adults, older adults had longer stays (an average of 6.8 days compared with only 5.5 days for younger persons) and twice as many contacts with physicians. Approximately 25% of the prescription drugs dispensed each year go to older Americans

KEY TERMS

food insecurity: occurence of times when an individual does not have physical and economic access to sufficient food to meet the needs for a productive and healthy life

dementia: organic loss of intellectual function

depression: psychiatric syndrome consisting of dejected mood, psychomotor retardation, insomnia, and weight loss

and two thirds of older persons take more than one prescription drug (Council on Scientific Affairs, 1990). The most frequently prescribed drugs are antibiotics, diuretics, antihypertensive agents, nonsteroidal antiinflammatory agents, cardiotonics, antiarrhythmics, steroids, tranquilizers, antidepressants, lipid-lowering drugs, and anticoagulants.

Because of multiple chronic health problems, *polypharmacy,* or the administration of many drugs together, is a real concern in older adults. The elderly are likely to take multiple prescription medications, perhaps from more than one healthcare provider, and may also use several over-the-counter products. Polypharmacy is a concern because drugs are likely to have greater potency in an older person because of increased brain and organ sensitivity, lower body water and blood volume, changes in body composition, and declining kidney and liver function, which decrease metabolism and excretion. Problems with management of medications and over-the-counter drugs may be dismissed as a sign of aging and not recognized as a more serious issue of overuse of medication and interaction among medications. Often no one person providing healthcare knows the full scope of the elderly individual's drug usage, making side effects almost impossible to identify and correct.

Foods or specific nutrients can affect drug action by altering digestion, absorption, distribution, metabolism, or excretion. Drugs, self-administered or prescribed, may influence the nutrition status of an individual in several ways, including changing energy and nutrient needs, reducing food ingestion, or altering nutrient absorption, metabolism, and excretion. The risk of adverse side effects increases with the number of drugs taken and the duration of exposure to drugs.

Alcohol

Although age does not affect the rate of absorption or elimination of alcohol, the decline in lean body mass and corresponding decrease in total body water volume means that alcohol is distributed over less area. Therefore an identical amount of alcohol will result in a higher blood alcohol concentration in an older adult than in a younger individual of the same size and sex (Dufor and Fuller, 1995).

Alcohol use by older adults is common, yet the risk or benefits of drinking are not well understood. It is estimated that 2% to 10% of adults age 60 years and older may abuse alcohol or have a drinking problem (AMA Council on Scientific Affairs, 1996). Moderate alcohol consumption (1 to 2 drinks per day) may increase feelings of freedom from care while lessening inhibitions, stress, and depression, and it may actually enhance appetite for some individuals. However, with reduced energy intake, calories from alcoholic beverages have the potential to displace more nutrient-dense sources of energy. The relationship of moderate alcohol consumption with reduced total and cardiovascular mortality that has been well documented in middle-aged populations appears to occur in older populations as well. A study of more than 6000 men and women age 65 years and older found that low to moderate alcohol consumption was associated with statistically significant lowering of total and cardiovascular mortality (Scherr et al., 1992). A more recent study of population-based sample of 2235 noninstitutionalized elderly persons found that increasing levels of moderate alcohol consumption were associated with a decreasing risk of heart failure (Abramson et al., 2001).

An important concern about alcohol use by older adults is the potential for interactions with both prescription and over-the-counter medications. In a random sample of community-dwelling older adults, the majority (57%) reported using alcohol. In addition 25% of drinkers took one or more other drugs, most commonly over-the-counter pain medications, for many of which alcohol could exaggerate or negate the effect. This fact placed them at potential risk for drug-related interactions (Forster et al., 1993). In addition consumption of alcoholic beverages may exacerbate cognitive impairment and dementias of other etiology. Heavy drinking is a well-established risk factor in causing disability and excessive mortality at all ages. It appears that for older adults, even modest alcohol consumption can contribute to disability and poorer health (Oslin, 2000).

Cigarette Smoking

Cigarette smoking is the number one avoidable cause of mortality in the United States. In addition to the well-known health risks associated with smoking, older smokers were found to be weaker and had poorer balance and poorer performance on measures of integrated physical function than nonsmokers (Nelson et al., 1994). For smokers the decrease in function (muscle strength, agility, coordination, gait) was 50% to 100% as great as that associated with a 5-year increase in age and most measures grew worse with increasing number of years the individual smoked.

ENERGY AND NUTRIENT NEEDS

- *How do energy and nutrient needs change with aging?*
- *How have energy and nutrient needs been established for older adults?*

Over several decades the changes of aging can influence energy and nutrient needs, patterns of food intake, and physical activity. In the past Recommended Dietary Allowances (RDAs) most of the nutrient recommendations for older persons were derived by extrapolation of data from younger adults (Food and Nutrition Board, 1989). In the decade since the tenth edition of the RDA, numerous studies addressed the nutrition requirement of older adults.

As discussed in Chapter 1, the dietary standards being formulated for individuals in the United States and Canada, the Daily Reference Intakes (DRIs) are being released in multiple reports. To date, the four reports covering vitamins and micro elements are available (Institute of Medicine, 1997, 1998, 2000, 2001).

In the process of formulating the DRIs, specific issues related to nutrient needs of older adults have been addressed in several ways. One important change was the age categories for the recommendations. The 1989 RDAs provided one set of recommendations for adults age 51 years and older. However, the heterogeneous nature of the older population makes it impossible to generalize from one established recommendation. The physiologic and health status of persons who are 60 years old is very different from that of persons who are 80 years old or 90 years old. For these reasons the DRIs (RDAs and Adequate Intake Levels) are reported for men and women age 50 years to 70 years and over age 70 years (see inside front cover of this text for DRIs for vitamins and minerals). Reference heights and weights for the DRIs were derived from NHANES III. Reference heights and weights for men are 176 cm (69 in) and 76 kg (166 lbs) and for women they are 163 cm (64 in) and 61 kg (133 lbs), respectively. Because there is no evidence that weight should change as adults age if activity is maintained, the reference weights for adults age 19 years through 30 years are applied to all adult age groups (Institute of Medicine, 1997). Therefore the levels for energy and protein discussed here are based on the 1989 RDA. The report for energy and micronutrients is scheduled to be released late in 2002. Be sure to check with your instructor about the report on energy and macronutrients and fiber.

Energy Needs

Energy is required for metabolic processes at the cellular level, for maintaining homeostasis of turnover processes (mainly protein turnover), and for muscular work. Energy needs decline with age in association with decreased body size, a loss of lean body mass, and a diminution of physical activity. The 1989 RDAs for energy intakes are 2300 kcal for the reference 77 kg older male and 1900 for the 65 kg older female (Food and Nutrition Board, 1989). These levels are approximately 30 kcal/kg per day, representing a reduction from the 33 kcal/kg to 34 kcal/kg per day that are the bases for younger adults.

Although body fat increases through middle age, after age 65, fat typically decreases even in healthy individuals (Roberts, 2000). The causes of weight loss in later life are poorly understood and data from NHANES III have suggested that low dietary energy intake is widespread even among healthy elderly individuals (Davis et al., 2000). Energy needs decline, but requirements for many nutrients may increase. That means older adults require a careful selection of nutrient-dense foods to meet their nutritional needs in fewer kilocalories. Physical activity is important compensation for decreased energy intake because it increases energy expenditure and food intake, delays lean body mass decline, and improves independence.

Protein

The RDA for protein, 0.8 g/kg body weight per day, has been assumed to be adequate for older adults when energy intakes exceed 30 kcal/kg per day. However, at usual energy intakes for older individuals, that level may be insufficient to attain nitrogen balance. Studies have documented a requirement of approximately 1 g or more of protein per kg of body weight (Campbell, 1996) per day to establish nitrogen **equilibrium.** Lower intakes have been shown to compromise lean tissue, immune response, and muscle function (Castaneda et al., 1995) and increase bone loss (Hannan et al., 2000). A protein intake 1.0 g/kg to 1.25 g/kg of high-quality protein per day is generally accepted to be an adequate and safe level.

Micronutrients

The DRIs for vitamins and minerals have been published in four reports and levels for older

Table 13-4 DIETARY REFERENCE INTAKES FOR VITAMINS AND MINERALS FOR OLDER ADULTS

Nutrient	Females 51-70 years	Females >70 years	Males 51-70 years	Males >70 years
Calcium, mg	*1200*	*1200*	*1200*	*1200*
Phosphorus, mg	**700**	**700**	**700**	**700**
Magnesium, mg	**45**	**45**	**45**	**45**
Fluoride, mg	*3*	*3*	*4*	*4*
Vitamin D, µg	*10*	*15*	*10*	*15*
Thiamin, mg	**1.1**	**1.1**	**1.2**	**1.2**
Riboflavin, mg	**1.1**	**1.1**	**1.3**	**1.3**
Niacin, mg	**14**	**14**	**16**	**16**
Vitamin B_6, mg	**1.5**	**1.5**	**1.7**	**1.7**
Folate, µg	**400**	**400**	**400**	**400**
Vitamin B_{12}, µg	**2.4**	**2.4**	**2.4**	**2.4**
Pantothenic Acid, mg	*5*	*5*	*5*	*5*
Biotin, µg	*30*	*30*	*30*	*30*
Choline, µg	*450*	*450*	*550*	*550*
Vitamin C, mg	**75**	**75**	**90**	**90**
Selenium, µg	**55**	**55**	**55**	**55**
Vitamin E, mg	**15**	**15**	**15**	**15**
Vitamin A, µg	**700**	**700**	**900**	**900**
Vitamin K, µg	*90*	*90*	*120*	*120*
Chromium, µg	*20*	*20*	*30*	*30*
Copper, mg	**900**	**900**	**900**	**900**
Iodine, µg	**150**	**150**	**150**	**150**
Iron, mg	**8**	**8**	**8**	**8**
Manganese, mg	*1.8*	*1.8*	*2.3*	*2.3*
Molybdenum, µg	**45**	**45**	**45**	**45**
Zinc, mg	**8**	**8**	**11**	**11**

Adapted with permission from the following Institute of Medicine publications: Dietary reference intakes for calcium, phosphorus, magnesium, vitamin D, and fluoride (1997); Dietary reference intakes for thiamin, riboflavin, niacin, vitamin B_6, folate, vitamin B_{12}, pantothenic acid, biotin, and choline (1998); Dietary reference intakes for vitamin C, vitamin E, selenium, and carotenoids (2000); and Dietary reference intakes for vitamin A, vitamin K, arsenic, boron, chromium, copper, iodine, iron, manganese, molybdenum, nickel, silicon, vanadium, and zinc (2001), Washington, DC, National Academy Press.
RDAs are printed in bold type; AIs are printed in italics.

adults are summarized in Table 13-4. The discussion of vitamins and minerals in this chapter is organized according to the grouping of the reports.

Calcium, Phosphorus, Fluoride, and Vitamin D

Bone formation involves approximately 99% of the calcium in the body. The process requires protein for the collagen matrix, phosphorus, and magnesium to be incorporated in the hydroxyapatite structure. Fluoride, when incorporated in bone, strengthens the crystalline structure. Bone mass continues to increase up to the third decade of life and then plateaus. Inadequate calcium during the growth period may result in failure to reach peak bone mass, contributing to decreased skeletal integrity and fracture in older adulthood. In later decades, adequate calcium intake is needed to maintain or minimize bone loss. Serum calcium levels are maintained via the parathyroid hormone. A decrease in blood calcium triggers a release of the parathyroid hormone, which increases serum calcium levels by increasing resorption of calcium from bone. In the absence of adequate intakes of calcium, bone resorption will exceed bone formation, resulting in decreased bone mass.

Surveys of food habits of older Americans reveal that most women and many men do not ingest sufficient quantities of calcium to meet needs. Accumulating scientific evidence indicates that calcium needs of the aging populations are greater than those for younger adults (Russell, 2000). Vitamin D_3 is hydroxylated to 25-cholecalciferol in the liver and to its active form, 1,25-hydroxyl cholecalciferol, in the kidney. Age brings a decline in the hydroxylation in the kidney and vitamin D receptors in the gastrointestinal tract (Harris et al., 1999), which may contribute to a deficiency. In addition intestinal calcium absorption is often reduced because of the effects of estrogen deficiency in women. Recommendations for calcium are 1200 mg for adults over the age of 50 years. Blood levels of 25-hydroxyvitamin D are reduced with age. In addition to decreased exposure to sunlight and use of sunscreens, older persons have a decreased capability to synthesize vitamin D_3 in the skin.

In some populations of older adults with limited exposure to sunlight, vitamin D intakes of 10 μg to 20 μg were necessary to maintain adequate vitamin D status (O'Dowd et al., 1993). This finding has resulted in recommendations of 10 μg (400 IU) per day for adults from 50 to 70 years and 15 μg (600 IU) for those older than 70 years. For the homebound elderly, those in nursing homes, and others who may have limited exposure to sunlight, this level would need to be supplied in fortified foods or supplements.

Food sources include vitamin D-enriched milk, fish oils, and liver. In the United States and Canada, the principal food source for vitamin D is fortified milk. However, the amount of vitamin D in milk is variable and some skim milks contain no vitamin D at all (Hollick, 1994).

B Complex Vitamins

For most water-soluble vitamins there has been increased evidence for age-related changes in needs, especially for vitamin B_6, vitamin B_{12}, and folate (see Table 13-4). Older adults tend to be at greater risk of vitamin B_6 deficiency. Serum B_6 levels decrease with age, suggesting that metabolic utilization is less efficient and that the requirement for vitamin B_6 may be higher for older individuals (Pannemans et al., 1994). Impaired cell-mediated immune responses have been associated with vitamin B_6 deficiency.

Low serum or plasma vitamin B_{12} levels are twice as common in older adults as in young adults (Lindenbaum et al., 1994). A low intake, especially among the poor elderly, and impaired absorption from atrophic gastritis may be important factors. In addition bacterial overgrowth in the small bowel may lead to competition for vitamin B_{12}. Anemia occurs in the most severely vitamin B_{12}-depleted individuals and neuropsychiatric manifestations and metabolic abnormalities often occur before low serum concentrations are observed (Allen and Casterline, 1994). The decrease in hydrochloric acid secretion may reduce absorption of dietary folate.

Given that 10% to 30% of individuals ages 51 years and older may have reduced absorption of

KEY TERMS

equilibrium: intake equal to output

vitamin B_{12}, the Institute of Medicine recommends that people in this age group should consume 2.4 μg in its synthetic form in fortified foods or supplements (Institute of Medicine, 1998). Recently Russell and colleagues (2001) reported that vitamin B_{12} in fortified bread and milk is well absorbed and would be a means by which to ensure vitamin B_{12} adequacy in older adults.

Vitamin B_6, vitamin B_{12}, and folate have been associated with epidemiologic observations that an elevated blood level of homocysteine is an independent risk factor for cardiovascular disease (Panchararuniti et al., 1994) and cerebrovascular disease (Selhub et al., 1995). Recently there have been suggestions that elevated homocysteine levels may be associated with loss of neurocognitive function with advancing age (Nicolas et al., 2001). It has been suggested that increased dietary intakes of these vitamins will normalize homocysteine levels and may reduce risk of atherosclerotic disease.

Antioxidant Nutrients

Vitamin E, vitamin C, and beta carotene. There is considerable interest in the antioxidant role that vitamin E (tocopherol) may play in aging or prevention of chronic disease. No deficiency of vitamin E has been reported in healthy older adults. However, vitamin E supplements have been shown to improve immune responses (Meydani et al., 1995) and decrease the risk of cardiovascular disease in older adults (Hodis, 1995).

Dietary antioxidants are one means of fighting against reactive oxygen species and protecting many body tissues and compounds. With aging, the balance between free radicals and antioxidants may be altered because of overproduction and a less efficient protection system.

Substantial evidence suggests that oxidative stress is important in the pathogenesis of Alzheimer's disease and cognitive decline and suggest that antioxidants may reduce the effect (Christen, 2000; Perkins et al., 1999). Clinical trials are currently underway.

Vitamin A, Iron, Zinc, and Other Minerals

Vitamin A. Vitamin A is rapidly absorbed and slowly cleared. The RDAs for vitamin A for women 51 years of age and older is 700 μg retinol equivalents and for men in this age category, 900 μg retinol equivalents. Current evidence supports a decreased requirement for preformed vitamin A in this age in this age group (Russell, 2000). This reduction is associated with age-related increases in absorption and delays in the clearance of dietary vitamin A by the liver and other peripheral tissues. Accumulation of vitamin A increases the risk of bone resorption and decreased bone formation contributing to osteoporosis (Brinkley and Krueger, 2000). On the other hand, beta carotene and other provitamin carotenoids, because of their antioxidant properties, may have health benefits related to cardiovascular disease, cataracts, and cancer (Gerster, 1993). Therefore it is important that a large fraction of the vitamin A intake come from the carotene-containing fruits and vegetables.

Iron. Iron absorption per se does not appear to decline significantly with age and iron stores appear to increase. However, iron deficiency still occurs in the elderly from inadequate iron intake or reduced nonheme iron absorption secondary to the hypochlorhydria of atrophic gastritis. In the NHANES I and II (National Center for Health Statistics, 1979; National Center for Health Statistics, 1983) studies, the prevalence of iron deficiency anemia in older adults was low and was most often attributable to chronic conditions such as infection, rheumatoid arthritis, cancer, and renal failure rather than to iron deficiency, indicating that the RDA of 8 mg for older adults is adequate. Iron supports the work of numerous proteins in the body, including metalloenzymes.

Zinc. Older adults may be at risk for low zinc intakes, which may contribute to reduced immune function.

Water

For adults daily water intake should approximate 30 mL/kg body weight (or about 1.9 liters for the reference woman and 2.3 liters for the man) to compensate for usual losses through skin, lungs, kidneys, and bowel. Additional amounts may be necessary to compensate for unusual losses from excessive perspiration, fever, diarrhea, vomiting, or hemorrhage.

Fluid balance deserves particular attention in older adults because dehydration often goes unrecognized in this group. In part, dehydration may be the result of decreased thirst sensitivity and older adults need to be encouraged to consume about 1.5 liters to 2.0 liters of fluid each day. Inadequate water intake can lead to dehydration, hypertension, elevated body temperature, constipation, nausea and vomiting, dryness of the mucosa, decreased urinary excretion, and mental confusion. In fact adequate fluid is so important, Tufts University researchers have modified the Food Guide Pyramid for people 70 years and older to include at least 8 servings of water, juice, or other source of fluid (Tufts University Health and Nutrition Letter, 1999).

In summary, to meet their energy and nutrient needs, the healthy members of the aging population need to consume a balanced, nutrient-dense diet containing a variety of foods of moderate to low fat content. In addition an adequate intake of fluids and regular moderate physical activity (strength training and aerobic exercise) are recommended to maintain a healthy, vigorous life for as long as possible.

DIETARY INTAKES AND PHYSICAL ACTIVITY PATTERNS OF OLDER ADULTS

Dietary Intakes

Major national surveys reporting the dietary intakes of older persons include NHANES I and II surveys (National Center for Health Statistics, 1979; National Center for Health Statistics, 1983). The NHANES I and II data were limited to individuals younger than 75 years of age. Therefore they offer no information regarding intakes of adults 75 years and older. Reports from NHANES III that was designed to have no upper age limit and will provide data on the very old are beginning to provide information about older adults.

Several studies have documented a progressive decline in energy intakes with advancing age. Men and women age 65 years to 74 years who were followed in NHANES II consumed an average of approximately 1800 kcal and 1400 kcal per day, respectively, as did individuals over age 65 in the U.S. Dietary Association Continuing Survey of

Table 13-5 Mean Daily Total Food-Energy Intake (TFEI), Percentages from Dietary Fat, and Saturated Fat

Age Group (Years)	Sample Size	TFEI	TFEI from Dietary Fat (%)	TFEI from Saturated Fat (%)
MALES				
60-69	546	2110	33.3	11.3
70-79	444	1887	33.8	11.6
≥80	296	1776	33.3	11.4
FEMALES				
60-69	560	1578	32.8	11.0
70-79	407	1435	32.3	10.8
≥80	313	1329	31.3	10.8

From Third National Health and Nutrition Examination Survey, Phase I, 1988-91, MMWR Morb Mortal Weekly Rep 43:117, 1994.

Food Intake of Individuals (CSFII) (Gerrior, 1999). As shown in Table 13-5, data from the national survey confirm and extend the reported downward trend in energy intakes for individuals in their 70s and 80s. The range of 31.3% to 33.8% of energy from dietary fat represents a decrease from previous surveys, but is still above levels recommended in the Dietary Guidelines.

Studies that have measured dietary intakes of healthy community-dwelling older adults show that mean intakes for most nutrients approached the level of the 1989 RDA. Older persons may consume less than the RDA for calcium, magnesium, zinc, folate, vitamin E, and vitamin B_6. More recent data from CSFII found that nutrient intakes of vitamin C, vitamin B_6, folate, magnesium, and zinc were below recommendations (Gerrior, 1999). Loss of autonomy in such individuals is associated with increased risk of nutritional problems (Payette et al., 1995) and older adults who are homebound are at high risk of inadequate intake of protein and energy (Gray-Donald, 1995).

Use of Supplements

Americans are users of supplements. Nowhere is this more apparent than in older adults. Studies indicate that 35% to 70% of older Americans use nutritional supplements regularly (Payette et al., 1995). In addition many older adults are taking more than one supplement each day; some take as many as 20 or 30 tablets, pills, capsules, or drinks each day. Women tend to take supplements more than do men. As with other age groups, the older adults who take supplements are often the ones who have the best diets and the least need for supplements to meet nutritional needs. Many older people are motivated to use dietary supplements promoted for their purported ability to slow aging, improve health, increase energy levels, or prevent chronic diseases.

Although a single multivitamin supplement may be appropriate for older individuals, the cost-benefit ratio of using multiple supplements must be questioned. Excess intake of vitamins and minerals can occur in elderly adults who regularly use single or small groups of vitamins or minerals as supplements.

Exercise

The peak of physical fitness and performance for most people occurs between the late teens and early thirties. At some point after the age of 30 years, there is usually a gradual decline in the components of fitness, including cardiorespiratory values, flexibility, strength, lean body mass, and bone density (see Chapter 15). Whether regular exercise delays this normal decline and whether exercise training can reverse these declines are current topics of investigation, especially in older adults (Evans, 1996; Fiatarone et al., 1994; Lemon, 2000).

Research in older men and women has demonstrated numerous benefits from exercise and specifically from strength training. For instance, strength training results in increased muscle mass, strength, muscle endurance, and bone mineral density in elderly subjects. Additionally improvements in glucose tolerance, insulin resistance, total body fat, and abdominal fat occur when older individuals participate in strength training (Hurley and Roth, 2000). The natural decreases in strength of about 12% to 14% per decade after the age of 50 have been reversed in groups of strength-training elderly subjects after just 2 months of heavy resistance training (Lemmer, Hurlbut, and Martel, 2000). The biggest benefit of strength training cited by older individuals is the fact that they find it easier to complete everyday tasks. Aerobic exercise training in elderly subjects, however, is beneficial, but does not affect the ADLs as much as strength training (Pendergast, Fisher, and Calkins, 1993).

Although some studies of strength-trained elderly men or women have not reported the same level of improvement (most likely from differences in amount and frequency of weight lifted), most of the work continues to suggest that age-related declines in function can be reversed with strength training (Evans, 1996; Fiatarone et al., 1994; Hurley and Roth, 2000). This is a great benefit for frail nursing home residents, whose walking speed and endurance improved after strength training, resulting in greater independence (Fiatarone et al., 1994; Fontera et al., 1991). Unfortunately ceasing the fitness program in these same individuals resulted in a loss of strength (Fiatarone et al., 1994) and other physiologic functions (Hurley and Roth, 2000). For this reason many experts suggest that weekly exercise (or some form of physical activity) be regularly incorporated into the life-styles of individuals of all ages.

Research has shown that many risk factors for chronic diseases may be ameliorated with exercise. For instance, in elderly individuals who exercise, serum total cholesterol (TC), low-density lipoprotein cholesterol (LDL-C), and triglycerides decreased while high-density lipoprotein cholesterol (HDL-C) increased (Tran and Weltman, 1985). Exercise has also been shown to increase insulin sensitivity and improve glucose tolerance, which may prevent or delay the onset of type II diabetes (Rosenthal et al., 1983). Additionally regular exercise contributes to weight maintenance and, as noted earlier, delays muscle loss in the aging individual.

Whether overall dietary intake or that of a specific nutrient has an impact on the outcomes of strength or aerobic training in older adults is less well studied and defined. However, early studies are beginning to confirm the importance of meeting energy and protein requirements for physically active older men and women. Most nutritional recommendations for individuals over 50 years of age had been extrapolated from the data for younger adults. This changed for vitamins and minerals and can be expected to change to be based on research with older adults when the DRI for energy and macronutrients are published (Russell, 2000). Energy requirements are thought to decline with reductions in lean body mass and BMR. However, there is evidence that regular aerobic exercise, resistance exercise, or both can sustain lean mass and energy requirements (Bunyard et al., 1998).

A concern for physically active elderly persons is meeting fluid requirements from the decline in body water and thirst sensation. It is recommended that active individuals acclimate themselves to the heat by decreasing the amount of work they do when the weather gets hot. Rosenbloom (2000) recommends that active older persons drink more fluid and drink it more frequently to stay hydrated, use common sense about staying cool in hot weather, recognize symptoms of dehydration and heat illnesses, and make sure they understand any dehydration-related side effects of medications that they use.

ASSESSMENT OF NUTRITION STATUS

- *How well nourished are older adults?*
- *Why is nutrition an essential component of geriatric assessment?*
- *How and by whom can nutrition screening be initiated?*
- *How does nutrition assessment of older adults differ from that for younger individuals?*

Undernutrition

Undernutrition in older adults is conventionally defined as an unintentional weight loss of 1% to 2% per week, 5% per month, or 10% over a period of 6 months. Clinical features of early protein-energy undernutrition include confusion and low levels of serum albumin, total lymphocytes, and hemoglobin.

Undernutrition has been reported in 17% to 65% of older persons in hospitals and in 26% to 59% of those in long-term care institutions (Morley and Solomon, 1994). The incidence of undernutrition in free-living adults is lower, but less well defined. A 1992 study in New England that screened a random sample of Medicare beneficiaries age 70 years and older identified 24% as being at high nutritional risk and found that 38% had intakes of less than 75% of the RDA for three or more nutrients (Posner et al., 1994).

Nutrition Screening

Because of skyrocketing healthcare costs and because the average personal healthcare expenditure for those over 65 years of age is four times that for younger individuals, geriatric assessment has become an integral component of healthcare services for older adults. In general, geriatric assessment has concentrated on issues relating to polypharmacy, functional status, cognitive problems, depression, and incontinence (Reuben et al., 1995). There is substantial evidence that geriatric assessment and rehabilitation improve functional status in some older persons and reduces mortality rates (Stuck et al., 1993).

Because of the integral relationship between nutrition and health status in aging, nutrition has become an essential part of geriatric assessment. Undernutrition develops in a fairly predictable fashion and evidence of marginal or poor dietary intake and nutrition status can be detected long before clinical signs and symptoms occur. Screening for risk factors allows implementation of preventive measures before the overt manifestations of nutritional problems appear.

Nutrition screening and early intervention are primary steps in the development of a system of healthcare that is affordable or accessible to all older adults (White, 1994). The Nutrition Screening Initiative (NSI) is an intensified effort to promote screening, identification, and aggressive nutrition support. A collaborative effort of numerous health professional organizations, the NSI began in 1990 with identification of potential risk factors, major indicators of poor nutrition status, and development and validation of tools for screening.

The NSI is a community-based collaborative project to improve nutrition status of older adults through three levels of screening. An initial tool for identifying nutritional risk is the "DETERMINE" checklist ("Determine Your Nutritional Health"; see Figure 2-2, page 45). It is designed as a public awareness tool for self-assessment by older adults or for assessment by friends, loved ones, and caregivers. The Level I screen, to be completed by a social service or healthcare professional, is designed to identify warning signs of nutritional risk (Figure 13-4). Individuals identified as at risk using the Level I screen would be further assessed using the Level II screen (Figure 13-5), which includes more specific diagnostic information. Level II screening is a nutrition assessment to be completed in a healthcare setting such as a physician's office, a hospital, or a nursing home.

The inclusion of nutrition screening in an overall geriatric assessment identifies individuals at risk so that intervention can be initiated early. Such intervention can alleviate remediable problems or control or ameliorate those problems that cannot be prevented. Priorities for nutrition intervention concentrate on social services, oral health, mental health, medication use, nutrition education and counseling, and nutrition support (NSI, 1991).

Assessment of Nutrition Status

In aging uncomplicated by disease, older individuals have nutrition reserves and nutrition status similar to those of younger adults. However, with aging, an increasing proportion of older persons deplete their reserve capacity and have increased nutrition risk. Assessment of older adults is based on anthropometric, laboratory, clinical, and dietary indicators, as discussed in Chapter 2. Box 13-5 outlines major indicators of poor nutrition status identified in the NSI. Most often undernutrition is secondary to physical, economic, and psychosocial factors, which are compounded by the numerous physiologic changes that occur at different rates as individuals age. This is further complicated by the stresses of disease, multiple medications, and trauma.

Anthropometry

Generally height declines by approximately 0.5 cm to 1.5 cm per decade with aging because of vertebral collapse or compaction. It may be difficult to measure an upright individual accurately because of **kyphosis**, bowing of the legs, or other loss of the ability to stand erect. Stature cannot be measured accurately in nonambulatory older individuals, but height can be estimated from recumbent length, knee height, or arm length (see Appendix F1) (Chumlea et al., 1994). A recorded height that is 2 inches to 3 inches less than that recalled by the individual may precede the development of osteoporosis by several years.

The limitations of the Metropolitan Height and Weight tables were discussed in Chapter 2. These tables may be less appropriate for older adults because they are based on weight data for individuals between 20 years and 59 years of age. Descriptive anthropometric reference data for Americans 50 years and older based on NHANES III have been published (Kuczmarski et al., 2000). The NHANES III population included 1861 persons age 50 years to 59 years and 5700 persons age 60 years and older. Tables in Appendix F give fifteenth, fiftieth, and eighty-fifth percentiles by age, sex, and ethnicity for weight, height, weight-for-height, Body Mass Index (BMI), mid-upper-arm circumference, triceps fatfold thickness, and arm muscle circumference.

An important predictor of risk is involuntary weight loss (Wallace et al., 1995). Extremes of high and low BMI confirm increased risk of mortality, but there is a broad range for BMI over which mortality does not vary.

Midarm circumference and fatfold measurements are less reliable in persons over 65 years of age than in younger adults because of difficulty in accurately locating anatomic landmarks, increased compressibility of subcutaneous adipose tissue, age-related loss of skin elasticity, and changes in hydration status. As people age, the thickness of adipose tissues decreases on the arms and legs and increases on the trunk.

KEY TERMS

kyphosis: abnormally increased convexity in the curvature of the spine; hunchback

Level I Screen

Body Weight

Measure height to the nearest inch and weight to the nearest pound. Record the values below and mark them on the Body Mass Index (BMI) scale to the right. Then use a straight edge (ruler) to connect the two points and circle the spot where this straight line crosses the center line (body mass index). Record the number below.

Healthy older adults should have a BMI between 24 and 27.

Height (in): ____________________

Weight (lbs): ____________________

Body Mass Index: ____________________

(number from center column)

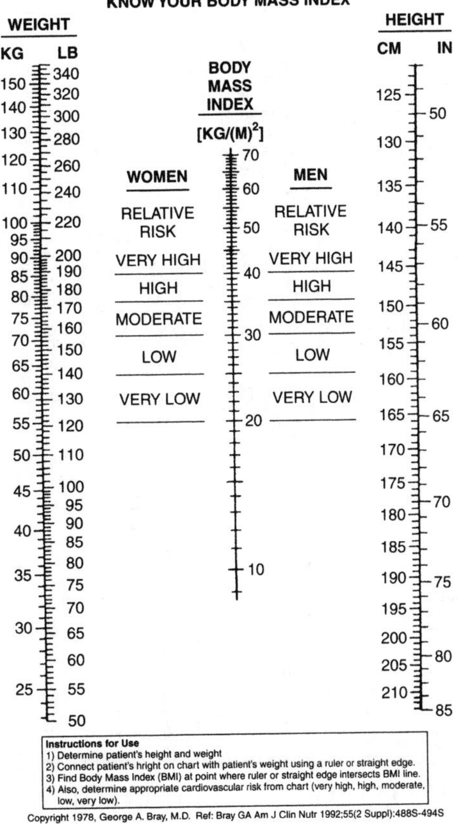

Check any boxes that are true for the individual:

- ❑ Has lost or gained 10 pounds (or more) in the past 6 months.
- ❑ Body mass index <24
- ❑ Body mass index >27

For the remaining sections, please ask the individual which of the statements (if any) is true for him or her and place a check by each that applies.

Eating Habits

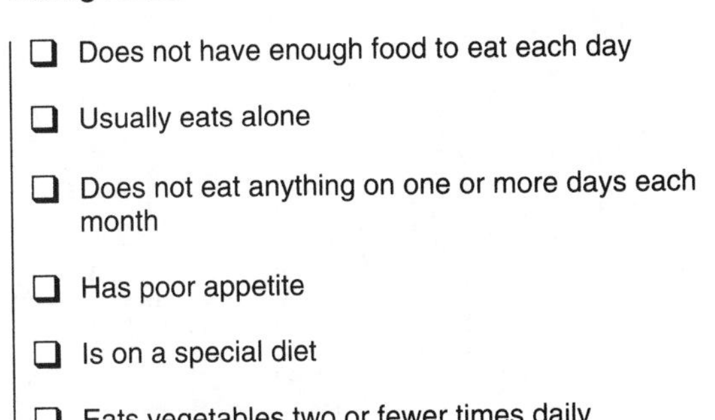

- ❑ Does not have enough food to eat each day
- ❑ Usually eats alone
- ❑ Does not eat anything on one or more days each month
- ❑ Has poor appetite
- ❑ Is on a special diet
- ❑ Eats vegetables two or fewer times daily

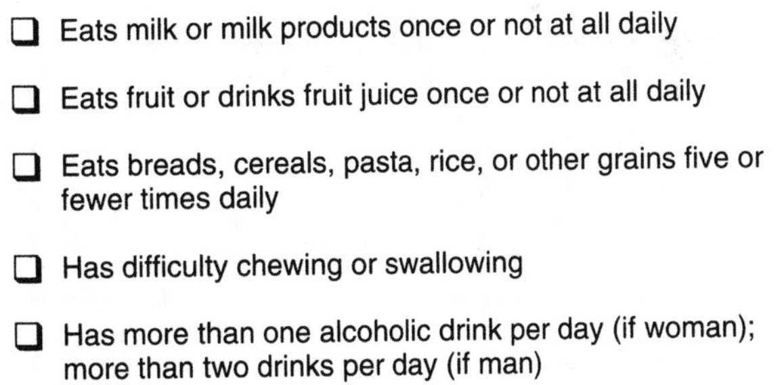

- ❑ Eats milk or milk products once or not at all daily
- ❑ Eats fruit or drinks fruit juice once or not at all daily
- ❑ Eats breads, cereals, pasta, rice, or other grains five or fewer times daily
- ❑ Has difficulty chewing or swallowing
- ❑ Has more than one alcoholic drink per day (if woman); more than two drinks per day (if man)
- ❑ Has pain in mouth, teeth, or gums

Level I Screen Name: Date:

Figure 13-4 Level I screen developed by the Nutrition Screening Initiative. When completed by social service or health care professionals, this form identifies older people who need further assessment for nutritional status or interventions to improve nutritional health. *(Reprinted with permission by the Nutrition Screening Initiative, a project of the American Academy of Family Physicians, the American Dietetic Association and the National Council on the Aging, Inc., and funded in part by a grant from Ross Products Division, Abbott Laboratories.)*

Level II Screen | Name: | Date:

Level II Screen

Complete the following screen by interviewing the patient directly and/or by referring to the patient chart. If you do not routinely perform all of the described tests or ask all of the listed questions, please consider including them but do not be concerned if the entire screen is not completed. Please try to conduct a minimal screen on as many older patients as possible and please try to collect serial measurements, which are extremely valuable in monitoring nutritional status. Please refer to the manual for additional information.

Anthropometrics

Measure height to the nearest inch and weight to the nearest pound. Record the values below and mark them on the Body Mass Index (BMI) scale to the right. Then use a straight edge (paper, ruler) to connect the two points and circle the spot where this straight line crosses the center line BMI. Record the number below; healthy older adults should have a BMI between 24 and 27; check the appropriate box to flag an abnormally high or low value.

Height (in): ____________
Weight (lbs): ____________
Body Mass Index (weight/height²): ____________

Please place a check by any statement regarding BMI and recent weight loss that is true for the patient.

- ❑ Body mass index <24
- ❑ Body mass index >27
- ❑ Has lost or gained 10 pounds (or more) of body weight in the past 6 months

Record the measurement of midarm circumference to the nearest 0.1 centimeter and of triceps skinfold to the nearest 2 millimeters.

Midarm Circumference (cm): ____________
Triceps Skinfold (mm): ____________
Midarm Muscle Circumference (cm): ____________

KNOW YOUR BODY MASS INDEX

WEIGHT (KG / LB): 150/340, 140/320, 130/300, 120/280, 110/260, 100/240, 95/220, 90/200, 85/190, 80/180, 75/170, 70/160, 65/150, 60/140, 55/130, 50/120, 45/110, 40/100, 35/95, 30/90, 25/85 … 80, 75, 70, 65, 60, 55, 50

BODY MASS INDEX [KG/(M)²]: 70, 60, 50, 40, 30, 20, 10

WOMEN — RELATIVE RISK: VERY HIGH, HIGH, MODERATE, LOW, VERY LOW

MEN — RELATIVE RISK: VERY HIGH, HIGH, MODERATE, LOW, VERY LOW

HEIGHT (CM / IN): 125, 130, 135, 140, 145, 150, 155, 160, 165, 170, 175, 180, 185, 190, 195, 200, 205, 210 / 50, 55, 60, 65, 70, 75, 80, 85

Instructions for Use
1) Determine patient's height and weight
2) Connect patient's hright on chart with patient's weight using a ruler or straight edge.
3) Find Body Mass Index (BMI) at point where ruler or straight edge intersects BMI line.
4) Also, determine appropriate cardiovascular risk from chart (very high, high, moderate, low, very low).

 Ref: Bray GA Am J Clin Nutr 1992;55(2 Suppl):488S-494S

Refer to the table and check any abnormal values:

- ❑ Midarm muscle circumference <10th percentile
- ❑ Triceps skinfold <10th percentile
- ❑ Triceps skinfold >95th percentile

Note: midarm circumference (cm)-{0.314 × triceps skinfold (mm)} = midarm *muscle* circumference (cm)

For the remaining sections, please place a check by any statements that are true for the patient.

Laboratory Data

- ❑ Serum albumin below 3.5 g/dl
- ❑ Serum cholesterol below 160 mg/dl
- ❑ Serum cholesterol above 240 mg/dl

Drug Use

- ❑ Three or more prescription drugs, OTC medications, and/or vitamin/mineral supplements daily

Clinical Features

Presence of (check each that apply):

- ❑ Problems with mouth, teeth, or gums
- ❑ Difficulty chewing
- ❑ Difficulty swallowing
- ❑ Angular stomatitis
- ❑ Glossitis
- ❑ History of bone pain
- ❑ History of bone fractures
- ❑ Skin changes (dry, loose, nonspecific lesions, edema)

Eating Habits

- ❑ Does not have enough food to eat each day
- ❑ Usually eats alone
- ❑ Does not eat anything on one or more days each month
- ❑ Has poor appetite
- ❑ Is on a special diet
- ❑ Eats vegetables two or fewer times daily
- ❑ Eats milk or milk products once or not at all daily
- ❑ Eats fruit or drinks fruit juice once or not at all daily
- ❑ Eats breads, cereals, pasta, rice, or other grains five or fewer times daily
- ❑ Has more than one alcoholic drink per day (if woman); more than two drinks per day (if man)

Living Environment

- ❑ Lives on an income of less than $6000 per year (per individual in the household)
- ❑ Lives alone
- ❑ Is housebound
- ❑ Is concerned about home security
- ❑ Lives in a home with inadequate heating or cooling
- ❑ Does not have a stove and/or refrigerator
- ❑ Is unable or prefers not to spend money on food (<$25-30 per person spent on food each week)

Percentile	Men 55-65 y	Men 65-75 y	Women 55-65 y	Women 65-75 y
Arm circumference (cm)				
10th	27.3	26.3	25.7	25.2
50th	31.7	30.7	30.3	29.9
95th	36.9	35.5	38.5	37.3
Arm muscle circumference (cm)				
10th	24.5	23.5	19.6	19.5
50th	27.8	26.8	22.5	22.5
95th	32.0	30.6	28.0	27.9
Triceps skinfold (mm)				
10th	6	6	16	14
50th	11	11	25	24
95th	22	22	38	36

From Frisancho AR. New norms of upper limb fat and muscle areas for assessment of nutritional status. Am J Clin Nutr 1981; 34:2540-2545. © 1981 American Society for Clinical Nutrition.

Functional Status

Usually or always needs assistance with (check each that apply):

- ❑ Bathing
- ❑ Dressing
- ❑ Grooming
- ❑ Toileting
- ❑ Eating
- ❑ Walking or moving about
- ❑ Traveling (outside the home)
- ❑ Preparing food
- ❑ Shopping for food or other necessities

Mental/Cognitive Status

- ❑ Clinical evidence of impairment, e.g., Folstein <26
- ❑ Clinical evidence of depressive illness,e.g., Beck Depression Inventory >15, Geriatric Depression Scale >5

Patients in whom you have identified one or more major indicator (see p. 2) of poor nutritional status require immediate medical attention; if minor indicators are found, ensure that they are known to a health professional or to the patient's own physician. Patients who display risk factors (see p. 2) of poor nutritional status should be referred to the appropriate health care or social service professional (dietitian, nurse, dentist, case manager, etc.).

Figure 13-5 Level II screen developed by the Nutrition Screening Initiative. *(Reprinted with permission by the Nutrition Screening Initiative, a project of the American Academy of Family Physicians, the American Dietetic Association and the National Council on the Aging, Inc., and funded in part by a grant from Ross Products Division, Abbott Laboratories.)*

Box 13-5 Major Indicators of Poor Nutrition Status

Significant loss of weight over time
- 5% of body weight in 1 month
- 7.5% or more in 3 months
- 10% or more in 6 months
- Unintended weight loss of more than 10 pounds

Significantly low weight-for-height
- MRW <80%

Significant change in functional status
- Change from independence to dependence in two of the self-care skills (activities of daily living)
- Change from independence to dependence in nutrition-related skills

Significant reduction in serum protein measures serum albumin <3.5 g/dL

Significant and sustained reduction of nutritional intake below RDA
- 3 months or more when intake is below the minimum from one or more of the five food groups

Significant reduction in midarm circumference <10th percentile

Significant increase or decrease in the triceps skinfold measurement <10th or >95th percentile

Significant obesity
- MRW >120%
- BMI ≥27

Nutrition-related disorders
- Osteoporosis
- Osteomalacia
- Folate deficiency
- Vitamin B_{12} deficiency

From The Nutrition Screening Initiative. Report of Nutrition Screening I: Toward a common view. Washington, DC: 1991. Reprinted with permission by the Nutrition Screening Initiative, a project of the American Academy of Family Physicians, the American Dietetic Association and the National Council on the Aging, Inc., and funded in part by a grant from Ross Products Division, Abbott Laboratories.

Biochemical

The most commonly used biochemical indicators of protein status are serum proteins that are synthesized in the liver. Serum albumin has prognostic value for subsequent mortality and morbidity in older adults (Ferguson et al., 1993). Proteins and smaller body pools with shorter half-lives, such as prealbumin, transferrin, and retinol-bending protein are better suited to monitor status during acute illness and convalescence. Although total lymphocyte count (TLC) values for older adults are somewhat below the base for younger individuals, a TLC less than 1500/cm^3 indicates deficit and the need for further assessment.

Because vitamin B_{12} deficiency is more common among older adults, especially those with atrophic gastritis, periodic screening of serum levels for vitamin B_{12} status is recommended after age 55 years to 60 years (Allen and Casterline, 1994).

Clinical Signs

Subjective global assessment completed by a trained observer is appropriate for nutrition assessment in older adults. Physical signs that suggest possible nutritional deficiency were outlined in Table 2-8. Clinical signs of malnutrition may be "softer" in older adults in that they are more difficult to identify because of age-related changes in hair, skin, nails, and body fat distribution. They may not correlate well with dietary intakes or even serum levels in older adults.

Dietary Assessment

In some ways, collecting dietary information from older adults can be easier than for other age groups because the dietary patterns of the elderly tend to be less variable than are those of younger adults. Many older adults concerned about nutrition and health are eager to share information about their dietary intakes and can be very conscientious about maintaining dietary records. However, age-associated decline in short-term memory may make self-reported intakes, especially the 24-hour dietary recall, unreliable. A dietary history method, although time-consuming, may be an effective means to estimate usual or typical dietary patterns (van Staveren et al., 1994). In some instances it may be necessary to gather dietary information from caregivers and family members. Accurate assessment includes information about appetite, eating or chewing problems, problems with swallowing or bowel function, food avoidances, and alcohol and tobacco use, and health problems and use of prescription and nonprescription drugs that may influence appetite or nutrient uptake. Because older adults tend to use more dietary supplements with greater frequency than other population groups, it is important to include this information in dietary assessment.

PROMOTING NUTRITION FOR OLDER ADULTS

- *What are the health and nutrition guidelines for optimum health for older adults?*
- *What community resources are available for older adults at nutritional risk?*

Consuming a nutritionally adequate diet and maintaining physical activity contribute significantly to the maintenance of health and well-being among older adults and may delay the decline of functional capacity that accompanies the normal process of aging. In addition diet is important in the treatment of chronic disease. Recommended intakes for older adults follow the Food Guide Pyramid and the Dietary Guidelines for Americans (see Chapter 1). Because caloric intakes decline with age, particular attention must be given to the nutrient density of the diet.

The Interventions Roundtable convened by the NSI identified interventions that are appropriate for the nutrition concerns identified with the DETERMINE checklist and the Level I and II screens. The interventions can be classified into the six following areas:

1. Obtain, prepare, and eat appropriate diets.
2. Maintain adequate oral health.
3. Maintain mental health.
4. Use medications appropriately.
5. Be aware of changing eating habits.
6. Provide nutrition support for individuals who cannot eat an adequate diet.

Identification of nutrition risk in older adults is significant only if steps are taken to improve status. Intervention must be individualized to use specific resources available to meet the unique needs of the older individual. Access to adequate quantity and quality of food is essential. Community-based resources can provide assistance with shopping for food and access to food assistance programs, including home-delivered meals. These services may be accessed through health maintenance organizations, healthcare agencies, and a series of community volunteer organizations. Nutrition services for older adults are available from a variety of resources at the community level, particularly from programs supported by Title III of the Older Americans Act (see the Application at the end of the chapter).

CHRONIC HEALTH CONCERNS

- *What chronic diseases occur more frequently in older adults?*
- *What changes in dietary habits can minimize the effects of chronic diseases?*
- *Identify one chronic disease and outline appropriate interventions for an older adult.*

Health status of older adults is complex. They frequently have multiple subclinical and clinical diseases and consequent disabilities. It is rare for a single aspect of health status to be the sole predictor of adverse outcomes, including mortality, in older adults. Food habits can contribute to the development of some of these diseases. In addition nutrition may be critically important to the treatment of chronic diseases of aging. Nutrition therapy is particularly appealing for those over 65 years of age because it is relatively inexpensive compared with medications and has no side effects.

Overall 7 of every 10 Americans who die are elderly. Most of the deaths among older adults may be attributed to cardiovascular disease, cancer, or stroke. These diseases are also the principal causes of morbidity, impaired mobility, and decreased cognitive function.

Excess body weight is associated with an increased risk of developing diabetes and cardiovascular disease. Avoidance of obesity and moderate increases in physical activity have been associated with longevity in middle-aged men (Paffenbarger et al., 1993) and have positive health benefits for older adults. The relationship between mortality and body weight is a J-shaped curve, with the greatest risk at the extremes of leanness and obesity. For older adults weight loss often becomes a critical predictor of morbidity and mortality (Fried et al., 1998).

Research Update

Alzheimer's Disease

Few public health problems have captured the attention of both the biomedical and general public as has Alzheimer's disease (Selkoe, 2000). Alzheimer's disease, the most common cause of dementia, is the epitome of the fears expressed by older people when they say they don't want to become a burden to their families. Nearly 10% of persons age 65 years and older suffer from it; 50% of those over 85 years of age are affected. Alzheimer's disease is one of the most frequent obstacles to healthy aging in this country and is more common in women than in men. Because women with Alzheimer's disease live longer than men with Alzheimer's disease, there are almost twice as many women as men with the disorder. Over a span of 5 years to 7 years, until death from complications such as pneumonia, the disease robs victims of their memory, thinking ability, normal behavior, and often their life savings as they become unable to care for themselves.

Alzheimer's disease is an abnormal progressive deterioration of the brain. Unfortunately the cause is mysterious and there are no signs of the disease's progression until substantial brain damage has occurred. It begins with cognitive deficiencies that gradually become worse. Diagnosis is difficult, but characteristic symptoms are gradual loss of memory and reasoning, loss of the ability to communicate, loss of physical capabilities, and eventually loss of life. The only conclusive diagnosis is examination of the brain at autopsy.

Alzheimer's disease is characterized neuropathologically by the presence of amyloid beta-peptide (A-beta)-containing plaques, referred to as "sticky protein gunk," and neurofibrillary tangles composed of abnormal tau protein. Considerable controversy exists as to whether the extent of accumulation of A-beta correlates with dementia and whether alterations of A-beta precede or follow changes in tau protein.

It appears that normal neurons release A-beta peptide and that overproduction of the peptide results in the accumulation of insoluble paired helical filaments. **Beta amyloid** protein has been demonstrated to be neurotoxic to rodent brain cell cultures, resulting in memory loss for recently acquired events in senescence-accelerated mice. Continuing studies have indicated that a number of small peptides may inhibit the **amnestic** effect of the A-beta peptide.

> **beta amyloid:** a fragment from a large, normally occurring protein called beta amyloid precursor protein
> **amnestic:** causing loss of memory

A number of studies of the nutrition status of individuals with Alzheimer's disease have reported weight loss that occurs even when energy content of the diet is considered adequate. It cannot be explained by food intake or physical activity (Renvall et al., 1993; Wolf-Klein and Silverstone, 1994). There is scientific speculation that the causes of weight gains and losses in Alzheimer's disease are associated with neuroendocrine disorders and atrophy of the brain cortex.

In the last several years there has been major interest in folic acid and vitamin B_{12} and their role in the elevation of blood levels of homocysteine, a known independent risk factor for vascular disease. This speculation has been extended by the observation of increased levels of homocysteine in some Alzheimer's disease patients, leading to a hypothesis that hyperhomocysteinemia may contribute to cognitive impairment. A study by Clark and coworkers (1998) has provided support for this thesis. This study found that the 164 Alzheimer's disease patients had higher serum homocysteine levels than the 108 controls. Scores on cognitive assessment measurements were significantly lower for the 164 Alzheimer's disease patients than the controls. The differences between homocysteine levels and scores on cognitive tests were even greater for 76 patients in the Alzheimer's disease group whose disease was confirmed on postmortem examination. Differences were more significantly different from the controls in that group. This study and work of other researchers support a relationship between hyperhomocysteinemia and Alzheimer's disease and are consistent with the emerging hypothesis that vascular disease may play a significant role in the pathogenesis of Alzheimer's disease (Miller, 2000).

Cardiovascular Disease

Because most new coronary heart disease (CHD) events and most coronary deaths occur in persons older than 65 years of age, a high LDL-C and a low HDL-C predict development of CHD. Recognizing that cardiovascular disease is the leading cause of death among older people, the National Cholesterol Education Program (NCEP) panel has recommended application of its lipid screening and management guidelines to management of older individuals (see Chapter 12) (Expert Panel on Detection, Evaluation, and Treatment of High Blood Cholesterol in Adults, 2001). The recommendations are for primary prevention via dietary changes and physical activity. Recommendations are to follow the Dietary Guidelines for Americans. Chapter 12 outlined cholesterol-lowering drugs, which are recommended when persons are at high risk because of multiple risk factors or advanced subclinical atherosclerosis and when diet and exercise alone are not totally effective.

Application of the NCEP guidelines to elderly persons in particular has been criticized. Several analyses have found a positive association between serum cholesterol and coronary disease risk among older adults, but the observed risk was smaller than that among younger individuals (Manolio et al., 1992; Wilson et al., 1998). Others have found that elevated serum TC or low HDL-C levels were not significant risk factors for all-cause mortality, CHD mortality, or hospitalization for myocardial infarction in persons older than 70 years (Krumholz et al., 1994). An analysis of data collected from 5209 men and women who were enrolled in the Framingham Heart Study from 1948 through 1980 found that the relationship between TC level and all-cause mortality was positive at age 40 years, negligible at ages 50 years to 70 years, and negative at age 80 years (Krommal et al., 1993). The relationship of TC to CHD mortality was positive at ages 40 years, 50 years, and 60 years, but attenuated with age until the relationship was insignificant at ages 70 years and 80 years. For non-CHD mortality, cholesterol was negatively related for ages 50 years and above. Thus it appears that for older adults, serum TC and LDL-C concentrations should be interpreted with caution and initiation of cholesterol-lowering treatment in men and women above 65 years to 70 years of age should be reconsidered.

In epidemiologic studies, hypocholesterolemia has been associated with increased mortality from noncardiovascular causes (Goichot et al., 1995). It may be that low cholesterol concentration is a nonspecific feature of poor health status that is independent of nutrient or energy intake.

Hypertension

A J-shaped curve illustrates the relationship between blood pressure and mortality in older persons, where both low blood pressure and high blood pressure are associated with increased risk of death. In older adults, low blood pressure is often associated with overmedication, PEU, inadequate sodium intake, anemia, dehydration, or an adrenal disturbance. All are potentially treatable conditions that should be considered when an older person has low blood pressure.

Blood pressure tends to rise with increasing age. This elevation is related to many factors, including genetics, body weight, physical exercise, alcohol consumption, and cigarette smoking. **Hypertension,** a common problem in older persons, is present in approximately 60% of Hispanics and non-Hispanic whites and in 71% of non-Hispanic African Americans age 60 years or older.

Hypertension often has no symptoms of its own, but it is an established risk factor for coronary artery disease, congestive heart failure, transient ischemic attacks, kidney failure, and **retinopathy** (Joint National Committee on Detection, Evaluation, and Treatment of High Blood Pressure, 1993). Treatment of hypertension in men and women over 60 years of age reduces the incidence of stroke by about 40% and some trials have also shown reductions in coronary events (Fletcher and Bulpit, 1994).

The initial treatment for hypertension is likely to be life-style changes, which include weight loss, increased physical activity, and moderation of alcohol and sodium intake. Although there has been extensive research on the impact of various dietary components (fatty acids, calcium, sodium, potassium, chloride, and magnesium) on blood pressure, the data currently available do not offer definitive conclusions or evidence for dietary intervention, except for weight loss and moderation of alcohol consumption (Reusser and McCarron, 1994). The most accepted dietary approach to hypertension is the Dietary Approaches to Stop Hypertension (DASH) diet, which has been associated with significant decreases in blood pressure when used alone (Colin, 1997) or in conjunction with sodium restriction (Svetkey et al., 1999). The eating plan incorporates high amounts of fruits, vegetables, and low-fat dairy foods (see Chapter 12).

Treatment of hypertensive older adults with **diuretics** and **beta-blockers** produces a significant benefit overall. A meta-analysis of nine major clinical trials involving more than 15,000 individuals older than 59 years found that, overall, treatment reduced all-cause mortality by approximately 12%, stroke mortality by 36%, and CHD mortality by 25% (Insua et al., 1994).

Antihypertensive drug therapy is carried out with caution because older persons may be more sensitive to decreases in fluid volume and sympathetic nervous system inhibition than are younger individuals. Treatment is usually initiated with smaller doses of the drugs and smaller increases in dosage spaced at longer intervals.

Osteoporosis

Most bone is made up of an outer layer of compact bone surrounding trabecular or cancellous bone structure. Bone loss occurs with age. The rate of loss is greatest in areas of cancellous bone—the vertebrae (the 33 bones of the spinal column), the proximal **femur**, and the distal **radius.**

Osteoporosis is a multifactorial disorder of the skeleton characterized by reduced bone mass resulting from an alteration in bone remodeling, the process in which bone is broken down or resorbed and replaced with new bone. It is characterized by increased osteoclastic activity, accelerated reduction in bone mass (Figure 13-6), and a consequent deterioration in the microarchitecture of bone leading to enhanced bone fragility and an increased risk of fracture. Osteoporosis is a major

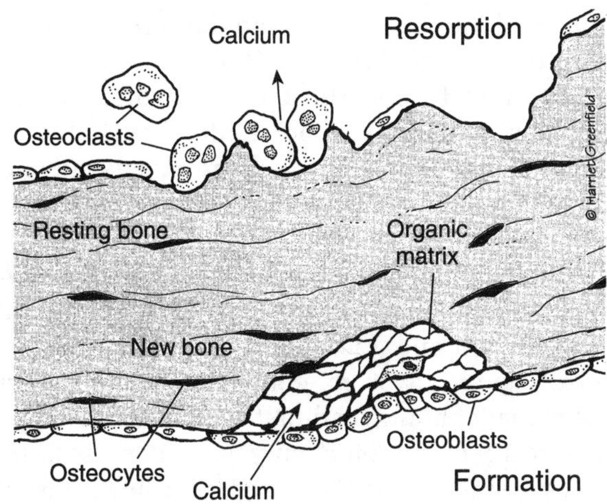

Figure 13-6 Bone is constantly remolded during osteoblastic and osteoclastic activity. *(Reprinted with permission. Copyright Harriet R. Greenfield, 1993.)*

public health problem in the United States. Based on data from NHANES III, 29.5% of women over 65 years of age and 5.7% of women under 65 years of age had bone mass density measurements that met the World Health Organization's definition for osteoporosis.

Osteoporotic fractures occur most frequently in the hips, vertebrae, and wrists. Hip fracture, usually the result of a fall, is a major cause of mortality and morbidity in older women. The incidence increases with age and between 12% and

KEY TERMS

hypertension: systolic blood pressure ≥140 mm Hg; diastolic blood pressure ≥90 mm Hg
retinopathy: a condition of the retina that can lead to blindness
diuretics: drugs that decrease blood pressure by increasing sodium and water loss through the kidney
beta-blockers: drugs that block responses of the sympathetic nervous system
femur: the bone that extends from the pelvis to the knee
radius: the bone along the forearm on the outer side when the hand is palm up

20% of all individuals with hip fracture die in the hospital of complications (Riggs et al., 1994). Approximately one third of survivors are left with some disability, which limits their independence. Wrist fractures, which are also usually incurred during a fall, generally heal completely with few lasting effects.

Vertebral fractures are often called *crush fractures* because they can lead to vertebral compression and a loss of height. When several vertebrae are involved, compression can distort the spinal column, leading to "dowager's hump" (Figure 13-7). As spinal curvature increases, the rib cage sinks toward the pelvis, causing internal organs to become cramped and consequently creating difficulties with breathing and gastrointestinal discomfort.

Risk Factors

Bone mass in old age depends on peak bone mass achieved in early adulthood and the rate of bone loss. Bone loss, although primarily from a reduction in the supply of estrogen, is influenced by many characteristics and behaviors that can predict the potential for osteoporotic fractures. Risk factors among osteoporotic women over age 65 years are summarized in Box 13-6.

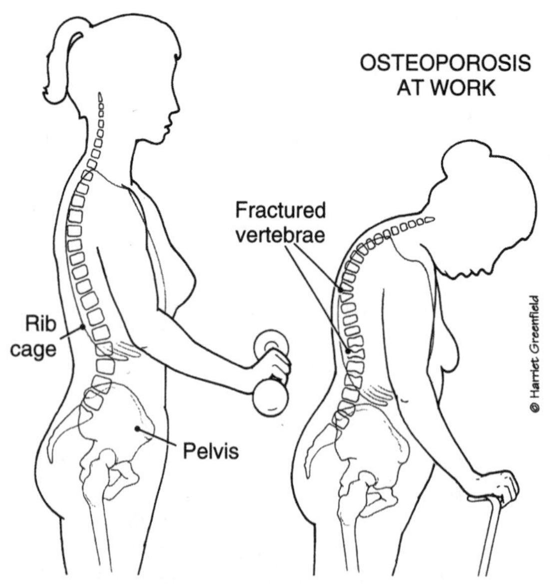

Figure 13-7 Compression fractures of the vertebrae lead to loss of height and forward bending of the upper spine. *(Reprinted with permission. Copyright Harriet R. Greenfield, 1993.)*

Detection

There are several techniques for estimating bone density. Single photon absorptiometry (SPA) and single X-ray absorptiometry (SXA) are used to assess mineral content of the forearm. They measure primarily cortical bone, in which tissue loss is not apparent until late in the course of the disease. Dual X-ray absorptiome-

Box 13-6 Risk Factors Linked to Osteoporosis

Gender: Women are at greater risk.
Age: Risk increases as bone loss increases with time.
Frame size: Women who are thin and have small frames are at greater risk.
Weight loss: Weight loss after age 50 is associated with lower bone mass.
Heredity: Women whose mothers had vertebral fractures seem to have less bone mass.
Race: Caucasians and Asians are at greater risk than Africans and African Americans.
Decreased estrogen: Postmenopausal women, women whose ovaries have been surgically removed, and young women with low body fat who have little estrogen and irregular menses are at greater risk.
Low dietary calcium: Low levels can increase bone resorption and lead to bone loss.
Inactivity: Lack of physical activity increases bone resorption.
Smoking: Cigarette smoking increases bone resorption.
Caffeine: Women who consume large amounts of caffeine regularly (3 or more cups of coffee per day) have lower bone density and more fractures.
Alcohol: Two or more drinks per day can accelerate bone loss.
Some drugs: Glucocorticoids such as prednisone (used to treat inflammatory diseases) and antiseizure drugs such as Dilantin can lead to bone loss.

try (DXA) gives a more accurate estimate of risk, measuring the mineral content of the total cortical and trabecular bones of the hip and spine and total bone mass. Radiation exposure for this procedure is less than that of a standard spine X-ray. Ultrasound uses high-frequency sound waves to make similar measurement.

Prevention

Prevention of osteoporosis is of the utmost importance. Approaches to prevention include maximizing peak bone mass in early life and reducing postmenopausal and age-associated bone loss.

Calcium and Vitamin D

Depending on body size, sex, and ethnicity, the human body contains approximately 1000 g to 1500 g of calcium, of which 99% is found as hydroxyapatite. Osteoporosis is not a disease resulting from obvious deficiencies in vitamin D, calcium, and phosphate, but subtle deficiencies may account for the ability of calcium and vitamin D supplements to have a beneficial effect on bone (Dawson-Hughes et al., 1997). Reduced calcium intake clearly can cause bone loss by necessitating the use of skeletal calcium to maintain a constant serum calcium level. When evaluating the effect of calcium on bone, clinicians should distinguish early (5 to 8 years after menopause) from late postmenopause (less than 8 years). In general calcium intervention studies conducted during the early postmenopausal period have shown small effects that were generally confined to cortical rather than trabecular bone. Although less effective than hormone replacement therapy (HRT), daily intakes of 1500 mg to 1700 mg of calcium with 5 mg to 10 mg (400 to 800 IU) of vitamin D in the early postmenopausal period have been shown to significantly retard bone loss from the lumbar spine (Reid et al., 1993) and proximal femur (Aloia et al., 1994) and to reduce the risk of hip and other nonvertebral fractures. However, the effect of dietary therapy is more pronounced in postmenopausal women than during early menopause. The combination of estrogen and dietary calcium is more effective than either alone in late menopausal women (Priestwood et al., 1994).

Exercise

The skeleton is subjected to weight-bearing stress of gravity and forces from muscle contraction. These forces change the shape of the bone. Bone mass increases in response to mechanical stress. Physical exercise enhances bone development and vigorous exercise augments bone mineral density. Physically active people appear to have higher bone density than those who are sedentary and some studies have reported a positive association between muscle strength and bone mass, especially in premenopausal women. In addition there is evidence that a variety of exercise programs have been associated with reduced risk of falls in older adults (Province et al., 1995).

Hormone Replacement Therapy

Many studies have shown that estrogen intervention, or HRT, reduces the rate of bone loss. (HRT is discussed in Chapter 12 on page 387). The effects of estrogen in preventing bone loss can be seen immediately after menopause, in women over 70 years old, and in those with established osteoporosis (Priestwood et al., 1994). Long-term estrogen use (more than 5 years) is associated with a reduction in the risk of fractures of the hip and distal radius and reduced risk of vertebral crush fracture (Kanis et al., 1992).

The mode of action of estrogen on bone is unclear. Recently estrogen receptors have been found in osteoblastic cells, suggesting a stimulation of bone synthesis. Estrogens may also influence calcium homeostasis in the body by increasing the hydroxylation of 25-hydroxyvitamin D to its active 1,25 form.

Many women who have osteoporosis or who are at high risk because of heredity, medication conditions, previous fractures, or the use of certain medications such as steroids will be unable to protect bone mass with the recommended exercise, calcium, and vitamin D regimen. For these women the Food and Drug Administration has approved bone remodeling medications that can help improve bone strength or help reduce bone loss (Kleerekoper and Schein, 2001). Table 13-6 describes the medications currently available.

Research Update

Are Calcium Supplements Safe?

The current DRI for calcium is 1200 mg per day for adults 51 years and older (Institute of Medicine, 1997). This is an amount difficult to obtain from food alone. According to the 1994 CSFII, mean daily intake of calcium of men over the age of 65 years is 778 mg per day; for women over 65 years of age it is 587 mg per day. Therefore intakes are approximately 75% of the recommendation for men, but only about 50% for women. Although it is preferable for calcium needs to be met using food sources, many older adults may be unable to attain this level without supplements.

There are more than a dozen commonly prescribed calcium supplements and hundreds of different formulations commercially available. The cost varies widely among different types of calcium preparations and among different brands of similar preparations. The most common and economical supplement, calcium carbonate, has the highest content of calcium—40% by weight. However, carbonate is a relatively insoluble form of calcium, especially at neutral pH, which may occur in the intestines of many older adults with atrophic gastritis and achlorhydria. Most other commercial calcium preparations contain 28% to 31% calcium by weight. Calcium supplement intake has increased. In addition many foods are now being fortified with calcium, including breakfast cereal, orange juice, and margarine.

An individual who opts for a calcium supplement should take it throughout the day on an empty stomach to enhance absorption. Although calcium supplements in the range of 1 g to 2 g per day are usually very well tolerated, some side effects are seen. Constipation, intestinal bloating, and excess gas are often reported. Supplemental calcium can suppress the absorption of other nutrients, especially iron and zinc, and may impede the absorption of concurrently administered drugs such as tetracyclines. Conversely calcium absorption is impaired by concurrent ingestion of aluminum-containing antacids, cholestyramine, and phosphate. The upper tolerable limit (UL) for calcium, 2500 g through diet and supplements, should not be exceeded for a prolonged period (Institute of Medicine, 1997).

Potential contamination of calcium supplements is a problem first recognized in the 1960s. Of concern are supplements that contain bone meal, dolomite, and fossilized oyster shells that may have biologically significant concentrations of lead. Other contaminants include aluminum, arsenic, mercury, and cadmium. Scelfo and Flegal (2000) determined the lead content of 136 bottles of calcium carbonate supplements and found that two thirds failed to meet standards for acceptable lead levels (1.5 μg per daily dose) of calcium.

Such an observation brings into question the safety of using some calcium supplements. Another group of researchers measured the lead content of 7 natural and 14 refined calcium carbonate formulations and found that 4 of the natural products and 4 of the 14 refined products had high lead content (Ross et al., 2000). Despite stringent limits on lead exposure, many calcium supplement formulations may contain lead and thereby pose an avoidable health risk. The issue of contamination in calcium supplements illustrates that the safety of a nutrient supplement is not limited to concerns about excess intake of the nutrient itself.

Recommendations

It is never too early or too late to initiate life-style changes to reduce loss of bone mass (Table 13-7). Adolescents and young adults can build maximal peak bone mass with exercise and a balanced diet containing 1200 mg of calcium and 5 μg of vitamin D. For older women, HRT can minimize bone loss and, in some instances, promote osteogenic activity. Weight-bearing physical activity has the potential not only to protect from further bone loss, but also to improve strength, mobility, flexibility, agility, and muscle strength, which may indirectly decrease the incidence of osteoporotic fractures by lessening the likelihood of falling (American

Table 13-6 FDA-Approved Drugs to Improve Bone Strength or Reduce Bone Loss

Medication	Use and Benefits	Risks and Side Effects
BISPHOSPHONATES		
• **Alendronate (Fosamax)** (Approved for once-a-week therapy, which is shown to have similar effects as daily administration.) • **Risedronate (Actonel)**	For prevention and treatment in women; for treatment only in men. Increases bone density at the spine and hip as compared with placebo. Lowers risk for spinal and hip fracture. Often prescribed for osteoporosis induced by glucocorticoids or seizure and thyroid medications.	Difficult to digest. May cause nausea, heartburn, or irritation of the esophagus or stomach if not taken properly. Take with water first thing in the morning; stay upright for 30 minutes. During this time, avoid ingesting anything else.
HORMONE-REPLACEMENT THERAPY (HRT)		
• **Various agents** (Premarin, Estrace, Ogen, Estratab, Premphase, Prempro, Femhrt, Estraderm, Activella, Cenestin, Menest, and Climara)	For prevention in women. Increases bone density at all sites as compared with placebo. Decreases risk for spinal fractures. (Also alleviates symptoms of menopause and improves blood lipids.)	Increases risk for breast cancer with 5 years or more of use. Rare side effects include blood clots and gallstones; more common side effects are breakthrough bleeding, breast tenderness, possible weight gain, and headaches.
SELECTIVE ESTROGEN RECEPTOR MODULATORS (SERMs)		
• **Raloxifene (Evista)**	For prevention and treatment in women. Increases bone density at spine, hip, and neck. Reduction in spinal fracture only.	Common side effects include hot flashes and leg cramps. Blood clots are a rare side effect.
CALCITONIN		
• **Miacalcin** • **Calcimar**	For treatment only in women. Under study for treatment in men. Decreases bone loss at the spine. Fracture data inconclusive. Reduces bone pain from osteoporosis-related fractures.	Injected form can cause allergic reaction, flushing of the face and hands, nausea, and skin rash. Nasal spray can cause a runny nose or nosebleeds.

College of Sports Medicine, 1995). Calcium and vitamin D are key dietary ingredients. Current recommendations (1200 mg calcium, 10 to 15 μg vitamin D) for these nutrients may be difficult to obtain through food alone. Supplements should be used with caution, though, because excess vitamin D can cause bone loss and neurologic problems. Other therapies, including fluoride, vitamin D analogs, and calcitonin, will undoubtedly have greater potential in the future.

Table 13-7 CHARACTERISTICS OF CALCIUM PREPARATIONS

Form of Calcium	Elemental Calcium (%)	Average Absorption (%)	Characteristics	Considerations
Calcium carbonate	40	26	Relatively insoluble, especially at neutral pH; do not take with food or milk	Absorption is very poor with achlorhydial constipation, gastric distention, flatulence
Calcium lactate	13	32-34	Contains lactose—milk yogurt	Less constipating than calcium carbonate
Calcium phosphate	38	28	Tend to be insoluble; contain substantial amounts of phosphate	
Dicalcium phosphate	31	28		
Calcium gluconate	8	26-34	More soluble than calcium carbonate—low calcium content	Less constipating than calcium carbonate
Calcium citrate	21	22	More soluble than calcium carbonate	
Calcium malate-citrate	21	34	More soluble than calcium carbonate	
Oyster shell	28-31	?	Relatively insoluble calcium carbonate	May contain many noncalcium compounds: lead, mercury, aluminum, cadmium
Bone meal	31	?	Less constipating than calcium carbonate	May contain noncalcium compounds: lead, mercury, aluminum, cadmium
Dolomite	22	?	Less constipating than calcium carbonate	May contain noncalcium compounds: lead, mercury, aluminum, cadmium

Concepts to Remember

- Aging is a process that is associated with functional decline, diminished physiologic reserves, and increased vulnerability to disease.
- Adults over the age of 65 years make up more than 12% of the American population and the number of persons in that age category increases daily.
- Older adults are a heterogeneous group of individuals who encounter age-related deficits at vastly different rates.
- "Being old" is less a chronologic age than a state of mind and physical status.
- The aging process is influenced by genetic and environmental factors.
- Aging is accompanied by numerous changes in physiologic status and body composition.

- The physiologic, social, economic, and health changes associated with aging are important determinants of an individual's ability to function independently and determine his or her quality of life.
- Although energy needs decline, requirements for most nutrients, except vitamin A, are equal to or greater than those of younger adults.
- Nutrition screening and assessment are essential components of geriatric assessment.
- Nutrition screening is important for identifying risk for poor nutrition at the community level and serves as a basis for intervention.
- Nutrition intervention is an important component of healthcare that allows older adults to maintain quality of life and independence.
- Older adults are more likely to have health problems and suffer from chronic diseases than are younger persons.
- Nutrition is important in the prevention and treatment of chronic diseases including osteoporosis, CHD, and hypertension.
- Multiple medications required by older adults may interfere with nutrition status and increase overall health risks.

REFERENCES

Abramson JL et al.: Moderate alcohol consumption and risk of heart failure among older persons, JAMA 285:1971, 2001.

Administration on Aging: A profile of older Americans, Washington, DC, 2000, U.S. Department of Health and Human Services, American Association of Retired Persons.

Allen LH and Casterline J: Vitamin B_{12} deficiency in elderly individuals: diagnosis and requirements, Am J Clin Nutr 60:12, 1994.

Aloia JF et al.: Calcium supplementation with and without hormone replacement therapy to prevent postmenopausal bone loss, Ann Intern Med 120:97, 1994.

AMA Council on Scientific Affairs: Alcoholism in the elderly, JAMA 275:797, 1996.

American College of Sports Medicine: ACSM position stand on osteoporosis and exercise, Med Sci Sports Exerc 227:i, 1995.

Baumgartner RN: Body composition in healthy aging, Ann N Y Acad Sci 904:437, 2000.

Birrer RB: Depression and aging too often do mix, Postgrad Med 104:143, 1998.

Bogden JD et al.: Daily micronutrient supplements enhance delayed-hyposensitivity skin test responses in older people, Am J Clin Nutr 60:437, 1994.

Brinkley N and Krueger D: Hypervitaminosis A and bone, Nutr Rev 58:138, 2000.

Brown L et al.: A prospective study of carotenoid intake and risk of cataract extraction in U.S. men, Am J Clin Nutr 70:517, 1999.

Bunyard LB et al.: Energy requirements of middle-aged men are modifiable by physical activity, Am J Clin Nutr 86:1136, 1998.

Campbell W: Dietary protein requirement of older people: is the RDA adequate? Nutr Today 31:192, 1996.

Carmeli E and Reznich AX: The physiology and biochemistry of skeletal muscle atrophy as a function of age, Proc Soc Exp Biol Med 206:103, 1994.

Castaneda C et al.: Elderly women accommodate a low-protein diet with losses of body cell mass, muscle function, and immune response, Am J Clin Nutr 62:30, 1995.

Chandra R: Nutrition and immunity in the elderly: clinical significance, Nutr Rev 53(Suppl):580, 1995.

Christen Y: Oxidative stress and Alzheimer's disease, Am J Clin Nutr 71:621S, 2000.

Chumlea WC et al.: Prediction of stature from knee height for black and white adults and children with application to mobility—impaired or handicapped persons, J Am Diet Assoc 94:1385, 1994.

Clark R et al.: Folate, vitamin B_{12} and serum total homocysteine levels in confirmed Alzheimer's disease, Arch Neurol 55:1449, 1998.

Colin PR: The dietary approaches to stop hypertension (DASH) clinical trial: implications for lifestyle and modifications in the treatment of hypertensive patients, Cardiol Rev 7:284, 1997.

Council on Scientific Affairs: American Medical Association white paper on elderly health, Ann Intern Med 150:2459, 1990.

Davis MA et al.: Living arrangements affect dietary quality for U.S. adults aged 50 years and older. NHANES III 1998-1994, J Nutr 130:2256, 2000.

Dawson-Hughes B et al.: Effects of calcium and vitamin D supplementation on bone density in men and women 65 years of age and older, N Engl J Med 337:670, 1997.

Dufor M and Fuller RK: Alcohol in the elderly, Annu Rev Med 46:123, 1995.

Evans WL: Effects of aging and exercise on nutrition needs of the elderly, Nutr Rev 54:S35, 1996.

Expert Panel on Detection, Evaluation and Treatment of High Blood Cholesterol in Adults: Executive summary of the third report of the National Cholesterol Education Program (NCEP), Adult Treatment Panel III, JAMA 185:2486, 2001.

Ferguson RP et al.: Serum albumin and prealbumin as predictors of clinical outcomes of hospitalized elderly nursing home residents, J Am Geriatr Soc 41:545, 1993.

Fiatarone M et al.: Exercise training and nutritional supplementation for physical frailty in very elderly people, N Engl J Med 330:1769, 1994.

Fletcher A and Bulpit C: Epidemiology of hypertension in the elderly, J Hypertens 12:S3, 1994.

Fontera WR et al.: A cross-sectional study of muscle strength and mass in 45- to 78-year-old men and women, J Appl Physiol 71:644, 1991.

Food and Nutrition Board: Recommended dietary allowances, ed 10, Washington, DC, 1989, National Academy Press.

Forster LE et al.: Alcohol use and potential risk for alcohol-related reactions among community-based elderly, J Community Health 18:225, 1993.

Fried LP et al.: Risk factors for 5-year mortality in older adults, JAMA 279:585, 1998.

Galanos AN et al.: Nutrition and function: is there a relationship between body mass index and the functional capabilities of community dwelling elderly? J Am Geriatr Soc 42:368, 1994.

Gerrior SA: Dietary changes in older Americans from 1977 to 1996: implications for dietary quality, Fam Econ Nutr Rev 12:3, 1999.

Gerster H: Anticarcinogenic effect of common carotenoids, Int J Vitam Nutr Res 63:93, 1993.

Goichot B et al.: Low cholesterol concentrations in free-living elderly subjects: relations with dietary intake and nutritional status, Am J Clin Nutr 62:547, 1995.

Gray-Donald K.: The frail elderly: meeting the nutritional challenge, J Am Diet Assoc 95:538, 1995.

Guo SS et al.: Aging, body composition, and lifestyle: the Fels Longitudinal Study, Am J Clin Nutr 70:40S, 1999.

Hannan MT et al.: Effect of dietary protein on bone loss in elderly men and women: the Framingham Osteoporosis Study, J Bone Miner Res 15:2504, 2000.

Harris SS et al.: Plasma 25-hydroxy vitamin D responses of younger and older men to three weeks of supplementation with 1800 IU of vitamin D, J Am Coll Nutr 18:470, 1999.

Hodis HN: Serial coronary angiographic evidence that antioxidant vitamin intake reduces progression of coronary artery atherosclerosis, JAMA 273:1849, 1995.

Hollick MF: Vitamin D—new horizons for the 21st century, Am J Clin Nutr 60:619, 1994.

Hollozy JO: The biology of aging, Mayo Clin Proc 75:53, 2000.

Holt PR and Balint JA: Effects of aging on intestinal lipid absorption, Am J Physiol 264:1, 1993.

Hurley BF and Roth SM: Strength training in the elderly: effects on risk factors for age-related diseases, Sports Med 30:249, 2000.

Institute of Medicine: Dietary reference intakes for calcium, phosphorus, magnesium, vitamin D, and fluoride, Washington, DC, 1997, National Academy Press.

Institute of Medicine: Dietary reference intakes for thiamin, riboflavin, niacin, vitamin B_6, folate, vitamin B_{12}, pantothenic acid, biotin and choline, Washington, DC, 1998, National Academy Press.

Institute of Medicine: Dietary reference intakes for vitamin C, vitamin E, selenium and carotenoids, Washington, DC, 2000, National Academy Press.

Institute of Medicine: Dietary reference intakes for vitamin A, vitamin K, arsenic, boron, chromium, copper, iodine, iron, manganese, molybdenum, nickel, silicon, vanadium and zinc, Washington, DC, 2001, National Academy Press.

Insua JI et al.: Drug treatment of hypertension in the elderly: a meta-analysis, Ann Intern Med 121:355, 1994.

Joint National Committee on Detection, Evaluation, and Treatment of High Blood Pressure: The fifth report of the Joint National Committee on Detection, Evaluation, and Treatment of High Blood Pressure (JNC V), Arch Intern Med 153:154, 1993.

Kanis JA et al.: Evidence for efficacy of drugs affecting bone metabolism in preventing hip fracture, BMJ 305:1124, 1992.

Kleerekoper M and Schein JR: Comparative safety of bone remodeling agents with a focus on osteoporosis therapies, J Clin Pharmacol 41:39, 2001.

Krause D et al.: Immune function did not decline with aging in apparently healthy well-nourished women, Mech Ageing Dev 112:43, 1999.

Krommal RA et al.: Total serum cholesterol levels and mortality risk as a function of age: a report based on the Framingham data, Arch Intern Med 153:1065, 1993.

Krumholz HM et al.: Lack of association between cholesterol and coronary heart disease mortality and morbidity and all-cause mortality in persons older than 70 years, JAMA 272:1335, 1994.

Kuczmarski MF et al.: Descriptive anthropometric reference data for older adults, J Am Diet Assoc 100:59, 2000.

Lee JS and Frongillo EA: Nutritional and health consequences are associated with food insecurity among U.S. elderly persons, J Nutr 131:2001, 2001.

Lemmer JT, Hurlbut DE, and Martel GF: Age and gender responses to strength training and detraining, Med Sci Sports Exerc 32:1505, 2000.

Lemon PWR: Beyond the zone: protein needs of active individuals, J Am Coll Nutr 19:513S, 2000.

Lindenbaum J et al.: Prevalence of cobalamin deficiency in the Framingham elderly population, Am J Clin Nutr 60:2, 1994.

Manolio TA et al.: Cholesterol and heart disease in older persons and women, review of NLIBI workshop, Ann Epidemiol 2:161, 1992.

Meydani SN et al.: Vitamin E enhancement of T cell-mediated function in healthy elderly: mechanism of action, Nutr Rev 53:S52, 1995.

Miller JW: Vitamin E and memory: is it vascular protection? Nutr Rev 58:109, 2000.

Morley JE and Solomon DH: Major issues in geriatrics over the last five years, J Am Geriatr Soc 42:218, 1994.

National Center for Health Statistics: Dietary intake source data, United States 1971-1974, PHS 79-1221, U.S. Department of Health, Education and Welfare, Hyattsville, Md, 1979, Public Health Service.

National Center for Health Statistics: Dietary intake source data, United States 1976-1980, PHS 83-1681, U.S. Department of Health and Human Services, Hyattsville, Md, 1983, Public Health Service.

Nelson HD et al.: Smoking, alcohol, and neuromuscular and physical function of older women, JAMA 272:1825, 1994.

Nicols A et al.: Successful aging and nutrition, Nutr Rev 59:588, 2001.
Nutrition Screening Initiative: Report of nutrition screening I: toward a common view, Consensus Conference, Washington, DC, 1991.
O'Dowd KJ et al.: Exogenous calciferol (vitamin D) and vitamin D endocrine status among elderly nursing home residents in the New York City area, J Am Geriatr Soc 41: 414, 1993.
Older Americans Report: Administration on Aging may get $5 million more: up from $872 million in FY '95, p. 315, 1994.
Oslin DW: Alcohol use in late life: disability and comorbidity, J Geriatr Psychiatry Neurol 13:134, 2000.
Paffenbarger RS et al.: The association of changes of physical activity level and other lifestyle characteristics with mortality among men, N Engl J Med 328:538, 1993.
Panchararuniti N et al.: Plasma homocysteine, folcite and vitamin B_{12} concentrations and risk for early-onset coronary artery disease, Am J Clin Nutr 59:940, 1994.
Pannemans DL et al.: The influence of protein intake on vitamin B_{12} metabolism differs in young and elderly humans, J Nutr 124:1207, 1994.
Payette H et al.: Predictors of dietary intake in a functionally dependent elderly population in the community, Am J Public Health 85:77, 1995.
Pendergast D, Fisher N, and Calkins E: Cardiovascular, neuromuscular and metabolic alterations with age leading to frailty, J Gerontol 48:61, 1993.
Perkins AJ et al.: Association of antioxidants with memory in a multiethnic elderly sample using the Third National Health and Nutrition Examination Survey, Am J Epidemiol 159:1313, 1999.
Posner B et al.: Nutritional risk in New England elders, J Gerontol 49:M123, 1994.
Priestwood KM et al.: The short term effects of conjugated estrogen on bone turnover in older women, J Clin Endocrinol Metab 79:366, 1994.
Province MA et al.: The effects of falls on elderly patients, a preplanned meta-analysis of the FICSIT trials: frailty and injuries: cooperative studies of intervention techniques, JAMA 273:1341, 1995.
Reid IR et al.: Effect of calcium on bone loss in postmenopausal women, N Engl J Med 328:460, 1993.
Renvall MJ et al.: Body composition of patients with Alzheimer's disease, J Am Diet Assoc 93:47, 1993.
Reuben DB et al.: Nutrition screening in older persons, J Am Geriatr Soc 43:415, 1995.
Reusser ME and McCarron DA: Micronutrient effects on blood pressure regulation, Nutr Rev 52:367, 1994.
Rhodus NL and Brown J: The association of xerostemia and inadequate intake in older adults, J Am Diet Assoc 90:1688, 1990.
Riggs BL et al.: Clinical trial of fluoride therapy in postmenopausal osteoporotic women: extended observations and additional analysis, J Bone Miner Res 9:265, 1994.
Roberts SB: Energy regulation and aging: recent findings and their implications, Nutr Rev 58:91, 2000.
Rosenberg IH and Miller JW: Nutritional factors in physical and cognitive functions of elderly people, Am J Clin Nutr 55:1237S, 1992.
Rosenbloom CA, editor: Sports nutrition: a guide for the professional working with active people, ed 3, Chicago, Il, 2000, American Dietetic Association.
Rosenthal M et al.: Demonstration of a relationship between level of physical training and insulin-stimulated glucose utilization in normal humans, Diabetes 32:408, 1983.
Ross EA et al.: Lead content of calcium supplements, JAMA 284:1425, 2000.
Rubenoff R and Hughes VA: Sarcopenia: current concepts, J Gerontol A Biol Sci Med Sci 55:M716, 2000.
Russell RM et al.: Older men and women efficiently absorb vitamin B_{12} from milk and fortified bread, J Nutr 131:291, 2001.
Russell RM: The aging process as a modifier of metabolism, Am J Clin Nutr 72:529S, 2000.
Scelfo GM and Flegal AF: Lead in calcium supplements, 108:309, 2000.
Scherr PA et al.: Light to moderate alcohol consumption and mortality in the elderly, J Am Geriatr Soc 40:651, 1992.
Seddon JM et al.: Dietary carotenoids, vitamins A, C, and E, and advanced age-related macular degeneration, Eye Disease Case-Control Study Group, JAMA 272:1413, 1994.
Selhub J et al.: Association between plasma homocysteine concentrations and extracranial carotid-artery stenosis, N Engl J Med 332:286, 1995.
Selkoe DJ: The origins of Alzheimer disease: a is for amyloid, JAMA 283:1615, 2000.
Singh MA: Combined exercise and dietary intervention to optimize body composition, Ann N Y Acad Sci 854:378, 1998.
Stevens J et al.: Attitudes toward body size and dieting: differences between elderly black and white women, Am J Public Health 84:1322, 1994.
Stuck AE et al.: Comprehensive geriatric assessment: a meta-analysis of controlled trials, Lancet 342:1032, 1993.
Svetkey LP et al.: The DASH Diet, Sodium Intake and Blood Pressure Trial (Dash-sodium rationale and design), DASH-Sodium Collaborative Research Group, J Am Diet Assoc 99:S96, 1999.
Tessari P: Changes in protein, carbohydrate, and fat metabolism with aging: possible role for insulin, Nutr Rev 58:11, 2000.
Tran ZV and Weltman A: Differential effects of exercise on serum lipid and lipoprotein levels seen with changes in body weight: a meta-analysis, JAMA 254:919, 1985.
Tufts University Health and Nutrition Letter: Food guide pyramid for people over 70 years, April 1999.
U.S. Bureau of the Census: Poverty levels in the United States, 1999, p. 60-210, 2000.
U.S. Census Bureau: Population division, population projections branch, www.census.gov/population projections/national, last update May 10, 2001.

van Staveren WA et al.: Assessing diets of elderly people: problems and approaches, Am J Clin Nutr 59:221S, 1994.

Vellas BJ et al.: Diseases and aging: patterns of morbidity with age: relationship between aging and age-associated diseases, Am J Clin Nutr 55:1225S, 1992.

Vita A et al.: Aging, health risk and cumulative disability, N Engl J Med 338: 1035, 1998.

Vitale S et al.: Plasma antioxidants and risk of cortical and nuclear cataract, Epidemiology 4:195, 1993.

Wallace JI et al.: Involuntary weight loss in outpatients: incidence and clinical significance, J Am Geriatr Soc 43:329, 1995.

White H et al.: The association of weight change in Alzheimer's disease with severity of disease and mortality: a longitudinal analysis, J Am Geriatr Soc 46:1123, 1998.

White JV: Risk factors for poor nutritional status, Prim Care 21:19, 1994.

Wilson PW et al.: Prediction of coronary heart disease using risk factor categories, Circulation 97:1837, 1998.

Wolf-Klein GP and Silverstone FA: Weight loss in Alzheimer's disease: an international review of the literature, Int Psychogeriatr 6:135, 1994.

Yung RL: Changes in immune function with age, Rheum Dis Clin Nirth Am 26:455, 2000.

APPLICATION

Health and Nutrition Programs for Older Adults

George was 67 years old when he joined the Senior Center of the local recreation department. He and his wife participated in many activities together until her death 4 years later. After that, George still came to play pool and he learned to play bridge. Sometimes he would go on sightseeing trips for seniors.

In his early 70s George developed hypertension and his physician prescribed a diuretic medication and recommended that he lose weight. George would take the medicine when he remembered, but made no attempt to lose weight. A couple of years later, George began to feel tired and had frequent headaches. His physician adjusted his medication, but insisted that he must get his weight down and referred him to the dietitian at the Community Senior Health Clinic where he could receive nutrition counseling for a sliding scale fee based on his income. When George appeared at the health clinic he was 74 years old. Five years earlier George had weighed 85 kg (188 lb), but his current weight, 96 kg (212 lb), had been stable for about a year. For his height, 180 cm (5′11″), his BMI was 30.

In the session with the dietitian, George reported that he took a number of food supplements, including garlic capsules, which he sometimes used in place of his antihypertensive medication to save money. The dietitian tried to convince him to stick to his prescribed medication and stop experimenting with supplements and panaceas. A 24-hour dietary recall revealed that George's diet consisted primarily of fast food and convenience foods, because, by his own admission, he did not like to cook. His consumption of fruits and vegetables was low. In fact for the previous day his only vegetable had been French fries. He considered the potatoes interchangeable with a cooked vegetable or a small green salad.

The dietitian suggested he eat foods of low caloric density for breakfast, such as cereal, skim milk, and fruit, which would require little preparation. She also suggested low-fat snacks to be eaten with his beer and substitutes for sweet snacks and desserts. George was resistant to changes in his eating habits, but when the dietitian reinforced the physician's claim that he would feel better, he agreed to try. George made an appointment to see the dietitian the following week to review his progress. Because of the sliding payment schedule he was able to see her regularly. After about three visits, George reported that the changes were not as bad as he expected. Breakfast was simple and he had begun to eat lunch at the local congregate-site meals program. The dietitian helped him plan simple evening meals and snacks. Gradually George began to lose weight. At the suggestion of the recreation leader at the senior center, he joined some other older adults in walking in the early morning at a local shopping mall.

> The congregate-site meals program for older adults is funded by the Elderly Nutrition Program (ENP) from the Administration on Aging.

With the assistance of the dietitian and the nurse at the senior health clinic, George learned to monitor his blood pressure and regulate his food intake, continuing to lose weight. As he began to feel better, he found he could do more. He even started going to dances at the senior center, something he had loved to do when he was younger.

The following year George developed a urinary tract infection. He didn't want to go all the way to his physician's office, so he went to the walk-in clinic near his house. The physician on duty prescribed a sulfa antibiotic without discovering that George was allergic to sulfa drugs. Two days later, George developed hives. He was so miserable that, at the suggestion of his neighbor, he went to her dermatologist, who prescribed an anti-itch medication for allergies of unknown origin. That drug controlled the hives, but caused central nervous system depression and lethargy. George became absent minded and withdrawn and lost interest in his usual activities, even declining to visit his grandchildren.

> Older adults often obtain medication from more than one source without the providers knowing the variety of medications taken.

George's children became concerned because his mind appeared to be "slipping" and wanted him to move in with one of them. George resisted because he did not want to leave his home. His daughter, who visited regularly to help him with some things around the house, continued to have the prescription for the anti-itch medication filled long after he had completed the course of sulfa because no one made the connections between the sulfa and hives or between the anti-itch drug and depression. George appeared to become more depressed, had no appetite, and was losing weight. His daughter became increasingly concerned and took him to the clinic at a local hospital. A third physician put him on medication for depression, promising he would feel better soon. Although he improved somewhat with this medication, George still didn't "perk up" and his family had him evaluated for home healthcare.

> Depression is often associated with decreased appetite and weight loss.

> Side effects of drugs are often unrecognized or misinterpreted.

A nurse from the senior community health program visited George at home to assess his case for home assistance. She discovered that he was taking multiple medications and suggested an appointment with a physician who specializes in geriatrics. This physician took George off all medication. The depression lifted as his mind cleared and he improved dramatically. Eventually the only medications George was taking were a diuretic for hypertension and aspirin for arthritis.

Almost 5 years later George, usually happy and active, began to lose weight and came to the senior center less often. He became fatigued just getting to the center or doing a small amount of grocery shopping. He complained of chest pain and shortness of breath. The diagnosis of advanced atherosclerotic disease resulted in a prescription for a lipid-lowering drug, cholestyramine, and medication to reduce chest pain, in addition to a stronger diuretic and an antiinflammatory agent for arthritis. A walker allowed him to get around more comfortably.

Although George's children encouraged him to move in with one of them, he still valued his independence and wanted to stay in his apartment. The physician's office referred the family to a community services agency of the county health department. Over a period of several weeks, arrangements were made for home nursing visits, assistance with shopping and housekeeping, and a home-delivered meals program on weekdays. Someone from the family would visit several times a week and to make sure George had suitable foods on hand for breakfast and dinner. A community services van took George to medical and dental appointments.

Older adults value independence. Community-based healthcare allows many to remain at home.

Home-delivered meals are essential to allow older adults to live independently. The program George had was near the same ENP site where he went to the congregate-site meals program.

George loved the meals program deliveries and looked forward to lunch and chatting with the driver who delivers his meals. He was much happier at home than anywhere else and the community-based services, including the meals program, allowed him an acceptable quality of life while permitting him to maintain some level of independence.

The volunteer is encouraged to spend some time with the elderly and to check on the welfare of the home-bound elderly and report any health or other problems noted during the visit.

For many older adults like George, the alternative to community-based long-term care is admission to a nursing home care or extended care facility. The high cost of nursing home care depletes the life savings of thousands of older persons every year. In addition the cost of extended healthcare has consumed an ever-growing portion of federal and state government budgets. There will be substantial increases in the need for long-term healthcare as the number of persons age 85 and over (the most frail population group) increases. Because of these growing expenditures, nursing homes can no longer be considered the best solution to meet the needs for services of a functionally compromised older population (Torres-Gil et al., 1995).

PROGRAMS FOR OLDER AMERICANS

Numerous food and nutrition programs and resources are available to support community-based long-term care for older persons. If elderly individuals meet the income guidelines, they are eligible for the regular federal food assistance available to all low-income individuals and families. These include the Food Stamp Program, which improves quality of the diet by increasing food-buying power, and the Surplus Agricultural Commodities Distribution Program, which provides direct food supplements and nutrition education. The surplus program can provide monthly food packages of staple food items, but it is not available in all areas.

Social Security celebrated its sixty-fifth anniversary in the new millennium and Medicare, Medicaid, and the Older Americans Act were 35 years old in 2000. These programs are important in providing services that improve the quality of life of older adults. Optimal nutrition status is essential to the well-being, health, independence, and quality of life for all older adults ranging from the healthy to the frail, vulnerable, and functionally impaired (American Dietetic Association, 1994). Nutrition programs and services do not function in isolation, however. They are an integral part of health and medical services and a broad, comprehensive system that encompasses social and supportive services that allow older adults to remain in their homes and communities.

The Nutrition Program for Older Americans (Title VII) of the Older Americans Act was authorized by Congress in 1972 to provide services such as outreach, escort and transportation, health, information, and referral, and health and welfare counseling and nutrition and consumer education. The 1978 amendments to the Older Americans Act included Title III, which provided funding from the U.S. Dietary Association for congregate and home-delivered meals operated through local area agencies on aging.

The Congregate Site Meals or Dining Program, created in 1965, was the first federal nutrition program specifically designed to improve the diets of older adults. It provides some food security to older Americans with nutritionally balanced meals at little or no cost. These meals are prepared at or delivered to a variety of centrally located public or private community facilities that are accessible to older people. Older persons gather for a nutritious noon meal and social interaction and nutrition education. Meals are usually available 5 days a week in urban settings and 2 to 3 days a week in rural communities, which may rotate the site throughout the county for better access. Depending on location, congregate meals participants have access to a variety of support services such as shopping assistance, medical assistance and referral, transportation, weatherization, and fuel assistance. Meals programs are often located in community facilities, which may provide access to other programs such as recreation, fitness, or even legal assistance.

The congregate-site meals or dining programs have numerous benefits:

- provide meals that meet one third of the daily dietary standards
- are available at little or no cost to the participant
- are served at centrally located sites
- promote social interaction
- allow access to a variety of support services

The average cost of a meal (including cost of volunteer time and donations):

- meal at congregate site: $5.17
- home-delivered meal: $5.31

For decades there have been home-delivered meals programs throughout the United States. Often referred to as Meals on Wheels, such programs frequently were operated by nonprofit community organizations that delivered hot meals to those unable to get out or to prepare meals for themselves. Usually the meals, delivered by volunteers, were prepared by the food service of local hospitals, nursing homes, schools, or churches. The Home Delivered Meals Program funded by Title III is designed to provide nutritious meals for homebound persons. Meals are delivered to the individual's home by couriers or volunteers. In addition to supporting nutritional needs for the older adult, the program provides regular human contact. The courier may be the only person the housebound individual sees during the day. In some locations a cold meal for supper or food for breakfast the next morning is delivered with the noon meal. For many older adults this program is essential to their ability to get an adequate diet and to continue to live independently.

Because resources are limited, the Meals programs strive to target higher-risk older persons. Risk is usually defined as advanced age (usually over age 80 years), low income, social isolation, minority status, mobility impairment, or limited ability to speak English. Many participants have a high level of risk for nutritional deficiency. A Congressionally mandated evaluation of the ENP found that its participants had higher daily intake of key nutrients than nonparticipants in similar circumstances and that participants had more social contacts as a result of the program (Neyman et al., 1996).

In 1998 the Federal Administration on Aging distributed almost $470 million to 57 states and territories and an additional $17 million to Indian tribes, earmarked for both congregate and home-delivered nutrition services (Administration on Aging, 2000). Funds from the United States Department of Agriculture Cash and Commodity Program, participant donations, and state and local sources added to Area Office on Aging (OAA) funding brought the total to over $1 billion a year for nutrition programs.

More than 240 million meals were served in 1998 through a network of more than 2200 Title III Elderly Nutrition Projects (Title III Elderly Nutrition Program Data, 2001). Of those meals, 45% were provided in the homes of the elderly. There were almost 16,000 meal sites in operation every day.

The ideal systems of long-term care are a continuum of home- and community-based services and institutional care, housing alternatives such as assisted living, transportation, nutrition, and other social services (Torres-Gil et al., 1995). Nutrition services, specifically meals delivered to those living at home, are a fundamental core service necessary for keeping functionally limited older people in their homes and in the community.

REFERENCES

Administration on Aging: A profile of older Americans, Washington, DC, 2000, U.S. Department of Health and Human Services, American Association of Retired Persons.

American Dietetic Association: Position of the American Dietetic Association: nutrition, aging and the continuum of health care, J Am Diet Assoc 94:80, 1994.

Neyman MR et al.: Effect of participation in congregate-site meal programs on nutritional status of the healthy elderly, J Am Diet Assoc 96:475, 1996.

Title III Elderly Nutrition Program Data: U.S. Administration on Aging, Washington, DC, OFO (OPCA) 98-63, Feb 14, 2001.

Torres-Gil FM et al.: Role of elderly nutrition in home and community-based care, Persp Appl Nutr 2:9, 1995.

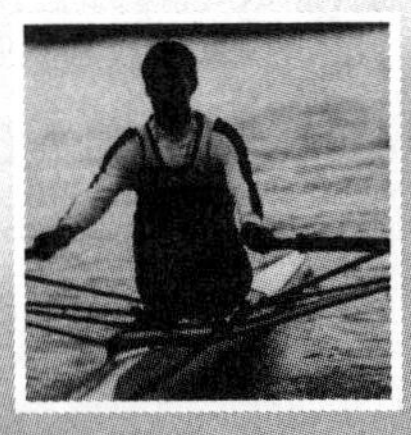

PART FIVE

SPECIAL CONCERNS ACROSS THE LIFE SPAN

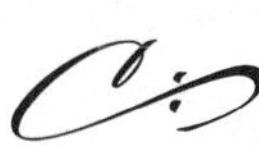

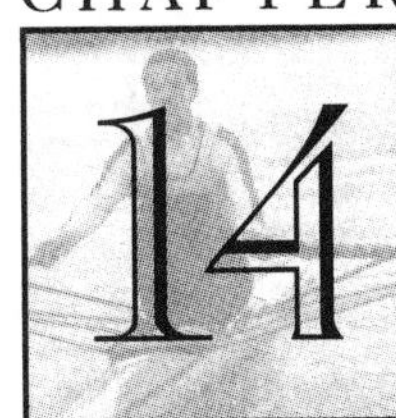

CHAPTER 14 Eating Dilemmas: Dietary Restraint, Binging, Purging, Excessive Consumption, and Excessive Exercise

Chapter Outline

Emily is a 35-year-old housewife who is 173 cm (68 in) tall and weighs 48 kg (106 lb; reference weight is 140 lb). She weighed 127 kg (280 lb) or more for most of her adult life, but she began to lose weight after her father died a year ago. Now she refuses to stop her weight-loss routine. Emily has numerous rituals that interfere with her life and that of her family. She has many cleaning compulsions. She does not allow guests in her home and, if someone visits unexpectedly, she spends hours cleaning after they leave. She insists on eating the same thing every day and at the same time and place. Her husband tolerates her peculiarities, but is concerned that she eats so little and has lost so much weight. Emily's last menstrual period was 8 months ago. She frequently complains of being cold, sleeps poorly at night, and thinks her hair is thinner. She spends at least 2 hours each day exercising, using two different aerobic tapes. If she feels fatter than usual, she exercises for an additional hour.

A typical dietary pattern for Emily is breakfast at 7:00 AM, consisting of one piece of dry whole-wheat toast and one cup of regular coffee. Lunch at noon is one piece of fruit (usually an apple or orange), 6 ounces of low-fat yogurt, and two glasses of diet cola. Emily is a good cook. She always prepares a balanced meal for her family and dinner is always at 6:00 PM. However, Emily eats only a slice of whole-wheat toast, one-half cup of cottage cheese, and a glass of water. At bedtime she allows herself two crackers and another piece of fresh fruit. Originally Emily planned to stop dieting when she reached 50 kg (110 lbs), but when she reached that point she refused to change her routine and rebuffed suggestions that she add more foods to her diet. She continued to lose weight. After reaching 110 lbs, it was apparent that her dieting was out of control. At the insistence of her physician, Emily began to see a counselor who attempted to involve her in psychotherapy to motivate her to eat. By that time, Emily was so cognitively impaired by starvation that she was unable to respond to the proposed therapy. When Emily reached 41 kg (90 lb) about 2 months later, she was hospitalized near death.

Eating is controlled by many factors, including appetite, food availability, family, peers, social and cultural practices, and attempts at voluntary control. At times initially voluntary behaviors such as eating small or large amounts of food move beyond control in some individuals. In the extreme, eating dilemmas evolve into severe disturbances in eating behavior, extreme and unhealthy reductions in food intake or severe overeating, and distress or extreme concern about body shape or weight. At any age mild deviations from the norm are common and occur with great variation. Eating disorders tend to be classified on the basis of their visible end result (extreme thinness or fatness) or on the basis of variations in eating patterns (fasting, food restriction, binge eating, excess exercise). The most common eating disorder is obesity (Figure 14-1). At the other end of the spectrum is anorexia nervosa, a disorder characterized by extreme thinness. Other disorders, such as bulimia nervosa, binge eating disorder (BED), or excess exercise may be associated with normal body weights, but represent behaviors characteristic of disordered eating.

Overweight and obesity are rapidly increasing in prevalence (Must et al., 1999) and are becoming major health problems in the United States (Mokdad et al., 1999). More than 50% of Americans are overweight and the preventable deaths attributed to obesity exceed 300,000 per year (Allison et al., 1999). The economic burden approximates $100 billion (Thompson et al., 1999). Current treatment approaches for obesity have not been very effective and many overweight and obese individuals attempt to achieve reduced weight with a wide variety of approaches, some nutritionally sound, others endorsing irrational and sometimes unsafe practices.

In affluent countries cultural perpetuation of slimness has created an unrealistic standard for **body image** for women and, to a lesser extent, for men (Abrams et al., 1994). Preoccupation with body weight and appearance contribute to food-related behaviors that range from dietary restraint to binging and purging.

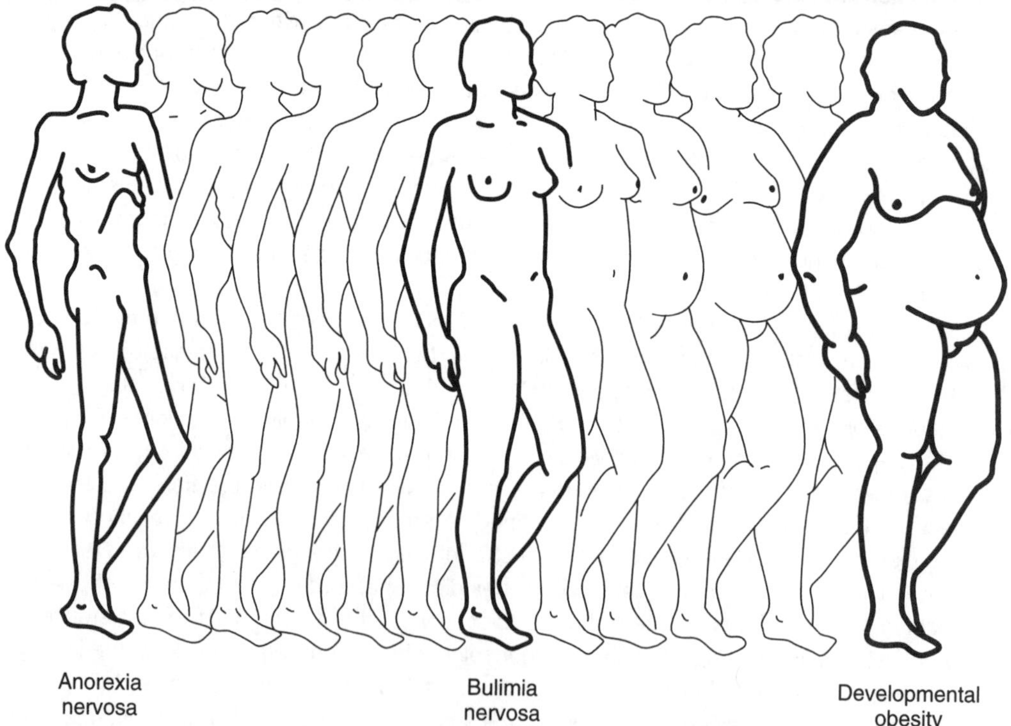

Figure 14-1 The spectrum of eating disorders. Although physical conditions vary, underlying phychologic characteristics are held in common across the spectrum. *(From Grodner M, Anderson SL, and DeYoung S: Foundations and clinical applications of nutrition: a nursing approach, ed 2, St. Louis, 2000, Mosby.)*

Excess concerns about body weight may be manifest in severe disturbances in eating behavior that may be associated with variations of body weight, but which, regardless of weight status, are characterized by behaviors classified as eating disorders. Among women an estimated 0.5% to 3.7% suffer from anorexia nervosa, 1.1% to 4.2% have bulimia nervosa, and 2% to 5% have binge-eating disorder in their lifetimes (National Institutes of Mental Health, 2001). It is estimated that 5% to 15% of people with anorexia or bulimia and 35% of those with binge eating disorder are male. Eating disorders frequently co-occur with other psychiatric disorders such as depression, substance abuse, and anxiety disorders. In addition persons with eating disorders may experience a wide range of physical health complications.

The American Psychiatric Association (1998) has established diagnostic criteria for eating disorders. The most recent edition of the *Diagnostic and Statistical Manual for Mental Disorders* (DSM-IV) includes anorexia nervosa and bulimia nervosa and subtypes within each group. A new provisional category, "eating disorders not yet specified," is reserved for disorders of eating that do not meet the criteria for anorexia nervosa or bulimia nervosa.

Eating disorders are not from a failure of will or behavior; rather they are real, treatable medical illnesses in which certain maladaptive patterns of eating take on a life of their own (American Psychiatric Association, 2000). Although various forms of **disordered eating** have been described, an individual is likely to manifest symptoms or characteristics of more than one disorder. For example 30% to 80% of those who meet diagnostic criteria for bulimia nervosa have a history of anorexia nervosa (Becker et al., 1999) and individuals with anorexia nervosa and bulimia nervosa often use excessive exercise as another method to control body weight.

ANOREXIA NERVOSA

- *What is anorexia nervosa?*
- *Do eating disorders serve a purpose for the individual?*
- *What factors predispose an individual to anorexia nervosa?*
- *What are the signs, symptoms, and complications of anorexia nervosa?*
- *How is anorexia nervosa treated? How successful is treatment?*

Definition and Incidence

Anorexia nervosa is characterized by self-imposed starvation resulting in excessive weight loss. The affected individual has a distorted body image and an intense fear of becoming fat even when underweight. The diagnostic criteria for anorexia nervosa established by the American Psychiatric Association are listed in Box 14-1. Traditionally the typical individual with anorexia nervosa has been described as a young, achievement-oriented, perfectionist female from a successful Caucasian middle- or upper-class family with high expectations of achievement for his or her offspring. Over the past decade, however, anorexia nervosa has been noted in males (Strober et al., 2001) and in all ethnic (Chamoro and Flores-Ortiz, 2000) and socioeconomic groups (Becker et al., 1999). An estimated 0.5% to 3.7% of women suffer from anorexia nervosa in their lifetimes (American Psychiatric Association, 2000).

Etiology

The etiology of anorexia nervosa is multifactorial, encompassing societal, biologic, psychologic, and familial factors. The role of society is the cultural focus on being slender, which drives a youngster to the pursuit of thinness. Anecdotal records of cases of anorexia nervosa indicate that restrictive food behavior can be triggered by

> **KEY TERMS**
>
> **body image:** a person's perception of the physical size and appearance of the body that includes the attitudes, feelings, and behavioral reactions of the individual regarding his or her body; body image is central to how individuals feel about themselves
>
> **disordered eating:** restrained eating, binge eating, fear of fatness, purging, and disordered body image

Box 14-1 DSM-IV Diagnostic Criteria for Anorexia Nervosa

A. Refusal to maintain body weight at or above a minimally normal weight for age and height (e.g., weight loss leading to maintenance of body weight less than 85% of that expected; or failure to make expected weight gain during period of growth, leading to body weight less than 85% of that expected)
B. Intense fear of gaining weight or becoming fat, even though underweight
C. Disturbance in the way in which one's body weight or shape is experienced; undue influence of body weight or shape on self-evaluation, or denial of the seriousness of the current body weight
D. In postmenarchal females, amenorrhea (i.e., the absence of at least three consecutive menstrual cycles). (A woman is considered to have amenorrhea if her periods occur only following hormone [e.g., estrogen] administration.)

SPECIFY TYPE:

Restricting type: During the episode of anorexia nervosa the person does not regularly engage in binge eating or purging behavior (i.e., self-induced vomiting or the misuse of laxatives or diuretics).

Binge eating/purging type: During the episode of anorexia nervosa, the person regularly engages in binge-eating or purging behavior (i.e., self-induced vomiting or the misuse of laxatives or diuretics).

something as small as a passing comment by a parent or peer suggesting the individual is heavy or overweight.

More than 3 decades ago persons with eating disorders were observed to have disturbances in perception and interpretation of visceral and emotional stimuli and a sense of ineffectiveness (Bruch, 1973). Recent studies have found that, unlike their peers not suffering from the disorder, adolescents with anorexia nervosa have low scores on measures of body- and self-image, social relationships, and sexual attitudes (Gupta and Johnson, 2000) and less self-liking and self-competence (Silver et al., 1998).

Many studies have shown relationships among anxiety, depression, and life stress and eating disorders (Lennkh et al., 1998). Adolescents with eating disorders have more first- and second-degree relatives with eating disorders and more first-degree relatives with depression and alcoholism.

Family dysfunction often exists for a long time before the onset of illness. Typical family characteristics are success orientation, rigidity, overprotectiveness, enmeshment, and avoidance of conflict. There is generally poor communication within the family, unrealistic expectations for achievement, and belittling, rejection, or neglect. Individuals with anorexia nervosa often struggle for autonomy, identity, self-esteem, and self-control. They feel out of control, insecure, and ineffective. Control of diet and body weight may give them a sense of control, confidence, and autonomy.

Characteristics

Emily is older than the "typical" anorexic, but the pattern of her behavior is representative of a sequence of events that might occur. The term anorexia is a misnomer. In actuality anorexics are preoccupied with thoughts of food and may be intensely hungry, but they are even more concerned with a terror of fat that causes high degrees of dietary restraint. Individuals with anorexia may repeatedly monitor body weight and engage in techniques to control body weight, such as intense exercise, purging by vomiting, abuse of laxatives, enemas or diuretics.

Psychologic Characteristics

Individuals with anorexia nervosa have a distorted image of their body. Although they can accurately perceive the relative body fatness of other individuals, they are unable to perceive themselves as anything but fat. Even a woman who is 170 cm (67 in) tall and weighs 39 kg (85 lb) with a body mass index (BMI) of 14 will maintain that she is too fat.

In addition to morbid fear of gaining weight and denial of the degree of emaciation, anorexia nervosa is characterized by obsessive-compulsive behaviors, some of which may relate to dietary intake, such as detailed calorie counting, ritualistic eating mannerisms, recipe collection, and food hoarding (Rosenvinge et al., 2000; Thiel et al., 1995). Persons with anorexia nervosa tend to be perfectionists who struggle to live up to performance standards, which are often self-imposed. Furthermore the anorexic is plagued by a pervasive sense of personal ineffectiveness. Distorted perceptions of stimuli arising in the body allow the individual to deny feelings of hunger and fatigue, resulting in semistarvation or exercising beyond the point of exhaustion for most individuals. Another characteristic, increasing social isolation, can be an early clue of potential problems for parents and teachers.

Physical Characteristics

Many characteristics distinguish anorexia nervosa from other eating disorders. The most significant characteristic is intentional, severe loss of body weight. The anorexic will refuse to eat and refuse to maintain a body weight that is within 15% of the expected weight-for-height.

Unchecked anorexia nervosa can result in a multitude of health problems and even death (Box 14-2). Anorexia nervosa has the highest mortality rate of any psychiatric disorder. The mortality rate among persons with anorexia has been estimated to be 0.56% per year, which is approximately 12 times the annual rate for all causes among girls and women 15 years to 24 years of age (Sullivan, 1995). Most of the complications of anorexia nervosa are the result of severe weight loss caused by inadequate food intake and, in some cases, purging. Starvation itself causes sleep disturbances, impaired concentration, irritability, anxiety, depression, and preoccupation with food (Garfinkel and Kaplan, 1985; Turner and Shapiro, 1992).

In early stages the complications of malnutrition are reversible with increased food intake and weight gain. The catabolic state of anorexia results in decreased body weight, decreased muscle mass, and declines in stores of body fat and depletion of liver and muscle glycogen. The decline in the basal metabolic rate is one of the body's mechanisms to maintain itself during the shortage of energy intake. A loss of the ability to regulate body temperature causes the individual to complain of feeling cold, especially in the extremities.

Severe weight loss results in decreased secretion of estrogen from the ovary and decreased secretion of the follicle-stimulating hormone (FSH) from the pituitary gland, which causes

Box 14-2 Complications of Eating Disorders

ANOREXIA NERVOSA

Dizziness, confusion
Dry skin
Dry, brittle hair
Lanugo-type hair
Low blood pressure, low pulse, bradycardia
Weight loss
Reduced metabolic rate and malnutrition
Muscle wasting, reduced body fat, hypothermia
Growth failure; delayed sexual maturation
Decreased estrogen secretion
Amenorrhea
Decreased bone mass
Decreased follicle-stimulating hormone secretion
Decreased kidney function (reduced glomerular filtration rate)
Dehydration
Delayed gastric emptying
Constipation; fecal impaction

BULIMIA NERVOSA

Frequent weight fluctuations
Irregular menses
WITH VOMITING
- Parotid (salivary) gland enlargement
- Erosion of dental enamel, dental caries
- Esophageal dysmotility, esophagitis, impaired gastric emptying
- Calluses on knuckles

WITH LAXATIVE ABUSE
- Alternating diarrhea, constipation

WITH VOMITING AND LAXATIVE OR DIURETIC ABUSE
- Hypokalemia
- Hypochloremia
- Metabolic alkalosis
- Dehydration
- Arrhythmia

amenorrhea (Stewart, 1992). With weight gain, normal cycles usually, but not always, return. A long-term complication of estrogen deficiency is **osteopenia**. Adolescents with anorexia nervosa accompanied by amenorrhea have deficits in bone mass of 10% to 30% compared with age- and sex-matched control subjects (Wong et al., 2001). Unfortunately the age at which anorexia most frequently occurs is a critical stage of development of maximum bone mass, which is related to long-term bone health (Matkovic, 1992).

Severe weight loss can have an effect on many body functions, including those of the heart, kidneys, and gastrointestinal tract. Cardiac manifestations include decreased cardiac output, **bradycardia**, **tachycardia**, arrhythmias, and hypotension. As kidney function decreases, the **glomerular filtration rate (GFR)** declines, resulting in increased levels of solutes in the blood and associated dehydration.

Chronic restriction of food intake can result in delays in gastric emptying and intestinal motility. In the absence of the stimulus of food, function of the colon may decline, resulting in chronic constipation and increasing the risk of **fecal impaction**. Some anorexics may induce vomiting or abuse laxatives or diuretics, which further complicates their medical condition. (Such abuse is discussed later in this chapter in the section on bulimia nervosa). Induction of vomiting, in addition to lowering body weight, can lead to fluid and electrolyte depletion and potentially to **alkalosis**, hypochloremia (low blood chloride), and hypokalemia (low blood potassium).

Treatment

Treatment of anorexia nervosa is complex and requires an ongoing, comprehensive plan to deal with multiple problems. Many individuals have lived with their illness for years and treatment involves a long-term commitment from both the patient and the treatment provider. Success of treatment can be predicted by certain prognostic signs (Box 14-3). Individuals with good prognostic signs may respond to outpatient treatment—usually a combination of individual and family psychotherapy and nutrition counseling. Those with poor prognostic signs are likely to require long-term treatment and possibly hospitalization if weight loss has been so prolonged or so rapid that life-threatening complications must be averted.

Box 14-3 Prognostic Signs for Recovery from Anorexia Nervosa

GOOD PROGNOSTIC SIGNS FOR RECOVERY

Young age of onset, recent onset
Normal premorbid weight
No bulimic symptomatology
Insignificant family pathology

POOR PROGNOSTIC SIGNS FOR RECOVERY

Late onset, long duration
Low body weight
Weight has decreased by 25%
Presence of bulimic symptoms
Disturbed relationships with family
Concomitant psychiatric illness
Severe metabolic disorders
Failed previous treatment
Greater social difficulties
Increased somatic or obsessional disorders

As eating disorders become more entrenched, the behaviors and their consequences become less reversible. It is hoped that the sooner the weight loss is stopped, the greater the chances are for a more complete recovery (Fisher et al., 1995).

The aims of treatment are to restore normal eating patterns, establish normal body weight, and resolve underlying psychologic conflicts. It is often easier to change eating behaviors than to correct psychologic problems, but long-term recovery depends on the resolution of the underlying conflicts. Currently the most successful early therapies are multidisciplinary approaches that incorporate weight restoration accompanied by individual and family psychotherapy (American Psychiatric Association, 2000).

Restoring Body Weight

Intervention involves nutrition education, counseling, and management (American Dietetic Association, 1994). The highest priority for treatment of anorexia nervosa is to reverse the individual's poor nutrition status. The first goal is cessation of weight loss. It is important to improve nutrition status even while the individual maintains a low weight and then to encourage gradual weight gain through self-feeding. It is essential to recognize that an anorexic in a state of starvation is cognitively impaired and a poor candidate for psychotherapy. Thus weight resolution is a prerequisite to other treatment modalities.

For the most severe cases, hospitalization and nutrition replacement via parenteral or nasogastric tube feeding may be appropriate to reverse potentially fatal self-starvation. Such feeding may increase medical and psychologic risks, and **refeeding** must be monitored carefully. Medical risks include fluid retention and changes in electrolyte and mineral status. Significant psychologic risks of rapid refeeding are associated with the patient's perceived loss of control, loss of identity, increased body distortion, and mistrust of the treatment team (American Dietetic Association, 1994).

Treatment involves a careful nutrition assessment, determination of caloric need, and design of an appropriate diet plan for weight maintenance followed by the gradual progression to meet weight gain expectations and, finally, design of a diet plan for maintenance of an acceptable weight. Guidelines for nutrition therapy appear in Box 14-4. Nutrition rehabilitation must be performed slowly. Treatment usually begins with a caloric level that is 130% of the resting energy expenditure (REE). When available, indirect calorimetry measurements of REE serve as the basis for energy intake calculations. If **indirect calorimetry** is not available, the Harris-Benedict equations for the prediction of REE, with an adjustment for the hypometabolic state, have been used with the following formulas:

Resting Energy Expenditure:

Females:

$$\text{REE (kcal)} = 655 + (9.56 \times \text{wt [kg]}) + (1.85 \times \text{ht [cm]}) - (4.68 \times \text{age [yr]})$$

Males:

$$\text{REE (kcal)} = 66.5 + (13.75 \times \text{wt [kg]}) + (5.0 \times \text{ht [cm]}) - (6.78 \times \text{age [yr]})$$

Using this formula for Emily at the point at which she was admitted to the hospital would yield the following:

$$\text{REE} = 655 + (9.56 \times 41) + (1.85 \times 173) - (4.68 \times 35)$$

$$\text{REE} = 655 + 392 + 320 - 164$$

$$\text{REE} = 1203 \text{ kcal}$$

The calculation is then adjusted for the hypometabolic rate as follows:

$$1.84 - \text{calculated REE (1193)} - 1435$$

$$2195 - 1435 = 760 \text{ kcal}$$

(adjusted REE for anorexia nervosa)

As the anorexic improves with refeeding, the resting metabolic rate increases beyond that which can be explained by the increased body mass alone (Obarzanek et al., 1994; Salisbury et al., 1995). Therefore caloric requirements for weight restoration may be greater than anticipated and monitoring of the response of the individual will be necessary to plan increases in dietary intake. The expected rate of weight gain varies among treatment programs, but a rate of 0.36 lb per day has been shown to be safe in adolescents with anorexia nervosa (Solanto et al., 1994). Successful refeeding programs can lead to

KEY TERMS

osteopenia: reduced bone mass from a decreased rate of synthesis to a level insufficient to compensate for breakdown

bradycardia: abnormally slow heart rate

tachycardia: abnormally rapid heart beat

glomerular filtration rate (GFR): rate at which the kidney filters blood; when the rate is decreased, the blood may contain substances ordinarily filtered out by the normal kidney

fecal impaction: a collection of hardened feces in the rectum or sigmoid colon

alkalosis: a condition resulting from accumulations of base or a decrease of acid (hydrogen ion) in body fluids characterized by an increase in pH

refeeding: the introduction of regular table foods

indirect calorimetry: measurement of oxygen used or carbon dioxide exhaled by the body to estimate energy expenditure

Box 14-4 Guidelines for Nutrition Therapy in Anorexia Nervosa and Bulimia Nervosa

ANOREXIA NERVOSA

Energy

1.3 × REE* for weight gain
Initial caloric prescriptions: generally in the range of 1000 kcal to 1400 kcal per day
Additional kcal for physical activity
Increase daily caloric prescription to promote steady weight gain: 100 kcal increments in early treatment; 200 kcal increments in late treatment

Macronutrients

Protein: minimum 0.8 g/kg target body weight
Carbohydrate: 50%-55% kcal
Encourage dietary fiber to reduce constipation
Fat: 25%-30% kcal

Micronutrients

100% DRI (RDA or AI)
Multivitamin supplement may be necessary

BULIMIA NERVOSA

Energy

Weight maintenance
1.2 × REE for sedentary activity
1.3 × REE for moderate activity
Monitor anthropometric status and adjust caloric prescription for weight maintenance.
Avoid weight reduction diets until eating patterns and body weight have stabilized.

Macronutrients

Protein: minimum 0.8 g/kg target body weight
Carbohydrate: 50%-55% kcal
Encourage water-soluble fiber to reduce constipation
Fat: 25%-30% kcal

Micronutrients

100% DRI (RDA or AI)
Multivitamin supplement may be necessary

Adapted with permission from Luder E, Schebendach J: Nutrition management of eating disorders, Top Clin Nutr 8(3):59-60, 1993. © 1993 Aspen Publishers, Inc.
*REE, resting energy expenditure. Can be measured by indirect calorimetry or calculated using the Harris-Benedict equation.

significant increases in body weight of which up to 50% may be fat (Probst et al., 2001).

Dietary education, counseling, and management are important components of overall treatment for anorexia nervosa. Nutrition therapy for eating disorders is usually a lengthy process (American Dietetic Association, 1994). It can be divided into an education phase and an experimental phase (Box 14-5). The primary focus of the education phase is to provide nutrition information and patient interaction is limited. The experimental phase is based on a long-term counseling relationship between the client and the registered dietitian (RD), who is part of the multidisciplinary treatment team. The experimental phase requires a dietitian with training and experience in the area of eating disorders.

Initial use of small quantities of food may meet the psychologic need of a person with anorexia nervosa who is fearful of gaining weight rapidly and becoming fat. Dietary patterns usually consist of three meals a day plus snacks. Oral liquid supplements may be of value in meeting caloric needs, because the person suffering from anorexia nervosa typically has problems consuming the increased amounts of food required for weight gain.

Treating Psychologic Disturbances

For the individual with anorexia nervosa to develop autonomy, he or she must identify feelings and their relationship to behavior. Individual psychotherapy facilitates personal growth, helping individuals to take responsibility for themselves. Counseling is likely to be required for several years. Issues specific to adolescents involve assertiveness, educational achievement, social skills, family interaction, substance use, and sexual behavior.

Behavior modification. The behavioral component of treatment provides the structure needed for anorexics to interfere with their self-destructive behaviors. It usually begins with strict monitoring of behavior. As an individual is better able to contain the deleterious behavior, the amount of autonomy and responsibility received increases. In this system the client agrees to a

Box 14-5 Phases of Nutrition Therapy for Eating Disorders

EDUCATION PHASE

The dietitian educates the client about his or her eating disorder. The dietitian:

- Collects relevant information.
- Establishes a collaborative relationship with the client.
- Defines and discusses relevant principles and concepts of food, nutrition, and weight regulation.
- Presents examples of typical hunger patterns, food intake patterns, and caloric intakes of someone who has recovered.
- Works to educate the family.

EXPERIMENTAL PHASE

The dietitian helps the client make changes in food- and weight-related behaviors in a safe environment. The client:

- Separates food- and weight-related behaviors from feelings and psychological issues.
- Makes gradual, incremental changes in food behaviors until food intake patterns are normalized.
- Slows increase or decrease in weight.
- Learns to maintain a weight that is healthful for the individual without using abnormal food- and weight-related behaviors.
- Learns to be comfortable in social eating situations.

From The American Dietetic Association: Position of the American Dietetic Association: nutrition intervention in the treatment of anorexia nervosa, bulimia nervosa and binge eating, J Am Diet Assoc 94:900, 1994. Copyright The American Dietetic Association. Reprinted by permission from Journal of the American Dietetic Association.

contract with a predetermined target weight to be rewarded with a variety of privileges. Initially physical exercise is kept to a minimum to avoid increases in energy expenditure.

Family Therapy

It is important for adolescents to identify the underlying dysfunctional family patterns that have prohibited development of independence. Involving parents is essential in building an alliance between the treatment team and the family and client because young adolescents are not emotionally or situationally autonomous. Later in the course of treatment, family therapy should center on separation and autonomy, family expression of feelings, and conflict resolution.

Achieving Long-Term Remission

Use of psychotropic medication in people with anorexia nervosa should be considered only after weight gain has been established and when the psychologic effects of undernutrition are resolving. Undernourished patients may be less responsive to medication and more prone to side effects. Certain serotonin reuptake inhibitors have been helpful for weight maintenance and resolving mood and anxiety symptoms associated with anorexia. No single medication has proven to be especially effective for treating anorexia nervosa (Fisher et al., 1995).

Prognosis

Anorexia nervosa is a chronic condition that requires long-term treatment programs to prevent **relapse**. For treatment to be successful, the chronic nature of the disorder must be considered. Follow-up studies of seriously ill anorexics show that 40% to 50% recovered. Another 25% showed some improvement, but for approximately 30%, the illness is chronic and marked by a relapsing course that requires repeated hospitalization (Mayer, 2001). Criteria of recovery were normal stable body weight (within 15% of recommended levels) and establishment of regular menses. Studies of milder cases of anorexia nervosa indicate as many as two thirds of recovering anorexics still worried about body shape and had persistent abnormal eating behavior years after "recovery."

KEY TERMS

relapse: return of symptoms at least weekly for a minimum of 2 months

Sue is 163 cm (64 in) tall and weighs 50 kg (109 lb). Her reference weight range is 51 kg to 58 kg (113 to 128 lb). Sue weighed about 55 kg (120 lb) when she was 15 years old. She started dieting when her best friend suggested she would look really great if she were thinner. During her senior year in high school, Sue discovered that if she ate and immediately vomited, she could achieve almost the same effect as her restrictive diet.

Her daily intake pattern is to skip breakfast. If her mother insists that she eat before going to school, she vomits before she leaves. Lunch is a diet cola or a piece of fruit. Sue has cheese and crackers or a candy bar before tennis practice and she eats a large evening meal. She snacks most of the evening while studying or watching television. She usually vomits before going to bed. In addition she takes laxatives, usually 3 to 4 every night, unless she feels really fat, in which case she may take up to 30. Sue really likes the new freedom she has found to eat, but she doesn't like the fact that she feels bad most of the time. She is chronically depressed and spends less time with friends because her binging rituals take up a great deal of time. Frequently she feels faint after long spells of vomiting or during her nightly diarrhea. Although Sue wants to stop the binging/purging pattern, she desperately wants to keep her weight under control and is not sure she can stop. She feels miserable most of the time.

BULIMIA NERVOSA

- *What are the signs and symptoms of bulimia nervosa? Who is at greatest risk?*
- *Describe binging and purging.*
- *What are the biologic, social, and emotional factors that predispose an individual to bulimia nervosa?*
- *What are the health risks of bulimia nervosa?*
- *How is bulimia nervosa treated?*

Definition and Incidence

In contrast to anorexia nervosa, individuals with bulimia nervosa have recurrent episodes in which they **binge** on copious amounts of food. Because of guilt over that extreme consumption, they tend to have recurrent inappropriate compensatory behaviors including **purging**, fasting, or excessive exercise to get rid of the excess food or calories they have consumed. They will use a variety of inappropriate **compensatory behaviors** to prevent weight gain. Current diagnostic criteria for bulimia nervosa established by the American Psychiatric Association (1998) appear in Box 14-6. This disorder is estimated to affect between 1.1% and 4.2% of women sometime during their lifetime (American Psychiatric Association, 2000). Bulimia nervosa occurs much less frequently in males (less than 5%) and is often associated with a history of sexual identity concerns, obesity, defensive dieting, or dieting in relation to sports participation (Carlat and Camargo, 1991).

Etiology

Although the causes of bulimia nervosa have been elusive and uncertain, it has been proposed that bulimic behavior may serve to reduce tension, help regulate the self, and provide stimulation needed to dampen feelings of emptiness. Biologic, psychologic, and environmental factors appear to be related to the development of bulimic behavior. Underlying issues are societal pressures, lack of **self-esteem**, and perceptions of body image and appearance.

Restrictive dieting produces abnormal eating behaviors, which may disturb intake and satiety regulation mechanisms. It may be related to dieting and its associated hunger and emotional precipitants, which lead to binging and then, eventually, to purging. The cycle perpetuates a caloric deficit, and biology drives overeating. Several theories have been postulated to explain the biologic mechanism of disordered satiety associated with bulimic behaviors. A decrease in the secretion of **cholecystokinin** in in-

Box 14-6 DSM-IV Diagnostic Criteria: Bulimia Nervosa

A. Recurrent episodes of binge eating. An episode of binge eating is characterized by both of the following:
   1. Eating, in a discrete period (e.g., within any 2-hour period), an amount of food that is definitely larger than most people would eat during a similar period and under similar circumstances.
   2. A sense of lack of control over eating during the episode (e.g., a feeling that one cannot stop eating or control what or how much one is eating).

B. Recurrent inappropriate compensatory behavior to prevent weight gain, such as self-induced vomiting; misuse of laxatives, diuretics, or other medications; fasting; or excessive exercise.

C. The binge eating and inappropriate compensatory behaviors both occur, on average, at least twice a week for 3 months.

D. Self-evaluation is unduly influenced by body shape and weight.

E. The disturbance does not occur exclusively during episodes of anorexia nervosa.

SPECIFY TYPE:

Purging type: During the current episode of bulimia nervosa, the person has regularly engaged in self-induced vomiting or the misuse of laxatives, diuretics, or enemas.

Nonpurging type: During the current episode of bulimia nervosa, the person uses other inappropriate compensatory behaviors, such as fasting or excessive exercise, but does not regularly engage in self-induced vomiting or the misuse of laxatives, diuretics, or enemas.

dividuals with bulimia nervosa may contribute to decreased satiety and the consequent binging behavior.

Other possible contributors to disordered satiety involve neurotransmitters (serotonin, catecholamines, opiates) of the central nervous system. Most research has focused on serotonin and its dietary precursor, the amino acid tryptophan. It may be that low levels of 5-hydroxyindoleacetic acid, a metabolite of serotonin, contribute to diminished activity of satiety-related pathways regulated by serotonin, thereby contributing to bulimic symptoms. Additional evidence for such an effect is the fact that antidepressant medications that increase available serotonin have met with success in the treatment of bulimia nervosa.

In bulimia nervosa, self-concept and self-esteem play critical causal roles. Adolescents particularly experience significantly lower self-esteem, more self-regulating difficulties, frustration intolerance, and impaired ability to express feelings compared with adolescents without eating disorders. The psychologic component may also be associated with food restriction, which leads to a decreased frustration tolerance and a decreased sense of well-being. Symptoms of anxiety and depression are more common among those with clinical and subclinical bulimia nervosa.

Characteristics

Bulimia nervosa is characterized by alternating episodes of binging and purging. Figure 14-2 illustrates a cycle of events that is characteristic of bulimia: anxiety, binge eating, guilt, purging, semistarvation, obsession, hunger, and binging.

The individual has a sense of being unable to control eating once a binge begins. A binge is terminated only by abdominal pain, sleep, social interruption, or vomiting. The loss of control results

KEY TERMS

binge: rapid consumption of large quantities of food

purging: self-induced vomiting, overuse of laxatives or other medications, or use of diuretics or enemas

compensatory behaviors: purging, starvation, and excessive exercise

self-esteem: confidence and satisfaction with one's self

cholecystokinin: a hormone that stimulates release of bile and produces satiety in humans

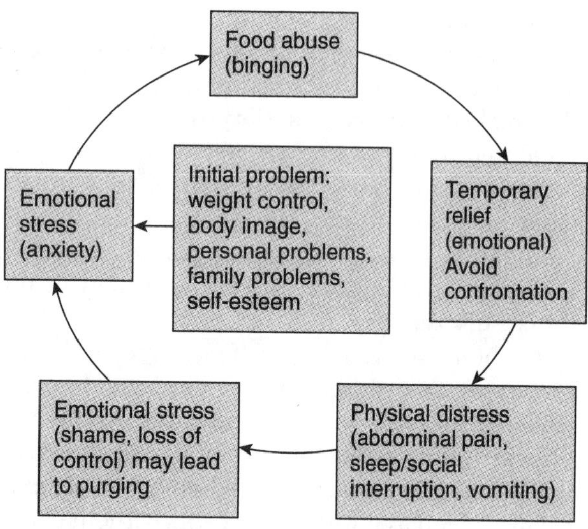

Figure 14-2 The dynamics of the food abuse process.

in shame and guilt, which in turn are usually followed by purging. In many instances, guilt for having lost control results in severe dietary restraint until stress, hunger, or both again precipitate a binging and purging episode. These behaviors have many medical consequences (see Box 14-2).

Bulimic individuals are aware that their eating pattern is abnormal, but for most bulimics binging episodes are secret and they deny the presence of the problem to other people. There are two major differences between bulimia nervosa and anorexia nervosa; that is, the individual with bulimia nervosa does not feel as personally ineffective as the individual with anorexia nervosa and is more aware of his or her emotions, even if unable to control them.

Purging

A variety of behaviors may be used to purge excess calories to control body weight, including vigorous exercise, use of diuretics, induction of vomiting, use of laxatives, and use of **sorbitol** to cause diarrhea. Purging behaviors have major health consequences (see Box 14-2).

Vomiting

About 60% to 80% of bulimics vomit repeatedly to rid themselves of huge quantities of food. Some use the **emetic ipecac**, which can cause dry heaves for several hours, to induce vomiting. Because ipecac has a long half-life, it may accumulate in the body with use on a regular basis and may become cardiotoxic. Repeated vomiting may lead to dental disease and perimolysis, in which the teeth are progressively decalcified and dissolved from contact with hydrochloric acid during regurgitation. The enamel layer of teeth gets thinner, causing sensitivity to hot, cold, and acid substances. In some instances, fillings become loose as the tooth structure to support them diminishes.

Perioral trauma may be associated with vomiting. The **parotid gland** may enlarge, giving a puffy, chipmunk-like facial appearance. The cause is unknown, but this enlargement is associated with malnutrition and chronic stimulation by the repeated ingestion of very large amounts of carbohydrate.

Esophageal disorders induced by repeated retching and vomiting include a painful sore throat, esophagitis, esophageal ulcers, and esophageal bleeding and rupture. **Aspiration** is always a danger with regurgitation. Acute dilation and rupture of the stomach after binge eating episodes have been reported. Many individuals develop calluses on their knuckles from using their fingers to induce vomiting. Severe metabolic complications of vomiting include hypokalemia and hypochloremia, which may lead to **metabolic acidosis** and, if severe, arrhythmias and sudden death.

Laxative Abuse

As many as 40% to 60% of those with bulimia nervosa use laxatives and diuretics regularly. The laxative abuse syndrome is associated with excess use of one or several of the stimulant type **cathartics**. Laxative abuse leads to watery diarrhea, which can cause dehydration and may exaggerate electrolyte depletion. Acute episodes of laxative abuse may be associated with nonspecific symptoms such as pain and vomiting. However, chronic use can lead to more severe problems such as cathartic colon. Symptoms characteristic of **cathartic colon** are alternating diarrhea and constipation, but the individual may also experience nausea, vomiting, and weight loss.

Diuretic Abuse

Diuretics are substances that increase kidney output. They vary from caffeine to alcohol to prescription drugs. However, many diuretics increase the excretion of other nutrients, especially potassium and magnesium. Diuretic abuse results in major losses of electrolytes, which may lead to severe metabolic imbalances, including hypokalemia and hypocalcemia. The combination of the abuse of laxatives and abuse of diuretics is particularly dangerous.

Treatment

People with bulimia nervosa can become so obsessive that the victims literally cannot stop their self-destructive behavior without professional help. Treatment is often difficult because of denial and the need for the individual to acknowledge the problem before treatment can begin. The biopsychosocial nature of bulimia nervosa indicates a need for interdisciplinary approaches. Intervention strategies include cognitive, behavioral, psychodynamic, and pharmacologic approaches in individual settings, group settings, or both (Gendall et al., 1999).

The goals of treatment of bulimia nervosa are to reduce or eliminate binge eating and purging behaviors and to normalize perceptions of body build and shape. Treatment early in the course of the disorder provides the most likelihood of recovery (Woodside, 1995). Establishment of a pattern of regular, nonbinge meals, encouragement of healthy (but not excessive) exercise, and resolution of co-occurring conditions such as mood or anxiety disorders are core among specific aims. Treatment includes psychotherapy, especially cognitive-interpersonal psychotherapy. Hospitalization is seldom necessary except for those who do not make progress or who have concurrent drug or alcohol abuse problems or other severe medical problems (American Psychiatric Association, 2000).

Nutrition Intervention

Appropriate nutrition therapy for the treatment of bulimia nervosa (see Box 14-4) will be implemented using the education and behavioral strategies outlined in Box 14-5. The primary goal is to structure eating patterns. The individual cannot diet or lose weight while learning to normalize eating habits. Dietary modifications include spreading kilocalories throughout the day and avoiding fasting. Techniques are learned to develop alternatives to eating to get past boredom, anxiety, and restlessness and to isolate and manage foods that trigger binging episodes. Therapy encourages establishing strategies, substituting, and sublimating to increase "free days" (days free of binging or purging) and broaden coping strategies.

Psychotherapy

Most treatment for bulimia nervosa is based on the cognitive-interpersonal approach in which habits and attitudes are the key targets (Gendall et al., 1999). The goal is to change the bulimic's attitude to change behavior. This treatment is similar to that of other indulgent behaviors such as use of alcohol, nicotine, and cocaine, which are associated with short-term gratification and long-term punishment.

Bulimics have a high rate of **comorbid** mood, anxiety, and personality disturbances and unresolved conflicts. Many recovering bulimics may require extended psychotherapy or psychoanalysis that addresses these intrapsychic and

KEY TERMS

sorbitol: alcohol from sugar that is used as a sweetener in some food products
emetic: something that causes vomiting
ipecac: dried roots of the plant *Cephaelis ipecacuanha* or *C. acuminata* used as an emetic
parotid gland: a gland located near the ear
aspiration: breathing vomitus or mucus into the respiratory tract
metabolic acidosis: a condition resulting from a depletion of the alkaline resins (bicarbonate) in body fluids characterized by a decrease in pH
cathartics: agents that cause evacuation in the bowels by increasing motor activity of the intestine
cathartic colon: thinning of the colon wall and structural defects associated with changes in motility
comorbid: occurring concurrently

intrapersonal issues, which come into focus as binge/purge-associated systems abate (Crow and Mitchell, 1994).

Pharmacology

Psychotropic medications, primarily the antidepressants, which are selective serotonin uptake inhibitors, have been found especially helpful for individuals with significant symptoms of depression, anxiety, obsession, or impulse disorder symptoms or for individuals who have failed previous attempts at appropriate psychosocial therapy (Agras, 1997). It may help to prevent relapses.

Prognosis

Although limited data are available on the success of treatment of bulimia nervosa, several studies have reported relapse rates ranging from 30% to 40% at 6 months to 8 months after recovery to 63% at 18 months after recovery (Olmsted et al., 1994). Frequency of continued vomiting appears to be an important prognostic indicator of relapse (Olmsted et al., 1994). Reiss and others (1995) reported that development of a stable, satisfactory social relationship was associated with a good outcome. One 10-year follow-up of persons treated for bulimia nervosa found that more than one half had full recovery (Collings and King, 1994). Although the remainder continued to experience some symptoms, only 9% continued to suffer the full syndrome.

Prognosis is much better for adolescents with bulimia nervosa than for adults (Fisher et al., 1995). This finding supports the value of early aggressive treatment in adolescents with eating disorders.

BINGE EATING DISORDER

- *What are the characteristics of individuals with BED?*
- *Why has binge eating been given a provisional category as an eating disorder?*
- *What are the health implications of BED? How is it treated?*

Binge eating, first described in 1959, has long been recognized as a serious clinical problem in obesity (Stunkard, 2000). Often referred to as compulsive overeating, binging occurs without the regular use of inappropriate compensatory purging behaviors. The DSM-IV includes BED as a provisional category warranting further study (American Psychiatric Association, 1998). Research criteria for this disorder appear in Box 14-7.

Box 14-7 Research Criteria for Binge Eating Disorder

Recurrent episodes of binge eating. An episode of binge eating is characterized by both of the following:

1. Eating in a discrete period (e.g., within any 2-hour period), an amount of food that is definitely larger than most people would eat in a similar period under similar circumstances
2. A sense of lack of control over eating during the episodes (e.g., a feeling that one cannot stop eating or control what or how much one is eating)

The binge-eating episodes are associated with three (or more) of the following:

1. Eating much more rapidly than normal
2. Eating until feeling uncomfortably full
3. Eating large amounts of food when not feeling physically hungry
4. Eating alone because of being embarrassed by how much one is eating
5. Feeling disgusted with oneself, depressed, or very guilty after overeating

Marked stress regarding binge eating is present.

The binge eating occurs, on average, at least 2 days a week for 6 months.

Note: The method of determining frequency differs from that used for bulimia nervosa; future research should address whether the preferred method of setting a frequency threshold is counting the number of days on which binges occur or counting the number of episodes of binge eating.

The binge eating is not associated with the regular use of inappropriate compensatory behaviors (e.g., purging, fasting, excessive exercise) and does not occur exclusively during the course of anorexia nervosa or bulimia nervosa.

Definition and Incidence

Although it has only recently been recognized as a distinct condition, BED is probably the most common eating disorder. Most people with BED are obese, but people of normal weight can be affected. Its prevalence has been estimated at approximately 2% to 5% of all adults, or 1 million to 2 million Americans (U.S. Public Health Service, 1993). Binge eating disorder occurs in approximately 10% to 15% of mildly obese people in self-help or commercial weight-loss programs and in 20% to 50% of those enrolled in medically supervised weight loss programs. In general BED affects three women for every two men (U.S. Public Health Service, 1993).

Characteristics

Binge eating disorder is characterized by eating an excessive amount of food within a discrete period and by a sense of lack of control over eating during the episode. Binge eating has been likened to drug abuse because both behavioral syndromes involve intense cravings and loss of control followed by disgust or guilt after over eating. Drewnowski and others (1995) have suggested that food preferences and binge episodes may be influenced by endogenous **opiate** peptides. They observed that a drug that blocked opiate function reduced the consumption of sweet and high-fat foods among women who had a history of binge eating, but did not have that affect in nonbinging women.

Individuals with BED share many characteristics with those who suffer from anorexia nervosa and bulimia nervosa. They have impaired social functioning and undue concerns about body weight (Spitzer et al., 1993). Obese binge eaters have been shown to have more psychopathologic problems (e.g., major depression, panic disorder, or borderline personality disorders) than normal-weight or obese individuals who do not binge (Antony et al., 1994), but less psychiatric disturbance than normal-weight women with bulimia nervosa. A study of almost 200 individuals with BED found that males appear to have a less emotional response to a binge (DiGioacchino et al., 1999).

Treatment

Many obese individuals with BED are able to lose weight with traditional diet, exercise, and behavioral self-management methods, but the effects are short-term and most regain virtually all the weight within a few years. Long-term treatment goals and strategies for binge-eating disorder are similar to those for bulimia nervosa.

Researchers are still trying to determine which method or combination of methods is most effective in controlling BED. Options currently being used center on cognitive-behavioral therapy, which teaches clients techniques for monitoring and changing eating habits, and interpersonal psychotherapy, which assists them in developing skills to cope with feelings of inadequacy, lack of self-esteem, and relationships with family and friends. Success of such programs can be predicted by the frequency of binge eating (Peterson et al., 2000).

Disordered eating is a society-wide concern that has major health consequences (Neumark-Sztainer, 1995). Preoccupation with body weight and concern about dieting begin early. In one study the weight-related concerns of 457 boys and girls between 9 years and 11 years of age revealed that children are concerned about body image and with food and weight control (Gustafson-Larson and Terry, 1992). Almost two thirds of the children reported they desired to be thinner and 80% reported that they avoided foods they felt would make them fat. A similar study of adolescent girls and young women (Moore, 1998) found that 67% were dissatisfied with their weight and that 54% were dissatisfied with their body image. Binging, dieting, and fasting to control body weight were reported by more than one third of these subjects.

The large numbers of children and adolescents with abnormal attitudes toward body image and

KEY TERMS

recovery: abstinence from or substantial decrease in binge eating or purging
opiate: any compound that induces sleep

Research Update

Can You Exercise Too Much?

About 2 years ago, Judy, a 32-year-old health-care professional, was exercising at least 4 hours a day. She didn't have a VCR, so she listened to exercise tapes. She'd play them again and again. Then, when others might be ready to relax, she went to the health spa, convinced that if she went one day without following this regimen, she would gain weight. Exercise became as much an addiction for her as food is for the binge eater. The more involved she became, the more rituals she developed. She was at the spa at 9 AM every day, even when she had a cold or developed the flu.

Gradually Judy developed a pattern. At first she was getting the exercise out of the way so she could enjoy something, such as meals. Then she cut herself to two meals, then to one, then to a carton of yogurt. As she cut herself off from food, she also avoided the rest of the world. She stopped seeing her friends. The spa came first, and she was too busy to make time for friends. By this time the 157 cm (62 in) Judy weighed 35 kg (78 lb). Other problems developed when she had to have intestinal surgery for an unrelated illness. Although she was told not to exercise after the surgery, she felt she had to. She ripped open her incision and had to undergo surgery again. Judy was scared and she finally realized she had a problem.

Decades of epidemiologic research have established a consensus that regular physical activity provides a number of benefits, reducing both mortality and morbidity of coronary heart disease, hypertension, and osteoporosis. However, that healthful practice can get out of control. For some individuals, excessive or compulsive exercise becomes a means to control body weight and emotional frustrations. Often such exercise is expressed by intensive and highly ritualized daily activities such as performing a specified number of sit-ups, swimming a set number of laps, or running set distances. Rituals become more pronounced and involved as the individual becomes "exercise dependent." "Excessive" has not been defined for exercise, but some researchers suggest that criteria include the following: exercise 2 hours to 3 hours a day, exercising despite injury or pain, and symptoms of withdrawal without activity after 24 hours to 36 hours.

Clearly there is harm in too much exercise. Body fat stores become depleted and continuing to exercise will cause degradation of muscle to meet energy needs. Low body weight may contribute to decreased bone mass and eventually to osteoporosis. Those who overexercise may experience more stress fractures and when they exercise despite injuries, they develop more serious injuries.

There is considerable overlap between compulsive athleticism and eating disorders. Both are associated with patterns of distorted self-esteem, distorted body image (Beumont et al., 1994; Sundgot-Borgen, 2002), depression (Specker et al., 1994), and obsessive-compulsive behavior personality disorders such as perfectionism. One study of 88 men and 97 women found a strong relationship between exercise and weight preoccupation among men and women and between exercise and obsessive-compulsiveness among men.

The overexerciser may need assistance in recognizing and acknowledging the problem before it can be confronted or treatment can be initiated. Treatment may be especially difficult because controlling the exercise may be only part of the problem. Former overexercisers often turn to other weight control methods and they may become bulimic. Treatment approaches are similar to those used for eating disorders. Beumont and others (1994) have developed an exercise program to be incorporated into the treatment of eating-disordered individuals that includes behavior modification, education, and shared responsibility.

eating make the issue of early prevention and intervention particularly pertinent (Fisher et al., 1995). It is essential for healthcare professionals to encourage parents and their children to develop healthy attitudes about their weight, body image, and self-esteem and to ameliorate the sociocultural influences that promote eating disorders.

OVERWEIGHT AND OBESITY

- *How are overweight and obesity assessed? What is the prevalence of these conditions?*
- *What are the risks of excess body weight and fat?*
- *Describe the genetic, physiologic, social, cultural, and psychologic factors that contribute to excess body weight.*
- *What are appropriate treatment modalities and programs for those who are overweight or obese?*
- *Discuss the advantages of weight reduction.*
- *How can the onset or progression of obesity be prevented or delayed?*

Increased life expectancy in the United States and many parts of the world is associated with an increase in chronic diseases, obesity, hypertension, diabetes, cardiovascular disease, and some forms of cancer, often referred to as the diseases of affluence. And yet treatment of these diseases is costly and only marginally effective. Every year overweight status and obesity contribute to substantial morbidity and mortality and are responsible for billions of dollars in medical costs and lost productivity (Wolf and Colditz, 1998). In affluent societies excess body weight is the most common nutrition-related health problem. Obesity is a complicated disordered condition or group of conditions that has physiologic, psychologic, and social consequences. Unfortunately the precise etiologies of obesity are poorly understood, and treatment programs are characterized by high rates of **recidivism**.

There is no question that the only really effective treatment for being overweight or obese is prevention through permanent changes in life-style factors. *Healthy People 2010* is a major initiative to improve the health of Americans (see Chapter 1). The list of 10 Leading Health Indicators was derived from the goals and objectives to be met by the year 2010. They are divided into life-style indicators and health system indicators. Obviously a major life-style indicator is associated with being **overweight** or **obese** and encompasses goals for life-style changes in nutrition and physical activity.

Assessment

Overweight status and obesity have traditionally been defined in terms of excess body weight and reported as a percentage of the reference weight, usually the Metropolitan Height-Weight Tables or percentiles reported from the National and Nutrition Examination Surveys (NHANES) (see Appendix B). There are sophisticated methods to determine body fat that are impractical for general clinical use.

Because obesity is defined in terms of fatness, fatfolds (skinfolds) may be useful for assessment. The thickness of the fatfold measurement increases and decreases when an individual gains or loses body fat. The distribution of body fat is an important determinant of health risks. An excessive amount of fat on the trunk and abdominal area (android fat) compared with gluteo-femoral (gynoid) fat is associated with increased risk for a variety of illnesses and increased overall mortality. The Guide for Identification, Evaluation, and Treatment of Overweight and Obesity in Adults from the National Institutes of Health (2000) recommends two surrogate measures to assess body fat: (1) BMI and (2) waist circumference (Table 14-1). The BMI provides a more accurate total body fat than weight alone. However, it will overestimate body fat in persons who are very muscular. Waist circumference is a practical tool to eval-

KEY TERMS

recidivism: tendency to relapse into a previous condition or mode of behavior
overweight: weight that exceeds reference weight based on height
obese: an excess accumulation of body fat

Table 14-1 Classification of Overweight and Obesity by BMI, Waist Circumference, and Associated Disease Risk

	BMI (kg/m2)	Obesity Class	Disease Risk* (Relative to Normal Weight and Waist Circumference) Men ≤40 in (≤102 cm) Women ≤35 in (≤88 cm)	>40 in (>102 cm) >35 in (>88 cm)
Underweight	<18.5		—	—
Normal[†]	18.5-24.9		—	—
Overweight	25.0-29.9		Increased	High
Obesity	30.0-34.9	I	High	Very High
	35.0-39.9	II	Very High	Very High
Extreme Obesity	≥40	III	Extremely High	Extremely High

From National Heart, Lung, and Blood Institute: The practical guide. Identification, evaluation, and treatment of overweight and obesity in adults. NIH Pub #00-4084, Oct. 2000. (Adapted from Preventing and managing the global epidemic of obesity. Report of the World Health Organization consultation of obesity. WHO, Geneva, June 1997.)
*Disease risk for type 2 diabetes, hypertension, and cardiovascular disease.
[†]Increased waist circumference can also be a marker for increased risk even in persons of normal weight.

uate abdominal fat before and during weight loss. It is an independent predictor of risk over and above BMI.

Prevalence

A *Healthy People 2000* objective for health promotion was to reduce the prevalence of overweight status (BMI >25) to no more than 20% of people age 20 years and older. Unfortunately rather than decreasing, the prevalence of overweight status in adults in the United States has increased. According to data from NHANES III (1988 to 1994), 54% of all American adults are classified as overweight (Mokdad et al., 1999; National Heart, Lung, and Blood Institute [NHLBI], 1998) (Figure 14-3). Minority populations are affected disproportionately, especially minority women. Nearly 50% of African-American women, Mexican-American women, and Native American women are overweight (NHLBI, 1998). Poverty and lower educational attainment increase the susceptibility to obesity and its progression (Kumanyika, 1994).

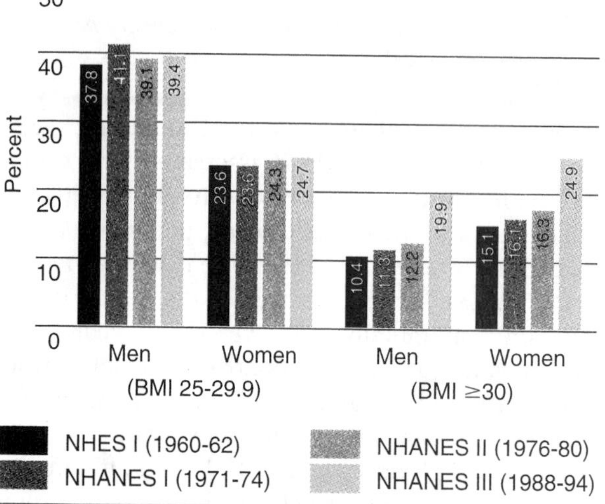

Figure 14-3 Age-adjusted prevalence of overweight (BMI 25 to 29.9) and obesity (BMI ≥30). *(From National Heart, Lung, and Blood Institute: The practical guide. Identification, evaluation, and treatment of overweight and obesity in adults. NIH Pub # 00-4084, Oct. 2000.)*

Health Risks

The NHLBI Expert Panel on Identification, Evaluation, and Treatment of Overweight and Obesity in Adults (1998) concluded that a BMI greater than 25 increases health risks. The consensus Development Conference on Obesity concluded that a BMI greater than 27.8 for boys or men or greater than 27.2 for girls or women has adverse affects on health and longevity. Box 14-8 lists the most common risks of excess body

Box 14-8 Health Risk Factors Associated with Obesity

- Increased mortality
  - >30% of weight-for-height, especially in younger age groups
- Respiratory difficulties
  - Pickwickian syndrome
- Cardiovascular disease
  - Coronary artery disease
    - Myocardial infarction
    - Hypercholesterolemia
  - Hypertension
- Cerebrovascular disease
- Endocrine difficulties
  - Non–insulin-dependent diabetes
  - Irregular menstrual cycles
  - Infertility
- Increased obstetric risk
  - Macrosomic infants
  - Prolonged labor, delivery complications
  - More gestational diabetes
- Higher risk with surgery
  - Requirement that fat layer be dissected first
  - Longer duration of request for anesthesia
  - Difficulty finding blood vessel for intravenous infusion
  - Increased sepsis and wound rupture
- Gallbladder disease
- Musculoskeletal problems
  - Gout
  - Osteoarthritis
- Some skin disorders
- Some forms of cancer
  - Males: colon, rectum, prostate
  - Females: gallbladder, breast, cervix, uterus, ovaries, endometrium
- Psychologic problems

weight. Optimum body weight for health is a subject of debate, but morbidity and mortality increase as weight increases. Among the most significant risks are increases in blood pressure and blood lipid levels, which generally decrease with weight reduction.

Mortality

The relationship between body weight and mortality is well established (Table 14-2). An excess body weight of 30% is associated with an increase of 25% to 42% in mortality and mortality increases with increasing body weight (Kushner, 1993). For those instances in which increased risk occurred with underweight individuals, it is uncertain if that risk is related to leanness or to unhealthy life-style habits, preclinical disease processes, or other unidentified factors.

Lee and others (1993) at Harvard University conducted a follow-up of 17,297 healthy men who completed health questionnaires in 1962 and 1966. After 27 years, the lowest mortality occurred among those who weighed approximately 20% below the U.S. average for men of comparable age and height. A similar observation from the longitudinal Nurses Health Study was the finding that for middle-age women, mortality was lowest when they weighed at least 15% less than the average weight for women in the United States (Manson et al., 1995).

Morbidity

Much of the morbidity associated with obesity is from an increase in the occurrence of hypertension, hyperlipidemia, and non-insulin-dependent diabetes mellitus (NIDDM), all of which contribute to an increased risk of cardiovascular disease (Denke et al., 1993; Sjostrom, 1992). Moreover the health risks from these comorbidities increase with the duration and severity of the obesity although the morbidity of obesity is not as prominent in women as in men. The association of obesity with cardiovascular disease is as strong in women as men, particularly with weight gains of more than 20 lbs. Excessive weight also increases the risk for gallbladder disease, **gout**, pulmonary and orthopedic problems (particularly osteoarthritis), and some types of cancer (Sjostrom, 1992).

KEY TERMS

gout: a form of arthritis characterized by excess uric acid in the urine and recurrent attacks of acute arthritis involving a peripheral joint followed by complete remission

Table 14-2 RISK FACTORS OR COMORBIDITIES ASSOCIATED WITH OBESITY

High Risk	Increased Risk—Not Life Threatening	Three or More of the Following Confer High Absolute Risk
Established coronary heart disease Other atherosclerotic diseases Type 2 diabetes mellitus Sleep apnea	Osteoarthritis Gallstones Stress incontinence Gynecological abnormalities such as amenorrhea	Hypertension Cigarette smoking High low-density lipoprotein cholesterol Impaired fasting glucose Family history of cardiovascular disease Age (male > 45 years, female > 55 years)

From National Heart, Lung, and Blood Institute. National Institutes of Health: The practical guide. Identification, evaluation, and treatment of overweight and obesity in adults. NIH Pub #00-4084, Oct. 2000.

The pattern of adipose tissue distribution can alter the health risks of obesity independent of total body fat. Excessive accumulation of intraabdominal fat is linked with other metabolic complications such as hyperinsulinemia and **insulin resistance** and hypertension, which are known risk factors for cardiovascular disease. The clustering of these abnormalities has been referred to as syndrome X (Reaven et al., 1993). In fact abdominal obesity is as strong a predictor of **myocardial infarction** as are the leading risk factors, hypercholesterolemia, hypertension, and smoking.

Excess body weight has substantial socioeconomic and psychologic ramifications that can impair the day-to-day functioning of an obese person. For example it has been observed that women who were overweight in adolescence were less likely to be married, completed fewer years of school, had lower household incomes, and had a higher incidence of poverty than those who were lean. In a society with strong psychologic and social pressures to maintain slimness, there is an unfortunate tendency to assume obesity is the result of self-indulgence and to view obese individuals negatively. This is often reflected in discrimination toward those with excess body weight.

Etiology

The fundamental basis of obesity is imbalance between energy intake and expenditure, but underlying origins are multifactorial, reflecting genetic, environmental, metabolic, cultural, socioeconomic, and psychologic factors.

Genetics

The observation that the adult weight of twins who have been raised in separate homes is very similar suggested heredity is a strong determinant of body weight. Specific genes responsible for excessive fatness have been identified in animals. Researchers at Rockefeller University identified a gene, called the ob gene, that regulates energy balance in the mouse. This gene directs the production of leptin by fat tissue that acts on the brain to affect a person's appetite and metabolism. It appears that *leptin* helps prevent starvation by regulating a person's appetite, emotional desire for food, and metabolism. When fat stores drop, leptin levels also drop. In response, appetite and desire for food increase and metabolism decreases, leading to an increase in body fat storage. This finding suggests a leptin resistance (Considine et al., 1996). Weight loss is associated with a decrease in circulating leptin. It would appear that at least some obese persons lack receptors for leptin or have a problem with its transport to the brain (Rink, 1994).

Regulation of Food Intake

Food intake appears to have both internal and external controls, which act jointly to control hunger, satiety, and eating behavior (Figure 14-4).

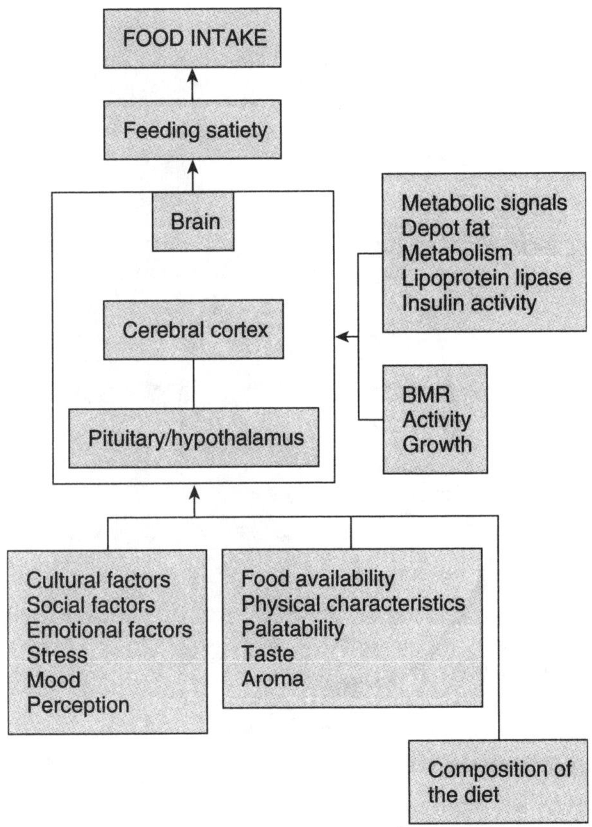

Figure 14-4 An overview of factors that regulate food intake.

These controls are integrated by the **cortex** of the brain. Internal controls are concerned with physiologic changes that signal depletion and the need to ingest food or satiation and cessation of eating. External controls reflect a learned association between external stimuli and food intake that may modify the internally regulated eating behavior. Internal control of body fat appears to involve a relationship between long-term feeding regulation, which maintains the nutrient stores of the body, and short-term feeding regulation, which is concerned with hunger and satiety.

Short-term control. The **hypothalamus** is believed to be the internal physiologic regulator for hunger and satiety. The ventromedial nucleus appears to be the satiety center, whereas the lateral hypothalamic area acts as the feeding center. Signals from the body reach the hypothalamus via various neurotransmitters and **brain peptides,** which may stimulate, inhibit, or modulate feeding. The hypothalamus regulates the release of certain pituitary hormones that influence food intake via stimulation of the **autonomic nervous system.**

Within the biologic system, the control of hunger and satiety involves postdigestive signals from the gastrointestinal tract and the release of hormones when food is processed. Postprandial sensations of satiety appear to respond to the activity of intestinal nutrient receptors. Cholecystokinin, released by the duodenum in response to dietary lipids and peptides, causes satiety by desensitizing gastric nerves (Read et al., 1994).

Long-term control. Depot fat appears to be primary in the long-term control of food intake, but the mechanisms by which this occurs are not clear. Recent research indicates that the activity

KEY TERMS

insulin resistance: a condition in which insulin is present in the blood and does facilitate glucose uptake by cells, but very slowly

myocardial infarction: blockage of an artery to the heart resulting in tissue damage

cortex: a thin layer of gray matter on the surface of the cerebral hemisphere that is responsible for higher mental functions, general movement, visceral functions, perception, and behavioral reactions for the association and integration of these functions

hypothalamus: a small gland in the midbasal brain area that controls and integrates peripheral autonomic mechanisms, endocrine activity, and many somatic functions, such as regulation of food intake, water balance, body temperature, and sleep

brain peptides: a chain of amino acids that can influence feeding functions, such as opioids, calcitonin, gastrin-releasing peptide, bombesin, cholecystokinin, thyrotropin-releasing hormone, and neurotensin

autonomic nervous system: autonomic, self-controlling, functionally independent; the portion of the nervous system concerned with regulation of the activity of cardiac muscles, smooth muscle, and glands

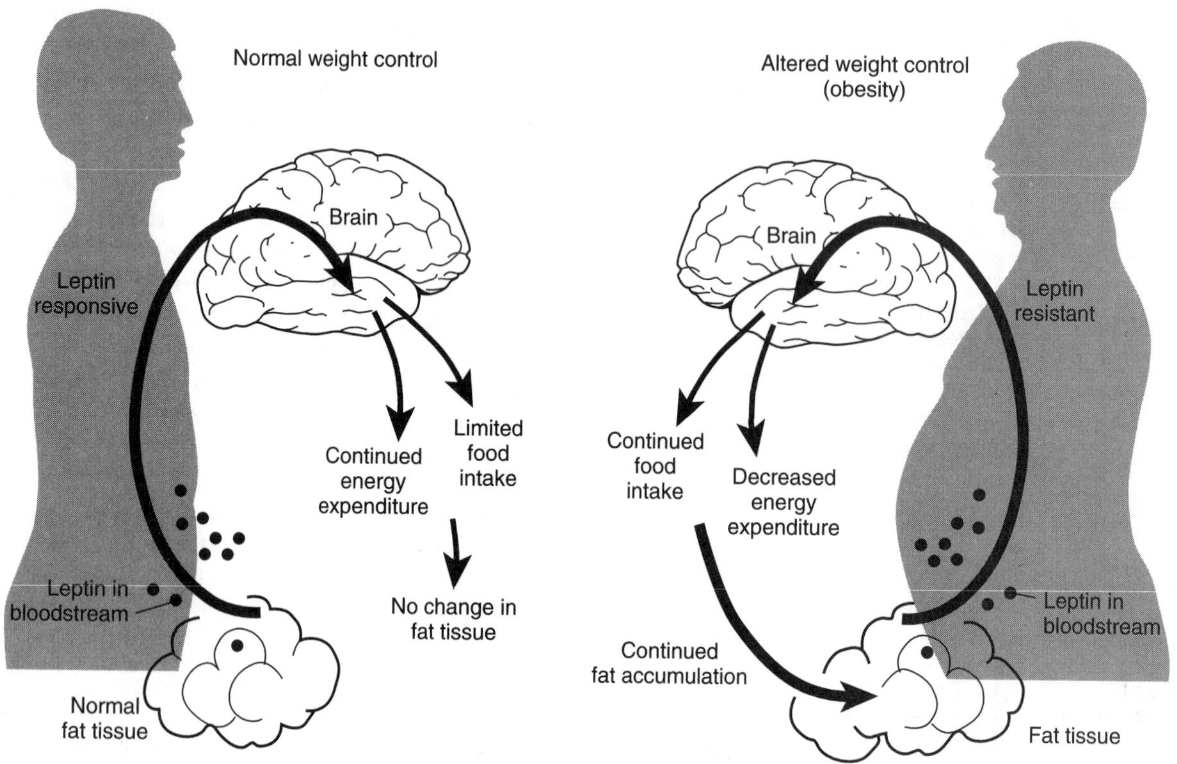

Figure 14-5 Leptin metabolism. *(From Weigh less, live longer, strategies for successful weight loss, a special health report, Boston, 2001, Harvard Health Publications. Copyright Harriet R. Greenfield, 2001.)*

level of adipose tissue **lipoprotein lipase (LPL)** is a regulator of body fat cell mass. It facilitates fat storage. The LPL levels are elevated in obesity, which may be a primary defect that promotes the development of obesity or a defect secondary to the enlarged fat cells that develop as the result of obesity. The activity of LPL rises with weight loss and returns to lower values when weight is regained. This elevation of LPL with weight loss acts to enhance triglyceride storage. The net effect may be rapid regain of lost weight and greater difficulty with succeeding attempts at weight loss.

Adipocytes. If energy balance is continuously positive, adipocytes gradually increase in size. When fat accumulation reaches a certain point, the adipocytes' ability to store fat is diminished. Additional excess energy will trigger adipocyte proliferation and cell number begins to rise. Overall there is approximately a fivefold increase in fat cell number from infancy to adulthood. It appears that in severely obese people (those with a BMI greater than 40), hyperplasia of adipocytes may continue as long as positive energy balance continues. Weight loss will diminish the size of adipocytes, but not the number. Refeeding of animals that have lost weight seems to continue until fat cells return to their original size. Thus adipose tissue appears to exert a regulatory function in energy intake. Leptin originates in adipose tissue and may act as a long-term satiety hormone that defends the level of depot fat (Figure 14-5).

Insulin resistance. Excess body weight, especially abdominal fat, is associated with the development of NIDDM (Goodpaster et al., 2000). Obesity may be an important environmental determinant of the manifestation of diabetes in genetically susceptible individuals. This condition is characterized by insulin resistance. When fat cells enlarge, their response to insulin is diminished, even when insulin concentrations are high. Excess body fat is related to low levels of insulin receptors on the outer cell membrane and intracellular defects in glucose metabolism (Abate et al., 1995).

Energy Expenditure

The REE of obese persons expressed per kilogram of body weight generally is lower than that of lean individuals. Although differences in REE among individuals may seem to be small, a low REE and total 24-hour energy expenditure are significant predictors of gains in body weight, especially of regain of lost weight.

The most variable component of energy expenditure is that spent on physical activity. Data from the Health Professionals Follow-Up Study found that among 222,076 men, low levels of physical activity were significantly related to the development of obesity (Ching et al., 1996). Nearly two thirds of the adult population of the United States report engaging in little or no leisure-time physical activity. Sedentary behaviors become important factors in the development of overweight and obesity.

Energy Density

Over time many components of the diet have been investigated for possible contributions to changes in body fat. Some researchers have suggested that effect of fat is related to its impact on satiety and therefore on food intake. A popular theory has been that a diet high in carbohydrates results in a spontaneous reduction in total energy intake. However, individuals fed isocaloric diets of varying levels of fat tended to gain weight on high fat intakes. More recently emphasis has been on **energy density**. Energy density can be influenced by the amount of fat, fiber, water, and type of sweetener and the volume of food consumed affects satiety (Rolls et al., 1998). Studies of compliance with low-fat regimens suggest a tendency to compensate for low-ED foods by consuming a greater volume of food, particularly when the fat content is low. Efforts to reduce energy density translates into reduction in dietary fat intake and increases in fiber and low-calorie sweeteners. Low-calorie sweeteners are important because recent epidemiologic studies demonstrate consistently higher rates of cardiovascular disease and type 2 diabetes in individuals who deserve a high percentage of energy from refined grains and sugars.

A review of studies of individuals consuming diets of low and high energy density revealed that weight loss occurred consistently with low energy density (Yao and Roberts, 2001). In general however, weight losses were less than that expected from reducing dietary fat content alone. These reviewers suggest that general dietary recommendations to consume more "low fat" may result in lower compliance than more specific prescriptions for changes in dietary habits. Overall these reviewers concluded that the studies reviewed suggest that low-energy density diets low in fat and high in fiber result in equivalent compliance satiety and reduced energy intake in short-term studies (Yao and Roberts, 2001).

Although there is substantial evidence of a genetic predisposition and aberrations in metabolic controls for obesity, environmental and behavioral factors play a significant role in the development of obesity (Roberts and Greenberg, 1996).

Intervention

Obesity is a chronic disorder with substantial comorbidities. Because of current limitations of treatment, increasing prevalence, high rate of recidivism, and significant associations with morbidity and mortality, intervention becomes a challenge. The report of the NHLBI (2000) has concluded that a combination of diet modification, increased physical activity, and behavior therapy can be effective in accomplishing and maintaining weight loss.

KEY TERMS

lipoprotein lipase (LPL): an enzyme located at the lining of the capillaries that promotes breakdown of circulating triglycerides and cell uptake of fatty acids

energy density: amount of energy available per unit of weight or volume

Macroenvironment for Behavior Change

Dietary and physical activity behaviors have a major impact on body weight and overall health. In turn these factors are influenced by a variety of factors. Obesity prevention and treatment strategies for targeting these behaviors are viewed as the most useful and the most feasible for implementation. Recently there has been an increased recognition that individual success in behavior changes is dependent on factors of personal environment, which, in turn, is shaped by community, governmental, educational, economic, and industrials structures of our society (Booth et al., 2001). Success in helping Americans become healthier via dietary change and increased physical activity will require strategies for partnerships with community, education, economic leaders and government, and industry to promote success. Figure 14-6 presents a framework for determinants of physical activity and eating behavior represents a model of collaboration or intervention that may be successful in changing food intake and physical activity and may potentially result in such desirable outcomes as prevention and reduction of obesity. In this diagram the center of the framework represents a psychobiologic core that is genetically determined. The second and third ring represent cultural and social influences of behavior. The middle layers refers to the immediate environment in which individuals live and function. The outer layers encompass enablers of choice and beyond that are physical and social settings in which physical activity and eating behaviors take place and choices are made. The outer two layers represent leverage points in controls of the structure and features of the microenvironment that affect behavior choices. The outer layers encompass all behavior settings and macroenvironments and are influenced by additional layers of factors that may control products and goods that consumers purchase or are exposed to along with laws, policies, economics, and politics. These distal leverage points also include multidimensional factors that pervade all levels that shape attitudes, beliefs, and knowledge. It has been suggested that working with all of these levels to create an environment for successfully assisting individuals to meet goals related to physical activity and diet (Booth et al., 2001).

Benefits of Weight Reduction

National recommendations for weight loss establish a goal of 5% to 10% of body weight (NHLBI, 1998). Individuals who lose even small amounts of weight are likely to improve their health by reducing the risk of comorbidities associated with obesity (Institute of Medicine, 1995). Specifically these guidelines make sense for several reasons: most obese or overweight persons have difficulty achieving their reference weight, the weight lost by obese and overweight persons often returns, and evidence supports the benefit of weight loss for reducing risk (blood pressure, lowering blood glucose, and improving blood lipid levels) (NHLBI, 2000).

Of adults with NIDDM, 80% to 90% are obese. If weight loss is maintained, insulin sensitivity improves and the need for oral hypoglycemic agents or insulin diminishes (Colditz et al., 1995). Similarly overweight hypertensive individuals who lose weight have a significant reduction in both systolic and diastolic blood pressure that is proportional to weight loss (NHLBI, 1998). Among obese individuals, total serum cholesterol levels decrease in proportion to the amount of weight lost (NHLBI, 1998). In one study a decrease of 5% to 6% in BMI was associated with reductions of 16% in total cholesterol and 12% in low-density lipoprotein (LDL) cholesterol, decreasing the risk of cardiovascular disease (Seim and Holtmeier, 1992).

Weight loss results in improved functional status and greater ease in daily activities such as climbing stairs, getting in and out of an automobile, or moving on and off a bus. Improved mobility allows the individual to participate in more physical activities, which may improve overall energy expenditure and health.

Treatment Approaches

The 2000 Dietary Guidelines recommend weight loss to the general public for the categories of BMI of 25 or greater. If weight reduction is a primary goal, a plethora of weight loss programs are available. They vary in intensity of treatment, cost, nature of interventions, and degree of involvement of healthcare professionals. An individual may

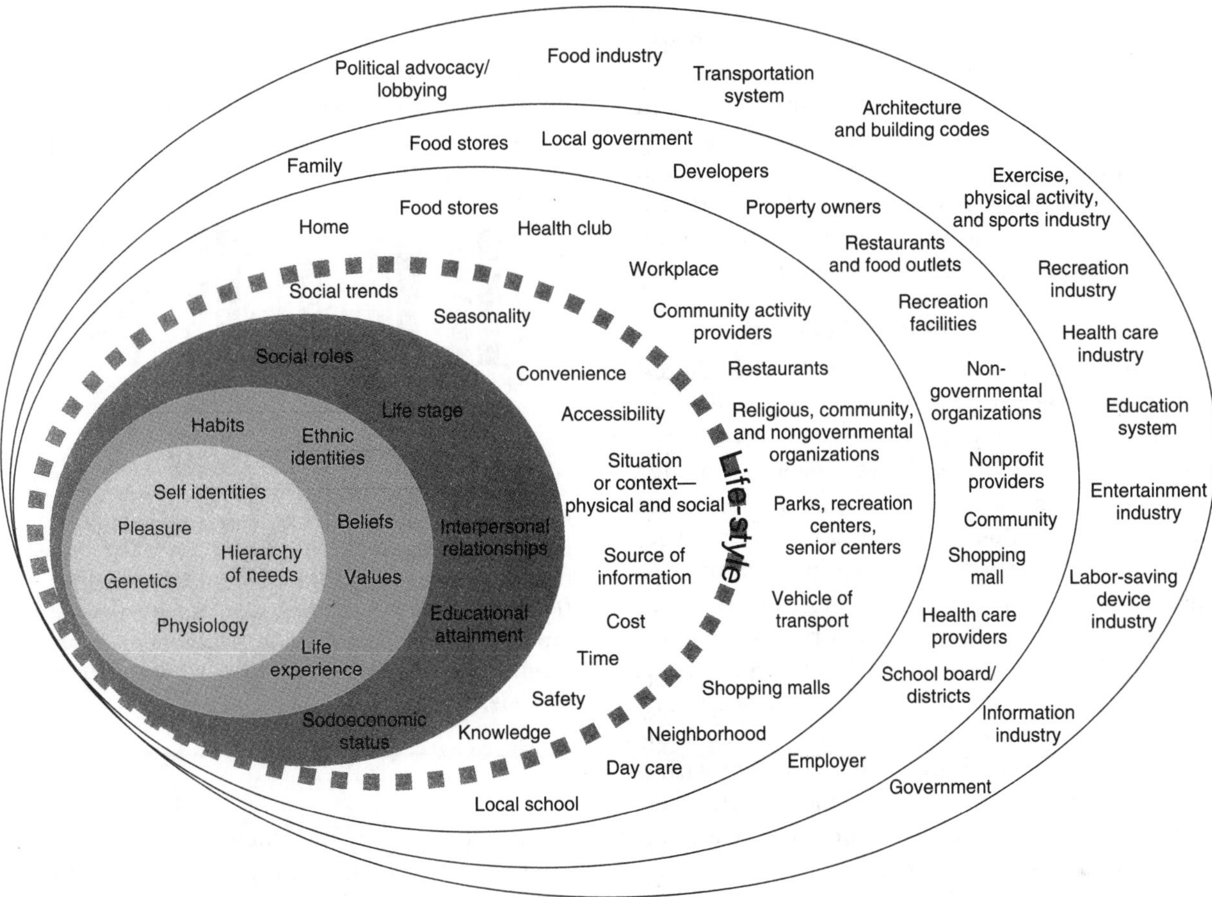

Beginning at the core, the inner circles represent:

1. Psychobiologic core: genetically program metabolism and behavior
2. Cultural: personal life experience, values and beliefs, self-identity within immediate social/cultural surroundings
3. Societal: role and relationships, acquired values and beliefs
4. Enablers of choice: most proximal factors affecting choices that are commonly identified as enhancers or barriers
5. Life-style: visible physical activity and eating behavior choices made by the individual

The three outer circles represent:

Inside circle: behavioral settings—physical and social settings in which physical activity and eating behaviors take place and choices are made

Middle circle: proximal leverage points—controllers of the structure and features of the microenvironment that affect the physical activity and eating behavior choices

Outer circle: distal leverage points—additional layers of factors that influence behavior, either directly or indirectly. May include controllers of raw materials, finished goods that consumers purchase, and laws, policies, economics, and politics that affect controllers.

Figure 14-6 Framework for determinants of physical activity and eating behavior. *(From Booth SI et al.: Environmental and societal factors affect food choice and physical activity: rationale, influences and leverage points, Nutr Rev 59(3):S21-S39, 2001.)*

initiate his or her own program, join a commercial program, or enter clinical programs in which services are provided by licensed health professionals. Treatment has been divided into five broad approaches: (1) diet, (2) physical activity, (3) behavior modification, (4) pharmacotherapy, and (5) **gastric surgery** (Institute of Medicine, 1995). See Table 14-2 for these approaches, their characteristics, and considerations related to nutrition.

Treatment of Overweight and Obesity

An estimated 97 million adults in the United States are overweight or obese. Overweight and obesity are rapidly increasing in prevalence (Must et al., 1999) and are becoming major health problems in the United States (Mokdad et al., 1999). More than 50% of Americans are overweight and the preventable deaths attributed to obesity exceed 300,000 per year (Allison et al., 1999). The economic burden approximates $100 billion (Thompson et al., 1999). Current treatment approaches for obesity have not been very effective and many overweight and obese individuals attempt to achieve reduced weight with a wide variety of approaches, some nutritionally sound, other procedures endorsing irrational and, sometimes, unsafe practices.

In 1998 the NHLBI published *Clinical Guidelines on the Identification, Evaluation, and Treatment of Overweight and Obesity in Adults: The Evidence Report* (NHLBI, 1998). The follow up to this report is *The Practical Guide* (NHLBI, 2000). The aim of this guide is to provide useful advice on how to achieve weight reduction and weight management to maintain a lower body weight. The guidelines emphasize that obesity is a chronic disease and successful management requires lifelong effort. The report emphasizes the importance of tailoring treatment to the individual and promotion of gradual weight loss using a variety of strategies. The initial strategies center on reducing total caloric intake by improved dietary intakes, increasing physical activity in the context of behavioral modification strategies that promote behavior change and support its maintenance.

Current treatment recommendations for an overweight or obese person begins assessment of degree of obesity and overall health risk status.

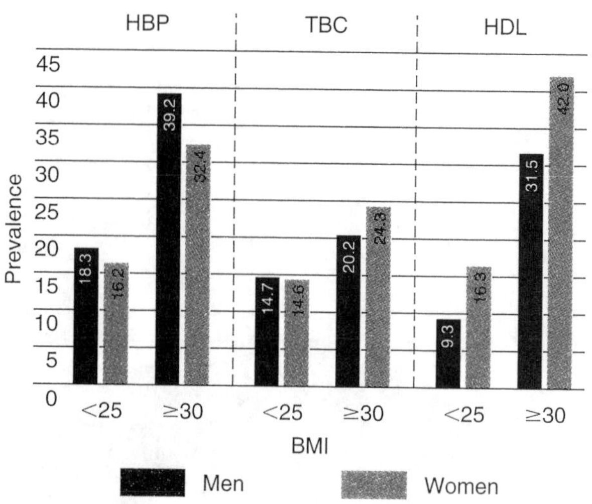

Figure 14-7 NHANES III age-adjusted prevalence of high blood pressure (HBP), high total blood cholesterol (TBC), and low HDL by two BMI categories. *(From National Heart, Lung, and Blood Institute: The practical guide. Identification, evaluation, and treatment of overweight and obesity in adults. NIH Pub # 00-4084, Oct. 2000.)*

Intervention or management involves multiple strategies for maintenance of body weight and promotion of weight loss. Assessment involves evaluation of BMI and waist circumference based on classification in Table 14-1 and overall health risk based on factors associated with obesity listed in Table 14-2 (NHLBI, 2000). To emphasize the importance of risk factors, Figure 14-7 illustrates the age-adjusted prevalence of hypertension, hypercholesterolemia, and low HDL when BMI exceeds 30.

Readiness to Lose Weight

An individual's readiness to make life-style changes is essential to successful weight loss. Evaluation of readiness should include reasons and motivation for weight loss, previous attempts at weight loss, support expected from family and friends, understanding of risk and benefits, attitudes toward physical activity, time availability, potential barriers including financial limitations to the person's adoption of change.

Prevention of weight gain may be appropriate for some individuals for whom weight loss is not achievable. A goal for these people should be prevention of further weight gain, especially for people with a BMI of 25 to 25.9 who have no other significant risk factors.

Weight loss therapy is recommended for individuals with a BMI over 30 and for individuals with a BMI between 25 and 25.9 or a high-risk waist circumference and two or more risk factors.

Goals for therapy are to reduce body weight and maintain a lower body weight for the longer term; the prevention of further weight is the minimum goal. An initial weight loss of 10% of body weight achieved over 6 months is a recommended target. An appropriate rate of weight loss is 1 to 2 pounds each week. Greater rates of weight loss do not achieve better long-term results. After the first 6 months of weight loss therapy, the priority should be weight maintenance achieved through combined change in diet, physical activity, and behavior. Further weight loss can be considered after a period of weight maintenance.

Diets

Balanced energy deficit diets. Balanced energy deficit diets provide 1200 kcal per day or more (22 to 25 kcal/kg of reference weight). These diets can be nutritionally adequate when the minimum number of servings in each group of the Food Guide Pyramid are included. For a 500 kcal per day energy deficit, weight loss would be approximately 0.25 kg per week. By normalizing food patterns, such diets have the potential for promoting permanent changes in eating patterns.

Low-calorie diets. Low-calorie diets (LCD) provide approximately 1000 kcal to 1200 kcal per day for most women and 1200 kcal per day to 1600 kcal per day for men and women who weigh 165 pounds or more who exercise regularly. Some diets use regular foods; others are based on formulated or fortified products or prepackaged foods designed as meal replacements. For diets using limited amounts of food, a vitamin-mineral supplement may be necessary to meet nutrient recommendations. Weight loss averages 0.5 kg to 1.5 kg per week, or about 8.5 kg in 20 weeks. Physician approval and supervision from health-care persons is desirable.

Very-low-calorie diets. Very-low-calorie diets (VLCDs) are modified fasts that provide less than 800 kcal per day. Programs using VLCDs are based in hospitals or clinics and include commercial products. They are supervised and administered by a multidisciplinary team of health-care professionals. Most of the formula products used provide 400 kcal to 700 kcal, most of which is protein (0.8 to 1.5 g/kg reference weight) and up to 100 g of carbohydrate. These programs are usually restricted to individuals who are moderately to severely obese (BMI >30) and who have been unsuccessful in more traditional weight loss approaches or those with BMIs between 27 and 30 when comorbidities are present. In the short term these severely restricted diets generate a rapid weight loss, but long-term maintenance of that loss is limited. However, clinical trials show that LCDs are as effective as VLCDs in producing weight loss after 1 year (Wadden et al., 1994). The comprehensive VLCD programs can be very expensive compared with other treatment modalities.

Physical activity. Depending on the survey, 23% to 40% of adults in the United States report no leisure time physical activity (Triano et al., 2001). If energy expenditure can be increased by physical activity while energy intake is kept constant, body weight will be reduced. The more vigorous the activity, the more energy stores are used. The amount of weight loss depends on the time and intensity of each activity. Success in improving physical fitness depends on selecting activities that appeal to the individual and fit into the individual's life-style constraints. Exercise has beneficial effects independent of weight loss, including improved cardiovascular fitness and increased high-density lipoprotein (HDL) cholesterol levels (Blair, 1995). Inclusion of resistance

KEY TERMS

gastric surgery: consists of surgical banding or stapling of the stomach to reduce capacity or creation of a small gastric pouch that empties into the jejunum

Table 14-3 Behavior Treatment Components for Obesity

Component	Description	Examples
Self-Monitoring	Recording of target behaviors and factors associated with behaviors.	Keeping records of food and exercise behaviors and environment associated with overeating or not exercising, noting mood.
Stimulus Control	Restricting environmental factors associated with inappropriate behaviors.	Keeping away from high-fat foods by not bringing them home. Setting a time and place of exercise.
Contingency Management	Rewarding appropriate behaviors.	Giving prizes or treats for achieving exercise goals. Using a nonfood reward for not overeating.
Changing Behavior Patterns	Directly altering target behavior topology.	Using stairs instead of elevators. Slowing down eating.
Cognitive-Behavior Modification	Changing thinking patterns related to target behaviors.	Changing social environment to reduce temptation to diet or avoid exercise.

training can increase lean body mass (LBM). Exercise can be an important adjunct to other weight-reduction strategies and may diminish the tendency for rapid postprogram weight gain (Zelasko, 1995). In 2000, for the first time, the Dietary Guidelines included a recommendation related to fitness: "Aim for Fitness" and "Be Physically Active Each Day." Noting that persons of all ages benefit from regular physical activity, the specific recommendation is that adults accumulate 30 minutes or more of moderate-intensity physical activity daily (NHLBI, 2000).

Behavior modification. Behavior treatment of obesity focuses on gradual changes to modify eating behavior and physical activity habits. It can be undertaken alone or through group or individual sessions, under the guidance of professional or lay personnel, or in conjunction with other approaches. Specific behavioral strategies include self-monitoring, stimulus control, contingency management, stress management, changing behavior parameters, cognitive-behavior strategies, and social support (Table 14-3). A typical behavior modification program takes about 16 weeks to 20 weeks and can generate a 0.5 kg to 0.75 kg per week weight loss. Behavior modification is a method that supports other treatment approaches. Appropriate questions for behavioral assessment for a weight-loss program appear in Box 14-9.

Box 14-9 Brief Behavioral Assessment for Weight Reduction Therapy

- Has the individual sought weight loss on his or her own initiative?
- What events have led the individual to seek weight loss now?
- What are the individual's stress level and mood?
- Does the individual have an eating disorder in addition to obesity?
- Does the individual understand the requirements of treatment or believe that he or she can fulfill them?
- How much weight does the individual expect to lose? What other benefits does he or she anticipate?

Pharmacotherapy

Recent recognition of obesity as a chronic disease has resulted in increased interest in medication to treat it (Table 14-4). Weight loss drugs approved by the FDA for long-term use may be

Table 14-4 WEIGHT LOSS DRUGS*

Drug	Dose	Action	Adverse Effects
Sibutramine (Meridia)	5, 10, 15 mg 10 mg po qd to start, may be increased to 15 mg or decreased to 5 mg	Norepinephrine, dopamine, and serotonin reuptake inhibitor.	Increase in heart rate and blood pressure
Orlistat (Xenical)	120 mg 120 mg po tid before meals	Inhibits pancreatic lipase, decreases fat absorption.	Decrease in absorption of fat-soluble vitamins; soft stools and anal leakage.

From National Heart, Lung, and Blood Institute. The practical guide. Identification, evaluation and treatment of overweight and obesity in adults. NIH Publ #00-4084. Oct, 2000.

*Ephedrine plus caffeine and fluoxetine have also been tested for weight loss, but are not approved for use in the treatment of obesity.

Mazindol, diethylpropion, phentermine, benzphetamine, and phendimetrazine are approved for only short-term use for the treatment of obesity. Herbal preparations are not recommended as part of a weight-loss program. These preparations have unpredictable amounts of active ingredients and unpredictable, and potentially harmful, effects.

useful adjuncts to diet and physical activity for individuals with a BMI ≥30 without concomitant obesity-related risk factors. Drug therapy may also be useful for persons with a BMI ≥27 who have concomitant health risk factors (NHLBI, 2000). Currently two drugs are approved by FDA: Sibutramine and Orlistat (see Box 14-9). Sibutramine inhibits the **reuptake** of the neurotransmitter epinephrine and serotonin into the neuron, thus suppressing appetite.

A second drug, Orlistat, was approved by the FDA in 1999. Orlistat works by inhibiting pancreatic lipase, the major fat digesting enzyme, reducing fat absorption. It can cause a variety of intestinal symptoms and has best acceptability if individuals consume diets with relatively small amounts of fat. Pharmaceutical companies have active research programs striving to develop a drug that will safely increase energy expenditure, decrease food intake, and accomplish weight loss with no side effects or acceptable side effects.

Gastric surgery. Surgery to accomplish weight reduction is an option for individuals with clinically severe obesity (BMI >40 or a BMI >35 with comorbid conditions). In general weight loss surgery is reserved for individuals for whom other methods of treatment have failed and have clinically severe obesity.

Currently two surgical procedures are used that reduce gastric capacity (Figure 14-8). The vertical banded **gastroplasty** is a procedure in which the upper portion of the stomach is surgically banded, creating a small pouch for food that severely reduces gastric volume. The second procedure limits food intake and alters digestion by creating a pouch in the upper part of the stomach that is connected to the small intestine so food is moved to the jejunum.

Complications associated with the surgery will vary with the overall health of the individual. Mortality rates vary from 1% to 4% and operative complications occur in less than 10% of patients (Pories et al., 1995). Long-term studies indicate that persons with diabetes and hyper-

KEY TERMS

reuptake: after a neurotransmitter is released from a neuron and performs its transmitting function, it is removed within seconds by breakdown or reuptake into the cell

gastroplasty: surgical revision of the stomach

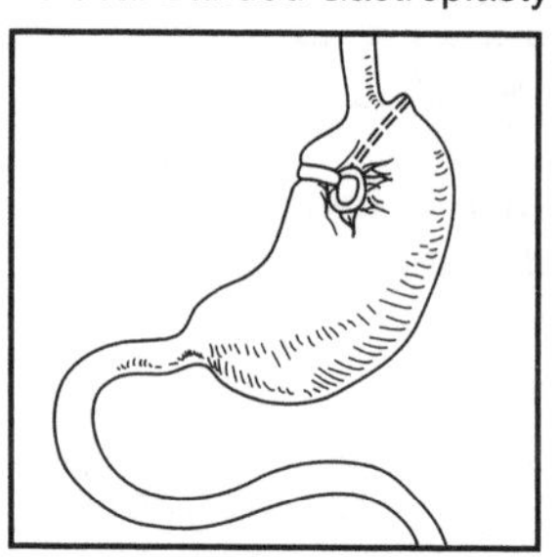

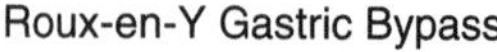

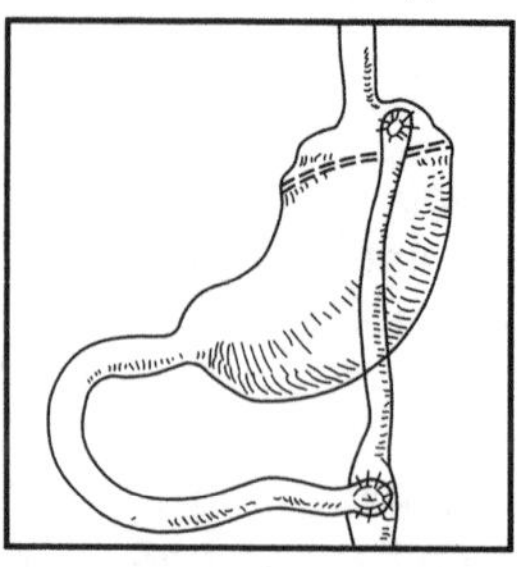

Figure 14-8 Surgical procedures in current use. *(From National Heart, Lung, and Blood Institute. The practical guide. Identification, evaluation and treatment of overweight and obesity in adults. NIH Publ #00-4084. Oct, 2000.)*

tension have marked improvement in mobility and quality of life (NHLBI, 2000).

These surgeries require lifelong monitoring. A program that provides guidance on diet, physical activity, and psychosocial concerns before and after surgery is necessary. Patients who do not follow dietary recommendations to maintain adequate intake may develop deficiencies of vitamin B_{12} and iron. Surveillance should include indices of nutrition.

Selecting a treatment approach. The 2000 Dietary Guidelines for Americans and *Healthy People 2010* objectives encourage maintenance of a healthy weight. In both instances the recommendations include dietary changes and increases in regular physical activity. Success of a program cannot be measured just by the amount of weight lost during a relatively short period. Appropriate goals are long-term amelioration of medical problems and health risks and improved quality of life with or without weight loss (Jeffery et al., 2000). Approaches should be health oriented and related to life-style changes.

The potential benefits to be accrued from weight loss and an individual's potential to maintain such a loss should be considered carefully before a program is initiated. For example if two women 163 cm (64 in) tall with a reference weight of 57 kg (125 lb) weighed 100 kg (220 lb), they would have a twofold increase in mortality risk. If the first woman was 60 years of age with osteoarthritis, she would benefit from some weight loss to decrease the physical discomfort of standing and walking. However, because of her limited ability to exercise, she would have difficulty attaining her reference weight and might not accrue benefits from such weight loss. By contrast, if the second woman were 20 years old with a family history of diabetes and hypertension, reducing to her reference weight could have lifetime benefits, and, because of her age and mobility, she would be much more apt to succeed.

EXCESS WEIGHT ACROSS THE LIFE SPAN

- *What are the problems and risks associated with excess body weight during growth and aging?*
- *What are the appropriate treatment modalities for young children whose BMIs exceed the eighty-fifth percentile on the CDC growth chart?*
- *Describe a circumstance in which an older adult with a BMI of 27 may be advised to undertake a weight loss program and one for an older adult with the same BMI who would not have weight loss recommended.*

Obesity in Childhood and Adolescence

In the United States overweight and obesity affects 25% to 30% of children (U.S. Public Health Service, 1994) and 27% of adolescents (Himes and Dietz, 1994). Of even greater concern is evidence that the prevalence of obesity is increasing. This trend is greater among children in low-income populations (Okamoto et al., 1993) and those subjected to parental neglect (Sorenson et al., 1992). Critical periods for development of obesity appear to occur during infancy, ages 5 years to 7 years, and adolescence (Dietz, 1994).

Assessment

Difficulty of determining obesity in childhood and adolescence is compounded by increases in height and weight and the changes in body composition associated with growth. BMIs at the eighty-fifth and ninety-fifth percentiles of BMI distribution on CDC growth charts at various ages are often used as criteria for overweight and obesity, respectively. It is important to monitor weight changes over time.

A triceps fatfold that exceeds the eighty-fifth percentile is a common definition of obesity. A more definitive measurement of childhood obesity would be a combination of triceps and subscapular fatfolds that exceeds the eightieth percentile and a weight greater than the seventy-fifth percentile (Rocchini, 1993). Obesity in adolescents is often defined as a weight greater than the ninety-fifth percentile and a BMI greater than 30 (Himes and Dietz, 1994).

Health Risks

Risk of becoming obese adults. The longer the duration of obesity, the greater is the likelihood that excess body weight will be sustained into adulthood. Although less than 10% of infants who are obese become obese adults, the risk increases to approximately one third for obese preschool children, 50% for school-age children (Serdula et al., 1993), and 70% to 80% for obese adolescents (Kolata, 1986). In addition the more severe the disease in childhood, the greater the chance of persistence into adulthood (Guo et al., 1994; Serdula et al., 1993). Risk of obesity in adolescents is associated with early maturation (van Lenthe, Kemper, and van Mechelen, 1996). There are some sex differences in the effect of childhood weight on adult weight. A 50-year follow-up of individuals who were enrolled in the Harvard Growth Study of 1922 to 1935 at ages 13 years to 18 years found that the BMI in childhood and adolescence was a predictor of body size in middle-age men, but not in women (Casey et al., 1992) and increased risk of morbidity and early death among men, but not women.

Immediate health effects. Various somatic changes accompany obesity in youth. Height and bone age are increased above the norms expected for children of the same age and sex. The LBM is increased to support the additional weight and may account for as much as 50% of the excess weight in obese adolescents.

Some of the greatest concerns about obesity in childhood center around increased health risks. As many as 80% of obese adolescents have been found to have elevated systolic or diastolic blood pressure and 97% already had known risk factors for heart disease, including elevated serum triglyceride and cholesterol levels and decreased HDL cholesterol levels (Becque et al., 1988). The relationship of intraabdominal fat to insulin resistance, hypertension, and hyperlipidemia, which is observed to increase risk in adults, is present in obese adolescent girls (Caprio et al., 1996).

There is strong prejudice against obese persons regardless of age, sex, race, and socioeconomic status. Such discrimination may be particularly devastating for children, who have little control over their own environments. Obese children experience discrimination by teachers and even parents, but that manifested by peers can be particularly damaging to the child's self-esteem (Hill and Silver, 1995). Children as young as 5 years of age, when asked to describe silhouettes of obese youngsters, characterized them as lazy, stupid, ugly, cheats, and liars and consistently ranked them as less desirable than children with other handicaps (Hill and Silver, 1995).

Etiology of Obesity during Growth

Multiple factors contribute to excess body fat in childhood. In addition to dietary intake and physical activity patterns, the development of obesity in childhood may be influenced by a breakdown in family interactions that precipitates inappropriate food behavior.

Children generally eat best when their parents are neither overmanaging nor overpermissive (Burroughs and Terry, 1992). Birch and others (1981) observed that mothers of fatter 4-year-old to 8-year-old children talked less to their children during mealtimes, were less responsive, gave less approval, and made fewer efforts to control inappropriate behavior during mealtime. If the parent is too involved or attempts to manipulate the child's eating, the child may feel uncomfortable and overeat. Uninterested parents who fail to provide guidance, or who are so enmeshed that they can't say no, may inadvertently promote overeating.

It has been observed that obese youngsters expend more total energy than their leaner peers on a daily basis (Bandini et al., 1990), but expenditure per kilogram of body weight is comparable (Maffels et al., 1993). When energy expenditure was calculated on the basis of LBM, there were no differences between obese and nonobese youths. Such observations have led to suggestions that obese children are less physically active than are leaner children.

It has been observed that 6- to 9-year-old children who were less physically active (based on reports of parents and teachers) tended to have thicker fatfolds (Pate et al., 1990). However, such observations must be interpreted cautiously. It may be that physical inactivity causes greater adiposity. It is also possible that higher levels of adiposity predispose youngsters to a less active life-style.

Two large-scale surveys have assessed the behavior of American children and adolescents related to physical activity. The first, using self-reported frequency and duration, determined that most youngsters between the ages of 10 years and 17 years of age had 1 hour to 2 hours of moderate to vigorous physical activity per day (Pate et al., 1990). However, 20% to 30% of the youths reported averaging less than one-half hour of physical activity per day. In a study of high school students, Sallis (1993) reported that girls tended to be less physically active than boys and there was a consistent decline in physical activity over the school years.

Prevention and Treatment

Therapy for or prevention of obesity in childhood or adolescence is complicated and must be sensitive to the child's needs—physical, nutritional, and emotional. A major concern in controlling gains in body weight or fat during growth is that long-term growth might be impaired. A recent study reported that moderate energy restriction in children age 6 years to 12 years did not negatively influence long-term growth after 10 years (Epstein et al., 1993).

The most practical intervention to prevent obesity in youngsters is to modify the environment in terms of habitual physical activity and food intake. It is vital that tactics be moderate and positive and promote realistic changes while doing no harm. The essential task is to create a structure in which the child's natural ability to regulate food intake is distorted as little as possible by outside influences and to encourage the child to respond to physiological cues for eating. The second guideline is to encourage physical activity, especially those that can be continued over time.

Benefits of treatment. There are several benefits to reducing obesity in childhood. In the long term, the most important is the prevention of adult obesity and related hypertension, cardiovascular disease, and diabetes. Short-term benefits include improved fitness, decreased blood pressure and glucose, and a more favorable lipid profile (Sutter and Hawes, 1993).

Physical activity as a singular intervention can have a beneficial effect on body composition in obese youngsters, but that intervention is more likely to be effective if dietary changes and behavior modification techniques are used in combination with increased physical activity.

Family therapy. Parents are very important in determining the behavior of their children. Family therapy assumes that children need parental support and family cohesion to make changes in eating and physical activity habits (Mellin and Frost, 1992). A focus on the family system attempts to modify how the family solves problems and resolves conflicts. It involves teaching children to connect with people rather than food when they are distressed. Support from the entire family promotes long-term changes in behavior such as diet and exercise. In a study that involved diet and exercise with and without family therapy, it was observed that adding family therapy to intervention programs improved outcomes as measured by weight, fatfolds, and physical fitness (Floodmark et al., 1993).

Older Adults

There is a growing prevalence of obesity among older persons. A decision regarding treatment of obesity in older adults will be based on potential benefits of weight reduction to improve day-to-day function and cardiovascular risk (Visser et al., 1998a). The association of excess body weight with mortality and morbidity decreases as aging progresses. Data from the NHANES II show that overweight adults age 45 years to 75 years have a lower risk of hypertension and diabetes and higher serum cholesterol levels than those younger than 45 years (Van Itallie, 1985). Although such observations have resulted in higher relative weight standards for older adults, avoidance of obesity and moderate increases in physical activity are associated with longevity in middle-age men (Paffenbarger et al., 1993).

Excess body weight in older adults means greater stress on joints that are often arthritic and greater demand on the respiratory and cardiovascular systems. However, it may be exceedingly difficult for older persons to lose weight because of decreased energy expenditure associated with lower basal metabolic rates and reduced activity levels. Women over 65 years are at greater disadvantage than are men because of lower energy requirements. It is important that the weight control program meet the needs of the individual and preserve body cell mass and its function (Visser et al., 1998b).

Concepts to Remember

- Behaviors associated with eating disturbances cover a spectrum from semistarvation to unhealthy dietary practices to binging and purging to compulsive overeating.
- Eating disturbances have potentially serious negative psychologic and physiologic consequences.
- The etiology of eating disorders (anorexia nervosa, bulimia nervosa, and BED) is complex and has biologic, social, psychologic, and environmental parameters.
- Success in treating eating disorders is related to the severity and duration of the disorder and to family circumstances. Therefore multidisciplinary approaches for prevention, early recognition, and intervention are important.
- Obesity, the most common nutrition-related health problem of Americans, has substantial psychologic, social, physiologic, and health consequences.
- Obesity is a chronic disease for which long-term treatment approaches are needed.
- Treatment programs for obesity must be individualized to meet the needs and life-styles of the individual.
- Initial treatment for overweight and obesity emphasizes dietary moderation, increased activity, and behavioral modification to promote behavior change and support its maintenance.
- Medications can be used as an adjunct to diet, exercise, and behavior modification for some individuals.
- For individuals with a BMI >40 or a BMI >35 with comorbidities, surgery may be appropriate to accomplish weight reduction.
- For very obese individuals, pharmacotherapy and gastric surgery may be treatment alternatives.
- Obesity is a health concern across all stages of the life span.

REFERENCES

Abate N et al.: Relationships of generalized and regional adiposity to insulin sensitivity in men, J Clin Invest 96:88, 1995.

Abrams KK et al.: Disordered eating attitudes and behaviors, psychological adjustment, and ethnic identity: a comparison of black and white female college students, Int J Eat Disord 14:49, 1994.

Agras WS: Pharmacotherapy of bulimia nervosa and binge eating disorders: long term outcomes, Psychopharm Bull 33:437, 1997.

Allison DB et al.: Annual deaths attributable to obesity in the United States, JAMA 282:1530, 1999.

American Dietetic Association: Position of the American Dietetic Association: nutrition intervention in the treatment of anorexia nervosa, bulimia nervosa and binge eating, J Am Diet Assoc 94:902, 1994.

American Psychiatric Association: Practice guidelines for eating disorders, Am J Psychiatry 150:212, 1993.

American Psychiatric Association: Diagnostic and statistical manual for mental disorders (DSM-IV), ed 4, Washington, DC, 1998, American Psychiatric Association Press.

American Psychiatric Association: Work Group on Eating Disorders: practice guideline for the treatment of patients with eating disorders (revision), Am J Psychiatry 157:1S, 2000.

Antony MM et al.: Psychopathology correlates of binge eating and binge eating disorder, Compr Psychiatry 35:386, 1994.

Bandini LG et al.: Energy expenditure in obese and nonobese adolescents, Pediatr Res 27:198, 1990.

Becker AE et al.: Eating disorders, N Engl J Med 340:109, 1999.

Becque MD et al.: Coronary risk incidence of obese adolescents: reductions with exercise plus diet intervention, Pediatrics 81:605, 1988.

Beumont PJV et al.: Excessive physical activity in dieting disorder patients: proposals for a supervised exercise program, Int J Eat Disord 15:21, 1994.

Birch LL et al.: Mother-child interaction patterns and the degree of fatness in children, J Nutr Educ 13:17, 1981.

Blair SN: Diet and activity: the synergistic merger, Nutr Today 30:108, 1995.
Booth SL et al.: Environmental and societal factors affect food choice and physical activity: rationale, influences, and leverage points, Nutr Rev 59:521, 2001.
Bouchard C and Perusse L: Genetics of obesity, Annu Rev Nutr 13: 337, 1993.
Bruch H: Eating disorders, New York, 1973, Basic Books.
Burroughs ML and Terry RD: Parents' perspectives toward their children's eating behavior, Clin Nutr 8:45, 1992.
Caprio S et al.: Fat distribution and cardiovascular risk factors in obese adolescent girls: importance of the intraabdominal fat depot, Am J Clin Nutr 64:12, 1996.
Carlat D and Camargo C: Review of bulimia nervosa in males, Am J Psychiatry 148:831, 1991.
Casey VA et al.: Body mass index from childhood to middle age: a 50 year follow-up, Am J Clin Nutr 56:14, 1992.
Chamoro R and Flores-Ortiz Y: Acculturation and disordered eating patterns among Mexican American women, Int J Eat Disord 28:125, 2000.
Ching PLYH et al.: Activity level and risk of overweight in male health professionals, Am J Public Health 86:25, 1996.
Colditz GA et al.: Weight gain as a risk factor for clinical diabetes mellitus in women, Ann Int Med 122:481, 1995.
Collings S and King M: Ten-year follow-up of 50 patients with bulimia nervosa, Br J Psychiatry 164:80, 1994.
Considine RV et al.: Serum immunoreactive-leptin concentrations in normal weight and obese humans, N Engl J Med 334:292, 1996.
Crow SJ and Mitchell JE: Rational therapy of eating disorders, Drugs 48:372, 1994.
Denke MA et al.: Excess body weight: an under-recognized contributor to high blood cholesterol levels in white American men, Arch Intern Med 153:93, 1993.
Dietz WH: Critical periods in childhood for the development of obesity, Am J Clin Nutr 59:955, 1994.
DiGioacchino RE et al.: Gender differences among those exhibiting characteristics of binge eating disorder, Eat Weight Disord 4:76, 1999.
Drewnowski A et al.: Nalopone, an opiate blocker, reduces the consumption of sweet high-fat foods in obese and lean female binge eaters, Am J Clin Nutr 61:1206, 1995.
Epstein LH et al.: Effect of weight loss by obese children on long-term growth, Am J Dis Child 147:1076, 1993.
Fisher M et al.: Eating disorders in adolescence: a background paper, J Adolesc Health 116:420, 1995.
Floodmark CE et al.: Prevention of progression to severe obesity in a group of obese schoolchildren treated with family therapy, Pediatrics 91:880, 1993.
Garfinkel PE and Kaplan AS: Starvation-based perpetuatory mechanisms in anorexia nervosa and bulimia, Int J Eating Dis 4:651, 1985.
Gendall KA et al.: Body weight in bulimia nervosa, Eat Weight Disord 4:157, 1999.
Goodpaster BH et al.: Thigh adipose tissue is associated with insulin resistance in adiposity and type 2 diabetes, Am J Clin Nutr 71:885, 2000.
Guo S et al.: The predictive value of childhood body mass index values for overweight at age 35 years, Am J Clin Nutr 59:810, 1994.
Gupta MA and Johnson AM: Nonweight-related body image concerns among female eating-disordered patients and nonclinical controls: some preliminary observations, Int J Eat Disord 27:304, 2000.
Gustafson-Larson AM and Terry RD: Weight-related behaviors of fourth-grade children, J Am Diet Assoc 92:818, 1992.
Hill AJ and Silver EK: Fat, friendless and unhealthy: 9-year old children's perception of body shape stereotypes, Int J Obes Relat Metab Disord 19:423, 1995.
Himes JH and Dietz WH: Guidelines for overweight in adolescent preventive services: recommendations from an expert committee, Am J Clin Nutr 59:307, 1994.
Horm J and Anderson K: Who in America is trying to lose weight? Ann Intern Med 119:672, 1993.
Institute of Medicine: Weighing the options: criteria for evaluating weight-management programs, Food and Nutrition Board, Washington, DC, 1995, National Academy Press.
Jeffery RW et al.: Long-term maintenance of weight loss: current status, Health Psychol 19:5, 2000.
Kanders BS and Blackburn GL: Very low calorie diets for the treatment of obesity. In Blackburn GL and Ganders BS, editors: Obesity: pathophysiology, psychology and treatment, New York, 1993, Guilford Press.
Knip M and Nuutinen O: Long-term effects of weight reduction in serum lipid and plasma insulin in obese children, Am J Clin Nutr 57:490, 1992.
Kolata G: Obesity in children: a growing problem, Science 232:20, 1986.
Kumanyika SK: Obesity in minority populations, Obes Res 2:166, 1994.
Kushner RF: Body weight and mortality, Nutr Rev 51:127, 1993.
Lee I et al.: Body weight and mortality: a 27-year follow-up of middle aged men, JAMA 270:2823, 1993.
Lennkh C et al.: Comorbidity of obsessive compulsive disorder in patients with eating disorders, Eat Weight Disord 3:37, 1998.
Maffels C et al.: Resting metabolic rate in six- to ten-year-old obese and nonobese children, J Pediatr 122:556, 1993.
Manson JE et al.: Body weight and mortality among women, N Engl J Med 333:677, 1995.
Matkovic V: Calcium intake and peak bone mass [editorial], N Engl J Med 327:120, 1992.
Mayer L: Body composition and anorexia nervosa: does physiology explain psychology? Am J Clin Nutr 73: 851, 2001.
Mellin LM and Frost L: Child and adolescent obesity: the nurse practitioner's use of the SHAPEDOWN method, J Ped Health Care 6:187, 1992.

Mokdad AH et al.: The spread of the obesity epidemic in the United States, 1991-1998, JAMA 282;1519, 1999.

Moore DC: Body image and eating behavior in adolescent girls, Am J Dis Child 142:1114, 1988.

Must A et al.: The disease burden associated with overweight and obesity, JAMA 282:1523, 1999.

National Heart, Lung and Blood Institute: Clinical guidelines on the identification, evaluation and treatment of overweight and obesity in adults: the evidence report, Obes Res 6(suppl 2):51S-210S, 1998.

National Institutes of Mental Health: Eating disorders: facts about eating disorders and the search for solutions, nih.gov/publicat/eatingdisorder.cfm#ed4 (accessed May 7, 2001).

National Institutes of Health, National Heart, Lung, and Blood Institute: The practical guide. Identification, evaluation, and treatment of overweight and obesity in adults, NIH Pub # 00-4084, 2000.

Neumark-Sztainer D: Excessive weight preoccupation, Nutr Today 30:68, 1995.

Obarzanek E et al.: Resting metabolic rate of anorexia nervosa patients during weight gain, Am J Clin Nutr 60:66, 1994.

Okamoto E et al.: High prevalence of overweight in inner-city school children, Am J Dis Child 147:155, 1993.

Olmsted MP et al.: Rate and prediction of relapse in bulimia nervosa, Am J Psychiatry 15:738, 1994. Osterman J et al.: Serum cholesterol profiles during treatment of obese outpatients with a very low calorie diet: effect of initial cholesterol levels, Int J Obes Relat Metab Disord 216:49, 1992.

Paffenbarger RS et al.: The association of changes of physical activity level and other life-style characteristics with mortality among men, N Engl J Med 328:538, 1993.

Pate RR et al.: Associations between physical activity and physical fitness in American children, Am J Dis Child 144:1123, 1990.

Peterson CB et al.: Predictors of treatment outcome for binge eating disorder, Int J Eat Disord 28:131, 2000.

Prewitt ET et al.: Changes in body weight, body composition and energy in lean women fed high- and low-fat diets, Am J Clin Nutr 54:304, 1991.

Probst M et al.: Body composition of anorexia nervosa patients assessed by underwater weighing and skinfold-thickness measurements before and after weight gain, Am J Clin Nutr 73:190, 2001.

Ravussin E and Swinburn A: Pathophysiology of obesity, Lancet 340:404, 1992.

Read N et al.: The role of the gut in regulating food intake in men, Nutr Rev 52:1, 1994.

Reaven FM et al.: Insulin resistance and hyperinsulinemia in individuals with small, dense low density lipoprotein particles, J Clin Invest 92:141, 1993.

Reiss D et al.: Bulimia nervosa: 5-year social outcome and relationship to eating pathology, Int J Eating Dis 18:127, 1995.

Rink TJ: In search of a satiety factor, Nature 372:406, 1994.

Rising R et al.: Decreased ratio of fat to carbohydrate oxidation with increasing age in Pima Indians, J Am Coll Nutr 15:309, 1996.

Roberts SB and Greenberg AS: The new obesity genes, Nutr Rev 54:41, 1996.

Rocchini AP: Adolescent obesity and hypertension, Pediatr Clin North Am 40:81, 1993.

Rolls BJ et al.: Volume of food consumed affects satiety in men, Am J Clin Nutr 67:1170, 1998.

Rosenvinge JH et al.: The comorbidity of eating disorders and personality disorders: a meta-analytic review of studies published between 1983 and 1998, Eat Weight Disord 5:52, 2000.

Rumpler WV et al.: Energy-intake restriction and diet composition effects on energy expenditure in men, Am J Clin Nutr 53:430, 1991.

Salisbury JJ et al.: Refeeding, metabolic rate, and weight gain in anorexia nervosa: a review, Int J Eating Dis 17:337, 1995.

Sallis JF: Epidemiology of physical activity and fitness in children and adolescents, Crit Rev Food Sci Nutr 33:403, 1993.

Sasaki J et al.: A long-term aerobic exercise program decreases the obesity index and increases the high density cholesterol concentration in obese children, Int J Obes Relat Metab Disord 11:339, 1987.

Schlicker SA et al.: The weight and fitness status of United States children, Nutr Rev 52:11, 1994.

Schotte DE and Stunkard AJ: The effects of weight reduction on blood pressure in 301 obese patients, Arch Intern Med 150:1701, 1990.

Seim HC and Holtmeier KB: Effects of a six-week, low-fat diet on serum cholesterol, body weight, and body measurements, Fam Pract Res J 12:411, 1992.

Serdula MK et al.: Do obese children become obese adults? A review of literature, Prev Med 22:167, 1993.

Silver DH et al.: Self-esteem and eating disorders: differential effects of self-linking and self-competence, Eat Weight Disord 3:95, 1998.

Sjostrom L: Morbidity of severely obese subjects: mortality of severely obese subjects, Am J Clin Nutr 55 (suppl):508S, 516S, 1992.

Solanto MV et al.: Rate of weight gain in patients with anorexia nervosa under two behavioral contracts, Pediatrics 93:989, 1994.

Sorenson TIA et al.: Childhood body mass index: genetic and familial environmental influences assessed in a longitudinal adoption study, Int J Obes Relat Metab Disord 16:705, 1992.

Specker S et al.: Psychopathology in subgroups of obese women with and without binge eating disorder, Compr Psychiatry 35:185, 1994.

Spitzer RL et al.: Binge eating disorder: its further validation in a multisite study, Int J Eat Disord 13:137, 1993.

Stevens SA: Weight loss intervention in phase I of the Trials of Hypertensive Prevention, Arch Intern Med 153:849, 1993.

Stewart DE: Reproductive functions in eating disorders, Ann Med 24:287, 1992.

Strober M et al.: Males with anorexia nervosa: a controlled study of eating disorders in first degree relatives, Int J Eat Disord 29:263, 2001.

Stunkard AJ: Two eating disorders: binge eating disorder and the night eating syndrome, Appetite 34:333, 2000.

Sullivan PF: Mortality in anorexia nervosa, Am J Psychiatry 152:1073, 1995.

Sundgot-Borgen J et al.: The effect of exercise, cognitive therapy and nutritional counseling in treating bulimia nervosa, Med Sci Sports Exerc 34:190, 2002.

Sutter E and Hawes MR: Relationship of physical activity, body fat, diet and blood lipid profile in youths 10-15 years, Med Sci Sports Exerc 25:748, 1993.

Thiel A et al.: Obsessive compulsive disorder among patients with anorexia nervosa and bulimia nervosa, Am J Psychiatry 152:72, 1995.

Thompson D et al.: Life-time health and economic consequences of obesity, Arch Intern Med 159:2177, 1999.

Turner MSJ and Shapiro C: The biochemistry of anorexia nervosa, Int J Eating Dis 12:179, 1992.

U.S. Public Health Service: Binge eating disorder, Washington, DC, 1993, National Institutes of Health.

U.S. Public Health Service: Prevalence of overweight among adolescents-United States, 1988-91, MMWR Morb Mortal Wkly Rep 43:818, 1994.

Van Itallie TB: Health implications of overweight and obesity in the United States, Ann Intern Med 103:983, 1985.

van Lenthe FJ, Kemper HCG, and van Mechelen W: Rapid maturation in adolescence results in greater obesity in adulthood: the Amsterdam Growth and Health Study, Am J Clin Nutr 64:18, 1996.

Visser M et al.: Body fat and skeletal muscle mass in relation to physical disability in very old men and women in the Framingham heart study, J Gerontology 53A:M214, 1998a.

Visser M et al.: High body fatness and skeletal muscle mass in relation to physical disability in older men and women: the cardiovascular health study, Am J Clin Nutr 68:584, 1998.

Williamson DF: "Weight cycling" and mortality: how do the epidemiologists explain the role of intentional weight loss? J Am Coll Nutr 15:6, 1996.

Williamson DF et al.: Weight loss attempts in adults: goals, duration, and rate of weight loss, Am J Public Health 82:1251, 1992.

Wing RR et al.: Effects of a very low-calorie diet on long-term glycemic control in obese type II diabetic subjects, Arch Intern Med 151:1334, 1991.

Wolf AM and Colditz GA: Current estimates of the economic cost of obesity in the United States, Obes Res 6:97, 1998.

Wong JC et al.: Bone mineral density in adolescent females with recently diagnosed anorexia nervosa, Int J Eat Disord 29:11, 2001.

Woodside DD: A review of anorexia nervosa and bulimia nervosa, Curr Prob Pediatr 25:67, 1995.

Yao M and Roberts SB: Dietary energy density and weight regulation, Nutr Rev 59:247, 2001.

Zelasko CJ: Exercise for weight loss: what are the facts? J Am Diet Assoc 95:1414, 1995.

APPLICATION

Managing Body Weight

Fred is a 30-year-old manager for a chain of hotels. He is 178 cm (70 in) in height, has a medium frame, and weighed 80 kg (170 lb) when he was 21. During high school and college, he was active with part-time jobs and played tennis and soccer. As his job responsibilities became more demanding, Fred had less time for exercise and his weight began to creep up because he loved to eat. He noticed he often needed to buy new clothes and he had begun to accumulate a closet full of clothes that were too tight. Now he weighs 95 kg (210 lb).

Last year Fred vowed to get physically fit and go on a diet. To lose weight he would skip breakfast and have a cup of yogurt for lunch. By dinnertime he was ravenous and later he would raid the refrigerator for snacks. He signed up to play tennis in a league, but he dropped out because he was embarrassed to be seen in a large pair of tennis shorts. Although Fred did lose a few pounds, he became increasingly frustrated with his semistarvation/gorging diet pattern and regained the weight quickly. Now Fred is very self-conscious about his weight and sometimes avoids social activities because of it.

Vicki is a 54-year-old junior-high school teacher. At a party on New Year's Day, she looked around the room and suddenly "felt fat." She weighed 190 pounds at the time and had accumulated a wardrobe of large sizes. Vicki's New Year's resolution was to lose weight. The next morning she made an appointment to see a dietitian at a clinic affiliated with the community hospital.

Vicki started to follow a meal pattern that provided approximately 1200 kilocalories per day and began to exercise at least an hour a day—usually to a video before going to school each morning. By the first of September, Vicki had lost 46 pounds. She had learned a lot about diet and exercise and was feeling much better. Her legs didn't hurt anymore and the pains in her back had subsided. She found friends who walked with her at lunchtime for exercise. She wants to lose 10 more pounds, but is thrilled by the improvement in how she feels and looks. To Vicki, it is important to maintain how she feels now.

WILL FRED EVER LOSE WEIGHT? CAN VICKI SUSTAIN HER WEIGHT LOSS?

Being obese or overweight is a common health problem and its prevalence has increased dramatically in the past 30 years. Currently one half of all U.S. adults are overweight (BMI >25) or obese (BMI >30). Excess weight is associated with an increased risk for numerous health problems, including dyslipidemia, hypertension, cardiovascular disease, type 2 diabetes, and some cancers. An estimated 325,000 deaths per year in the United States are attributable to obesity (Klem, 2000).

The goal of treatment of overweight and obese individuals should be focused on maintaining a **healthy weight** rather than on weight loss (American Dietetic Association, 1997). Recent evidence-based guidelines have recognized clinical benefits of even moderate weight loss (5% to 10%), which is achievable using a variety of interventions (Weiss, 2000).

Fred and Vicki are characteristic of millions of overweight and moderately obese adults who struggle to lose weight and whose lives become dominated by restrictive eating to control body weight. Although a combination of diet, exercise, and behavior modification can result in substantial success in achieving weight loss, only a small percentage of individuals who complete a comprehensive weight-reduction program maintain that weight loss after 5 years.

healthy weight: the best possible weight for the individual given overall health; for some it may be attainment of a reference weight, but for others it may be loss of 5% or 10% of current body weight, which will improve health and reduce severity of comorbidities

BEHAVIORAL APPROACHES TO OBESITY

Any intervention that causes negative energy balance is guaranteed to be efficacious in producing weight loss, which will continue while negative energy balance is maintained. In clinical practice compliance is rarely 100%, so the efficiency of even the most efficacious treatment is usually low.

A variety of approaches to managing body weight focus on life-style changes or behavior modification. Characteristics common to such programs are listed on page 510. A major advantage of this approach is the fact that it diminishes emphasis on dieting and the frustration associated with failure to control eating behavior (Wadden and Sarwer, 1998). A life-style approach that uses strategies to modify behaviors related to eating and exercise, group support, and longer treatments have reported better long-term success when emphasis was removed from calorie restriction and placed on normalizing eating habits (Foreyt and Goodrick, 1993).

Concepts basic to behavioral approaches center on self-acceptance and nondieting. An important component of self-acceptance is acceptance of one's size. Size acceptance rejects the negative concept of fatness, the assumption that obesity constitutes a major problem requiring change. The basic premise of nondieting is to avoid perpetuation of the physiologic and psychologic consequences of restrained eating. The

Characteristics common to body weight management programs focused on life-style changes or behavior modification:

- Eat in response to internal cues for hunger and satiety.
- Avoid restrictive dieting.
- Avoid binge eating.
- Recognize that there are no good or bad foods.
- Focus on psychologic and physical health rather than appearance.
- Focus on self-acceptance—enjoy one's strengths and dispassionately view limitations or weaknesses.
- Develop self-esteem.
- Use family and social support.
- Emphasize exercise that is within ability and enjoyed.
- Identify eating that is a response to emotional or environmental factors.
- Develop alternatives to emotional eating responses.

focus is on adopting behaviors that enhance quality of life and support eating in response to internal cues for hunger and satiety.

These approaches are especially helpful for binge eaters and others who believe their eating is out of control or guided by emotions or environmental factors rather than internal cues. Nondieting programs help individuals focus on health and well-being by breaking away from these old responses and developing new behaviors. Various methods are used to facilitate this approach, including psychologic, educational, cognitive, behavioral, and social techniques.

ARE BEHAVIORAL APPROACHES TO BODY FATNESS SUCCESSFUL?

Traditional weight control programs are evaluated based on loss of weight or fat, increases in physical fitness, and changes in blood pressure or levels of blood glucose or lipids. Behavioral programs, on the other hand, emphasize factors related to self-esteem, eating behavior, and quality of life. Several short-term group programs have reported significant improvements in self-acceptance (Omichinski and Harrison, 1995), eating style, dietary behavior, self-esteem, and physical activity (Carrier et al., 1994).

Most of the reports of behavioral programs have positive weight loss outcomes, which were maintained for more than a year. This approach may be very promising for individuals like Fred who have fallen into a restrictive eating/binging pattern. These programs are relatively inexpensive to operate and easy to initiate because they can use available techniques. In addition the behavioral approaches avoid the physiologic and psychologic risks associated with chronic dieting. Although weight loss is not a primary goal of such programs, small changes may be a benefit of normalized eating patterns, and modest weight loss can improve the risk profile for diabetes mellitus, hypertension, and coronary heart disease.

In the last 20 years, evaluation of weight control techniques has resulted in dramatic improvements in short-term treatment efficacy, but has been less successful in improving long-term success. Extending treatment length and putting more emphasis on energy expenditure have resulted in modest improvements in long-term weight loss (Jeffery et al., 2000).

CAN WEIGHT LOSSES BE MAINTAINED OVER THE LONG TERM?

Most long-term studies of weight loss tend to focus on programs that combine weight loss (usually completed in 1 to 6 months) and variable weight maintenance (Lean, 2000). Few studies have adopted specific and separate strategies for weight loss and maintenance of weight loss. Any serial dieter knows losing weight is easy compared with keeping it off in the long run. The goal is to determine how successful weight losers maintain their reduced weight.

Recently researchers have begun to address issues of long-term maintenance of weight loss. For example one study documented maintenance of weight loss in twins from the ongoing study of Finnish Twin Cohort (Sarlio-Lahteenkrova et al., 2000). Participants had lost at least 5% of their body weight between 1975 and 1981 and had maintained that loss for 9 years to 15 years until

1990. Predictors of weight loss maintenance were somewhat different for women and men, but both were related to health status. In men weight loss maintenance was associated with a low level of stress and health-promoting behaviors and to a lesser extent to the presence of medical problems. For women weight loss maintenance was associated with low initial well-being and health-compromising behaviors that improved after weight loss.

In North America, the National Weight Control Registry is the largest study of individuals successful at long-term maintenance of weight loss (Klem, 1997). It was created by recruiting individuals who had lost at least 30 pounds and kept it off for 1 year or more. Currently there are more than 3000 people on the registry. Each year these men and women complete questionnaires about their diets, exercise, and other health-related factors. Several studies have investigated various factors associated with individuals who have maintained weight loss.

A number of studies based on members of the National Weight Control Registry have reported on various factors associated with loss of body weight and maintenance of that weight loss. There are two questions these studies hope to answer: (1) what was successful in achieving weight loss? and (2) what are the characteristics or behaviors that indicate maintenance of that weight loss?

Members of the registry reported losing weight on their own, through organized programs, and through use of a liquid formula. However, regardless of the methods used, the behavioral strategies for weight maintenance were similar among groups—they, like Vicki, consumed diets low in energy and engaged in high levels of physical activity.

Two studies included 874 enrollees who had histories of being overweight. Individuals in one group had lost an average of 30 kg (66 lbs) and maintained the weight loss for 5.1 years (Shick et al., 1998); those in the other group had maintained a 13.6 kg weight loss for 5 years (Klem et al., 1997). Over one half of the individuals in these programs had lost weight through formal programs and the remainder had lost weight on their own. Both groups reported having used diet and exercise to lose weight and nearly three quarters of the individuals in these studies reported that a triggering event (often a medical concern) had preceded their successful weight loss. These weight loss maintainers reported mean caloric intakes of 1350 kcal per day for women and 1685 kcal per day for men. The energy from fat was approximately 24%. Their energy and fat intakes were less than those of the participants in NHANES III (Shick et al., 1998). Also members appear to be highly active. They reported expending approximately 2815 kcal per week through physical activity (Klem et al., 1997). One encouraging observation was the fact that 42% of participants reported that maintaining their weight loss was less difficult than losing weight. Nearly all indicated that weight loss had led to improvements in their level of energy, physical mobility, general mood, self-confidence, and physical health.

These findings weren't all that surprising. The enrollees did the things health professionals had been telling them to do, so it's not surprising that successful losers would follow the same methods to keep their weight down. What the authors of these research studies wanted to know was how they keep at it, shunning dessert and sweating through a daily workout, year after year after year.

Successful losers tended to have four factors in common. Most, if not all, weighed themselves frequently and ate breakfast every day. More importantly, they consumed a low-fat diet and exercised regularly.

Behaviors of weight maintainers:

- Weighed themselves frequently
- Ate breakfast almost daily
- Consumed a diet low in fat
- Exercised regularly

To sort out some of the factors influencing weight maintenance, McGuire and colleagues (1999) compared the eating, exercise, self-weighing, and dietary restraint characteristics of weight-loss maintainers with those of individuals who had lost weight and regained it, and against those of individuals whose weight had been stable within the last 5 years. Weight-loss maintainers reported using more behavioral strategies to control dietary fat intake, higher levels of strenuous activity, and greater frequency of self-weighing than weight-loss regainers or weight-stable individuals. For psychologic factors, the weight-loss maintainers reported less endorsement for medical causes of obesity, cited greater endorsement for psychologic consequences, and indicated that they had been motivated to lose weight for psychologic reasons (Ogden, 2000). These results suggest weight-loss maintainers use more behavioral strategies to control their weight than do either regainers or weight-stable controls.

In a similar study, McGuire et al. (1999) collected behavior and psychologic information after 1 year of weight maintenance from long-term weight-loss maintainers and gainers. Risk factors for weight regain included more recent weight losses and higher levels of depression, dietary disinhibition, and binge eating levels at entry into the registry. Over the year of follow-up, gainers reported greater decreases in energy expenditure and greater increases in percentage of calories from fat. Gainers also reported greater decreases in restraint and increases in hunger, dietary inhibition, and binge eating. This study suggests that several years of successful weight maintenance increase the probability of future weight maintenance and that weight gain is because of, at least in part, failure to maintain behavior changes. Reestablishing behavior techniques successful in weight loss becomes an important factor in maintaining weight loss in the long term.

Risk factors for weight regain:
- Weight loss <2 years
- Weight loss >30% of maximum weight
- Higher levels of depression
- Decreased dietary restraint
- Binge eating

REFERENCES

American Dietetic Association: Position of the American Dietetic Association: weight management, J Am Diet Assoc 97:71, 1997.

Carrier KM et al.: Rethinking traditional weight management programs: a 3-year follow-up evaluation of a new approach, J Psychol 128:517, 1994.

Foreyt JP and Goodrick GK: Weight management without dieting, Nutr Today 28:4, 1993.

Jeffery RW et al.: Long-term maintenance of weight loss: current status, Health Psychol 19:5, 2000.

Klem ML et al.: A descriptive study of individuals successful at long-term maintenance of substantial weight loss, Am J Clin Nutr 66:239, 1997.

Klem ML: Successful losers. The habits of individuals who have maintained long-term weight loss, Minn Med 83:43, 2000.

Lean ME: Is long-term weight loss possible? Br J Nutr 83:S103, 2000.

McGuire MT et al.: What predicts weight regain in a group of successful weight losers? J Consult Clin Psychol 67:177, 1999.

Ogden J: The correlates of long-term weight loss: a group comparison study of obesity, Int J Obes Relat Metab Disord 24:1018, 2000.

Omichinski L and Harrison K: Reduction of dietary attitudes and practices after participation in a non-diet lifestyle program, J Can Diet Assoc 56:81, 1995.

Sarlio-Lahteenkorva S et al.: A descriptive study of weight loss maintenance: 6 and 15 year follow-up of initially overweight adults, Int J Obes Relat Metab Disord 24:116, 2000.

Shick SM et al.: Persons successful at long-term weight loss and maintenance continue to consume a low-energy, low-fat diet, J Am Diet Assoc 98:408, 1998.

Wadden T and Sarwer DB: Behavioral treatment of obesity: new approaches to an old disorder. In Goldstein D, editor: The management of eating disorders, Totowa, NJ, 1998, Humana Press.

Weiss D: How to help your patients lose weight: current therapy for obesity, Cleve Clin J Med 67:739, 2000.

CHAPTER

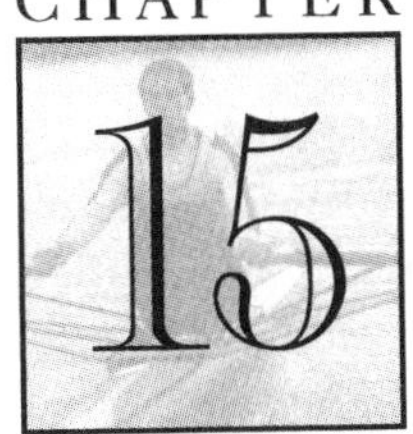

Nutrition, Physical Activity, and Performance

Diane L. Habash

Chapter Outline

Kristen could not wait to begin college and to finally be independent. As she began her freshman year, she developed friendships with other freshmen girls. This was when she first heard about the "freshman 15" weight gain. Kristen, a former high school cheerleader, is 66 inches in height and weighs 135 pounds. She, like many other high school students, remained physically fit because her coach expected it. On her own she is not as likely to be physically fit or even active. Her hobbies include dancing, listening to music, and using the Internet. After her first semester Kristen noticed that she had gained about 5 pounds and, along with another friend, she planned to ride a stationary bike for 30 minutes 5 days each week for 2 months. However, physical activity is not the only aspect that Kristen should confront in her attempt to maintain a healthy body weight. She often eats only once a day, with snacks at night while she is studying. She says the cafeteria food is not as appealing as it once was and now she eats sweetened cereal and milk with every cafeteria meal. Her friends often ask her to go to parties several times a week, where there is always plenty of beer and pizza. Her sleep habits are different from her high school sleep patterns and her study hours are often late at night when the dorm is quiet. In essence, college life, although full of independence, has little routine and is actually challenging Kristen to establish better eating, sleeping, studying, and activity habits.

The author wishes to acknowledge the NIH Grant M01RR00034 for time to prepare this manuscript.

Daily life in the industrialized world has become more sedentary. A sedentary life-style has been directly linked to elevated risks of chronic diseases, such as diabetes, obesity, heart disease, and cancer (Blair et al., 1995; Blair et al., 2001; Bouchard and Despres, 1995; National Institutes of Health Consensus Conference, 1996). The relationship between physical inactivity and chronic disease is so significant that Americans of all ages are strongly urged to become more active (Blair et al., 1996b; National Institutes of Health Consensus Conference, 1996). This is especially true because over 60% of Americans do not obtain sufficient weekly exercise to derive health benefits and about 25% of Americans do not get weekly exercise at all (Williams, 1999). Some of these health benefits include improvements in blood lipid profile, carbohydrate metabolism, blood pressure, body weight, and mortality rate. This chapter addresses the relationship between nutrition and physical activity with particular attention to this relationship in college-age adults.

PHYSICAL FITNESS

- *What is physical fitness and how is it assessed?*
- *What are the benefits of improved physical fitness?*
- *What are some of the recommendations for improving physical fitness?*

The set of characteristics or attributes that a body requires to perform the physical activities of daily life is known as **physical fitness** (American College of Sports Medicine [ACSM], 1998). Some individuals are more fit than others and are capable of performing routine daily activities and unplanned activities of increased intensity and duration. On an individual basis physical fitness can be viewed as a continuum. One extreme represents the attributes needed to perform only the routine daily tasks of living without any reserve for unplanned events; the other extreme represents attributes that are necessary to perform activities of daily life and unplanned events plus those required for participation in a competitive sport or activity.

Regardless of the level of physical fitness and whether an individual's daily activities involve sitting all day, jogging through the neighborhood, shoveling snow, planting a garden, moving furniture, competing in a marathon, or watching television, the attributes or components that make up physical fitness are similar for all individuals.

Components of Physical Fitness

The primary components of physical fitness include flexibility, muscle strength, muscle endurance, cardiorespiratory endurance, and body composition (Table 15-1) (ACSM, 1998). To estimate an individual's level of fitness, health professionals can measure each of these components for that person and compare those measurements with norms established as a result of data collected from large population groups. Suggestions can then be made for improving specific components of fitness for the purpose of reducing risk of chronic disease (ACSM, 1998).

Flexibility

Flexibility, or the range of motion around a joint, depends on muscle temperature, muscle viscosity (stiffness), and the amount of stretch in the muscle, ligaments, and tendons associated with joints. The most common test of flexibility, the sit-and-reach test, measures the ability to bend at the hips (trunk flexion). This test determines the flexibility of the muscles in the lower back and hamstring areas (ACSM, 1998).

Flexibility is important to physical fitness because a person with a limited range of motion eventually has to reduce daily activities associated with the affected joints, which could result in total dependence on others. Aging is associated with a decline in flexibility. When stretching and warm-up exercises are used, flexibility can improve by 20% to 50%, regardless of gender or age, and great improvements in independent living have been noted in elderly individuals who participate in stretching exercise classes.

Muscle Strength

Muscle strength refers to the ability of a muscle to generate **force**, or tension, in a maximal effort. It depends on the anatomic location of the muscle, muscle size, speed of contraction, type of muscle action, and the flexibility of the joint associated with that particular muscle or muscle

Table 15-1 COMPONENTS OF PHYSICAL FITNESS

Component	Definition
Flexibility	The range of motion around a joint
Muscle strength	The ability of a muscle to generate force or tension
Muscle endurance	The ability of a muscle to generate force or tension in a submaximal effort over a sustained period
Cardiorespiratory endurance	The ability to complete moderate- to high-intensity aerobic activity for more than a few minutes
Body composition	The percentage of the body composed of fat versus the percentage composed of lean mass

group. Tests used to measure muscle strength are diverse. For instance one common strength test includes the use of a single movement such as a pull-up, another involves lifting a maximal amount of weight with weight-lifting equipment for one repetition (1 repetition maximum [RM]), and a third involves lifting a maximal weight throughout an entire range of motion on equipment that regulates and controls speed. The best measure of muscle strength is assessed with a combination of these methods (ACSM, 1998).

Although the events of daily life may not require significant muscle strength, a loss of strength or a decline with age would be most obvious when individuals try to accomplish unusual and infrequent tasks. College students move into their dorms or apartments at least once a year and good muscle strength for them and those helping (such as parents) will make the job much easier. Improvements in and maintenance of muscle strength can be obtained by **resistance** training, or weight training, which progressively overloads the muscle (works the muscle against an increasing amount of opposing force). Because muscle strength is known to decline with aging, it is easy to understand its importance for persons of all ages who live independently. Resistance training improves not only muscle strength, but also muscle endurance, a third component of physical fitness.

Muscle Endurance

Muscle endurance is the ability to generate force or perform work in a **submaximal** capacity over a sustained period until fatigue occurs. A test of muscle endurance measures the total number of repetitions of an exercise that can be completed within a timed interval, such as the 60-second sit-up or push-up test (ACSM, 1998).

To improve muscle endurance, **calisthenics** and weight training are often suggested. A physically fit individual would have the muscle endurance to shovel several inches of snow from a driveway and still be capable of performing usual daily activities.

Cardiorespiratory Endurance

Cardiorespiratory endurance is the one component of physical fitness that is familiar to most people. It represents the ability to perform moderate- to high-intensity activities for a prolonged period and relies on the efficiency of oxygen and carbon dioxide exchange at the lung and

KEY TERMS

physical fitness: the group of features needed for the body to perform physical activity
force: the effort needed to resist or maintain a muscular movement
resistance: an opposing force; in the case of resistance training it is typically a form of weight lifting in which muscles move against some force
submaximal: below maximal effort
calisthenics: exercises completed without the use of exercise equipment to increase heart rate and strength; examples are jumping jacks, sit-ups, and push-ups

the muscle. The best estimator of cardiorespiratory endurance is obtained by measuring the maximum volume of oxygen consumed (VO_{2max}) during a graded exercise test that proceeds until the client reaches fatigue or exhaustion. An example would be having the individual run on a treadmill set at 6 mph as the grade (slope) is increased 2% every 2 minutes until the person reaches exhaustion.

However, measurement of maximal oxygen consumption is not practical for all individuals. Conveniently scientists have validated correlations between heart rate, oxygen consumption, and performance in running and cycling aerobic tests to predict VO_{2max}. Some of these tests, which include the 12-minute run and the 1-mile walk, can be more easily administered to various individuals or groups and do not require a maximal effort (ACSM, 1998). In the preceding case study Kristen will be working to improve her cardiorespiratory endurance by increasing the duration and frequency of aerobic exercise on a stationary bicycle.

Body Composition

The final component of physical fitness, body composition, is most simply defined in terms of two compartments—fat versus fat-free (lean) masses. The techniques most commonly used to measure body composition include anthropometry (fatfolds) and bioimpedance analyses. Many more sophisticated techniques exist; however, they are used predominantly with clinical and research populations. In general all techniques estimate the amount of body fat and muscle and some also estimate fat in various locations of the body or fat distribution. The location of body fat has been linked with the risk of some chronic diseases. For instance evidence suggests that as abdominal fat increases, the risk of coronary heart disease also increases. This finding does not suggest that abdominal fat should be extremely minimal, as many college-age women might believe. Fat in the body serves a purpose and, like muscle, is an essential component.

Experts have recommended ranges for a healthy percent of body fat for adults. For men the range is 13% to 19% body fat; for women a healthy range is 19% to 25% (Sizer and Whitney, 1994). A body fat percentage at or above 25% for men and 32% for women is considered excessive body fat (Lohman, 1992). This level of fat is associated with greater risk of diseases associated with obesity. On the other hand an extremely low level of body fat, such as below 5% in men and 8% in women, increases risk of diseases associated with undernutrition.

Body composition alone, like the other components of physical fitness, is not the sole determinant of physical fitness. For instance several female swimmers who had more than 30% body fat swam the English Channel. Likewise elite marathon racers often have body fat below the minimal healthy recommendations. Body fat may vary depending on age, gender, genetic background, daily physical activity, and usual dietary intake. This explains why it is important for persons of all ages to use a multifaceted approach to maintain or improve their physical fitness.

Assessment of Physical Fitness

The ACSM suggests that fitness should be evaluated at least once before a person begins an exercise program (ACSM, 1998). Exercise trainers and other health professionals, using the guidelines, tests, and recommendations established by the ACSM, provide information to the individual on their level of fitness and the appropriate exercises needed for improvement (ACSM, 1998). The assessment of physical fitness may be quite extensive. It can include one or more of the following: medical, dietary, and activity histories and opinion questionnaires; a physical examination by a physician; an analysis of coronary artery disease risk profile; numerous diagnostic exercise tests (for the components of fitness previously mentioned); and perhaps advanced cardiac diagnostic testing.

Benefits of Physical Fitness

An increase in daily physical activity promotes fitness and health by affecting the components of fitness. Flexibility, muscle endurance, strength, cardiorespiratory capacity, and body composition are all improved with increased fitness, which is favorable for reducing the risk of chronic dis-

Mrs. B. is ecstatic. For years as a diabetic she had experienced what she perceived as a poor quality of life. Now she eagerly describes how wonderful she feels after 8 weeks of treadmill walking. "I sleep so much better now and feel rested when I awaken and the little things that used to bother me at home do not annoy me anymore! I have so much more energy now in the afternoons that I don't need to nap. You wouldn't believe what I am doing. I can do the grocery shopping myself, after my exercise, and I make dinner, clean up the dishes, and still feel good. My husband and sons are wondering, 'who is this woman?' I'm so happy to be a part of this diabetes exercise training study. Everyone should do this! Everyone should walk for 30 to 60 minutes 3 times every week."

eases. In one 8-year study of more than 13,000 people, individuals who walked briskly 30 minutes per day for 3 days each week significantly reduced their risk of dying from heart disease, cancer, and other causes compared with those who did not walk (Blair et al., 1989). In a follow-up of this study population, the authors concluded that low fitness levels were such great predictors of mortality that even the participants who smoked cigarettes, but remained moderately active, had significantly reduced mortality rates (Blair et al., 1996a). Interestingly, intense exercise is not necessarily required for these effects to occur. In a group of 17,000 male Harvard alumni, mortality rates were 21% lower for men who walked 9 miles per week compared with the rate for those who walked 3 miles or less per week (Paffenbarger et al., 1986).

Although increased physical activity improves health, no single recommendation for increasing exercise or daily activity has been adopted. Instead exercise recommendations have been made for enhancing health (i.e., lowering risk factors for chronic disease), for enhancing fitness (i.e., increasing VO_{2max}, muscle strength, flexibility, and endurance), or for a combination of both (ACSM, 1998).

For instance, ACSM recommends that to improve health, one should participate in activities that use large muscle groups of the legs and trunk (such as walking, jogging, skating, climbing stairs, rowing, or cycling) 3 days to 5 days each week for 15 minutes to 60 minutes per day at a low to moderate intensity (ACSM, 1998). (A general rule to characterize low- to moderate-intensity exercise is the finding that the exercising individual is breathing harder than at rest, but is quite capable of carrying on a conversation.) Three brief 10-minute periods of moderately intense exercise (or activity) throughout the day have also been suggested as an alternative to one longer period of exercise (DeBusk et al., 1990); however, a recent symposium of physical activity experts strongly suggest 60 minutes of at least light activity daily (Bouchard, 2001).

To improve fitness, an increase in exercise intensity, frequency, and duration is recommended. This amounts to exercise involving large muscle groups at least 5 times per week for 15 minutes to 60 minutes each time at a moderate to high intensity (ACSM, 1998). (At this intensity, breathing rate is increased above low-intensity levels and the individual should still be capable of some conversation.)

Whether the goal is to improve physical fitness or to enhance health, those who do exercise regularly, such as Mrs. B., may report some or all of the following benefits:

- Improved cardiovascular function
- Increased strength
- Reduced body fat and increased lean body mass
- Improved blood lipid profile
- Decreased risk of chronic disease
- Restful sleep
- Improvement in measures of diabetes, obesity, or hypertension, which include decreased blood glucose, weight loss, and decreased blood pressure

Increasing activity through structured exercise may result in many health benefits, but some of these same benefits can be achieved by increasing the daily activities of normal life, such as taking the stairs instead of the elevator, walking instead of driving, gardening, washing the car, and participating in recreational sports or activities.

Physical Inactivity

Despite the strong evidence that physical inactivity or a sedentary life-style is a risk factor for coronary heart disease, stroke, diabetes, cancer, hypertension, and other chronic diseases, over 60% of U.S. adults do not exercise at levels recommended to improve health. About 15% of adults exercise at levels intended for increasing fitness. Health professionals continue to express serious concern about the prevalence of sedentary life in the industrialized world (Blair et al., 1996b; Williams, 1999).

THE COMPONENTS OF MUSCLES AND HOW PHYSICAL ACTIVITY AFFECTS THEM

- *What are muscles composed of and how do they enlarge or change with training?*
- *How will aerobic training or anaerobic training affect muscles?*
- *What are reasonable expectations for improvements in strength and endurance after aerobic or anaerobic training?*

Participation in any physical activity requires muscular work. The work that a muscle is able to complete depends on the type and number of muscle fibers involved, the availability of energy to fuel that muscular work, and how well the muscle has been trained to perform that work.

Components of Muscle: Muscle Fiber Types

Skeletal muscles are large bundles of individual **muscle fibers** or cells. These fibers can be classified into one of three general fiber types—I, IIa, or IIb—based on structural and functional characteristics (Table 15-2). These characteristics affect the strength, endurance, and speed with which a muscle contracts (McArdle et al., 1994).

Structurally, one characteristic that distinguishes muscle fiber types from one another is

Ryan is a typical college junior from a middle-class family. He attends a large midwestern university and is working toward a major in business, like many in his family. He has two part-time jobs to support himself and to help pay for school. He spends most of his day in classes and at one of his jobs and he studies most nights and works his second job on weekends. Ryan enjoys apartment living and has four roommates. He has noticed that he is now 20 pounds heavier than when he played high school football. For the past 6 weekends, Ryan has gone to the gym on Saturday morning for 2 hours of pick-up basketball and then to the weight room on Sunday for 1 hour of lifting and 1 hour of treadmill running. After this weekend, Ryan realizes as he struggles to get out of bed for his 7:30 AM class that he has been sore and tired every Monday morning for the past 6 weeks. He thought by now he would feel better because he knows that staying physically active is supposed to make a person feel better. He notices that his right knee aches again like it did last Monday. As he drinks his fourth cup of coffee and gobbles the last three doughnuts from the weekend, he begins to think back over the past 6 weeks. He purposely took a vitamin and mineral supplement every day thinking that it would give him energy to exercise, based on what the label said. He admits to himself that he often eats fast food, especially beer and pizza on the weekends, while he is watching football games. Thinking that he is simply not as tough as he used to be in high school, Ryan vows to take more supplements and work even harder in the gym next weekend.

the variation in the concentration of **myoglobin**. Myoglobin is a protein that carries oxygen inside the muscle cell. With the mitochondria and blood capillaries, it influences the individual's capacity to supply oxygen and energy to the working muscle.

Functionally, muscle fibers are characterized by their ability to continue working and to resist **fatigue**. The speed of **contraction** and the amount of force generated during a contraction are also characteristics used to differentiate the fiber types. These functional characteristics can be attributed to the availability of the energy molecule (adenosine triphosphate [ATP]) in the fiber. The obvious link between physical activity and nutrition stems from the production and availability of ATP. It can be obtained only by oxidizing carbohydrate, fat, or protein. Based on all of the above characteristics, the three muscle fiber types are differentiated as described in Table 15-2.

In reality, all skeletal muscles are a mixture of the three fiber types. The proportion of each type is determined genetically and through physical training. Most sedentary individuals have a predominance (46 to 48%) of type I fibers. Trained elite athletes, on the other hand, have muscle fiber types that reflect their training (e.g., a prevalence of type IIb fibers with speed and strength training versus type I fibers with endurance training). Although fiber type may be altered in response to training, further research describing the prevalence, quantity, and time course of these changes is necessary.

Regardless of muscle fiber type, muscle contraction requires energy in the form of ATP. The contractile proteins in muscle, actin and myosin, are unable to move without it and the speed and force of contraction are greatest when ATP is most available. Like all cells, muscle cells

KEY TERMS

muscle fibers: individual muscle cells that are usually identified as type I, IIa, or IIb
myoglobin: the protein in muscle that combines with or "holds" oxygen so that it is available to be used in aerobic oxidation of fuels
fatigue: a physical state in which one is unable to continue muscular work at the same intensity
contraction: the shortening or lengthening of a muscle fiber, which results in the production or generation of force

Table 15-2 MUSCLE FIBERS AND THEIR STRUCTURAL AND FUNCTIONAL CHARACTERISTICS

Fiber Type/Names	Structural and Functional Characteristics
TYPE I Slow-twitch Slow-oxidative Fatigue-resistant Red	Have very high amount of myoglobin and mitochondria, increased capillary density, slow velocity of contraction, appear red in color. Predominant use of oxidative processes for ATP production.
TYPE IIA Fast-twitch A Fast-oxidative Fatigue-resistant Red	Have high amount of myoglobin and mitochondria, with many surrounding blood capillaries, so fibers appear red in color. Faster rate of ATP production so velocity of contraction is faster than type I. Somewhat less resistant to fatigue than type I fibers.
TYPE IIB Fast-twitch B Fast-glycolytic Fatigable White	Have little myoglobin and fewer mitochondria and blood capillaries than other muscle types so appearance is white. Relies on glycolytic- and phosphocreatine-derived sources of ATP, hence easily fatigued, but velocity of contraction is fast.

obtain ATP through intracellular **aerobic** or **anaerobic** metabolic pathways. The actual pathways used to produce ATP in muscle depend on the fiber type, the nutrients available, the intensity and duration of the muscular activity, and the physical fitness of the individual. Highly trained individuals optimize each of these areas to affect performance.

Producing Energy Inside the Muscle Fibers

There are four potential sources of energy or ATP within the cell. The working muscle uses ATP from the various sources in an overlapping and integrated sequence. The continued use of ATP from each source depends on the type of muscular activity, the supply of nutrients, the duration of the activity, and the fitness level of the person (Figure 15-1).

Free Adenosine Triphosphate

First a small amount of free ATP is available inside the muscle cell, which is used to fuel the initial 2 to 3 seconds of activity. This source of ATP is very limited and easily exhausted. Free ATP is used up in the first several seconds of a fast movement such as in a high jump, long jump, sprint, or lift. When this source of ATP is exhausted, the next immediate source of ATP is derived from the molecule phosphocreatine (PC).

Phosphocreatine Supply of Adenosine Triphosphate

Phosphocreatine has a high-energy phosphate group attached to it that can be used to convert adenosine diphosphate (ADP) to ATP within the cell. The PC-derived ATP lasts for only 6 to 8 seconds, but PC can be remade after a period of rest. This source of ATP, coupled with the free ATP, provides a 100-meter sprinter with 98% of the energy to get to the finish line (about 10 to 12 seconds) (Table 15-3). Both sources of ATP are used when the muscle is in need of very quick energy and when there is little time to use systems that require oxygen; therefore they are called anaerobic sources of ATP. Sports such as football that require short bursts of speed and strength depend on these systems (see Table 15-3). The average college student might use these for any quick, short bursts of muscle activity, such as running to class in the rain or sprinting up the steps to answer a ringing phone.

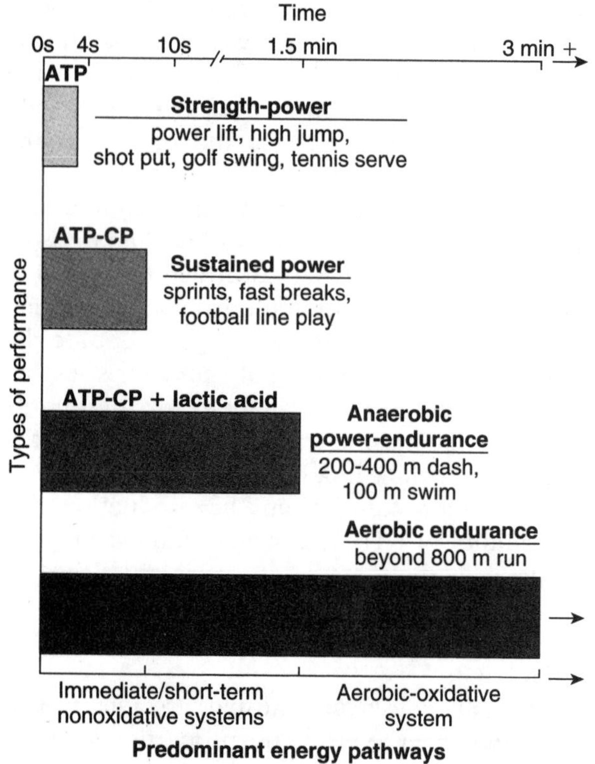

Figure 15-1 Predominant energy pathways. *(From McArdle WD et al.: Exercise physiology, energy, and human performance, ed 3, Philadelphia, 1991 Lea & Febiger.)*

KEY TERMS

aerobic: a metabolic process that requires oxygen to continue

anaerobic: a metabolic process that does not require oxygen

glycolysis: the breakdown of glucose to two pyruvate molecules

Glycolysis Supply of Adenosine Triphosphate

A third immediate source of ATP, also anaerobic, is **glycolysis**. For this process one glucose molecule is partially broken down to provide a few ATPs. However, this source of ATP lasts for only 1 to 2 minutes of a maximal effort (see Figure 15-1). Athletes who run 200 m to 800 m, swim

Table 15-3 Popular Sports and Their Associated Energy Systems

Sports or Sport Activity	Percentage of Emphasis According to Energy Systems		
	ATP-PC and LA*	$LA\text{-}O_2$†	O_2‡
Baseball	80	20	—
Basketball	85	15	—
Fencing	90	10	—
Field hockey	60	20	20
Football	90	10	—
Golf	95	5	—
Gymnastics	90	10	—
Ice hockey			
Forwards, defense	80	20	—
Goalie	95	5	—
Lacrosse			
Goalie defense, attack men	80	20	—
Midfielders, man-down	60	20	20
Rowing	20	30	50
Skiing			
Slalom, jumping, downhill	80	20	—
Cross-country	—	5	95
Pleasure skiing	34	33	33
Soccer			
Goalie, wings, strikers	80	20	—
Halfbacks or link men	60	20	20
Swimming and diving			
50 yd, diving	98	2	—
100 yd	80	15	5
200 yd	30	65	5
400, 500 yd	20	40	40
1500, 1650 yd	10	20	70
Tennis	70	20	10
Track and field			
100, 220 yd	98	2	—
Field events	90	10	—
440 yd	80	15	5
880 yd	30	65	5
1 mile	20	55	25
2 miles	20	40	40
3 miles	10	20	70
6 miles (cross-country)	5	15	80
Marathon	—	5	95
Volleyball	90	10	—
Wrestling	90	10	—

Adapted from Fox EL and Mathews DK: Interval training: conditioning for sports and general fitness, New York, 1974, Saunders College Publishing.

*Anaerobic (phosphagen system) (ATP-PC)

†Combination (lactic acid-oxygen) ($LA\text{-}O_2$) = Glycolsis-Krebs

‡Aerobic (oxygen) = Krebs

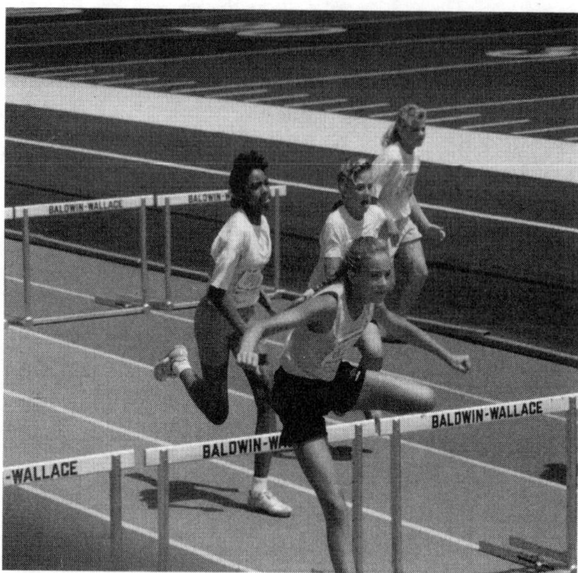

Figure 15-2 Glycolysis contributes energy for track athletes to jump hurdles.

200 m or more, run hurdles (Figure 15-2), or complete other events in 1 to 2 minutes rely primarily on glycolysis and the previously discussed systems of anaerobic ATP production. Glycolysis is also used in events beyond 2 minutes for sports such as football, soccer, hockey, or basketball, where short bursts of intense activity are interspersed with longer periods of low to moderate activity that could last for 1 to 4 hours. These athletes rely on a highly trained glycolytic system for a fast break, goal line defense, or touchdown run. The production of ATP from the glycolytic system becomes especially important in a team's final quarter of play, when the athletes are close to exhaustion, yet must maintain speed and strength.

Several limitations to glycolysis make it necessary for an exercising muscle to seek additional ATP from a fourth system. First, for glycolysis to continue, its byproduct (pyruvate) must not accumulate in the cell and must continue to be completely metabolized through the aerobic pathway of ATP production (Kreb's cycle, discussed later). If there is limited use of the aerobic pathway, pyruvate is converted to lactic acid (LA), which accumulates in the cell and impairs muscle contraction. This is evident in sedentary individuals who begin an exercise program, although it occurs to some degree in individuals of all fitness levels. Second, glycolysis requires a steady source of glucose. Sources of glucose might include glucose from the blood, muscle and liver glycogen, and compounds such as some amino acids (alanine, glutamine), glycerol, and LA that the liver can remake into glucose in a process called **gluconeogenesis.** Many of these sources of glucose are in limited supply and can be nearly exhausted after approximately 90 minutes of continuous exercise.

Krebs Cycle Supply of Adenosine Triphosphate

The fourth system of ATP production, which is used for exercise beyond 2 minutes, is the aerobic system known as the tricarboxylic acid cycle, or Krebs cycle. Unlike the other ATP producers, this system requires the presence of oxygen and mitochondria, produces relatively more ATP, and is less limited by the availability of a fuel source. Endurance activities, athletic events, and sports (see Table 15-3) that rely on the aerobic pathway include running (800 m or more), swimming (200 m or more), cross-country skiing, competitive cycling, and many others. Aerobic production of ATP is the source of ATP used to complete daily routine activities of living such as sitting, studying, shoveling snow, walking up steps, weeding the garden, or raking leaves.

In summary the production of ATP in a muscle fiber occurs in response to the need for energy and is related to the intensity and duration of the exercise, the types of muscle fibers involved, the person's level of training, and the availability of fuel (discussed later). Muscle fibers are classified by the features that relate to ATP production. Regardless of the level of training, the availability of these systems of energy production provides the versatility to meet the energy needs of the working muscle. Enhancing these energy production pathways is one key to improving several aspects of physical fitness and is the basis of how nutrition can affect physical performance.

Guidelines for Exercise Training and Typical Results from a Training Program

Athletes, coaches, and trainers develop programs, that enhance the energy production systems specific to their sport, event, or activity of interest. In other words a sprinter, power lifter, or lineman on a football team will use resistance training to increase the anaerobic processes of ATP production because quick powerful bursts of energy are important for their sports performance. The opposite is true for a marathon athlete, who will run between 50 miles and 120 miles each week to enhance the aerobic oxidative system and aerobic endurance (for sustained energy). However, as noted in Table 15-3, most sports require use of all systems of ATP production; therefore an individual may train both aerobically and anaerobically. Basketball, football, soccer, and ice hockey are examples of sports that require athletes to have quick start and stop movements, movements of enormous strength, and the endurance to maintain these activities for a prolonged period. These same principles can be applied to recreational athletes and college students who work out on their own to maintain their physical fitness, as noted earlier with Kristen or Ryan.

For specific sports, however, training regimens are individualized first for the athlete's level of fitness and second for performance of the specific sport. Muscles that are exercised and trained are not able to transfer their improvements to other muscles in the body. For example bicycle training may not make a person a better runner.

Aerobic Exercise Training

The basic requirement of an aerobic exercise training program for a sedentary individual is to exercise the large muscles of the body in a constant manner (as in walking, running, or cycling) for a minimum of 15 minutes 3 times per week at a moderate intensity. Moderate intensity is usually calculated as 60% to 80% of maximum heart rate (maximal heart rate = 220 minus age). In addition warm-up (10 minutes) and cool-down periods (10 to 20 minutes) should accompany each exercise session. These recommendations are based on large prospective and retrospective studies that determined that decreased rates of mortality from cardiovascular disease and cancer were associated with this minimal amount of weekly exercise (Blair et al., 1996b).

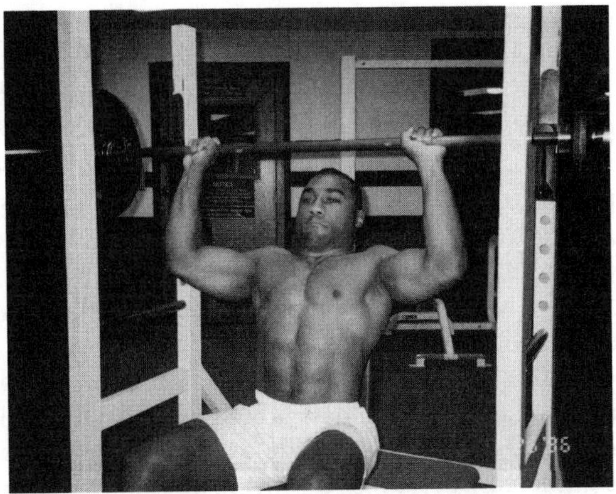

Figure **15-3** Muscle strength and size increase with resistance training. *(Photographer: Diane Habash.)*

Anaerobic Exercise Training

The premise of an anaerobic exercise program (e.g., weight lifting) is that strength will be increased by making the muscle work repeatedly to overcome resistance (Figure 15-3). This process is often referred to as overloading the muscle and can be accomplished by altering the resistance against which the muscle works, the number of repetitions completed, the speed of the repetition, or some combination of these factors. Three different methods of strength or resistance training can be used: (1) isotonic, (2) isometric, or (3) isokinetic training. These methods differ from one another based on the length of the muscle when it contracts and whether the opposing force on the muscle remains the same throughout the entire range of motion.

Isotonic training is completed when a muscle shortens or lengthens as it contracts. A common example is the bicep curl. Isometric training occurs when the muscle is not allowed to shorten or lengthen while contracting. Male gymnasts who

KEY TERMS

gluconeogenesis: a process in which some compound such as pyruvate, lactate, or an amino acid such as alanine is made into a glucose molecule

suspend their bodies in midair on the still rings use this form of resistance exercise. Isokinetic training occurs when the muscle shortens as it contracts; however, the speed with which the weight is moved and the force of resistance opposing the muscle remain the same throughout the entire range of motion (i.e., the movement is not faster or easier at any time during the lift). Isokinetic training is done with electronically sensitive, computer-aided equipment that is capable of setting, monitoring, and maintaining the speed and resistance against which the individual moves. In general strength exercises should be completed 2 to 3 times per week, allowing time for rest and recovery.

To increase the size of the muscle (or to hypertrophy the muscle), as a body builder might desire, resistance is greatly increased to near maximum as the number of repetitions is decreased. To obtain a greater increase in strength as opposed to the size of muscle, the resistance is lowered to 60% to 80% of maximum and the number of repetitions is increased. Repeated lifts of 90% to 100% of maximum, especially early in a training program, could cause damage to joints, tendons, and ligaments (which may be the problem of the college student Ryan, mentioned earlier). Such injuries often require complete rest and can severely impair motivation for further exercise training and performance. Patience is a necessary ally in any training program and successful performance can be more easily obtained with short-term realistic goal setting.

Results of Exercise Training

The changes and adaptations that occur in the body as a result of exercise training depend on the type and frequency of training completed, the state of physical fitness before training begins, and the intensity and duration of the training. Sedentary individuals who participate in exercise training will have more significant adaptations to the training than individuals who complete the same training program in a partially trained state.

Aerobic Exercise Adaptations

Adaptations resulting from aerobic exercise are related to the transport and use of oxygen and enhanced fuel use (to be discussed later in the chapter). The most significant change is the increase in the volume of blood pumped from the heart with each beat, known as stroke volume. Plasma volume also increases. These adaptations result in greater efficiency of the heart muscle and increased transport of oxygen to the body both during exercise and at rest. Other adaptations include improved oxygen uptake by the working muscle and increased ability to direct blood flow to the working muscle and away from areas of less importance, such as the gastrointestinal tract. This latter point has significance when trying to feed a person who exercises continuously for many hours.

Adaptations facilitating oxygen use occur because mitochondria increase in size and number and the enzymes of the Krebs cycle increase in activity. These changes contribute to a greater capacity to oxidize fat and carbohydrate for production of ATP. Aerobic exercise also results in reduced resting systolic and diastolic pressures, increased lung volumes, increased ability to dissipate body heat (or to cool more easily), and, over time, a reduced percentage of body fat.

The time of onset for these adaptations is variable, depending, to some extent, on the frequency, intensity, and duration of exercise training. Noticeable adaptations usually occur within 8 to 12 weeks of a 3-day per week program. However, some adaptations can occur more quickly. After beginning an intense daily running program, plasma volume in a group of men increased 10% to 20% within 4 to 5 days (Saltin et al., 1977). Body fat, on the other hand, may require many months of work before significant change is apparent.

Anaerobic Exercise Adaptations

With an anaerobic training program, the adaptations that occur are usually related to the enhancement of anaerobic ATP production and neural responses. Therefore enzymes of the PC and glycolytic systems increase in the ability to either recycle or produce ATP, respectively. Muscle fibers increase in a cross-sectional area, contraction time decreases, and tendon and ligament strength increase. Capillary density and mitochondrial size and number appear to decrease because muscle fiber area increases. Another result of resistance training is great enhancement of neural signaling to the trained muscles, which produces a much stronger and more powerful contraction.

Most individuals exhibit significant gains in strength after weight training 3 times per week for 6 to 8 weeks. However, a more sedentary individual has a greater potential for developing strength. Strength can be improved regardless of age. An average strength improvement of 174% was made in the thigh muscles of 10 subjects who were 90 years of age (Fiatarone et al., 1990). These 10 men completed a training program 3 days per week for a period of 8 weeks that included three sets of leg extensions with seven to nine repetitions per set at 80% of the maximum weight lifted by their legs. Although this level of improvement is greater than the 30% found in younger men and women (Duchateau and Hainaut, 1982) and in other studies of elderly men, the authors noted that it does indicate that the potential for improvements in strength are significant. For an aspiring college student, a 30% to 70% improvement in strength, depending on the type of training, can be expected in a 2- to 3-month period.

NUTRIENTS THAT FUEL PHYSICAL ACTIVITY

- *How does a person's nutrition affect his or her fitness and performance?*
- *What metabolic fuels are used for quick sprint activities versus endurance events?*
- *Should athletes or active individuals engaged in different sports eat distinctly different diets?*

For a person who must complete a physical task such as shoveling snow, running a race, or working a late-night job after a day of college classes, expectations about performance are related to physical attributes of strength, flexibility, and endurance. In addition a critical factor influencing performance is the amount and type of fuel used to provide the energy to complete the task.

Carbohydrates, fats, and proteins are the macronutrient fuels that are oxidized by the working muscle to produce ATP. The relationship between nutrition and physical activity centers on the use and regulation of these fuels during physical work. Figure 15-4 identifies these fuels, pathways of energy production, and their metabolic byproducts. Although each energy-yielding macronutrient is discussed individually, in reality, energy is obtained simultaneously from all nutrients during physical work. The contribution of each pathway toward total energy production is regulated by the intensity of effort, the availability of fuels, the hormones responsive to exercise and diet, and the physical fitness of the individual.

Carbohydrate

In general carbohydrates are the preferred fuel of a muscle cell during moderate- to high-intensity exercise (>50 to 60% maximal heart rate). This occurs because glucose (the form of carbohydrate most recognized by cells) is readily absorbed from the blood, is freely available in the muscle cell, is available from stored glycogen, and, as noted earlier, is a quick source of ATP through glycolysis. However, the use of carbohydrates during physical activity depends on the integration of many factors. For instance, at moderate- to high-intensity work in a poorly trained state, the use of stored carbohydrates is stimulated more readily. The process of using stored carbohydrate (liver glycogen, muscle glycogen, or both) is further controlled by nutrition status, physical fitness, and the intensity and duration of exercise. As the glycogen supply becomes exhausted (perhaps from a poor diet), the body must rely on other fuel sources. This deficit in glycogen can become more pronounced as exercise continues beyond 30 minutes from a relative rise in hormones (epinephrine, glucagon, and glucocorticoids), but also because of the preexercise meal, byproducts of glycolysis, muscle cell pH, and oxygen availability.

In an individual who is exercising, but has had minimal or inconsistent aerobic training, glycolysis would be used to produce ATP, but LA would increase and cause a decline in pH, which would slow glycolysis. As glycogen stores decrease and carbohydrate use declines, performance in high-intensity exercise is usually impaired and limited.

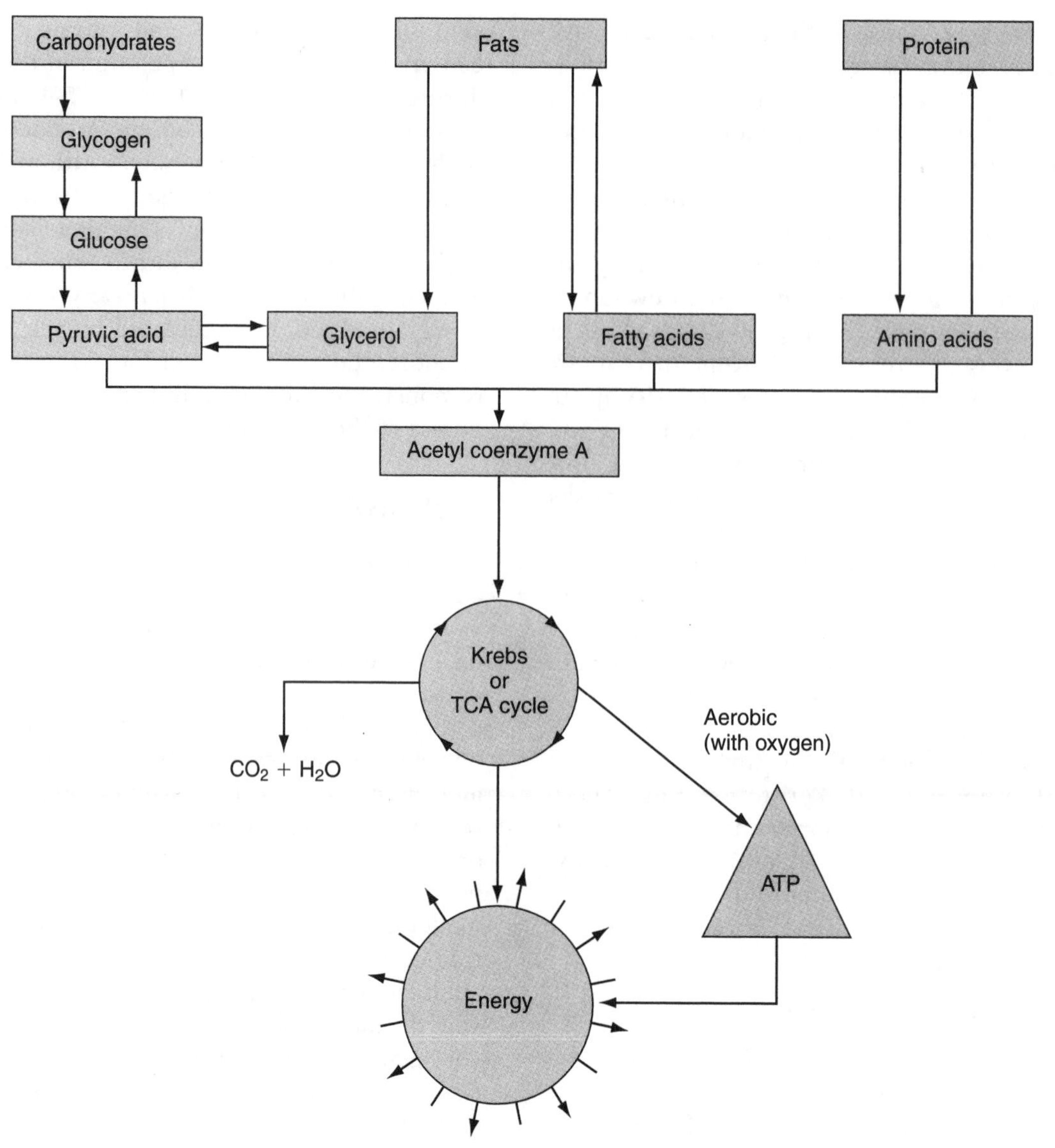

Figure 15-4 Oxidation processes to obtain ATP from nutrients: carbohydrate, protein, and fat.

The weekend athlete is an example of a person whose high-intensity performance often cannot be sustained because of declining carbohydrate use and inadequate aerobic training.

Lactic acid (a byproduct of glycolysis) is produced during exercise, regardless of intensity, and is chemically changed by the body. Aerobic exercise training teaches the body to get better at processing lactate. It is produced in greatest quantity during intense physical work when rapid movements of speed or strength are completed or during prolonged (>60 minutes) moderate- to high-intensity exercise. Lactic acid produced in the muscle cell enters the circulation, is taken up by the liver, and is made into glucose, which is then circulated back to muscles for use. This form of gluconeogenesis, called the Cori cycle, occurs predominantly in sports or during activities in which glycolysis provides the ATP for muscle work (see Table 15-3). Trained individuals can exercise at higher intensities for a longer time because their bodies are prepared to process the lactate.

Other factors, such as diet, influence carbohydrate use during exercise. These factors are discussed in greater detail as the chapter progresses. The general sequence of nutrient fuel utilization during exercise is illustrated in Figure 15-5. In this example an endurance-trained cyclist attempts to work at a relatively high intensity (70% VO_{2max}) for as long as possible. Initially, when ATP is needed quickly, glucose derived from muscle glycogen is the primary carbohydrate source of energy as long as it is available. Muscle glycogen provides approximately 50% of the total energy in the early stages of this cyclist's work. (Note that fat provides a significant portion of the energy also.) As the availability of muscle glycogen declines, the use of blood glucose begins to increase. Unless the athlete is getting glucose orally during exercise, the liver is primarily responsible for resupplying glucose to the blood and, thus, the working muscle. Glucose is stored in the liver in limited amounts and as the level of liver-derived glucose is exhausted, performance at this intensity also declines unless an outside or exogenous source of glucose, via the diet, is available. This is the basis of glucose feedings for many types of endurance activities beyond approximately 60 minutes of work.

During resistance exercise, blood glucose does not decline significantly after a 1-hour series of resistance exercises, and, it may actually increase slightly. Carbohydrate ingestion before and during resistance exercise may increase insulin levels, which may improve muscle glycogen stores and the size and growth of the muscle.

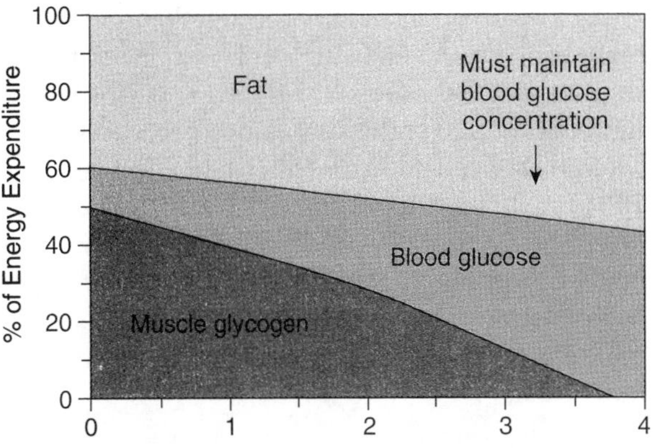

Figure 15-5 Glycogen depletion in cyclists. *(Adapted from Coyle EF and Montain SJ: Carbohydrate and fluid ingestion during exercise: are there trade-offs? Med Sci Sports Exerc 24:671, 1992. Reprinted by permission of Lippincott, Williams & Wilkins.)*

Fat

Fat is available to the muscle cell as fatty acids in the blood or as intracellular triglycerides. Hormones secreted in response to exercise, such as glucagon, norepinephrine, and epinephrine, stimulate **lipolysis**, making fatty acids available for the muscle cell to oxidize for energy. To obtain ATP, fatty acids are broken down to two-carbon units (called Acetyl-CoA) through **beta oxidation** and used in the Krebs cycle to make ATP. One fatty acid molecule can yield many more ATPs than one glucose molecule. However, for fatty acids to be used for energy, there must be a carbohydrate-derived compound (oxaloacetate) available in the Krebs cycle. The working muscle can access many sources of carbohydrate, as previously noted. The glycerol molecule, which is a part of a triglyceride, can be converted to glucose by the liver and made available for glycolysis. However, the amount of glucose available from this conversion is small and incapable of sustaining intense activity.

When individuals improve their aerobic endurance, their muscles use more fat as a fuel than when untrained. As noted in Figure 15-5, this can help to sustain intense activity by sparing carbohydrate use. This improvement in endurance occurs because there are more mitochondria and they are more capable of using fat for making ATP instead of having to rely on carbohydrate. In addition training may bring more intramuscular stores of triglycerides.

KEY TERMS

lipolysis: the breakdown of a triglyceride into three fatty acids and a glycerol molecule

beta oxidation: the process in which a fatty acid is broken down into two-carbon units that enter the Krebs cycle and are oxidized to yield ATP

As a result it has been suggested that endurance athletes consume diets high in fat to "load" the intramuscular fat stores and improve performance; however, this hypotheses has not been confirmed when tested scientifically (Sherman and Leenders, 1995). On the other hand, with resistance exercise, the increased concentration of free fatty acids in the blood could potentially elevate total fat oxidation, resulting in a decrease in body fat, a desirable outcome for the sedentary overweight individual.

Protein

The primary role of protein is to build, replace, repair, and maintain cellular structures and functional body proteins. This is no simple task when muscles are challenged with the daily physical stress of exercise. Because of this role, proteins are not the preferred fuel at rest or during exercise. However, when first beginning an intense training program, or when the intake of energy or carbohydrate before prolonged exercise is low, proteins may contribute up to 15% of the energy needs.

The metabolic processes in which proteins are used to produce energy in the muscle fiber are quite varied. Proteins must be degraded into their constituent amino acids and the nitrogen must be removed and excreted in urea. The remaining carbons can be converted to glucose by the liver or can be oxidized via glycolysis or the Krebs cycle to yield ATP. The metabolic direction taken by individual amino acids depends on their structure. When proteins are used to produce ATP, they cannot fulfill other roles, and ultimately, nitrogen balance can be compromised. A compromised nitrogen balance implies an overall net loss of body protein, which is not ideal for anyone.

In general recent research demonstrates that regularly training athletes require more dietary protein than the Recommended Dietary Allowance (RDA) of 0.8 g/kg per day, based on the primary role of protein in the body as opposed to protein's limited energy contribution. For athletes who regularly participate in vigorous aerobic exercise, the recommendation is 1.2 g/kg to 1.4 g/kg per day. For athletes attempting to build lean body mass with resistance types of exercise, 1.4 g/kg to 1.8 g/kg per day is recommended. Athletes who are just beginning an intense training program may have requirements of 1.2 g/kg to 2.0 g/kg per day (Carroll, 2000). However, as often noted by nutritionists, most Americans obtain this level of protein intake every day.

Recent research suggests that routinely training strength athletes may require a 1:3 protein: carbohydrate ratio to improve both nitrogen balance and glycogen synthesis during the recovery period (Tarnopolsky, 1998).

ADAPTATIONS IN NUTRIENT USE DURING PHYSICAL ACTIVITY

The pathways used to produce energy from carbohydrate, fat, and protein are interconnected, which enhances the response to a change in metabolism (see Figure 15-4). For instance, during rest, when energy is predominantly supplied by fatty acids, nutrients that are not used for fuel can be used for synthesis of body proteins, triglycerides, glycogen, or other cellular structures. When an individual engages in physical activity, the body must rely on more readily available sources of energy, most often carbohydrates. This is especially true during activities of high intensity where a greater proportion (60%) of energy comes from carbohydrates and less (40%) from fat (Coyle and Montain, 1992). In this manner the body can be selective of its fuel source.

Improvements in physical fitness result in adaptations in the use of these fuels. With exercise training, muscle cells begin to use fatty acids in increased proportions even at higher work intensities, conserving stored carbohydrate. Potentially this can delay the onset of fatigue because glycolysis is no longer the predominant source of energy. In addition fatigue is also delayed because of better processing of LA and other byproducts of glycolysis. (Fatigue, however, is not solely related to fuel use or LA production. Other factors such as declining neural function, metabolic waste accumulation, or the onset of conscious fatigue may be important.)

Exercise intensities, in general, must reach 55% to 65% of VO_{2max} in untrained individuals and approximately 80% of VO_{2max} in trained individuals before lactate accumulation in the blood impairs performance (McArdle et al., 1994). With aerobic exercise training, an individual produces less lactate at any relative intensity and is capable of improved performance. This adaptation is a result of improved fat use; increased lactate and alanine-derived gluconeogenesis in the liver; and more efficient oxygen delivery, uptake, and use at the muscle. These effects of training can be exploited to enhance exercise performance.

Enhancing Performance with Nutrient Fuels

An appreciation of how nutrition can enhance exercise performance is easily characterized by Astrand's classic study of diet and human performance. This study was conducted to determine the effect of varying carbohydrate intake on running performance. For several days before a timed treadmill run, three groups of equally trained runners were fed high-fat diets (94% of calories from fat), medium-carbohydrate diets (55% of calories from carbohydrates), or high-carbohydrate diets (83% of calories from carbohydrate). Figure 15-6 shows that a high-carbohydrate diet greatly improved the endurance time and performance in these. This study laid the groundwork for the current concept of carbohydrate loading, in which muscle cells, forced to store more glycogen before exercise, experience a delay in the onset of fatigue during endurance exercise (Astrand, 1968).

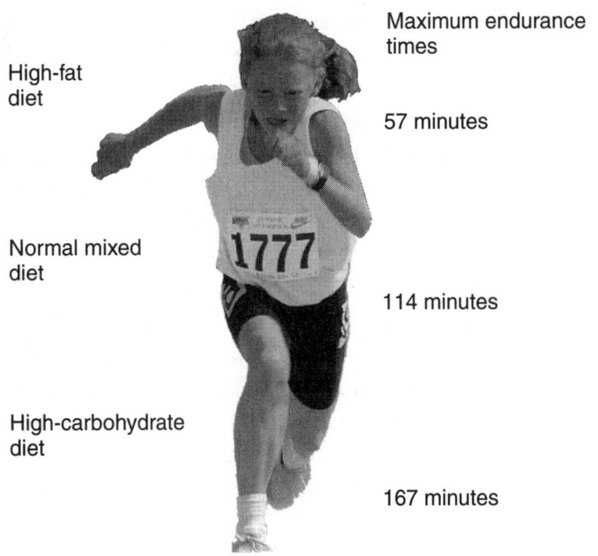

Figure 15-6 The effect of diet on exercise endurance. *(Photographer: Kirk Fisher.)*

The basic concept of carbohydrate loading involves depletion of muscle glycogen by exhaustive exercise and consumption of a high-fat, low-carbohydrate diet (60 to 120 g per day) followed by repletion of glycogen stores with a high-carbohydrate diet (55% or more) and low-intensity exercise. Some methods of carbohydrate loading may not be safe and have resulted in abnormal heart rhythms and ankle edema (McArdle et al., 1994). A safe method of carbohydrate loading begins with a 90-minute bout of high-intensity exercise (85% of VO_{2max}) completed 6 days before the day of competition. The athlete should exercise for the next 2 days at the same intensity, but for half the time (45 minutes). After days 2 and 3, there should be 2 days of even less exercise (20 minutes per day) and finally a day of rest just before competition. Carbohydrate intake, on the other hand, should be increased from 50% of calories on the first 3 days to 70% of total calories daily until competition (Sherman et al., 1981).

Other suggestions for increasing carbohydrate stores in the body include the following:

- Eat a high-carbohydrate diet every day ($\geq$55 to 60% kilocalorie [kcal] as carbohydrate, or 300 to 600 g per day for most individuals, or 7 to 10 g carbohydrates per kg body weight depending on hours of training per day). Those who train 1 hour per day should consume 6 g/kg to 7 g/kg, those who train 2 hours per day should consume 8 g/kg, those who train 3 hours per day should consume 10 g/kg, and those who train 4 or more hours per day should consume 12 g/kg to 13 g/kg (Coleman, 2001).
- Ingest carbohydrate liquids during endurance exercise because this form is better absorbed. Ingest 30 g to 60 g per hour or 200 g once after 90 minutes of exercise.

- Replace carbohydrates within 30 minutes of the end of exercise. Eat 50 g to 75 g of carbohydrate every 2 hours after exercise or until 500 g has been consumed.

In fact these suggestions form the basis for the nutrition recommendations for meals before, during, and after exercise that are noted later in this chapter. For athletes who compete in events that last less than 60 minutes or for those who participate in resistance exercise, a high-carbohydrate diet (55 to 60% or more of total energy) is sufficient to replete carbohydrate stores and increase insulin, which promotes the desired effect. For recreational athletes or those who want to be physically active, the recommendations would be similar.

MICRONUTRIENTS, WATER, AND PHYSICAL ACTIVITY

- *Does exercise increase dietary vitamin and mineral requirements?*
- *Does vitamin and mineral supplementation enhance exercise performance?*
- *What is the importance of hydration to performance? How is good hydration achieved?*

Vitamins, minerals, and water are essential nutrients for the human body regardless of activity level. The work of vitamins and minerals would have little meaning without the appropriate volume of water and electrolyte concentrations inside, outside, and between the cells. Figure 15-7 illustrates the point at which the water-soluble vitamins and minerals are required in energy production. Other functions of vitamins and minerals, such as those that offer antioxidant defense and those that assist in building new cells and repairing tissues, are also important for active individuals. Currently there is limited research to determine whether highly active individuals and athletes require greater amounts of vitamins and minerals in their diets.

Water-Soluble Vitamins

A study of the diets of more than 900 athletes, with at least 90 minutes training per day, indicated that the diets of those who ate less than 45 kcal/kg per day (i.e., 2000 kcal per day for typical female athletes and 2300 kcal per day for most male athletes) contained less than 70% of the RDA for vitamins B_{12}, thiamin, riboflavin, B_6, and several minerals. However, adequate energy intake did not necessarily result in adequacy of all vitamins and minerals. This may have been from the consumption of foods high in fat and simple sugars. Interestingly the majority of the athletes studied used a daily multivitamin supplement (Economos et al., 1993).

A 6-month multivitamin supplementation trial was conducted in athletes (Weight et al., 1988). They received either a multivitamin or a placebo for the first 3 months and crossed over to the opposing supplement in the second 3 months of the study. As long as the energy intake was adequate, there were significant increases only in blood levels of pyridoxine and riboflavin when the athletes used vitamin supplements. This may indicate an increased requirement of these vitamins with training. Although there were no measures of performance, no other effect of this supplementation was found. It is evident that more long-term studies need to be completed.

Of the limited research conducted, most indicated that as long as the athletes were eating adequate calories (some suggested 45 to 50 kcal/kg per day), there was little need for vitamin supplementation (Economos et al., 1993; Tiidus and Houston, 1995; Volpe, 2000). For instance after an 11-week dietary restriction (29 to 50% Dutch RDA) of thiamin, riboflavin, pyridoxine, and ascorbic acid in 24 healthy men, there was a significant decrease in aerobic power and anaerobic threshold (an indicator of LA accumulation) (van der Beek et al., 1994). The authors could not attribute these changes to any one of these vitamins, however. Many individuals may claim that "megadosing" with vitamins or minerals enhances performance. However, if an individual has a well-balanced diet, there is almost no research to support this claim (Lukaski, 1994; Manore, 2000; Weight et al., 1988).

With insufficient energy intake, marginal deficiencies may result in impaired performance (McDonald and Keen, 1988; Volpe, 2000). Long-term effects of poor vitamin status on performance have not been well studied.

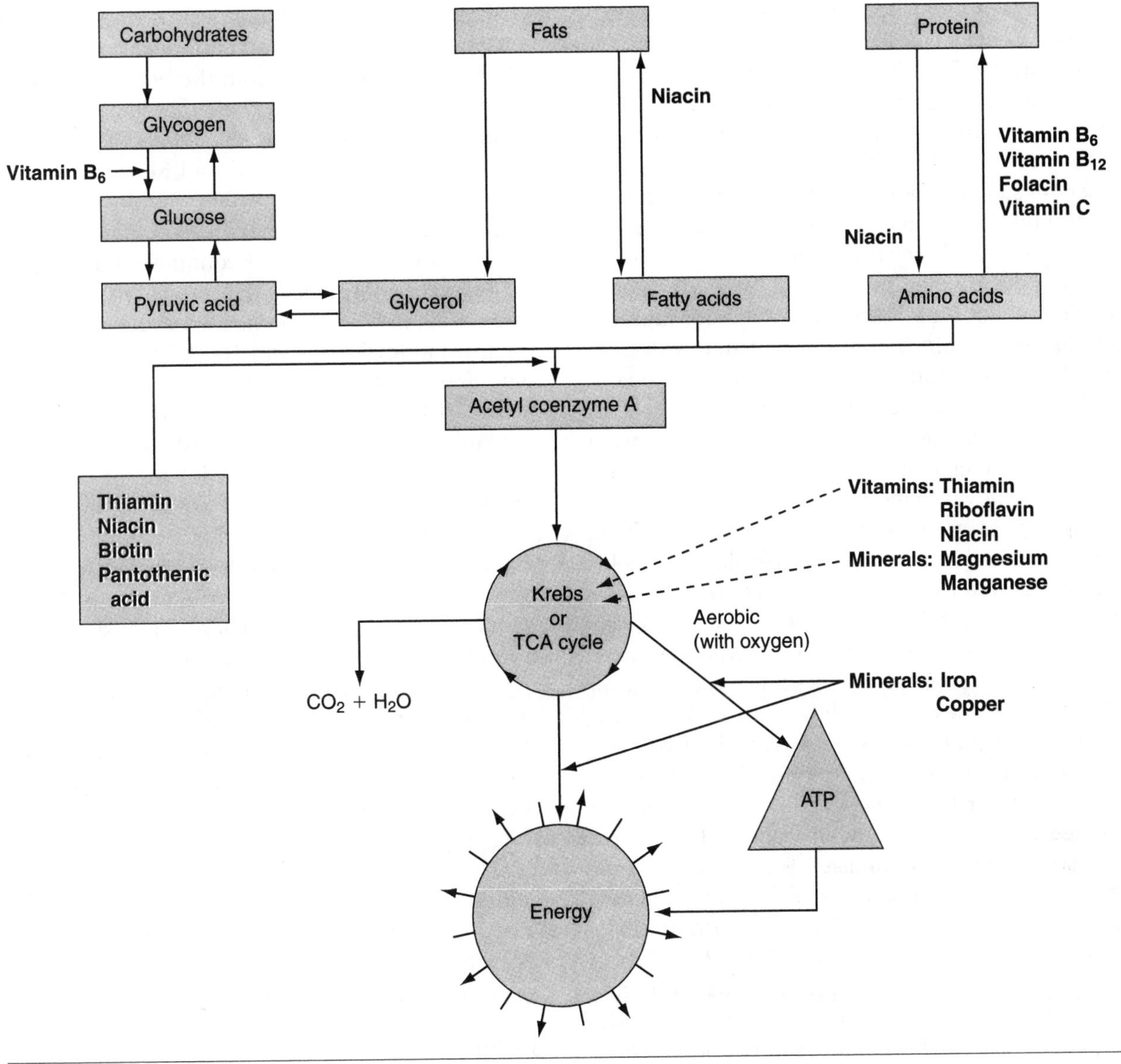

Figure 15-7 The integration of vitamins and minerals in metabolism.

Vitamin C may elicit some benefit for a well-fed athlete, especially during recovery from exercise, by slowing the peroxidative damage of exercise and by decreasing the loss of muscle contractile function (Jakeman and Maxwell, 1993; Williams, 1999). It was helpful in decreasing the onset of upper respiratory tract infections in runners (Peters et al., 1993). These benefits, though, are not consistently evident in all exercise studies using ascorbic acid supplementation (Dekkers et al., 1996), so recommendations for supplementation are not currently being made (Volpe, 2000).

Fat-Soluble Vitamins

Whether exercise increases the requirement for a specific fat-soluble vitamin is difficult to say, primarily because these vitamins are easily stored in body fat, which is in good supply even in lean individuals. Additionally assessing the effect of supplementation on performance is equally difficult because it is a challenge to produce even a marginally deficient state for testing (Tiidus and Houston, 1995; Volpe, 2000). Although supplementation with fat-soluble vitamins D and K does not appear to enhance performance in athletes (Weight et al., 1988), there is some debate over the effect of supplementation with vitamins A and E.

Vitamin A is known to have a role in glycogen synthesis, yet there was no effect on aerobic exercise performance in humans after a 6-month depletion diet. This is thought to be from the large storage of vitamin A in the liver (van der Beek et al., 1984). Vitamin E, an important antioxidant, decreases the oxidant substances that result from intense exercise and thus improves recovery from exercise-induced muscle damage; however, it has not been shown to increase performance.

During exercise, especially aerobic exercise, there is a normal increase (approximately 20 fold) in the amount of oxygen circulated to working cells (Dekkers et al., 1996). All but about 5% of this oxygen combines with hydrogen to produce water (McArdle et al., 1994). The small percentage of oxygen that does not combine with hydrogen instead forms **superoxides** and eventually hydrogen peroxide (H_2O_2) or other **free radicals**, which can be very destructive to a cell. The oxidative damage of free radicals can result in leaky mitochondria and cell membranes, damaged genes and DNA, and the general destruction of cellular proteins including cytochrome Q in the electron transport chain (McArdle et al., 1994; Sizer and Whitney, 1994).

Despite some indication that antioxidant vitamins may provide limited benefit in active individuals, supplementation does not appear necessary when the diet is adequate (Volpe, 2000).

Minerals

The research related to the mineral requirements of athletes suggests that, as with vitamins, those who consume an adequate energy intake will have adequate stores of minerals (Burke and Read, 1989; Economos et al., 1993). However, with an energy intake lower than approximately 45 kcal/kg per day, elite endurance athletes who exercised at least 90 minutes per day had low intakes of iron, zinc, copper, magnesium, and calcium (Economos et al., 1993).

Exercise, especially endurance exercise, may elevate requirements for minerals, based on either an increased loss from the body in sweat or urine or an increase in their metabolism during exercise (Economos et al., 1993; Hickson and Wolinsky, 1989; McDonald and Keen, 1988). An adequate well-balanced energy intake should be sufficient to meet the increased requirements (Burke and Read, 1989; Economos et al., 1993).

Sports performance, depending on how it is measured, may not be enhanced with mineral supplementation (Burke and Read, 1989; McDonald and Keen, 1988). For instance women who consumed 135 mg per day of zinc had an increase in isokinetic strength (Krotkiewski et al., 1982), yet rats who were zinc deficient for 3 weeks could perform equally well on a treadmill compared with a zinc-sufficient group of rats (McDonald and Keen, 1988) and blood levels of zinc in trained or untrained men did not correlate with VO_{2max} (Lukaski et al., 1983). These inconsistent research results are common for minerals, probably because of the variety of experimental designs and performance tests (Economos et al., 1993; McDonald and Keen, 1988). In addition supplementation of one mineral may impair the absorption and metabolism of another mineral (McDonald and Keen, 1988).

The minerals (other than the electrolytes sodium and potassium discussed later with water) that have received the most attention in the literature and that are most likely to affect sports performance are calcium and iron.

Calcium

Calcium intake levels of athletes and Americans of various levels of fitness have been found to be below the Dietary Reference Intake (DRI) (Clarkson and Haymes, 1995; Economos et al., 1993). Most susceptible to the effects of low calcium status are women who are involved in rigorous endurance training, who have 17% or less body fat, who have a low calcium and low energy intake, and who have a habit of practicing restrictive eating. These circumstances are collectively now recognized as the Female Athlete Triad, which involves disordered eating, menstrual dysfunction, and decreased bone mineral density. Highly active women exhibiting these

Donna had been crying again, as her best friend noticed. This was the third time she'd been running and found that her foot began to ache at the start of her 6 miles. She was painfully frustrated. She had been really watching what she ate because she thought her 110 pounds was too much for her 64-inch frame. She'd cut out breakfast and all snacking and had decreased her fat intake drastically, totally avoiding things like the pizza and chips that her friends often ate. In fact she often avoided meat if she could because she thought it was too fattening. Her parents wouldn't be happy with this, she knew, but she was determined to be the best distance runner at school. She worked out at least 30 minutes every day in the gym and she had run 40 to 80 miles per week for months. She had reminded her friend how thrilled she was not to be having a menstrual cycle over the last 6 months and thought that she should now be at her competitive peak. Instead she could hardly walk and when she finally told her parents and coach, the X-rays indicated two stress fractures and a low bone density for her age.

risk factors may experience **athletic amenorrhea** and **stress fractures** and they often exhibit compulsive behaviors with diet and exercise. The bone density of athletes and others in this circumstance may be so poor that it resembles that of a postmenopausal woman (Rencken et al., 1996; Sizer and Whitney, 1994). The amenorrhea that often results from hormonal shifts and food restriction may require many months to reverse when eating patterns and amounts resume. Some physicians recommend hormone replacement therapy; a decrease in training; a dietary intake of 1500 mg calcium per day; and nutrition counseling, psychiatric counseling, or both (American Academy of Pediatrics, 2000). The best treatment of this triad requires solutions to both the short-term hormonal, energy, and calcium deficits and the long-term aberrant eating and exercise behaviors.

Iron

Athletes may have difficulty maintaining adequate iron status for several reasons. Athletes lose iron through sweat and blood losses associated with their sport, such as the small amount of hemorrhaging that occurs in the feet of runners every day. Athletes expend more energy and thus have an increased demand for the iron-containing proteins of the electron transport chain (Sizer and Whitney, 1994). Athletes may have both poor absorption and poor intake of iron (Volpe, 2000). Finally female athletes lose iron monthly during their menstrual cycle (Haymes, 1987).

Three levels of iron deficiency in athletes have been described. Ranging from the mildest to the most severe, these include iron depletion, which is a reduction in serum ferritin (<12 to 20 μg/L); iron deficiency erythropoiesis, or an elevation in protoporphyrin, the protein that binds iron to facilitate erythropoiesis (>1.8 mmol/L); and iron-deficiency anemia, defined as hemoglobin values less than 14 g/dl in men and 12 g/dl in women (Clarkson and Haymes, 1995; McDonald and Keen, 1988; Weight, 1993).

Some of the difficulty in diagnosing iron deficiency anemia has been from the hemodilution of the blood that accompanies endurance exercise training, resulting in falsely low hemoglobin values

KEY TERMS

superoxides: oxygen-containing molecules that are free radicals

free radicals: unstable molecules with unpaired electrons in their outer shells that are trying to combine with other molecules to satisfy their electron configuration

athletic amenorrhea: the cessation of the menstrual cycle usually brought on by low body fat and excessive athletic training

stress fractures: fractures or breaks in bones resulting from stress related to exercise

(Casoni et al., 1985). This condition has been identified as a pseudoanemia, or false anemia, and continues to be reported as sports anemia, which some suggest is a misnomer (Eichner, 1988; Weight, 1993). The incidence of iron deficiency anemia in athletes has been severely overstated from this hemodilution problem (Clarkson and Haymes, 1995; Weight, 1993) and is actually no different from that in the general public when athletes consume balanced diets (Weight, 1993). Female athletes and those who purposely restrict energy intake, such as gymnasts and wrestlers, are predisposed to low iron stores.

Dietary recommendations for increasing iron absorption include consuming meat, fish, and poultry 3 to 4 times per week; increasing consumption of iron-fortified breads, cereals, and grains; and consuming foods high in vitamin C. In addition foods that inhibit iron absorption, such as tea, coffee, and bran, should be consumed in moderation (Volpe, 2000). Iron supplementation has been recommended in some cases of iron deficiency anemia (Eichner, 1988), but improved sports performance has been observed only during submaximal and not maximal exercise (McDonald and Keen, 1988).

Water

The importance of water to physical performance can never be stressed enough to an athlete or any active person, regardless of age or skill level (Convertino et al., 1996). Sixty percent of the body is water and a 5% depletion of body water could have serious consequences (Murray, 2000). The primary functions of water during activity are to transport nutrients in the blood, to participate in metabolic reactions, and, most importantly, to cool the body. This cooling effect of water occurs as the heat produced during exercise is dissipated through the blood and eventually to the skin, where sweat is produced. The amount of heat produced during sustained vigorous exercise is enough to raise core body temperature (i.e., that of the deep tissues) by approximately 1° C every 5 minutes (McArdle et al., 1991).

Adequate cooling is essential during exercise because the body can tolerate an increase of only about 5° C before sports performance is impaired (McArdle et al., 1991). Heat dissipation is especially critical in a hot, humid environment when the body's ability to sweat is reduced. Physically active individuals participating in outdoor activities such as mowing the lawn or playing a game of softball on humid days should be aware of the need to keep the body hydrated and cool. Likewise athletes in endurance events such as marathons (26.2 miles) and ultramarathons (50 or more miles) and athletes in other long sporting events that allow intermittent rest, such as football and basketball, must address these same issues.

Exercise or activity longer than about 60 minutes is likely to result in the production of 1 L to 1.5 L of sweat per hour (Hickson and Wolinsky, 1989; Noakes et al., 1988). Also sweating on a hot, humid day can also result in the loss of electrolytes such as sodium, potassium, and chloride, which influence fluid concentration in and around cells. With excess loss of sweat and electrolytes, core body temperature may increase and produce decreased performance and **heat exhaustion** and **heat stroke** (Murray, 2000).

In fact numerous studies, using body weight as a marker of water loss, have demonstrated that a decrease in body weight of 1% to 3% during a bout of exercise can significantly increase the risk of poor performance (Armstrong et al., 1985). The typical amount of water lost during activity was demonstrated in controlled experiments in which football athletes, dressed in full uniform, lost 1.8% of their body weight after 30 minutes of exercise (Matthews et al., 1969). Marathon athletes lost as much as 6% to 10% of their body weight during the 2- to 4-hour race (Pugh et al., 1966). These differences may be related to intensity and duration of exercise and hydration level before the start of exercise.

Fluid replacement

One of the first recommendations for fluid replacement is that athletes should never begin practice or competition in a poorly hydrated state. This problem can be avoided if the athlete drinks fluids before the event. In addition an athlete should determine his or her usual change in body weight (or sweat rate) associated with practice or competition and should replace flu-

Table 15-4 CONTENTS OF COMMON FLUID-REPLACEMENT BEVERAGES

Beverage	Carbohydrate Type	Carbohydrate g/8 oz (%)	Sodium mg	Potassium mg
Gatorade	Sucrose Glucose Fructose	14 (6)	110	30
Powerade	Fructose Glucose Polymers Maltodextrins	19 (8)	55	30
All Sport	High-Fructose Corn Syrup	19 (8-9)	55	55
Fruit Juice	Glucose Fructose Sucrose	25-30 (11-15)	0-15	60-150
Soft Drinks	High-Fructose Corn Syrup Sucrose	(10-11)	9-28	Trace
Water	None	0 (0)	Minimal	Minimal

The above information available at www.gssiweb.com/reflib/refs, accessed 12/27/01.

ids lost during the practice or competition so there is minimal weight change as a result of exercise (Murray, 2000).

However, some sports may not allow time for fluid replacement. In this case a general recommendation is that for each pound of weight lost during practice or competition, an athlete should consume 3 cups of fluid as soon as possible. Ideally an athlete should drink 4 to 8 oz every 15 to 30 minutes during the game or event (Murray, 2000).

The type of beverage to drink and perhaps the temperature of the fluid consumed by the athlete depend on the event, environmental conditions, and personal preferences. Carbohydrate-electrolyte replacement beverages are recommended when moderate to intense exercise continues for more than 60 to 90 minutes (Murray, 2000). For athletes who exercise for less than 60 minutes, either plain water or a carbohydrate-electrolyte beverage serves the purpose of cooling the body; personal preference is usually the deciding factor.

Sports drinks. Fluid, sodium, potassium, and chloride are the predominant minerals lost in sweat. Their replacement after 1 to 2 hours of moderate exercise can be easily accomplished with usual food intake. However, activity in hot conditions or by individuals who sweat excessively requires the use of a carbohydrate-electrolyte replacement beverage (Murray, 2000).

Table 15-4 lists numerous fluid-replacement beverages and compares the type and percentage of carbohydrate and concentration of electrolytes. Electrolytes in sports drinks, specifically sodium and potassium, are most beneficial because they are needed to maintain intracellular versus extracellular fluid balance. Ingesting them will not necessarily prevent the muscle cramping often

KEY TERMS

heat exhaustion: a state of dehydration in which body fluids have been depleted and body temperature may be slightly elevated >40° C, or 104° F); fluid replacement is necessary

heat stroke: a dangerous and acute reaction to the increase of body temperature; symptoms include dizziness, weakness, cessation of sweating, confusion, body temperature >40° C (104° F), and perhaps loss of consciousness; requires medical intervention

thought to be associated with prolonged exercise in the heat; however, one advantage to a glucose-salt drink is the fact that a weak salt solution enhances glucose absorption (Schedl et al., 1994). Also consumption of fluids is improved with a flavored sports drink. As suggested earlier in this chapter, sports performance during exercise that lasts longer than 60 minutes has been enhanced with the ingestion of glucose before the onset of fatigue (Coggan and Coyle, 1987) because endogenous sources of glucose alone cannot maintain blood glucose levels. With exercise lasting less than 60 minutes, there may be no benefit to these drinks except for hydrating purposes.

The carbohydrates in these drinks are supplied predominantly in the form of glucose; however, some beverages contain sucrose, fructose, or **glucose polymers**. Glucose polymers are not as sweet in taste and may be preferred by some people; however, when provided in concentrations of 10%, glucose polymers may inhibit fluid absorption.

Athletes should take care not to consume a concentrated beverage during an endurance event in the heat when the beverage could be too concentrated and draw water into the gastrointestinal system. In addition drinking a beverage with excessive caffeine may bring on or increase dehydration. Other beverages consumed during exercise by some recreational athletes, including beer and other alcoholic drinks, are dangerous because alcohol dehydrates the body and impairs performance.

PRACTICAL SUGGESTIONS FOR DIETS OF ACTIVE INDIVIDUALS

- *What should an active individual eat and drink before exercising?*
- *Can an active person improve recovery from an intense workout by consuming specific foods?*

KEY TERMS

glucose polymers: chains of glucose molecules attached to one another; also called maltodextrins; provide a decreased sweetness in sports drinks and may appeal to some athletes

Most of the guidelines for planning the diets of exercising individuals have been based on research specific to endurance athletes; limited nutrition-related work has been completed with resistance athletes (Rosenbloom, 2000) and virtually none can be found for recreational athletes. However, all individuals of varying fitness and activity levels can benefit from the following discussion and application because the information is based on both laboratory-controlled exercise performance studies and the literature used to set the RDA and the Food Guide Pyramid recommendations.

Training Diet

The foods and beverages athletes consume every day can affect their performance and this is true for individuals of all activity levels. Athletes of all fitness levels require fuel to perform their activities. The amount required varies depending on age, sex, body weight, and body composition, and type, duration, and intensity of the physical activity. To estimate total amount of energy, baseline kcals are added to kcals needed for both exercise and sedentary activities and kcals for the digestion and absorption of food. The total daily kcals required by most active individuals ranges from 3000 kcal to 6000 kcal (Rosenbloom, 2000). Tabular data that provide an estimate of the energy expended for various sports and other activities are available (McArdle et al., 1991). Studies of endurance athletes report that they consume about 45 kcal/kg to 50 kcal/kg per day.

Training diets have a purpose and should be nutritionally balanced, a task most easily accomplished by using the guidelines set up by the Food Guide Pyramid. Table 15-5 lists the approximate number of servings required from each food group with a menu for a diet of 2000 kcals versus 4000 kcals. Although obtaining a sufficient number of servings from each food group ensures balance, some active individuals find it very difficult to eat this much food while maintaining time for training and other commitments. For this reason many active individuals rely on kcals from sports

Table 15-5 NUMBER OF SERVINGS REQUIRED FOR 2000 KCAL AND 4000 KCAL DIETS

2000 kcal diet	4000 kcal diet
10 servings of starch	20 servings of starch/breads
4 servings of vegetables	7 servings of vegetables
5 servings of fruit	10 servings of fruit
6 ounces of meat	10 ounces of meat
3 servings of milk	6 servings of milk
7 servings of fat	11 servings of fat
Menu	
BREAKFAST	
1½ c apple juice	3 c apple juice
1 c oatmeal + butter	1½ c oatmeal + margarine
1 slice toast + 1 T jelly	2 slices toast + 2 T jelly
1 c milk	1 banana
MIDMORNING SNACK	
1½ c orange juice	2 c orange juice + bagel
LUNCH	
2 slices bread	4 slices bread (4 st)
2 oz turkey	4 oz turkey
1 oz cheese	½ sliced tomato
2 T low-fat mayonnaise	4 T low-fat mayonnaise
½ c baby carrots	2 oz cheese
½ c pretzels	1 c baby carrots
1 milk	12 gingersnaps
	2 c milk
DINNER	
3-4 oz chicken breast	6-8 oz chicken breast
1 c noodles + butter	1 c noodles + butter
1 c green beans	1½ c green beans
1 c salad	2 c salad
3 T low-fat salad dressing	5 T low-fat salad dressing
Iced tea	Iced tea
SNACK	
½ c low-fat frozen yogurt	1 c low-fat frozen yogurt
½ c sliced peaches	1 c sliced peaches
1 slice angel food cake	1 slice angel food cake

drinks or sports bars and take daily vitamin and mineral supplements.

Because carbohydrates are the preferred fuel of working muscles and because performance and endurance are enhanced with adequate stores of carbohydrate, it has been recommended that active individuals consume 55% to 70% of their energy intake from carbohydrates, with 10% of this total from simple sugars (Coleman, 2001; Conley and Stone, 1996). This total level of carbohydrate intake may be difficult to obtain consistently and perhaps this is the reason that dietary studies of athletes indicate they consume only 45% to 50% of their kcals from carbohydrates (Hawley et al., 1995).

The amount of dietary protein required by an athlete and other active individuals is often misunderstood and even controversial. Most recommendations are to obtain about 0.8 g/kg per day, or 10% to 12% of total calories from protein (National Research Council, 1998). However, some athletes who are involved in intense strength and endurance training may require more, or 1.0 g/kg to 2.0 g/kg per day (Lemon, 1996). Most Americans consume well above the RDA, so it is usually not a concern (Carroll, 2000; Lemon, 1996). Of course these recommendations are based on assumptions of adequate intake of energy and high-quality proteins in the training diet.

Proteins of high quality include meat, eggs, milk, and cheese, or a combination of these foods, and legumes, nuts, and seeds for the various types of vegetarians. Many athletes are convinced that they need additional protein (Slavin et al., 1988) and a high proportion of athletes use protein powders and supplements, which are not recommended as the best quality source of protein (Philen et al., 1992). Their mix of amino acids may not be absorbed and amino acids from foods and their concentrations of all the amino acids may not support growth and repair and the best food proteins. Additionally manufacturers lure individuals into purchasing protein supplements with sensational advertising, much of which has not been scientifically verified (Lemon, 1996; Williams, 1999).

Fat obtained from the diet should be about 30% or less of total kcal intake. Ideally saturated, polyunsaturated, and monounsaturated fatty acids should each represent about 10% of the total fat intake. Eating lean meats and drinking low-fat milk helps to ensure that athletes can obtain good sources of protein as they limit saturated fat intake.

Following the Food Guide Pyramid for a training diet allows active persons to obtain the recommended amounts of vitamin and minerals daily, especially if they are obtaining adequate kcal intake and get 5 or more servings of fruits and vegetables daily.

The training diet is extremely important, but should not be rigid. It should allow for a wide variety of foods and beverages because it is the source of all energy and nutrients for the working muscles of active individuals. Some attention should be given to the timing of the meals that surround the physical activity, especially intense exercise.

Preevent Foods

Before carbohydrate and exercise research, many believed that the meal eaten just before competition should be composed of high-protein foods such as steak and eggs. We now know that high-carbohydrate meals before competition or any physical activity are more advisable to promote performance and delay fatigue (Coggan and Coyle, 1987).

The purpose of the preevent meal is multifaceted. It should prevent symptoms of hypoglycemia such as light headedness and fatigue before the event, decrease hunger, and provide energy for working muscles and fluid for hydration. It should also fit the personal preferences and habits of the individual. The preevent meal should be easy to digest and should not remain in the stomach for longer than 3 to 4 hours. If an individual is prone to gastrointestinal distress from either a nervous stomach or the intake of high-fiber foods, the preevent meal should be adjusted. Foods that cause distress should be excluded from the diet on the day of competition or even several days before competition. Identification of these foods and food preferences can be accomplished with a training log in which the individual records foods and beverages that may cause gastrointestinal distress.

For athletic competition (including training), the time of day and the type of sport influence the timing of the preevent meal and the volume of food ingested. For morning competition, a small meal of cereal and milk, toast with jelly, or a liquid carbohydrate would be recommended 1 to 2 hours before the event. A high-carbohydrate dinner the night before an early morning exercise or competition is very important because some liver glycogen stores will be used by the body during the night. Eating a small meal before early morning exercise will help to replace glycogen used at night.

Afternoon athletic events allow a person to eat a breakfast with more carbohydrates. Regardless of the time of day, it is important that athletes drink plenty of fluids before an event to maintain hydration.

Those preparing for evening events or exercise can use the beginning of the day to refill their carbohydrate stores from the previous day and to become properly hydrated. Both breakfast and lunch should be high-carbohydrate meals, which could be followed by a light snack 1 to 2 hours before competition. A typical preevent meal for some athletes is 2 cups of spaghetti with 1 cup meat sauce, a salad, 2 or 3 dinner rolls, a glass of milk or juice, and water (approximately 1000 kcals).

Eating candy or drinking sugar-based beverages within 45 minutes of the start of exercise or a competitive event may cause feelings of sluggishness and premature fatigue in some individuals. This has been attributed to low blood glucose resulting from the release of insulin and the corresponding uptake of glucose from the blood. However, not all individuals are sensitive to glucose or sucrose ingestion within an hour of their event.

Glycemic index has been used to plan preevent meals. Foods with a low glycemic index (beans, milk, pasta) ingested before exercise trials that exercised a person to the point of exhaustion were found to provide a more steady and prolonged blood glucose level during exercise than foods with a high glycemic index (potatoes, sugar, bread, sports drinks, and candy).

Because much of the research regarding carbohydrate and performance has been performed in cycling athletes, it is important that all individuals experiment with preevent foods or beverages during training to determine whether performance is adversely affected by foods before competition or exercise.

Foods during Competition

Individuals who perform moderate to intense exercise for more than 60 minutes benefit from carbohydrate consumption during competition. Studies of cyclists have indicated that endurance performance was increased by 18% when 1 g carbohydrate/kg body weight was consumed after 60 to 90 minutes of exercise (Coggan and Coyle, 1987).

During intense exercise some athletes may prefer not to consume anything but water; however, sports drinks with sugar concentrations less than 8% are usually well tolerated, taste good, and offer advantages such as the maintenance of blood glucose and replacement of fluid and electrolytes. Some of these beverages are listed in Table 15-4.

Although blood flow to the abdominal organs is decreased during exercise and absorption is 60% to 70% of normal, some endurance athletes (cyclists, football and soccer players, ultramarathon runners) can also eat solid and semisolid foods while exercising. Carbohydrate gels and fruit/grain bars are currently popular during exercise. Recent limited research suggests that this may also be appropriate for improving performance of resistance athletes as well.

Postevent or Recovery Foods

Most recently, exercise and nutrition scientists have found that without adequate consumption of carbohydrate after exercise, glycogen stores and endurance in subsequent events are hindered (Coleman, 2001; Ivy, 1988). Many athletes do not feel like eating after exercise; however, it has been demonstrated that consumption of a carbohydrate beverage (50 to 100 g carbohydrate or 200 to 400 kcal) within 2 hours of the event aids recovery of muscle glycogen. Additionally a high-carbohydrate meal within 4 hours after the event is recommended (Coleman, 2001).

Suggestions for high-carbohydrate foods that provide 50 g to 100 g carbohydrate within the first 2 hours after exercise include one or several of the following:

- 32-oz sports beverage
- 1 to 2 sportsbars
- 1 bagel (36 g carbohydrate, 187 kcal)
- 1 oz raisins (22 g carbohydrate, 84 kcal)
- 8-oz orange juice (27 g carbohydrate, 112 kcal)
- 1 banana (27 g carbohydrate, 104 kcal)
- 1 low-fat granola bar (22 g carbohydrate, 110 kcal)

- 3 c air-popped popcorn (18 g carbohydrate, 93 kcal)
- 1 c pasta (40 g carbohydrate, 197 kcal)
- 1 c yogurt with fruit (43 g carbohydrate, 230 kcal)
- 1 large apple (32 g carbohydrate, 212 kcal)

Individuals who exercise regularly and are highly active, and those who are competitive athletes, benefit from balancing good nutrition and exercise training habits. Using sound principles of nutrition to consume adequate fluids, eat nutrient-dense foods, and satisfy energy requirements improves endurance and performance during exercise and enhances recovery after exercise.

BRIEF PRACTICAL SUGGESTIONS FOR THE INDIVIDUALS HIGHLIGHTED IN THIS CHAPTER

The first case study presented in this chapter involves Kristen, a college freshman who has been told by her peers that she will gain 15 pounds during her first college year. The actual weight gain noted in a study in the mid-1980s was about 8 pounds (Hovell, 1985). However, the incidence of overweight and fat adults in the U.S. population is increasing every year. The best advice for Kristen is that she follow her instincts to get about 30 minutes of moderate- to high-intensity activity 5 days per week and to use the Food Guide Pyramid as a basis for making good dietary choices (especially fruits and vegetables). She should try not to skip breakfast and she should use moderation in her consumption of alcohol, sweets, and fat. Kristen should also investigate the resources at her college such as student health services. Many colleges provide the assistance of a registered dietitian or nurse for answering nutrition and wellness questions or for providing other information. In addition she should investigate credible websites such as those provided by the American Dietetic Association for diet information (www.eatright.org) and the USDA's Center for Nutrition Policy and Promotion for interactive input on the quality of her diet (by clicking on Interactive Healthy Eating Index at www.usda.gov/cnpp).

The second case study involving Mrs. B. is a description of the benefits of exercise from a diabetic woman who entered an exercise training research study. The most important point to note is that although body weight changes are often the reason that most people start an exercise program, they are sometimes the last changes to occur with exercise training. In the exercise training study in which Mrs. B was a participant, very few diabetic subjects were able to lose weight with just 8 or 16 weeks of exercise. However, the most gratifying changes that they perceived were improvements in their sleep quantity and quality, improvements in their abilities to handle daily stressors, a better general outlook on life, declining fatigue levels, and the fact that their clothes fit more loosely. These kinds of benefits have been verified scientifically in recent studies (Dunn et al., 2001; Spirduso and Cronin, 2001).

The third case study is a description of a typical former athlete, Ryan, who is trying to get back into shape quickly, yet inconsistently. In high school Ryan did not have the pressures of a job, an independent life-style, college classes, and an unpredictable food source (his food was probably prepared at home). In high school he also had coaches who made him work out. To improve physically, Ryan should make better plans to get plenty of sleep, eat a high-quality diet (limited fast foods and more fruits and vegetables), and work out more consistently throughout the week. However, in light of his class and work schedule, he should work out at lower intensities while doing things that are fun. Finally he should also be patient and realize that getting his body in the shape he remembers from high school will take time. Short-term realistic goals which allow for the realities and demands of his current life-style are more likely to yield success.

The final case study describes Donna as she experiences all or most of the symptoms from the female athlete triad. She is lucky. Her stress fractures made this problem more evident. Her physician, coach, and parents should be sure to help

KEY TERMS

ergogenic: a term that implies "energy production" or "energy giving," but which typically has not been proven as such for products with which it is associated

Donna address this problem with a team of healthcare professionals. Many women deny having one or all of these symptoms. The physician can arrange for numerous meetings to address the nutritional, psychologic, hormonal, and medical aspects of her health. Some of the predominant nutrition-related issues to address include energy, protein, calcium (amount and quality), and vitamin D intake. Donna should be eating enough to compensate for her energy expenditure and she should get at least the recommended level of protein. There is still debate about the value of protein quality for this situation. Many specialists suggest that she should consume 1500 mg of calcium per day and adequate vitamin D. Hormone replacement therapy is now being used for individuals like Donna because an improved diet and decreased exercise does not necessarily result in recovery of lost bone density (American Academy of Pediatrics, 2000).

NUTRITION CONCERNS FOR ACTIVE PEOPLE ACROSS THE LIFE SPAN

- *Do age, sex, and level of physical fitness affect nutrition requirements for athletes and active individuals?*
- *Are ergogenic aids useful for enhancing performance? Who uses them?*

Active individuals of all levels have nutrition requirements that cannot be made into a "one-size-fits-all" program. Just as requirements for energy and nutrients are varied across the life span, the needs of active individuals are also varied. Specific needs and recommendations for the various stages of the life span are located in the respective chapters. The use and significance of **ergogenic** aids are addressed in the Application at the end of this chapter.

Concepts to Remember

- Physical fitness is defined as the set of attributes required to perform physical activity, including flexibility, muscular strength and endurance, cardiorespiratory endurance, and body composition.
- Exercise in which large muscle groups of the back and legs are used continuously for at least 15 minutes 3 times per week are beneficial for lowering the risk of chronic diseases such as cardiovascular disease, obesity, and diabetes.
- Muscle fibers respond to specific exercise training by adapting either aerobic or anaerobic energy production.
- All nutrients play an important role in the total performance of an active individual.
- A daily intake of carbohydrates at a level of 55% to 70% of total energy improves the aerobic endurance performance of an athlete.
- Working muscles prefer to use glucose as their primary fuel source, especially at higher intensities of work.
- Aerobic exercise training enhances the use of fatty acids and improves performance by sparing endogenous carbohydrate stores for later use.
- Resistance exercise training enhances lean body mass accretion and sustains or improves bone density.
- The best way to build more muscle is to eat a well-balanced diet and exercise the muscle with some form of resistance training.
- Active individuals will experience decreased performance if not properly hydrated.

REFERENCES

American Academy of Pediatrics: Committee on sports medicine and fitness. Medical concerns in the female athlete, Pediatrics 106:610, 2000.

American College of Sports Medicine: Resource manual. Guidelines for exercise testing and prescription, ed 3, Baltimore, 1998, Williams & Wilkins.

Armstrong LE et al.: Influence of diuretic-induced dehydration on competitive running performance, Med Sci Sports Exerc 17:456, 1985.

Astrand P: Something old and something new...very new, Nutr Today 9, 1968.

Blair SN et al.: Is physical activity on physical fitness more important in defining health benefits? Med Sci Sport Exerc 33:S379, 2001.

Blair SN et al.: Physical activity, nutrition, and chronic disease, Med Sci Sports Exerc 28:335, 1996a.

Blair SN et al.: Influences of cardiorespiratory fitness and other precursors on cardiovascular disease and all-cause mortality in men and women. JAMA 276:205, 1996b.

Blair SN et al.: Changes in physical fitness and all-cause mortality. A prospective study of healthy and unhealthy men, JAMA 273:1093, 1995.

Bouchard C: Physical activity and health: introduction to the dose-response symposium, Med Sci Sport Exerc 33:S347, 2001.

Bouchard C and Despres JP: Physical activity and health: atherosclerotic, metabolic, and hypertensive diseases, Res Quar Exerc Sport 66:268, 1995.

Burke LM and Read RSD: Sports nutrition: approaching the nineties, Sports Med 8:80, 1989.

Carroll C: Protein and exercise. In Rosenbloom CA, editor: Sports nutrition. A guide for the professional working with active people, Chicago, 2000, American Dietetic Association.

Casoni I et al.: Reduced hemoglobin concentration and red cell hemoglobinization in Italian marathon and ultramarathon runners, Int J Sports Med 6:176, 1985.

Clarkson PM: Nutrition for improved sports performance. Current issues on ergogenic aids. Sports Med 6:393, 1990.

Clarkson PM and Haymes E: Exercise and mineral status of athletes: calcium, magnesium, phosphorus, and iron, Med Sci Sports Exerc 27:831, 1995.

Coggan AR and Coyle EF: Reversal of fatigue during prolonged exercise by carbohydrate infusion or ingestion, J Appl Physiol 63:5, 1987.

Coleman E: Carbohydrate and exercise. In Rosenbloom CA, editor: Sports nutrition. A guide for the professional working with active people, Chicago, 2001, American Dietetic Association.

Conley MS and Stone MH: Carbohydrate ingestion/supplementation for resistance exercise and training, Sports Med 21:7, 1996.

Convertino VA et al.: American College of Sports Medicine position stand: exercise and fluid replacement, Med Sci Sport Exerc 28:I, 1996.

Coyle EF and Montain SJ: Carbohydrate and fluid ingestion during exercise: are there trade-offs? Med Sci Sport Exerc 24:671, 1992.

DeBusk RF et al.: Training effects of long versus short bouts of exercise in healthy subjects, Am J Cardiol 65:1010, 1990.

Dekkers JC et al.: The role of antioxidant vitamins and enzymes in the prevention of exercise-induced muscle damage, Sports Med 21:213, 1996.

Duchateau J and Hainaut K: Isometric or dynamic training: differential effect on mechanical properties of a human muscle, J Appl Physiol 6:296, 1982.

Dunn AL et al.: Physical activity dose-response effects on outcomes of depression and anxiety, Med Sci Sport Exerc 33:S587, 2001.

Economos CD et al.: Nutrition practices of elite athletes: practical recommendations. Sports Med 16:381, 1993.

Eichner ER: "Sports anemia": poor terminology for a real phenomenon, Gatorade Sports Science Institute. Sports Science Exchange, August 1988.

Fiatarone MA et al.: High-intensity strength training in nonagenarians: effects on skeletal muscle, JAMA 263:3029, 1990.

Hawley JA et al.: Nutritional practices of athletes: are they sub-optimal? J Sport Sci 13:S75, 1995.

Haymes EM: Nutritional concerns: need for iron, Med Sci Sports Exerc 19:S197, 1987.

Hickson JF and Wolinsky I: Nutrition in exercise and sport, Boca Raton, 1989, CRC Press.

Ivy JL: Muscle glycogen synthesis after exercise: effect of time of carbohydrate ingestion, J Appl Physiol 64:1480, 1988.

Jakeman P and Maxwell S: Effect of antioxidant vitamin supplementation on muscle function after eccentric exercise, Eur J Appl Physiol 67:426, 1993.

Krotkiewski M et al.: Zinc and muscle strength, Acta Physiol Scand 116:309, 1982.

Kuel J et al.: The effect of weight lifting exercise on heart rate and metabolism in experienced weightlifters, Med Sci Sports Exerc 10:13, 1978.

Lemon PWR: Is increased dietary protein necessary on beneficial for individuals with a physically active lifestyle? Nutr Rev 54:S169, 1996.

Lohman TG: Advances in body composition assessment. Current issues in exercise science series, Monograph No. 3., Champaign, IL, 1992, Human Kinetics.

Lukaski HC: Micronutrients (magnesium, zinc, and copper): are mineral supplements needed for athletes? Gatorade Sports Science Institute, November 1994.

Lukaski HC et al.: Maximum oxygen consumption as related to magnesium, copper, and zinc nutriture, Am J Clin Nutr 37:407, 1983.

McArdle WD et al.: Exercise physiology, energy, and human performance, ed 3, Philadelphia, 1991, Lea & Febiger.

McArdle WD et al.: Essentials of exercise physiology, Philadelphia, 1994, Lea & Febiger.

McDonald R and Keen CL: Iron, zinc, and magnesium nutrition and athletic performance, Sports Med 5:171, 1988.

Manore MM: Effect of physical activity on thiamine, riboflavin, and vitamin B_6 requirements, Am J Clin Nutr 72(Suppl):598S, 2000.

Matthews DK et al.: Physiological responses during exercise and recovery in a football uniform, J Appl Physiol 26:611, 1969.

Murray R: Fluid and electrolytes. In Rosenbloom CA, editor: Sports nutrition. A guide for the professional working with active people, Chicago, 2000, American Dietetic Association.

National Institutes of Health Consensus Conference: Physical activity and cardiovascular health, JAMA 276:241, 1996.

National Research Council: Dietary reference intake series, National Academy of Sciences, Washington, DC, 1997, 1998, 2000, 2001, National Academy Press.

Noakes TD et al.: The danger of inadequate water intake during prolonged exercise: a novel concept revisited, Eur J Appl Physiol 57:210, 1988.

Paffenbarger RS Jr et al.: Physical activity, all-cause mortality, and longevity of college alumni, N Engl J Med 314:605, 1986.

Peters EM et al.: Vitamin C supplementation reduces the incidence of post race symptoms of upper-respiratory tract infection in ultramarathon runners, Am J Clin Nutr 57:170 1993.

Philen RM et al.: Survey of advertising for nutritional supplements in health and bodybuilding magazines, JAMA 268:1008, 1992.

Pugh LCGE et al.: Rectal temperatures, weight losses and sweat rates in marathon running, J Appl Physiol 21:1251, 1966.

Rencken ML et al.: Bone density at multiple skeletal sites in amenorrheic athletes, JAMA 276:238, 1996.

Rosenbloom CA, editor: Sports nutrition: a guide for the professional working with active people, ed 3, Chicago, 2000, American Dietetic Association.

Saltin B et al.: Fiber types and metabolic potentials of skeletal muscles in sedentary man and endurance runners, Ann N Y Acad Sci 301:3, 1977.

Schedl HP et al.: Intestinal absorption during rest and exercise: implications for formulating an oral rehydration solution, Med Sci Sport Exerc 26:267, 1994.

Sherman WM and Leenders N: Fat loading: the next magic bullet? Int J Sport Nutr 5:S1, 1995.

Sherman WM et al.: Effect of exercise-diet manipulation on muscle glycogen and its subsequent utilization during performance, Int J Sport Nutr 2:114, 1981.

Sizer FS and Whitney EN: Nutrition and physical activity. In Sizer F and Whitney E, editors: Nutrition concepts and controversies, ed 6, Minneapolis, 1994, West Publishing Co.

Slavin JL et al.: Amino acid supplement: beneficial or risky? Physician and Sports Med 16:221, 1988.

Spirduso WW and Cronin DL: Exercise dose-response effects on quality of life and independent living in older adults, Med Sci Sport Exerc 33:S598, 2001.

Tarnopolsky MA: Influence of differing macronutrient intakes on muscle glycogen resynthesis after resistance exercise, J Appl Physiol 84:890, 1998.

Tarnopolsky M, MacDougall D, and Atkinson S: Influence of protein intake and training status on nitrogen balance and lean body mass, J Appl Physiol 64:187, 1988.

Tiidus PM and Houston ME: Vitamin E status and response to exercise training, Sports Med 20:12, 1995.

van der Beek EJ et al.: Effect of marginal vitamin intake on physical performance of man, Int J Sport Med 5S:28, 1984.

van der Beek EJ et al.: Thiamin, riboflavin and vitamin B6. Impact of restricted intake on physical performance in man, J Am Coll Nutr 13:269, 1994.

Volpe S: Vitamins and minerals for active people. In Rosenbloom CA, editor: Sports nutrition. A guide for the professional working with active people, Chicago, 2000, American Dietetic Association.

Weight LM: 'Sports anaemia,' does it exist? Sports Med 16:1, 1993.

Weight LM et al.: Vitamin and mineral status of trained athletes including the effects of supplementation, Am J Clin Nutr 47:186, 1988.

Williams MH: Nutrition for health fitness and sport, ed 5, Boston, 1999, WCB/McGraw-Hill.

APPLICATION

Are Ergogenic Aids Enhancers of Sports Performance?

Jordan is a college student who wants to participate in bodybuilding contests some day. He attends a Midwestern university where he was recruited to wrestle, but after suffering an injury last year, he has decided to take a year off and train in a more complete manner. He is not a novice to his sport. He has been wrestling and working out in the gym nearly all his life. His father started him in wrestling at the age of 6. Jordan religiously reads muscle and fitness magazines and, although he thinks his training and recovery are progressing quickly, he is always looking for a competitive edge. His goals are to get his injured shoulder back in shape and to increase his current weight from 185 to 195 while decreasing his body fat from 15% to 8%. Along with a rigorous weight training program, he plans to use a variety of ergogenic aids, supplements, or herbals—namely, creatine, hydroxy methyl butyrate (HMB), glutamine, branched chain amino acids (BCAAs), multivitamins, protein powder, and ginseng—to obtain his goals.

Athletically competitive individuals of all levels and ages want to be bigger, stronger, faster, leaner, or somehow more impressive than their opponents. Losing a gold medal by 0.01 seconds as Gwen Torrence did in the 100 m race in the 1996 Olympics is an often cited example of how and why athletes might use supplements to improve by even a tiny amount that might help them win. They will try almost anything to give them a competitive edge. Very often, despite a lack of scientific proof or the assurance of safety, athletes will spend a great deal of money to use ergogenic (work producing) aids, diet supplements, or herbals to stay at the top of their game (Ahrendt, 2001; Hawley et al., 1995; Krcik, 2001). This may be especially true for college and high school athletes whose coaches often believe that performance can be enhanced with these supplements (National Strength and Conditioning Association, 1998). However, athletes are not the only users of dietary supplements. In fact the use of supplements by all Americans has increased so dramatically that sales equaled $11.8 billion in 1997 (Nesheim, 1999).

One very popular type of ergogenic aid used by many college students is advertised as a "high energy drink." This drink is usually a carbonated beverage loaded with caffeine and an ephedra-like herb known as guarana. A recent internet search listed 33 brands of "high energy drinks" or "natural energy drinks" with this combination. Use of these products has become a concern for many professionals who provide health-care services at colleges and universities around the country. So far, one death has been reported using one of these energy drinks (Hinson, 2001).

The Dietary Supplement and Health Education Act of 1994 (DSHEA) allows vitamins, minerals, amino acids, herbs, protein powders, and other botanicals to be classified as dietary supplements. This means that the Food and Drug Administration (FDA) does not have to evaluate these products or enforce standards for them. Consequently, although DSHEA requests that manufacturers advertise only substantiated claims, the label can be inaccurate and claims of the contents of the bottle do not have to be verified.

Advertisers use citations of research studies from impressive-looking journals. Many of these scientific studies do not support the actual claim and may have serious flaws in design. Often the advertiser uses results from studies of individuals who began the study with a marginal nutritional status. In addition some claims rely on results from animal research (Clarkson, 1996; Sarubin, 1999; Williams, 1995). Very few of the supplements—that is, those not banned by athletic organizations or illegal—have been found to improve performance as the manufacturers claim. Random laboratory testing of the same supplement from different manufacturers indicated that the purity and concentration of the active ingredient was quite varied and unpredictable and not as claimed on the label (Tufts University Health and Nutrition Letter, 2000).

In general advertisers of supplements used for sports performance claim one or more of the following functions:

- Increase lean mass or promote muscle growth or strength
- Increase the hormones responsible for muscle growth (i.e., testosterone, insulin, growth hormone, anabolic steroids)
- Decrease body weight or mass
- Increase the body's ability to do work by increasing energy, aerobic capacity, or endurance
- Improve the body's ability to recover from strenuous exercise or rebuild/repair cells damaged during exercise
- Reduce anxiety, pain, or mental fatigue

Table 15-6 classifies ergogenic aids, nutrition supplements, and herbals by these proposed functions. Additionally the table indicates whether there has been some scientific evidence to support or refute the claim and, finally, the table indicates which of these substances are legal or banned by the International Olympic Committee (IOC) or the National Collegiate Athletic Association (NCAA).

A high priority of many individuals, especially men with an obsessive desire to be big (now termed biggerexia), is to increase lean body or muscle mass. This does not happen, appreciably, unless the muscle is stressed with resistance training and provided with sufficient nutrients (i.e., amino acids and energy) to make new muscle. Many investigators have shown that resistance training coupled with an adequate diet are the foundation for increasing lean body mass (Lemon and Nagle, 1981; Lemon et al., 1984; Tarnopolsky et al., 1988). Some supplements may assist these processes, but there may be some serious safety concerns and adverse effects as a result. One group of supplements boosts the growth signals (insulin, growth hormone, testosterone, steroids), but these supplements are illegal or banned by sports associations (Ahrendt, 2001; Lamb, 1989; NCAA Banned-Drug Classes, 2001). A second group increases the nutrients

Table 15-6 NUTRITION SUPPLEMENTS, ERGOGENIC AIDS, AND HERBS CATEGORIZED BY PROPOSED FUNCTION, SCIENTIFIC EVIDENCE (+) OR DENIAL (−) OF FUNCTION AND LEGALITY

Proposed Function	Supplements on Market That Claim This Proposed Function	Scientific Evidence of Function (positive/negative)	Supplements That Are Illegal or Banned by IOC or NCAA
Increase Lean Mass, Muscle Growth, and Strength	Anabolic steroids Androstenedione Beta$_2$ agonists Chromium Creatine D-ribose GHB Growth hormone Magnesium Protein Pyruvate Vitamin B$_6$ Vitamin B$_{12}$ Zinc	Anabolic steroids (+) Androstenedione (+/−) Creatine (+) Chromium (+ with deficiency only) GHB (−) Growth hormone (−) Magnesium (+ with deficiency only) Protein (+ with exercise training) Pyruvate (limited) B$_6$, B$_{12}$, zinc (+ only with deficiency)	Anabolic steroid Androstenedione Beta$_2$ agonists Growth hormone
Increase Endogenous Steroid Production or Hormones Responsible for Growth	Arginine Avena sativa Boron Chrysin DHEA GHB Glutamine Phytosterols Tribulus terrestris Yohimbine	Arginine (+/−) Avena sativa (−) Boron (−) Chrysin (−) DHEA (+/−) GHB (+/−) Glutamine (−) Phytosterols (−) Tribulus terrestris (−) Yohimbine (+/−)	DHEA GHB
Decrease Body Weight or Body Mass	Amphetamines Caffeine/ephedrine Diuretics Guarana Ma huang	Amphetamines (+) Caffeine/ ephedrine (+) Diuretics (+) Guarana/ ma huang (+)	Amphetamines Caffeine (>15 mg/mL) Ephedrine Diuretics Guarana Ma huang
Increase Fat Use and Metabolism	Aspartates Caffeine Carnitine Guarana Growth hormone	Aspartates (+/−) Caffeine (+) Carnitine (−) Guarana (+) Growth hormone (−)	Caffeine Guarana Growth hormone

DHEA = docosanexanoic acid; GHB = gamma-hydroxy butyrate; IOC = International Olympic Committee; NCAA = National Collegiate Athletic Association.

Continued

Table 15-6 NUTRITION SUPPLEMENTS, ERGOGENIC AIDS, AND HERBS CATEGORIZED BY PROPOSED FUNCTION, SCIENTIFIC EVIDENCE (+) OR DENIAL (−) OF FUNCTION AND LEGALITY—CONT'D

Proposed Function	Supplements on Market That Claim This Proposed Function	Scientific Evidence of Function (positive/negative)	Supplements That Are Illegal or Banned by IOC or NCAA
Increase Ability to Work:			
Increase Energy Production	Dimethylglycine Ephedrine Ephedrine/caffeine Guarana Ma huang Inosine Multivitamin Niacin Phosphates Thiamin Vitamin C	Dimethylglycine (−) Ephedrine (+) Ephedrine/caffeine (+) Guarana/ ma huang (+) Inosine (−) Multivitamin, niacin, thiamin, vitamin C (+ only with deficiency) Phosphates (−)	Ephedrine Ephedrine/ caffeine Guarana/ ma huang
Increase Aerobic Capacity	Blood doping CoEnzyme Q_{12} Erythropoietin Folic acid Inosine Iron Multivitamin Oxygen Thiamin Riboflavin, vitamin C Vitamin E, zinc	Blood doping (+) Coenzyme Q_{12} (−) Erythropoietin (+) Folic acid, iron, multivitamin, thiamin, riboflavin, vitamins C/E, and zinc (+ only with deficiency) Inosine (−) Oxygen (−)	Blood doping Erythropoietin
Increase Endurance	Bee pollen Caffeine Carbohydrates Choline Fat supplements Fluids Ginseng Glycerol Multivitamins Narcotics Niacin Phosphates Tryptophan Riboflavin	Bee pollen (−) Caffeine (+) Carbohydrates (+) Choline (+/−) Fat supplements (−) Fluids (+) Ginseng (+/−) Glycerol (+/−) Multivitamins, niacin, Riboflavin (+ only with deficiency) Narcotics (−) Phosphates (−) Tryptophan (−)	Caffeine Narcotics

IOC = International Olympic Committee; NCAA = National Collegiate Athletic Association.

Table 15-6 NUTRITION SUPPLEMENTS, ERGOGENIC AIDS, AND HERBS CATEGORIZED BY PROPOSED FUNCTION, SCIENTIFIC EVIDENCE (+) OR DENIAL (−) OF FUNCTION AND LEGALITY—CONT'D

Proposed Function	Supplements on Market That Claim This Proposed Function	Scientific Evidence of Function (positive/negative)	Supplements That Are Illegal or Banned by IOC or NCAA
Increase Ability to Work:—cont'd Improve Hydration	Fluid Glycerol orally	Glycerol (+) Fluid (+)	
Enhance Recovery and Boost Immunity	CoEnzyme Q_{12} Glucosamine Glutamine HMB Multivitamin Oxygen Pycnogenol Vanadyl sulfate	CoEnzyme Q_{12} (−) Glucosamine (−) Glutamin (+/−) HMB (+/−) Multivitamin (+ with deficiency only) Oxygen, V. Sulfate (−) Pycnogenol (+)	
Improve Antioxidant Status	CoEnzyme Q_{10} Pycnogenol Selenium Vitamin C Vitamin E	CoEnzyme Q_{10} (−) Pycnogenol (+) Selenium, vitamins C and E (+ with deficiency)	
Decrease Muscle Breakdown and Enhance Recovery	Aspirin BCAA Ginseng Glucosamine HMB Leucine Protein	Aspirin (−) BCAA (−) Ginseng (−) Glucosamine (+ as antiinflammatory) HMB, leucine (−) Protein (+ as part of regular diet)	
Delay Fatigue	Amphetamines Carbohydrates Sodium bicarbonate	Amphetamines (+) Carbohydrates (+) Sodium bicarbonate (+/−)	Amphetamines
Decrease Anxiety, Pain, or Mental Fatigue	Alcohol Aspirin Beta blockers BCAA Cocaine CoEnzyme Q_{10} Ephedra Ma huang Marijuana Narcotics Vitamin B_6	Alcohol (+) Aspirin (+) Beta blockers (+) BCAA (+/−) Cocaine (+/−) CoEnzyme Q_{10} (−) Ephedra/ma huang (+) Marijuana, narcotics (+) Vitamin B_6 (+ only with deficiency)	Alcohol Beta blockers Cocaine Ephedra Ma huang Marijuana Narcotics

BCAA = branched chain amino acids; HMB = hydroxy methyl butyrate; IOC = International Olympic Committee; NCAA = National Collegiate Athletic Association.

that participate in the building process or that are part of the muscle (amino acids, protein powders, multivitamins, D-ribose, creatine) and these products have met with some limited success, often because the people who use them may have very poor diets. Enhancing the recovery and thus depressing muscle breakdown after exercise (antioxidants, vitamins, HMB, pycnogenol) is a third type, which has had less testing and limited success. Each of these types of supplements, if taken in excessive doses, can have adverse effects. For instance, although creatine is an effective supplement for increasing body weight, muscle tears, severe cramping, and dehydration have been reported (Krcik, 2001; Poortmans and Francauz, 2000). Dehydration from creatine ingestion when coupled with high temperature and humidity could make a situation just right for heat stroke injury.

Competitive individuals are also eager to support their energy supply when they exercise. Several substances are used for increasing the feeling of more energy (ephedrine, ma huang, caffeine), but are banned. Others that seem to increase the energy or aerobic capacity of the user (blood doping, vitamins, minerals, CoEnzyme Q) are either banned or work only because of nutritional deficiency.

Promoting recovery of carbohydrate stores (as noted in the "Postevent or Recovery Foods" section earlier in this chapter) is a very recent topic for affecting performance, as is the decrease in mental fatigue during exercise. Supplements that claim success with the latter goal (alcohol, ephedrine, marijuana) affect pain perception and may be effective, but are either illegal or banned.

Most nutritionists prudently recommend that users of supplements be well informed about the claims, risks, and benefits of their supplement. Users should consult scientifically sound articles, legitimate websites, and knowledgeable medical professionals to stay informed and make the most appropriate choices (Rosenbloom, 2000; Rosenbloom and Storlie, 1998).

REFERENCES

Ahrendt DM: Ergogenic aids: counseling the athlete, Am Fam Physician 63:913, 2001.

Clarkson PM: Nutrition for improved sports performance: current issues on ergogenic aids, Sports Med 6:393, 1996.

Hawley JA et al.: Nutritional practices of athletes: are they sub-optimal? J Sports Sci 13:S75, 1995.

Hinson N: adacomm@taex001.tamu.edu, American Dietetic Association Listserve for College Healthcare Dietitians, July 17, 2001.

Krcik JA: Performance-enhancing substances: what athletes are using, Cleve Clin J Med 68:283, 2001.

Lamb DR: Abuse of anabolic steroids in sport. Gatorade Sports Science Institute, Sports Science Exchange April 1989.

Lemon P and Nagle F: Effects of exercise on protein and amino acid metabolism, Med Sci Sports Exerc 13:141, 1981.

Lemon P et al.: The importance of protein for athletes, Sports Med 1:474, 1984.

National Collegiate Athletic Association Banned-Drug Classes, 2000-01. http://www.ncaa.org/sports_sciences/drugtesting/banned_list.htr. Accessed January 20, 2001.

National Strength and Conditioning Association: Use of dietary supplements in sports training bulletin,19:1, 1998.

Nesheim MC: What is the research base for use of dietary supplements? Public Health Nutr 2:35, 1999.

Poortmans JR and Francauz M: Adverse effects of creatine supplementation, fact or fiction, Sports Med 30:155, 2000.

Rosenbloom CA, editor: Sports nutrition: a guide for the professional working with active people, ed 3, Chicago, 2000, American Dietetic Association.

Rosenbloom CA and Storlie J: A nutritionist's guide to evaluating ergogenic aids, PULSE: Sports, Cardiovascular, and Wellness Nutritionists Newsletter 17:1, 1998.

Sarubin A: The health professional's guide to popular dietary supplements, Chicago, 1999, American Dietetic Association.

Tarnopolsky MA et al.: Influence of protein intake and training status on nitrogen balance and lean body mass, J Appl Physiol 64:187, 1988.

Tufts University Health and Nutrition Letter (Special Supplement): Does the supplement you buy contain what its label says? October 2000.

Williams MH: Nutritional ergogenics in athletics, J Sports Sci 13:S63, 1995.

Williams MH: Nutrition for health fitness and sport, ed 5, Boston, 1999, WCB/McGraw Hill.

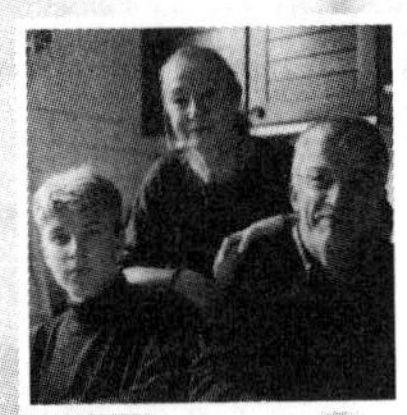

APPENDIXES

APPENDIX A

ESTIMATED SODIUM, CHLORIDE, AND POTASSIUM MINIMUM REQUIREMENTS OF HEALTHY PERSONS*

Age	Weight (kg)	Sodium (mg)*†	Chloride (mg)*†	Potassium (mg)‡
MONTHS				
0-5	4.5	120	180	500
6-11	8.9	200	300	700
YEARS				
1	11.0	225	350	1000
2-5	16.0	300	500	1400
6-9	25.0	400	600	1600
10-18	50.0	500	750	2000
>18§	70.0	500	750	2000

*No allowance has been included for large, prolonged losses from the skin through sweat.

†There is no evidence that higher intakes confer any health benefit.

‡Desirable intakes of potassium may considerably exceed these values (~3500 mg for adults).

§No allowance included for growth. Values for those below 18 years assume a growth rate at the 50th percentile reported by the National Center for Health Statistics and averaged for males and females.

APPENDIX B

REFERENCE DATA FOR ANTHROPOMETRIC MEASUREMENTS

Metropolitan Life Insurance Company Height-Weight Data, Revised 1983

Height-Weight Tables for Adults

Women					Men				
Height		Frame*			Height		Frame*		
Ft	In	Small	Medium	Large	Ft	In	Small	Medium	Large
4	10	102-111	109-121	118-131	5	2	128-134	131-141	138-150
4	11	103-113	111-123	120-134	5	3	130-136	133-143	140-153
5	0	104-115	113-126	122-137	5	4	132-138	135-145	142-156
5	1	106-118	115-129	125-140	5	5	134-140	137-148	144-160
5	2	108-121	118-132	128-143	5	6	136-142	139-151	146-164
5	3	111-124	121-135	131-147	5	7	138-145	142-154	149-168
5	4	114-127	124-138	134-151	5	8	140-148	145-157	152-172
5	5	117-130	127-141	137-155	5	9	142-151	148-160	155-176
5	6	120-133	130-144	140-159	5	10	144-154	151-163	158-180
5	7	123-136	133-147	143-163	5	11	146-157	154-166	161-184
5	8	126-139	136-150	146-167	6	0	149-160	157-170	164-188
5	9	129-142	139-153	149-170	6	1	152-164	160-174	168-192
5	10	132-145	142-156	152-173	6	2	155-168	164-178	172-197
5	11	135-148	145-159	155-176	6	3	158-172	167-182	176-202
6	0	138-151	148-162	158-179	6	4	162-176	171-187	181-207

Based on a weight-height mortality study conducted by the Society of Actuaries and the Association of Life Insurance Medical Directors of America. Metropolitan Life Insurance Company, revised 1983.

*Weights at ages 25 to 59 based on lowest mortality. Height includes 1-in heel. Weight for women includes 3 lb for indoor clothing. Weight for men includes 5 lb for indoor clothing.

Determination of Frame Size

The patient's right arm is extended forward perpendicular to the body, with the arm bent so the angle at the elbow forms 90° with the fingers pointing up and the palm turned away from the body. The greatest breadth across the elbow joint is measured with a sliding caliper along the axis of the upper arm, on the two prominent bones on either side of the elbow. This is recorded as the elbow breadth. The following tables give the elbow breadth measurements for medium-framed men and women of various heights. Measurements lower than those listed indicate a small frame size; higher measurements indicate a large frame size.

Men		Women	
Height in 1″-Heels	Elbow Breadth	Height in 1″-Heels	Elbow Breadth
5′2″-5′3″	2 1/2″-2 7/8″	4′10″-4′11″	2 1/4″-2 1/2″
5′4″-5′7″	2 5/8″-2 7/8″	5′0″-5′3″	2 1/4″-2 1/2″
5′8″-5′11″	2 3/4″-3″	5′4″-5′7″	2 3/8″-2 5/8″
6′0″-6′3″	2 3/4″-3 1/8″	5′8″-5′11″	2 3/8″-2 5/8″
6′4″	2 7/8″-3 1/4″	6′0″	2 1/2″-2 3/4″

From Metropolitan Life Insurance Company, 1983.

Norms for Triceps Fatfold (mm) from the Second National Health and Nutrition Examination Survey

Sex and Age	Percentile 5th	10th	15th	25th	50th	75th	85th	90th	95th
MALE									
6-11 months	6.5	7.0	7.0	8.0	10.0	12.0	14.0	15.0	16.0
1 year	6.5	7.0	7.5	8.5	10.0	12.0	13.0	14.0	15.5
2 years	6.0	7.0	7.0	8.0	10.0	12.0	13.0	14.5	15.0
3 years	6.5	7.0	7.5	8.0	9.5	11.5	12.5	13.0	15.0
4 years	6.0	6.5	7.0	7.5	9.0	11.0	12.0	13.0	15.0
5 years	5.5	6.0	6.5	7.0	8.0	10.5	11.5	12.5	14.5
6 years	5.0	5.5	6.0	6.5	8.0	10.5	12.0	13.0	17.5
7 years	5.0	5.5	6.0	6.5	8.5	11.0	12.0	15.0	17.5
8 years	5.5	6.0	6.0	7.0	9.0	12.0	16.5	17.0	22.0
9 years	5.0	5.0	6.0	7.0	9.0	12.5	16.0	19.0	23.0
10 years	5.0	6.0	6.5	7.5	11.0	16.5	20.0	22.0	26.0
11 years	4.5	5.5	6.0	7.5	10.5	17.0	22.0	25.0	30.0
12 years	5.0	6.0	6.0	8.0	11.0	15.0	18.0	21.5	26.5
13 years	5.0	5.5	6.0	7.0	9.0	12.5	16.5	20.5	22.5
14 years	4.0	5.0	5.5	6.0	9.0	13.0	15.0	17.0	23.0
15 years	5.0	5.0	6.0	6.0	7.5	11.0	14.5	18.0	22.0
16 years	4.5	5.0	5.5	6.5	8.0	13.0	18.5	20.5	25.5
17 years	4.0	4.5	5.0	5.5	7.0	10.5	12.5	15.0	18.0
18 years	4.0	5.0	5.0	6.0	9.5	14.5	17.5	19.0	22.5
18-24 years	4.5	5.0	6.0	6.5	10.0	15.0	17.5	20.0	24.5
25-34 years	4.5	5.5	6.5	7.5	11.5	16.5	20.0	23.0	26.0
35-44 years	5.0	6.0	7.0	9.0	12.5	17.0	20.0	23.0	27.0
45-54 years	5.5	6.5	7.0	9.0	12.0	16.5	20.0	22.0	25.5
55-64 years	5.0	6.0	7.5	9.0	12.0	16.0	19.5	21.5	25.5
65-74 years	5.0	6.0	7.0	8.0	11.5	16.0	18.5	21.0	25.0
FEMALE									
6-11 months	6.5	7.0	7.0	8.0	10.0	11.5	12.5	13.0	14.5
1 year	6.0	7.0	7.5	8.0	10.5	12.0	13.5	15.0	16.5
2 years	6.0	7.0	7.5	8.0	10.5	12.5	13.5	15.0	16.0
3 years	6.0	7.0	7.0	8.0	10.0	12.0	12.5	13.5	16.5
4 years	6.0	6.5	7.5	8.0	10.0	12.0	13.0	14.0	15.5
5 years	6.0	7.0	7.5	8.5	10.5	12.5	14.0	14.5	16.0
6 years	6.0	7.0	7.5	8.0	10.0	12.0	14.5	16.0	18.5
7 years	6.0	7.0	7.5	9.0	10.5	13.0	15.0	18.0	20.0
8 years	6.0	6.5	7.0	8.5	11.0	14.0	16.0	18.0	21.0
9 years	7.0	7.5	8.5	10.0	13.0	16.0	20.0	23.0	27.0
10 years	7.0	8.0	8.0	10.0	13.5	18.0	21.0	22.5	24.5
11 years	8.0	8.5	9.0	11.0	14.0	19.5	21.5	23.0	29.5
12 years	7.5	8.0	9.0	11.5	13.5	18.5	21.5	23.0	27.0
13 years	6.0	7.5	9.0	10.5	15.0	19.0	22.0	25.0	30.0
14 years	8.0	10.0	10.5	12.0	17.0	21.5	25.0	29.5	32.0
15 years	8.5	9.5	10.0	11.5	16.5	20.5	24.5	26.0	32.1
16 years	11.0	11.5	12.0	14.0	18.0	23.0	27.0	30.5	33.1
17 years	9.5	11.0	11.5	14.0	20.0	24.5	26.5	28.5	34.5
18 years	11.0	12.0	12.5	14.0	18.0	23.5	27.0	32.5	35.0
18-24 years	10.0	11.5	12.5	15.0	19.0	25.0	29.5	32.0	37.0
25-34 years	10.0	13.0	14.0	16.5	22.0	29.0	33.5	36.6	43.5
35-44 years	12.0	14.5	16.5	19.5	25.0	32.6	37.0	40.5	44.5
45-54 years	12.5	15.0	17.0	20.5	27.0	34.0	38.0	40.5	45.0
55-64 years	12.0	15.0	17.5	21.0	26.5	33.0	37.0	40.0	43.6
65-74 years	12.0	14.5	16.5	19.0	25.0	31.0	35.0	37.6	42.0

From Anthropometric Reference Data and Prevalence of Overweight, United States, 1976-80, Vital and Health Statistics Series 11, No 238, National Center for Health Statistics, 1987, U.S. Department of Health and Human Services.

Norms for Subscapular Fatfold (mm) from the Second National Health and Nutrition Examination Survey

Sex and Age	Percentile 5th	10th	15th	25th	50th	75th	85th	90th	95th
MALE									
6-11 months	4.0	5.0	5.0	5.5	6.0	7.5	8.0	8.5	9.0
1 year	4.0	4.5	5.0	5.0	6.5	7.5	8.0	9.0	10.5
2 years	3.5	4.0	4.0	5.0	5.5	7.0	7.5	9.0	10.0
3 years	4.0	4.0	4.0	4.5	5.5	6.5	7.0	7.5	9.0
4 years	3.5	3.5	4.0	4.0	5.0	6.0	7.0	7.5	9.0
5 years	3.0	3.5	4.0	4.0	5.0	6.0	6.5	7.0	8.0
6 years	3.5	3.5	4.0	4.0	5.0	6.0	8.0	10.0	16.0
7 years	3.5	4.0	4.0	4.0	5.0	6.0	7.0	7.5	11.5
8 years	3.5	4.0	4.0	4.5	5.0	6.5	8.0	11.0	21.0
9 years	3.5	4.0	4.0	4.5	6.0	7.0	10.0	12.0	15.0
10 years	4.0	4.0	4.5	5.0	6.0	9.5	11.5	17.0	22.0
11 years	4.0	4.0	4.5	5.0	6.5	10.0	17.5	25.0	31.0
12 years	4.0	4.5	4.5	5.0	6.5	10.0	15.5	19.0	22.5
13 years	4.0	4.5	5.0	5.0	7.0	9.0	13.0	15.0	24.0
14 years	4.5	5.0	5.5	6.0	7.0	9.0	12.0	13.5	20.0
15 years	5.0	5.5	6.0	6.0	7.5	10.0	12.0	16.0	24.5
16 years	5.0	6.0	6.5	6.5	9.0	12.5	14.5	21.5	25.0
17 years	5.5	6.0	6.5	7.0	8.5	11.5	14.0	17.0	20.5
18 years	6.0	7.0	7.0	8.0	10.0	14.0	16.0	18.0	24.0
18-24 years	6.5	7.0	7.5	8.5	11.5	16.0	20.0	23.0	30.0
25-34 years	7.0	8.0	9.0	10.0	15.0	22.0	25.5	29.0	34.0
35-44 years	7.0	8.5	10.0	12.0	17.0	24.0	28.0	30.5	37.0
45-54 years	7.5	9.0	10.0	12.5	18.0	25.0	29.0	31.0	36.0
55-64 years	7.5	9.0	10.0	12.5	18.0	24.0	27.0	30.0	34.5
65-74 years	7.0	8.0	9.5	11.0	16.0	23.0	27.5	30.5	35.1
FEMALE									
6-11 months	4.5	5.0	5.0	5.5	6.5	7.5	8.0	9.0	10.0
1 year	4.0	4.0	5.0	5.0	6.5	8.0	8.5	9.5	10.5
2 years	4.0	4.5	4.5	5.0	6.0	7.5	8.5	9.5	11.0
3 years	3.5	4.0	4.5	5.0	6.0	7.0	8.0	9.0	11.0
4 years	3.5	4.0	4.5	5.0	5.5	7.0	8.0	9.0	10.5
5 years	4.0	4.0	4.5	5.0	5.5	7.0	8.0	10.0	12.0
6 years	4.0	4.0	4.0	5.0	6.0	7.5	9.0	10.5	14.0
7 years	3.5	4.0	4.0	4.5	6.0	7.5	9.0	12.0	16.5
8 years	3.5	4.0	4.5	5.0	6.0	8.0	10.5	12.0	15.0
9 years	4.0	5.0	5.0	5.5	7.0	9.5	13.0	21.0	29.0
10 years	4.5	5.0	5.0	6.0	8.0	13.5	18.0	19.5	23.0
11 years	4.5	5.0	5.5	6.5	8.0	12.0	17.0	22.0	29.0
12 years	5.0	5.5	6.0	6.5	9.0	13.0	17.0	22.0	29.0
13 years	4.5	5.5	6.0	7.0	9.5	14.0	17.5	20.0	29.0
14 years	6.0	6.5	7.0	7.5	10.5	16.0	22.0	26.0	31.0
15 years	6.0	7.0	7.5	8.5	10.5	16.0	20.5	22.5	27.5
16 years	6.5	7.5	8.5	9.5	12.0	16.5	23.5	26.0	36.6
17 years	6.5	7.0	8.0	9.5	13.0	19.5	27.0	29.0	37.0
18 years	7.0	7.5	8.0	10.0	13.0	18.5	22.0	27.5	34.5
18-24 years	7.0	7.5	8.0	10.0	13.0	20.5	26.0	31.0	38.0
25-34 years	7.0	8.0	8.5	10.5	16.0	27.0	33.5	38.0	45.0
35-44 years	7.0	8.5	10.0	12.0	19.0	31.0	36.6	40.1	46.5
45-54 years	7.0	10.0	11.0	14.5	22.0	32.5	37.5	40.5	47.6
55-64 years	7.5	9.0	11.0	13.5	22.0	32.0	37.0	41.0	47.0
65-74 years	7.0	8.5	10.0	13.0	21.0	30.0	35.0	37.1	43.0

From Anthropometric Reference Data and Prevalence of Overweight, United States, 1976-80, Vital and Health Statistics Series 11, No 238, National Center for Health Statistics, 1987, U.S. Department of Health and Human Services.

Equivalent Fat Content, as Percentage of Body Weight, for a Range of Values for the Sum of Four Skinfolds*

	Men (age in years)				Women (age in years)			
Skinfolds (mm)	17-29	30-39	40-49	50+	16-29	30-39	40-49	50+
15	4.8	—	—	—	10.5	—	—	—
20	8.1	12.2	12.2	12.6	14.1	17.0	19.8	21.4
25	10.5	14.2	15.0	15.6	16.8	19.4	22.2	24.0
30	12.9	16.2	17.7	18.6	19.5	21.8	24.5	26.6
35	14.7	17.7	19.6	20.8	21.5	23.7	26.4	28.5
40	16.4	19.2	21.4	22.9	23.4	25.5	28.2	30.3
45	17.7	20.4	23.0	24.7	25.0	26.9	29.6	31.9
50	19.0	21.5	24.6	26.5	26.5	28.2	31.0	33.4
55	20.1	22.5	25.9	27.9	27.8	29.4	32.1	34.6
60	21.2	23.5	27.1	29.2	29.1	30.6	33.2	35.7
65	22.2	24.3	28.2	30.4	30.2	31.6	34.1	36.7
70	23.1	25.1	29.3	31.6	31.2	32.5	35.0	37.7
75	24.0	25.9	30.3	32.7	32.2	33.4	35.9	38.7
80	24.8	26.6	31.2	33.8	33.1	34.3	36.7	39.6
85	25.5	27.2	32.1	34.8	34.0	35.1	37.5	40.4
90	26.2	27.8	33.0	35.8	34.8	35.8	38.3	41.2
95	26.9	28.4	33.7	36.6	35.6	36.5	39.0	41.9
100	27.6	29.0	34.4	37.4	36.4	37.2	39.7	42.6
105	28.2	29.6	35.1	38.2	37.1	37.9	40.4	43.3
110	28.8	30.1	35.8	39.0	37.8	38.6	41.0	43.9
115	29.4	30.6	36.4	39.7	38.4	39.1	41.5	44.5
120	30.0	31.1	37.0	40.4	39.0	39.6	42.0	45.1
125	31.0	31.5	37.6	41.1	39.6	40.1	42.5	45.7
130	31.5	31.9	38.2	41.8	40.2	40.6	43.0	46.2
135	32.0	32.3	38.7	42.4	40.8	41.1	43.5	46.7
140	32.5	32.7	39.2	43.0	41.3	41.6	44.0	47.2
145	32.9	33.1	39.7	43.6	41.8	42.1	44.5	47.7
150	33.3	33.5	40.2	44.1	42.3	42.6	45.0	48.2
155	33.7	33.9	40.7	44.6	42.8	43.1	45.4	48.7
160	34.1	34.3	41.2	45.1	43.3	43.6	45.8	49.2
165	34.5	34.6	41.6	45.6	43.7	44.0	46.2	49.6
170	34.9	34.8	42.0	46.1	44.1	44.4	46.6	50.0
175	35.3	—	—	—	—	44.8	47.0	50.4
180	35.6	—	—	—	—	45.2	47.4	50.8
185	35.9	—	—	—	—	45.6	47.8	51.2
190	—	—	—	—	—	45.9	48.2	51.6
195	—	—	—	—	—	46.2	48.5	52.0
200	—	—	—	—	—	46.5	48.8	52.4
205	—	—	—	—	—	—	49.1	52.7
210	—	—	—	—	—	—	49.4	53.0

From Durnin JVGA and Womersley J. Br J Nutr 32:77-97, 1974.
*Biceps, triceps, subscapular, and suprailiac of men and women of different ages.

Percentiles for Upper Arm Circumference and Estimated Upper Arm Muscle Circumference of Whites in the United States Health and Nutrition Examination Survey I, 1971 to 1974*

Age Group	Arm Circumference (mm)							Arm Muscle Circumference (mm)						
	5th	10th	25th	50th	75th	90th	95th	5th	10th	25th	50th	75th	90th	95th
MALE														
1-1.9	142	146	150	159	170	176	183	110	113	119	127	135	144	147
2-2.9	141	145	153	162	170	178	185	111	114	122	130	140	146	150
3-3.9	150	153	160	167	175	184	190	117	123	131	137	143	148	153
4-4.9	149	154	162	171	180	186	192	123	126	133	141	148	156	159
5-5.9	153	160	167	175	185	195	204	128	133	140	147	154	162	169
6-6.9	155	159	167	179	188	209	228	131	135	142	151	161	170	177
7-7.9	162	167	177	187	201	223	230	137	139	151	160	168	177	190
8-8.9	162	170	177	190	202	220	245	140	145	154	162	170	182	187
9-9.9	175	178	187	200	217	249	257	151	154	161	170	183	196	202
10-10.9	181	184	196	210	231	262	274	156	160	166	180	191	209	221
11-11.9	186	190	202	223	244	261	280	159	165	173	183	195	205	230
12-12.9	193	200	214	232	254	282	303	167	171	182	196	210	223	241
13-13.9	194	211	228	247	263	286	301	172	179	196	211	226	238	245
14-14.9	220	226	237	253	283	303	322	189	199	212	223	240	260	264
15-15.9	222	229	244	264	284	311	320	199	204	218	237	254	266	272
16-16.9	244	248	262	278	303	324	343	213	225	234	249	269	287	296
17-17.9	246	253	267	285	308	336	347	224	231	245	258	273	294	312
18-18.9	245	260	276	297	321	353	379	226	237	252	264	283	298	324
19-24.9	262	272	288	308	331	355	372	238	245	257	273	289	309	321
25-34.9	271	282	300	319	342	362	375	243	250	264	279	298	314	326
35-44.9	278	287	305	326	345	363	374	247	255	269	286	302	318	327
45-54.9	267	281	301	322	342	362	376	239	249	265	281	300	315	326
55-64.9	258	273	296	317	336	355	369	236	245	260	278	295	310	320
65-74.9	248	263	285	307	325	344	355	223	235	251	268	284	298	306
FEMALE														
1-1.9	138	142	148	156	164	172	177	105	111	117	124	132	139	143
2-2.9	142	145	152	160	167	176	184	111	114	119	126	133	142	147
3-3.9	143	150	158	167	175	183	189	113	119	124	132	140	146	152
4-4.9	149	154	160	169	177	184	191	115	121	128	136	144	152	157
5-5.9	153	157	165	175	185	203	211	125	128	134	142	151	159	165
6-6.9	156	162	170	176	187	204	211	130	133	138	145	154	166	171
7-7.9	164	167	174	183	199	216	231	129	135	142	151	160	171	176
8-8.9	168	172	183	195	214	247	261	138	140	151	160	171	183	194
9-9.9	178	182	194	211	224	251	260	147	150	158	167	180	194	198
10-10.9	174	182	193	210	228	251	265	148	150	159	170	180	190	197
11-11.9	185	194	208	224	248	276	303	150	158	171	181	196	217	223
12-12.9	194	203	216	237	256	282	294	162	166	180	191	201	214	220
13-13.9	202	211	223	243	271	301	338	169	175	183	198	211	226	240
14-14.9	214	223	237	252	272	304	322	174	179	190	201	216	232	247
15-15.9	208	221	239	254	279	300	322	175	178	189	202	215	228	244
16-16.9	218	224	241	258	283	318	334	170	180	190	202	216	234	249
17-17.9	220	227	241	264	295	324	350	175	183	194	205	221	239	257
18-18.9	222	227	241	258	281	312	325	174	179	191	202	215	237	245
19-24.9	221	230	247	265	290	319	345	179	185	195	207	221	236	249
25-34.9	233	240	256	277	304	342	368	183	188	199	212	228	246	264
35-44.9	241	251	267	290	317	356	378	186	192	205	218	236	257	272
45-54.9	242	256	274	299	328	362	384	187	193	206	220	238	260	274
55-64.9	243	257	280	303	335	367	385	187	196	209	225	244	266	280
65-74.9	240	252	274	299	326	356	373	185	195	208	225	244	264	279

From Frisancho AR: New norms of upper limb fat and muscle areas for assessment of nutritional status, Am J Clin Nutr 34:2540, 1981.

*Percentiles are not yet available for the black population for upper arm circumference or arm muscle circumference.

Percentiles for Estimates of Upper Arm Fat Area and Upper Arm Muscle Area of Whites in the United States Health and Nutrition Examination Survey I, 1971 to 1974*

	Arm Muscle Area Percentiles (mm²)							Arm Fat Area Percentiles (mm²)						
Age Group	5th	20th	25th	50th	75th	90th	95th	5th	10th	25th	50th	75th	90th	95th
MALE														
1-1.9	956	1014	1133	1278	1447	1644	1720	452	486	590	741	895	1036	1176
2-2.9	973	1040	1190	1345	1557	1690	1787	434	504	578	737	871	1044	1148
3-3.9	1095	1201	1357	1484	1618	1750	1853	464	519	590	736	868	1071	1151
4-4.9	1207	1264	1408	1579	1747	1926	2008	428	494	598	722	859	989	1085
5-5.9	1298	1411	1550	1720	1884	2089	2285	446	488	582	713	914	1176	1299
6-6.9	1360	1447	1605	1815	2056	2297	2493	371	446	539	678	896	1115	1519
7-7.9	1497	1548	1808	2027	2246	2494	2886	423	473	574	758	1011	1393	1511
8-8.9	1550	1664	1895	2089	2296	2628	2788	410	460	588	725	1003	1248	1558
9-9.9	1811	1884	2067	2228	2657	3053	3257	485	527	635	859	1252	1864	2081
10-10.9	1930	2027	2182	2575	2903	3486	3882	523	543	738	982	1376	1906	2609
11-11.9	2016	2156	2382	2670	3022	3359	4226	536	595	754	1148	1710	2348	2574
12-12.9	2216	2839	2649	3022	3496	3968	4640	554	650	874	1172	1558	2536	3580
13-13.9	2863	2546	3044	3553	4081	4502	4794	475	570	812	1096	1702	2744	3322
14-14.9	2830	3147	3586	3963	4575	5368	5530	453	563	786	1082	1608	2746	3508
15-15.9	3138	3317	3788	4481	5134	5631	5900	521	595	690	931	1423	2434	3100
16-16.9	3625	4044	4852	4951	5753	6576	6980	542	593	844	1078	1746	2280	3041
17-17.9	3998	4252	4777	5286	5950	6886	7726	598	698	827	1096	1636	2407	2888
18-18.9	4070	4481	5066	5552	6374	7067	8355	560	665	860	1264	1947	3302	3928
19-24.9	4508	4777	5274	5913	6660	7606	8200	594	743	963	1406	2231	3098	3652
25-34.9	4694	4963	5541	6214	7067	7847	8436	675	831	1174	1752	2459	3246	3786
35-44.9	4844	5181	5740	6490	7265	8034	8488	703	851	1310	1792	2463	3098	3624
45-54.9	4546	4946	5589	6297	7142	7918	8458	749	922	1254	1741	2359	3245	3928
55-64.9	4422	4783	5381	6144	6919	7670	8149	658	839	1166	1645	2236	2976	3466
65-74.9	3973	4411	5031	5716	6432	7074	7453	573	753	1122	1621	2199	2876	3327
FEMALE														
1-1.9	885	973	1084	1221	1378	1535	1621	401	466	578	706	847	1022	1140
2-2.9	973	1029	1119	1269	1405	1595	1727	469	526	642	747	894	1061	1173
3-3.9	1014	1133	1227	1396	1563	1690	1846	473	529	656	822	967	1106	1158
4-4.9	1058	1171	1313	1475	1644	1832	1958	490	541	654	766	907	1109	1236
5-5.9	1238	1301	1423	1598	1825	2012	2159	470	529	647	812	991	1330	1536
6-6.9	1354	1414	1513	1683	1877	2182	2323	464	508	638	827	1009	1263	1436
7-7.9	1330	1441	1602	1815	2045	2332	2469	491	560	706	920	1135	1407	1644
8-8.9	1513	1566	1808	2034	2327	2657	2996	527	634	769	1042	1383	1872	2482
9-9.9	1723	1788	1976	2227	2571	2987	3112	642	690	933	1219	1584	2171	2524
10-10.9	1740	1784	2019	2296	2583	2873	3093	616	702	842	1141	1608	2500	3005
11-11.9	1784	1987	2316	2612	3071	3739	3953	707	802	1015	1301	1942	2730	3690
12-12.9	2092	2182	2579	2904	3225	3655	3847	782	854	1090	1511	2056	2666	3369
13-13.9	2269	2426	2657	3130	3529	4081	4568	726	838	1219	1625	2374	3272	4150
14-14.9	2418	2562	2874	3220	3704	4294	4850	981	1043	1423	1818	2403	3250	3765
15-15.9	2426	2518	2847	3248	3689	4123	4756	839	1126	1396	1886	2544	3093	4195
16-16.9	2308	2567	2865	3248	3718	4353	4946	1126	1351	1663	2006	2598	3374	4236
17-17.9	2442	2674	2996	3336	3883	4552	5251	1042	1267	1463	2104	2977	3864	5159
18-18.9	2398	2538	2917	3243	3694	4461	4767	1003	1230	1616	2104	2617	3508	3733
19-24.9	2538	2728	3026	3406	3877	4439	4940	1046	1198	1596	2166	2959	4050	4896
25-34.9	2661	2826	3148	3573	4138	4806	5541	1173	1399	1841	2548	3512	4690	5560
35-44.9	2750	2948	3359	3783	4428	5240	5877	1336	1619	2158	2898	3932	5093	5847
45-54.9	2784	2956	3378	3858	4520	5375	5964	1459	1803	2447	3244	4229	5416	6140
55-64.9	2784	3063	3477	4045	4750	5632	6247	1345	1879	2520	3369	4360	5276	6152
65-74.9	2737	3018	3444	4019	4739	5566	6214	1363	1681	2266	3063	3943	4914	5530

From Frisancho AR: New norms of upper limb fat and muscle areas for assessment of nutritional status, Am J Clin Nutr 34:2540, 1981. © Am J Clin Nutr. American Society for Clinical Nutrition.

*Percentiles are not yet available for the black population for arm fat areas.

One-Month Increments in Recumbent Length and Weight From Age 1 to 12 Months*

Age (months)	Recumbent Length (cm/month)		Weight (kg/month)	
	Boys	Girls	Boys	Girls
1-2	3.88	3.54	1.28	1.12
2-3	2.85	2.70	0.85	0.76
3-4	2.35	2.28	0.66	0.61
4-5	2.05	2.03	0.55	0.52
5-6	1.83	1.83	0.48	0.45
6-7	1.68	1.68	0.43	0.41
7-8	1.55	1.57	0.38	0.37
8-9	1.45	1.47	0.35	0.34
9-10	1.37	1.39	0.33	0.32
10-11	1.30	1.32	0.31	0.30
11-12	1.24	1.26	0.29	0.28

From Roche AF, Shumei G, and Moore MWM: Weight and recumbent length from 1 to 12 months of age: reference data for 1-mo increments, Am J Clin Nutr 49:599, 1989. © Am J Clin Nutr, American Society for Clinical Nutrition.

*Increments represent the 50th percentile from the Fels Longitudinal Study of Infants.

APPENDIX C

EXAMPLE OF A FOOD FREQUENCY QUESTIONNAIRE

PERSONAL INFORMATION, HABITS

1. When were you born? ____/____/____ (Month Day Year)
2. How old are you? ____ years
3. Sex: 1 ___ Male 2 ___ Female
4. Race or ethnic background:
   - 1 ___ White, not of Hispanic origin
   - 2 ___ Black, not of Hispanic origin
   - 3 ___ Hispanic
   - 4 ___ American Indian/Alaskan native
   - 5 ___ Asian
   - 6 ___ Pacific Islander
5. Please circle the highest grade in school you have completed:
   1 2 3 4 5 6 7 8 9 10 11 12 13 14 15 16+
6. What is your marital status? 1 ___ Single 3 ___ Widowed
   2 ___ Married 4 ___ Divorced/Separated
7. How many times have you moved or changed residences in the last 10 years? ___ times
8. Have you smoked at least 100 cigarettes in your entire life? 1 ___ No 2 ___ Yes **If Yes,** →

   IF YES: About how old were you when you first started smoking cigarettes fairly regularly? ___ years old
   On the average of the entire time you smoked, how many cigarettes did you smoke per day? ___ cigarettes per day
   Do you smoke cigarettes now? 1 ___ No 2 ___ Yes
   IF NO: How old were you when you stopped smoking? ___ years old
   IF YES: On the average, about how many cigarettes a day do you smoke now? ___ cigarettes

9. Have you ever smoked a pipe or cigars regularly? 1 ___ No 2 ___ Yes **If Yes,** →

   IF YES: For how many years? ___ years
   About how much? ___ pipes or cigars per ______________ (day or week) 1 2

10. During the past year, have you taken any vitamins or minerals?
    1 ___ No 2 ___ Yes, fairly regularly 3 ___ Yes, but not regularly **If Yes,** →

    What do you take fairly regularly? # of PILLS per DAY, WEEK, etc.

    Multiple Vitamins
    - One-a-day type _____ pills per _________
    - Stress-tabs type _____ pills per _________
    - Therapeutic, Theragran type _____ pills per _________

    Other Vitamins (How many milligrams or IUs per pill?)
    - Vitamin A _____ pills per _________ → _____ IU per pill
    - Vitamin C _____ pills per _________ → _____ mg per pill
    - Vitamin E _____ pills per _________ → _____ IU per pill
    - Calcium or dolomite _____ pills per _________ → _____ mg per pill

    Other (What?) 1 ___ Yeast 2 ___ Selenium 3 ___ Zinc 4 ___ Iron 5 ___ Beta-carotene
    6 ___ Cod liver oil 7 ___ Other ______________________

    Please list the brand of multiple vitamin/mineral you usually take: ______________________

Example of a Food Frequency Questionnaire *Continued*

11. Are you on a special diet?
 1 ___ No 2 ___ Weight loss 3 ___ For medical condition 4 ___ Vegetarian 5 ___ Low salt
 6 ___ Low cholesterol 7 ___ Weight gain
12. How often do you eat the following foods from *restaurants* or *fast food places?*

RESTAURANT FOOD	1 Almost every day	2 2-4 times a week	3 Once a week	4 1-3 times a month	5 5-10 times a year	6 1-4 times a year	7 Never, or less than once a year
Fried chicken							
Burgers							
Pizza							
Chinese food							
Mexican food							
Fried fish							
Other foods							

13. This section is about your *usual* eating habits. Thinking back over the past year, how often do you usually eat the foods listed on the next page?

 First, check (√) whether your usual serving size is small, medium, or large. (A small portion is about one half the medium serving size shown or less; a large portion is about one-and-a-half times as much or more.)

 Then, put a *NUMBER* in the most appropriate column to indicate *HOW OFTEN*, on the average, you eat the food. You may eat bananas *twice a week* (put a 2 in the "*week*" column). If you never eat the food, check "Rarely/Never." Please DO NOT SKIP foods. And please BE CAREFUL which column you put your answer in. It will make a big difference if you say "Hamburger once a day" when you mean "Hamburger once a week"!

 Some items say "in season." Indicate how often you eat these just in the 2-3 month time when that food is in season. (Be careful about overestimating here.)

 Please look at the *example* below. This person:

 1) eats a medium serving of cantaloupe once a week, in season
 2) has 1/2 grapefruit about twice a month
 3) has a small serving of sweet potatoes about 3 times a year
 4) has a large hamburger or cheeseburger or meat loaf about four times a week
 5) never eats winter squash

EXAMPLE:

	Medium Serving	Your Serving Size			How often?				
		S	M	L	Day	Week	Month	Year	Rarely/ Never
Cantaloupe (in season)	1/4 medium		√			1			
Grapefruit	(1/2)		√				2		
Sweet potatoes, yams	1/2 cup	√						3	
Hamburger, cheeseburger, meat loaf	1 medium					4			
Winter squash, baked squash	1/2 cup								√

PLEASE GO TO NEXT PAGE

Example of a Food Frequency Questionnaire *Continued*

	Medium Serving	Your Serving Size			How often?				
FRUITS & JUICES		S	M	L	Day	Week	Month	Year	Rarely/ Never
EXAMPLE—Apples, applesauce, pears	(1) or 1/2 cup		√			4			
Apples, applesauce, pears	(1) or 1/2 cup								
Bananas	1 medium								
Peaches, apricots (canned, frozen or dried, whole year)	(1) or 1/2 cup								
Peaches, apricots, nectarines (fresh, in season)	1 medium								
Cantaloupe (in season)	1/4 medium								
Watermelon (in season)	1 slice								
Strawberries (fresh, in season)	1/2 cup								
Oranges	1 medium								
Orange juice or grapefruit juice	6 oz. glass								
Grapefruit	(1/2)								
Tang, Start breakfast drinks	6 oz. glass								
Other fruit juices, fortified fruit drinks	6 oz. glass								
Any other fruit, including berries, fruit cocktail	1/2 cup								
VEGETABLES		S	M	L	Da	Wk	Mo	Yr	Nv
String beans, green beans	1/2 cup								
Peas	1/2 cup								
Chili with beans	3/4 cup								
Other beans such as baked beans, pintos, kidney beans, limas	3/4 cup								
Corn	1/2 cup								
Winter squash, baked squash	1/2 cup								
Tomatoes, tomato juice	(1) or 6 oz.								
Red chili sauce, taco sauce, salsa picante	2 Tblsp. sauce								
Broccoli	1/2 cup								
Cauliflower or brussel sprouts	1/2 cup								
Spinach (raw)	3/4 cup								
Spinach (cooked)	1/2 cup								
Mustard greens, turnip greens, collards	1/2 cup								
Cole slaw, cabbage, sauerkraut	1/2 cup								
Carrots or mixed vegetables containing carrots	1/2 cup								
Green salad	1 med. bowl								
Salad dressing, mayonnaise (including on sandwiches)	2 Tblsp.								
French fries and fried potatoes	3/4 cup								
Sweet potatoes, yams	1/2 cup								
Other potatoes, including boiled, baked, potato salad	(1) or 1/2 cup								
Rice	3/4 cup								
Any other vegetable, including cooked onions, summer squash	1/2 cup								
Butter, margarine, or other fat on vegetables, potatoes, etc.	2 pats								
MEAT, FISH, POULTRY & MIXED DISHES		S	M	L	Da	Wk	Mo	Yr	Nv
Hamburgers, cheeseburgers, meat loaf	1 medium								
Beef—steaks, roasts	4 oz.								
Beef stew or pot pie with carrots, other vegetables	1 cup								
Liver, including chicken livers	4 oz.								
Pork, including chops, roasts	2 chops or 4 oz.								
Fried chicken	2 sm. or 1 lg. piece								
Chicken or turkey, roasted, stewed, or broiled	2 sm. or 1 lg. piece								
Fried fish or fish sandwich	4 oz. or 1 sand.								
Tuna fish, tuna salad, tuna casserole	1/2 cup								
Shell fish (shrimp, lobster, crab, oysters, etc.)	(5) 1/4 cup or 3 oz.								
Other fish, broiled, baked	4 oz.								
Spaghetti, lasagna, other pasta with tomato sauce	1 cup								
Pizza	2 slices								
Mixed dishes with cheese (such as macaroni and cheese)	1 cup								

Example of a Food Frequency Questionnaire *Continued*

	Medium Serving	Your Serving Size			How often?				
					Day	Week	Month	Year	Rarely/ Never
LUNCH ITEMS		S	M	L					
Liverwurst	2 slices								
Hot dogs	2 dogs								
Ham, lunch meats	2 slices								
Vegetable soup, vegetable beef, minestrone, tomato soup	1 med. bowl								
Other soups	1 med. bowl								
BREADS/SALTY SNACKS/SPREADS		S	M	L	Da	Wk	Mo	Yr	Nv
Biscuits, muffins, burger rolls (incl. fast foods)	1 med. piece								
White bread (including sandwiches), bagels, etc., crackers	2 slices, 3 cracks								
Dark bread, including whole wheat, rye, pumpernickel	2 slices								
Corn bread, corn muffins, corn tortillas	1 med. piece								
Salty snacks (such as chips, popcorn)	2 handfuls								
Peanuts, peanut butter	2 Tblsp.								
Butter on bread or rolls	2 pats								
Margarine on bread or rolls	2 pats								
Gravies made with meat drippings, or white sauce	2 Tblsp.								
BREAKFAST FOODS		S	M	L	Da	Wk	Mo	Yr	Nv
High fiber, bran or granola cereals, shredded wheat	1 med. bowl								
Highly fortified cereals, such as Product 19, Total, or Most	1 med. bowl								
Other cold cereals, such as Corn Flakes, Rice Krispies	1 med. bowl								
Cooked cereals	1 med. bowl								
Sugar added to cereal	2 teaspn.								
Eggs	1 egg=small, 2 eggs=medium								
Bacon	2 slices								
Sausage	2 patties or links								
SWEETS		S	M	L	Da	Wk	Mo	Yr	Nv
Ice cream	1 scoop								
Doughnuts, cookies, cakes, pastry	1 pc. or 3 cookies								
Pumpkin pie, sweet potato pie	1 med. slice								
Other pies	1 med. slice								
Chocolate candy	small bar, 1 oz.								
Other candy, jelly, honey, brown sugar	3 pc. or 1 Tblsp.								
DAIRY PRODUCTS		S	M	L	Da	Wk	Mo	Yr	Nv
Cottage cheese	1/2 cup								
Other cheeses and cheese spreads	2 slices or 2 oz.								
Flavored yogurt	1 cup								
Whole milk and bevs. with whole milk (not incl. on cereal)	8 oz. glass								
2% milk and bevs. with 2% milk (not incl. on cereal)	8 oz. glass								
Skim milk, 1% milk or buttermilk (not incl. on cereal)	8 oz. glass								
BEVERAGES		S	M	L	Da	Wk	Mo	Yr	Nv
Regular soft drinks	12 oz. can or bottle								
Diet soft drinks	12 oz. can or bottle								
Beer	12 oz. can or bottle								
Wine	1 med. glass								
Liquor	1 shot								
Decaffeinated coffee	1 med. cup								
Coffee, not decaffeinated	1 med. cup								
Tea (hot or iced)	1 med. cup								
Lemon in tea	1 teaspn.								
Nondairy creamer in coffee or tea	1 Tblsp.								
Milk in coffee or tea	1 Tblsp.								
Cream (real) or half-and-half in coffee or tea	1 Tblsp.								
Sugar in coffee or tea	2 teaspn.								
Artificial sweetener in coffee or tea	1 packet								
Glasses of water, not counting in coffee or tea	8 oz. glass								

From National Cancer Institute, Division of Cancer Prevention and Control, National Institutes of Health

APPENDIX D

NUTRIENT CONTENT OF BREAST MILK AND SELECTED COMMERCIAL INFANT FORMULAS

	Nutrient Source								
	Breast Milk	Similac	Enfamil	Good Start	Prosobee	Isomil	Nutramigen	Alimenum	Progestimil
PROTEIN	lactalbumin, casein	casein, whey protein	reduced minerals, whey	reduced mineral whey	soy protein isolate	soy protein isolate	casein hydrolosate, added amino acids	casein hydrolysate, L-cysteine, L-tyrosine, L-tryptophan	protein hydrolysate, L-cysteine, L-tyrosine, L-tryptophan
FAT	human fat	soy, safflower, coconut, corn oil	palm, soy coconut, palm, safflower oil	palm, soy, coconut, safflower oil	palm, soy, coconut, sunflower oil	safflower, soy, coconut oil	corn oil	safflower, MCT, soy oils	MCT oil, corn, soy, high-oleic safflower oil
CARBOHYDRATE	lactose	lactose	lactose	lactose, corn, maltodextrin	corn syrup solids	corn syrup, sucrose	corn syrup, modified cornstarch	sucrose, modified tapioca	sucrose, modified tapioca starch

	Nutrients per 100 kcal (5 oz)								
	Breast Milk	Similac	Enfamil	Good Start	Prosobee	Isomil	Nutramigen	Alimenum	Progestimil
PROTEIN (G)	1.5	2.07	2.1	2.25	2.9	2.45	2.75	2.75	2.76
FAT (G)	6	5.49	5.3	5.1	5.2	5.46	5.55	5.54	5.55
LINOLEIC ACID (G)	0.55	1	0.86	.85	0.8	1.0	1.3	1.9	1.0
CARBOHYDRATE (G)	9.3	10.56	10.9	11.15	8.8	10.3	11	10.1	10.9
VITAMIN A (IU)	331	300	300	300	300	300	300	300	380
VITAMIN D (IU)	3	60	60	60	60	60	60	45	75
VITAMIN E (IU)	0.6	1.5	2	2	2	1.5	2	3	3.8
VITAMIN K (μG)	0.3	8	8	8.2	8	9	3	15	18.8
VITAMIN C (MG)	6	9	12	8	12	60	8	9	11.7
THIAMIN (μG)	31	100	80	60	80	60	80	60	78
RIBOFLAVIN (μG)	51	150	140	135	90	90	80	90	94
NIACIN (μG)	221	1050	1000	750	100	1350	1000	1350	1250
VITAMIN B_6 (μG)	30	60	60	75	60	60	60	60	63
VITAMIN B_{12} (μG)	0.07	0.25	0.3	0.22	0.3	0.45	0.3	0.45	0.31
FOLIC ACID (μG)	7	15	16	15	16	15	16	15	15.6
PANTOTHENIC ACID (μG)	265	450	500	450	500	750	60	750	470
BIOTIN (μG)	0.6	4.4	3	2.2	3	4.5	3	4.5	7.8
CHOLINE (μG)	14	16	12	12	12	8	12	8	13.3
CALCIUM (MG)	45	78	78	64	105	105	94	105	94
PHOSPHORUS (MG)	38	42	53	36	83	75	63	75	63
MAGNESIUM (MG)	5.1	6	8	6.7	11	7.5	11	7.5	10.9
IRON (MG)	0.04	1.8	1.8	1.5	1.8	1.8	1.8	1.8	1.88
ZINC (MG)	0.18	0.75	1	0.75	1.2	0.75	1	0.75	0.94
COPPER (MG)	37	90	75	80	75	75	15	75	94
IODINE (μG)	16	6	10	8	15	15	15	16	7
SODIUM	26	21.6	24.4	25	36	44	40	44	38
POTASSIUM	78	94	97	110	120	108	113	118	111
CHLORIDE	62	61	60	80	80	62	59	62	60

APPENDIX E

GROWTH CHARTS: UNITED STATES, CENTERS FOR DISEASE CONTROL AND PREVENTION (CDC)

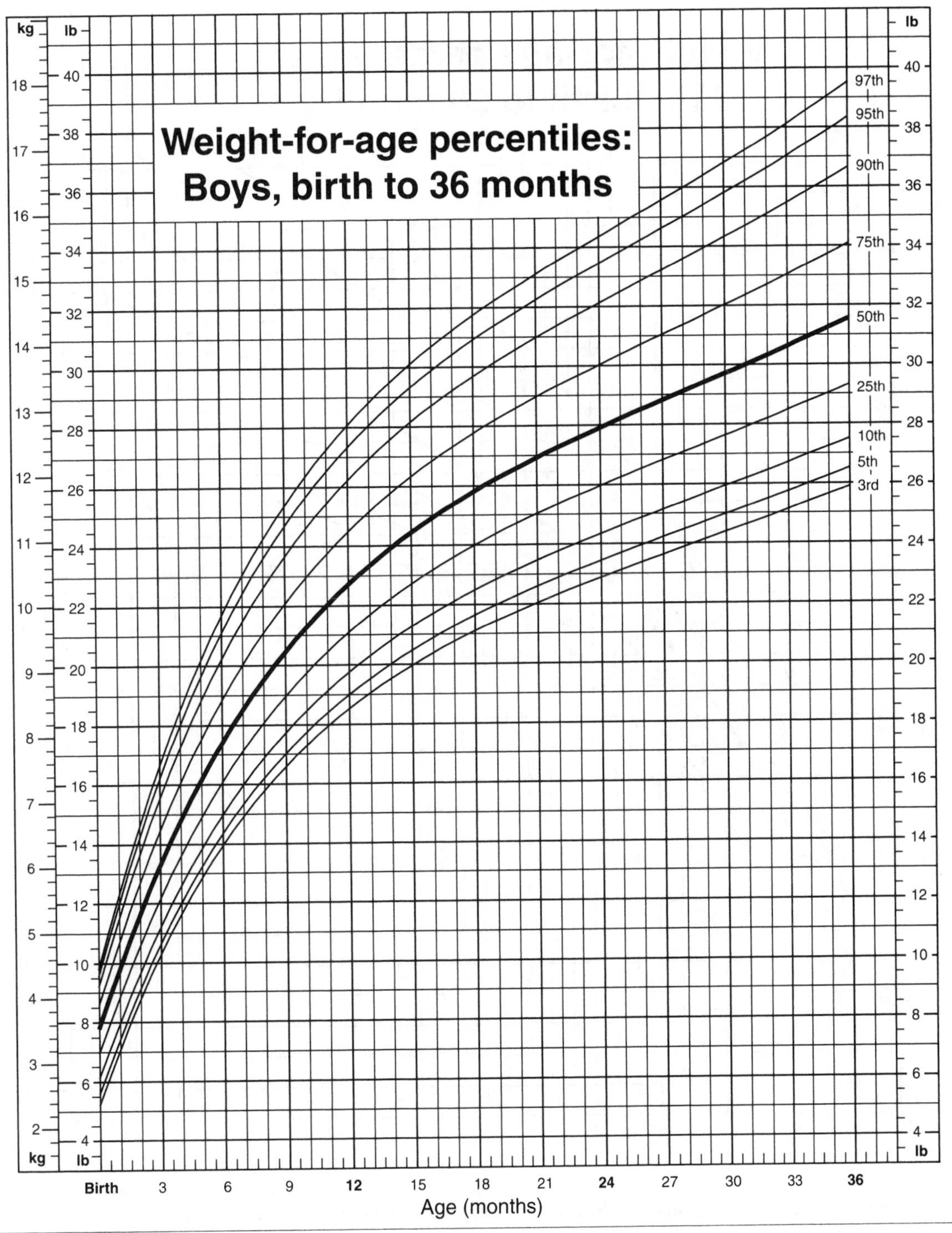

Weight-for-age percentiles, boys, birth to 36 months, CDC growth charts: United States. *(Source: Developed by the National Center for Health Statistics in collaboration with the National Center for Chronic Disease Prevention and Health Promotion (2000). From Kuczmarski RJ, Ogden CL, and Gummer-Strawn LM et al.: CDC growth charts: United States. Advanced data from vital and health statistics, no. 314, Hyattsville, Maryland, 2000, National Center for Health Statistics.)*

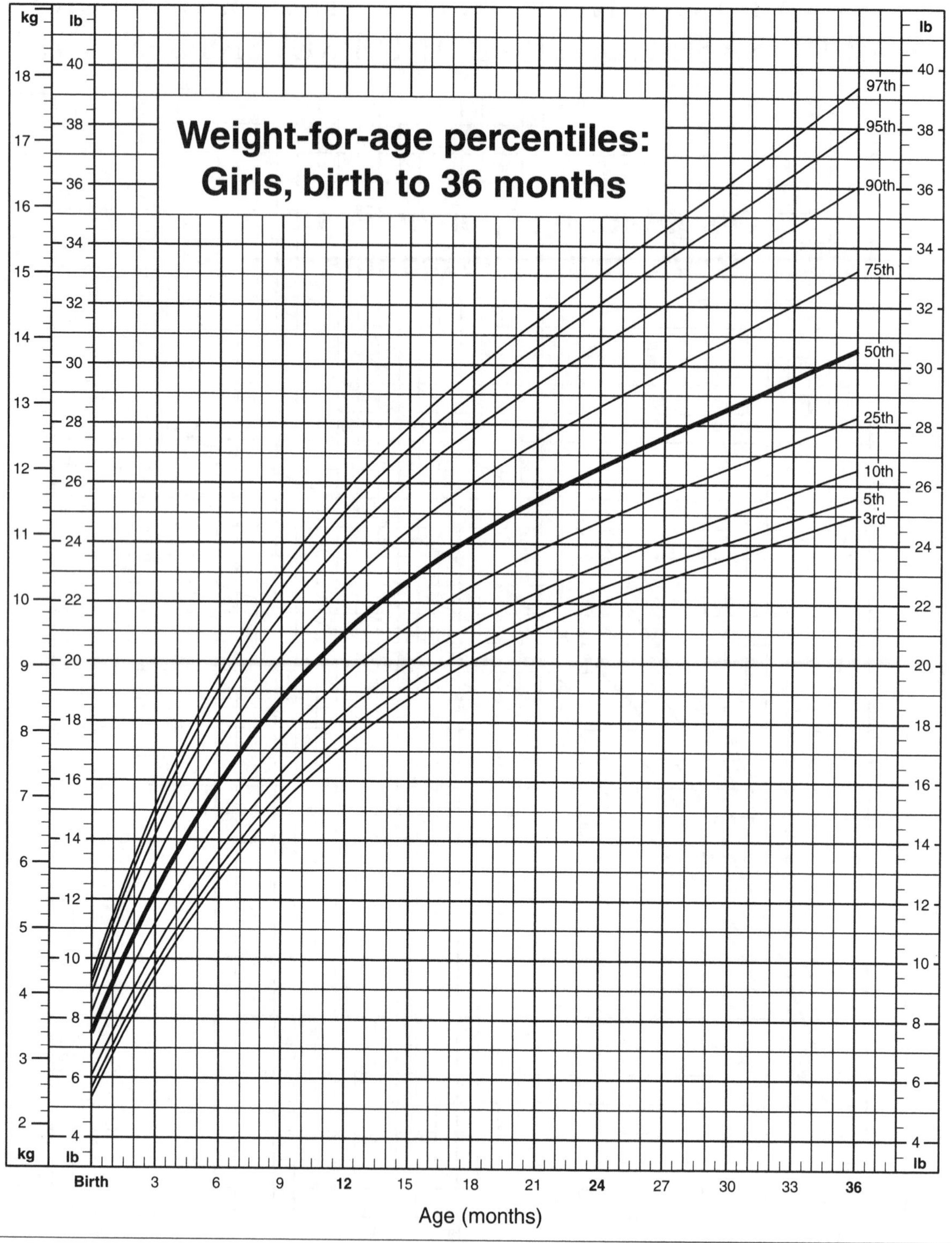

Weight-for-age percentiles, girls, birth to 36 months, CDC growth charts: United States. *(Source: Developed by the National Center for Health Statistics in collaboration with the National Center for Chronic Disease Prevention and Health Promotion (2000). From Kuczmarski RJ, Ogden CL, and Gummer-Strawn LM et al.: CDC growth charts: United States. Advanced data from vital and health statistics, no. 314, Hyattsville, Maryland, 2000, National Center for Health Statistics.)*

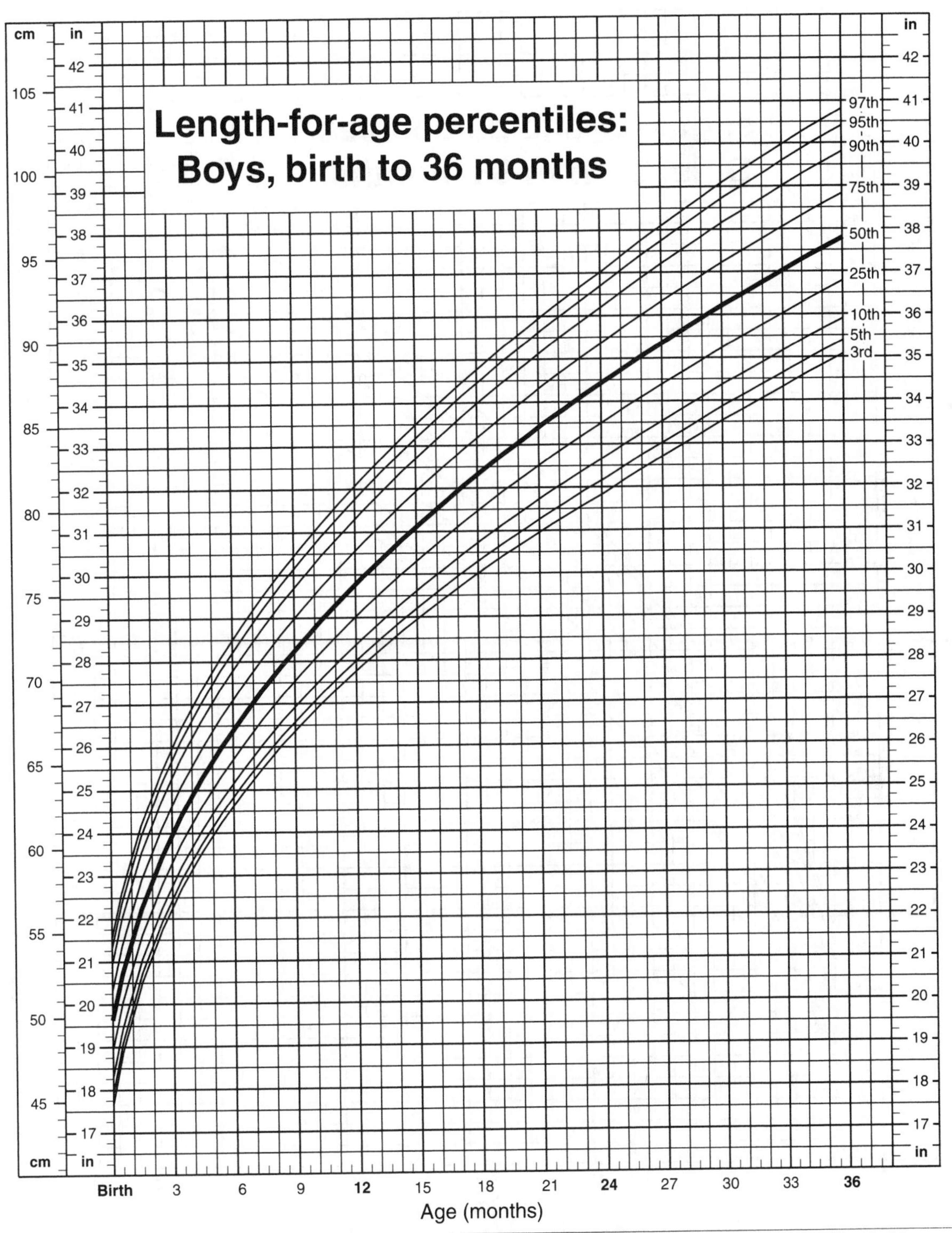

Length-for-age percentiles, boys, birth to 36 months, CDC growth charts: United States. *(Source: Developed by the National Center for Health Statistics in collaboration with the National Center for Chronic Disease Prevention and Health Promotion (2000). From Kuczmarski RJ, Ogden CL, and Gummer-Strawn LM et al.: CDC growth charts: United States. Advanced data from vital and health statistics, no. 314, Hyattsville, Maryland, 2000, National Center for Health Statistics.)*

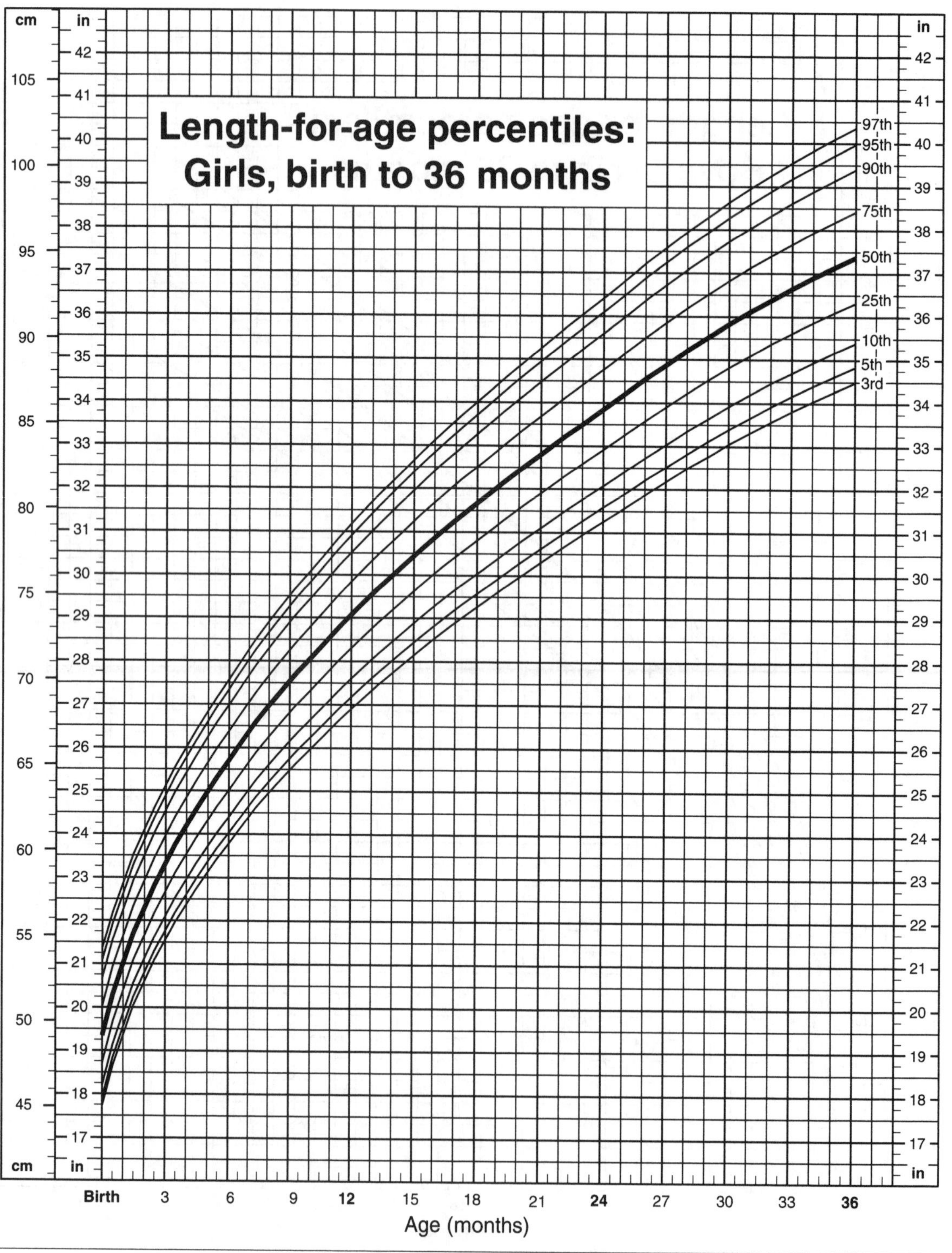

Length-for-age percentiles, girls, birth to 36 months, CDC growth charts: United States. *(Source: Developed by the National Center for Health Statistics in collaboration with the National Center for Chronic Disease Prevention and Health Promotion (2000). From Kuczmarski RJ, Ogden CL, and Gummer-Strawn LM et al.: CDC growth charts: United States. Advanced data from vital and health statistics, no. 314, Hyattsville, Maryland, 2000, National Center for Health Statistics.)*

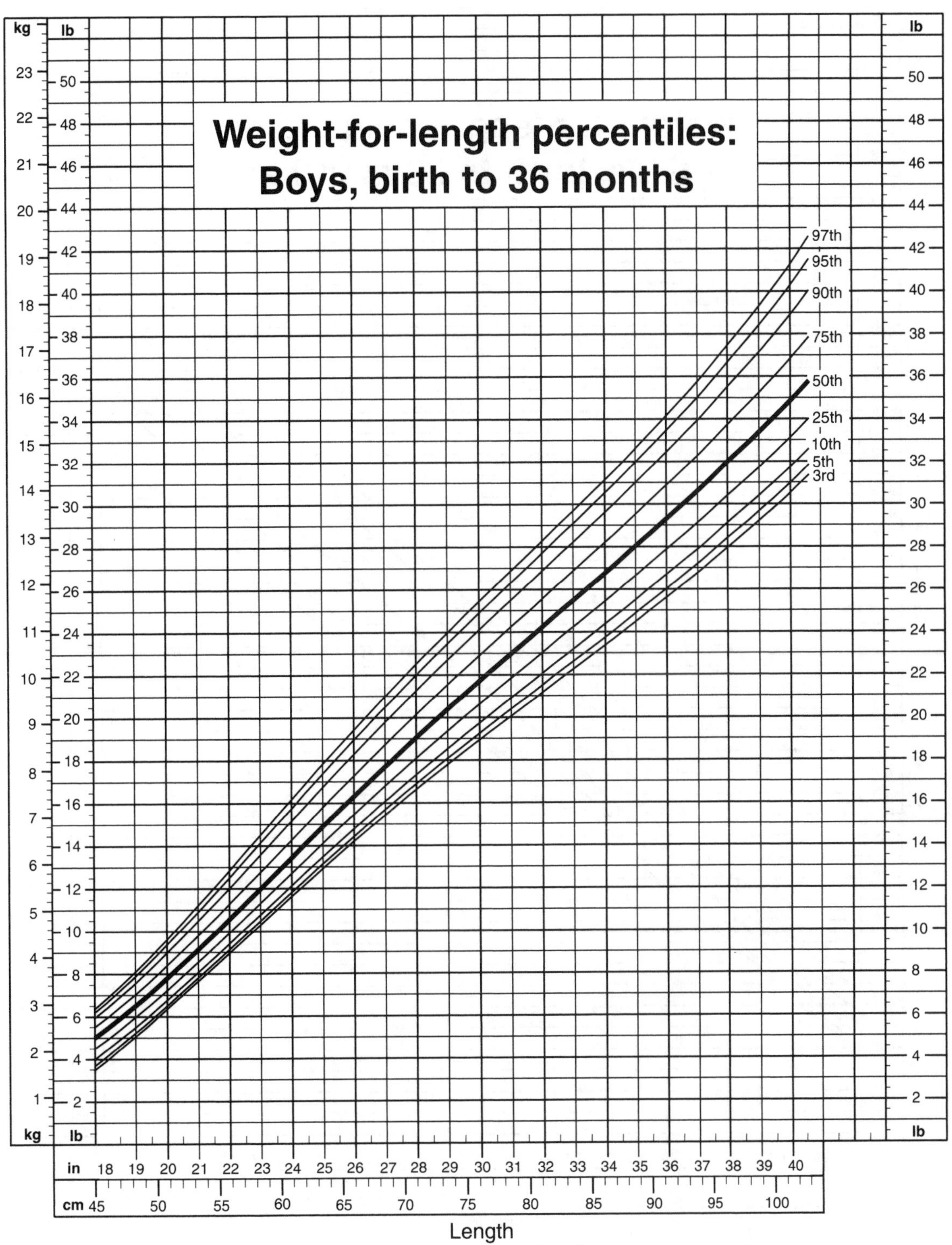

Weight-for-length percentiles, boys, birth to 36 months, CDC growth charts: United States. *(Source: Developed by the National Center for Health Statistics in collaboration with the National Center for Chronic Disease Prevention and Health Promotion (2000). From Kuczmarski RJ, Ogden CL, and Gummer-Strawn LM et al.: CDC growth charts: United States. Advanced data from vital and health statistics, no. 314, Hyattsville, Maryland, 2000, National Center for Health Statistics.)*

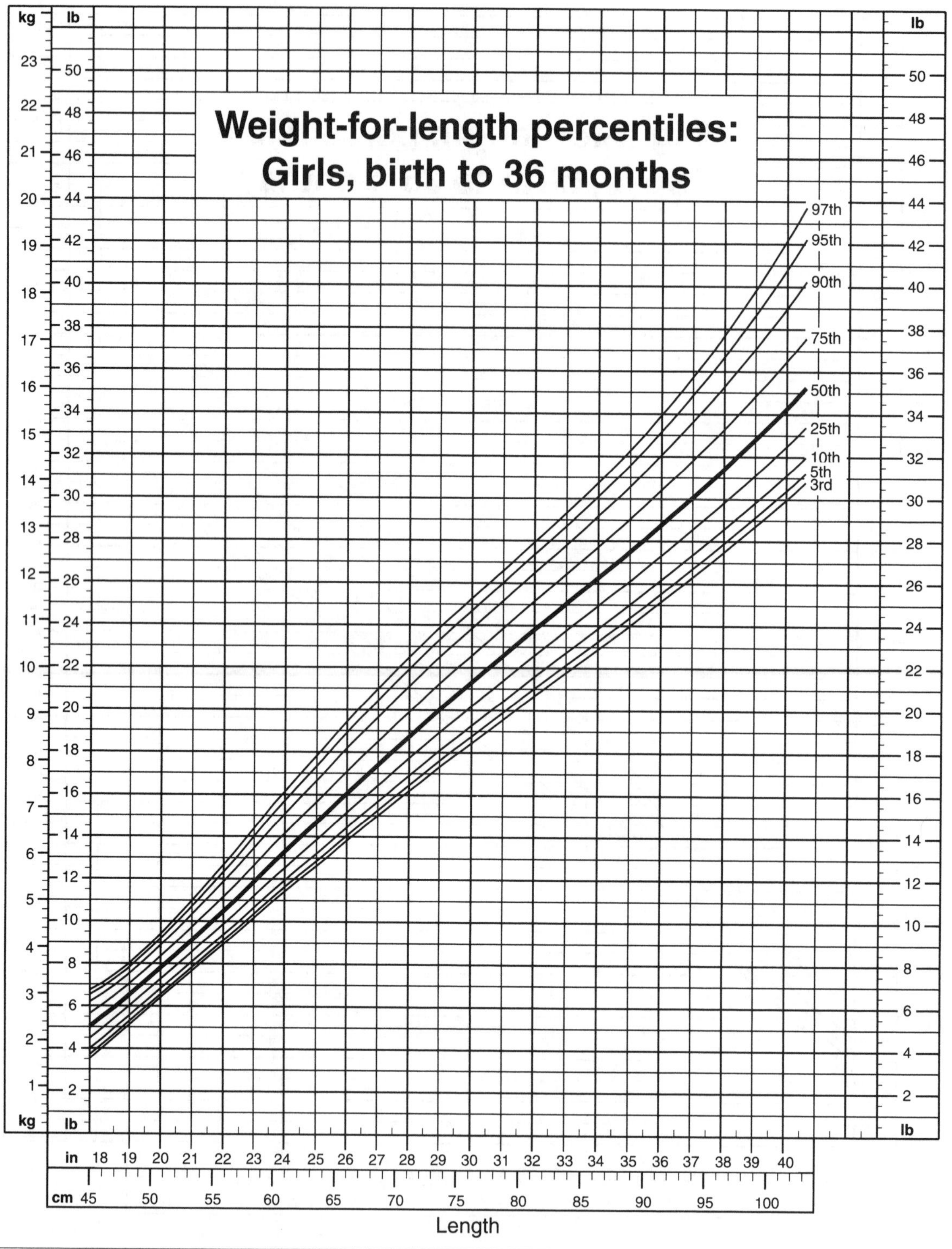

Weight-for-length percentiles, girls, birth to 36 months, CDC growth charts: United States. *(Source: Developed by the National Center for Health Statistics in collaboration with the National Center for Chronic Disease Prevention and Health Promotion (2000). From Kuczmarski RJ, Ogden CL, and Gummer-Strawn LM et al.: CDC growth charts: United States. Advanced data from vital and health statistics, no. 314, Hyattsville, Maryland, 2000, National Center for Health Statistics.)*

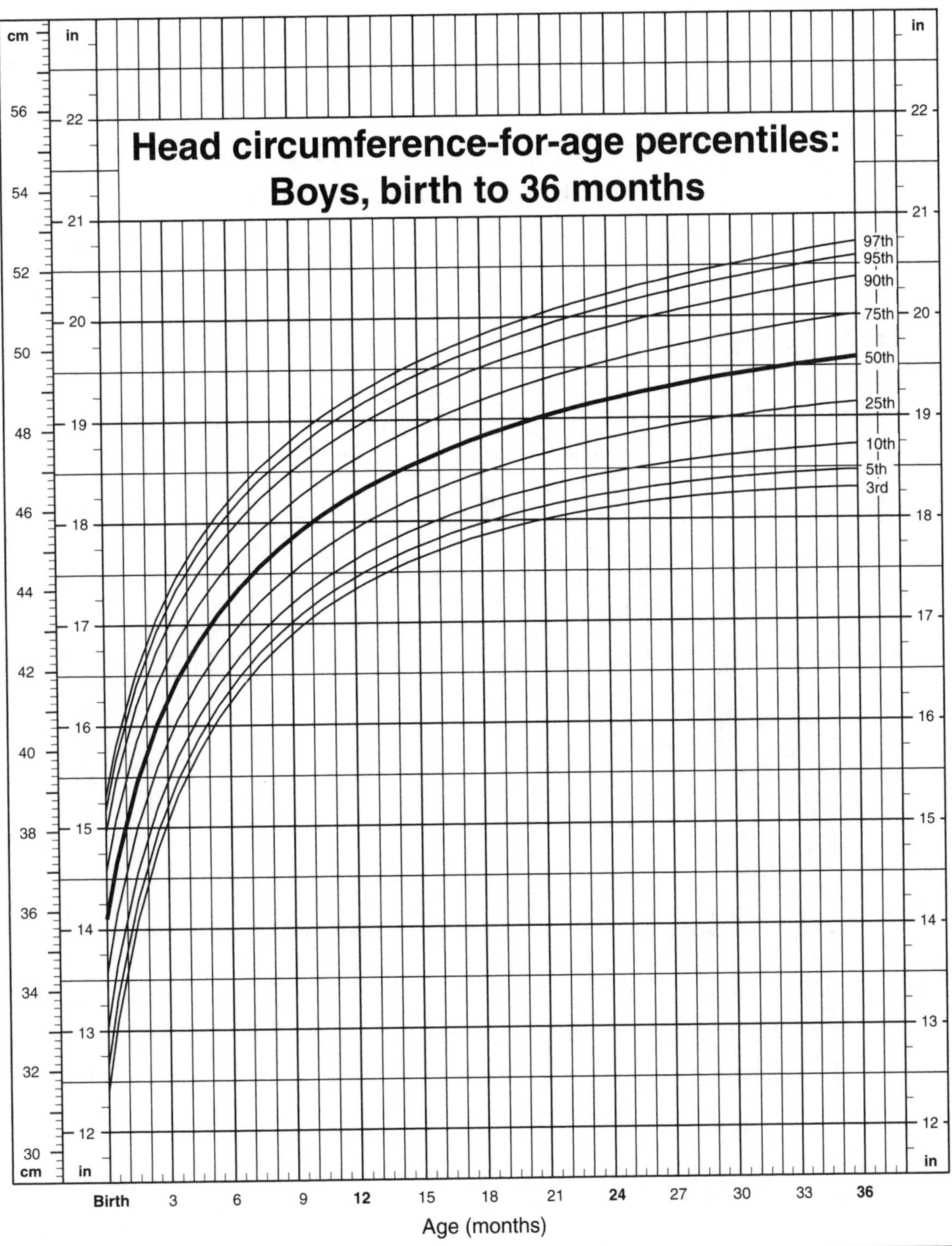

Head circumference-for-age percentiles, boys, birth to 36 months, CDC growth charts: United States. *(Source: Developed by the National Center for Health Statistics in collaboration with the National Center for Chronic Disease Prevention and Health Promotion (2000). From Kuczmarski RJ, Ogden CL, and Gummer-Strawn LM et al.: CDC growth charts: United States. Advanced data from vital and health statistics, no. 314, Hyattsville, Maryland, 2000, National Center for Health Statistics.)*

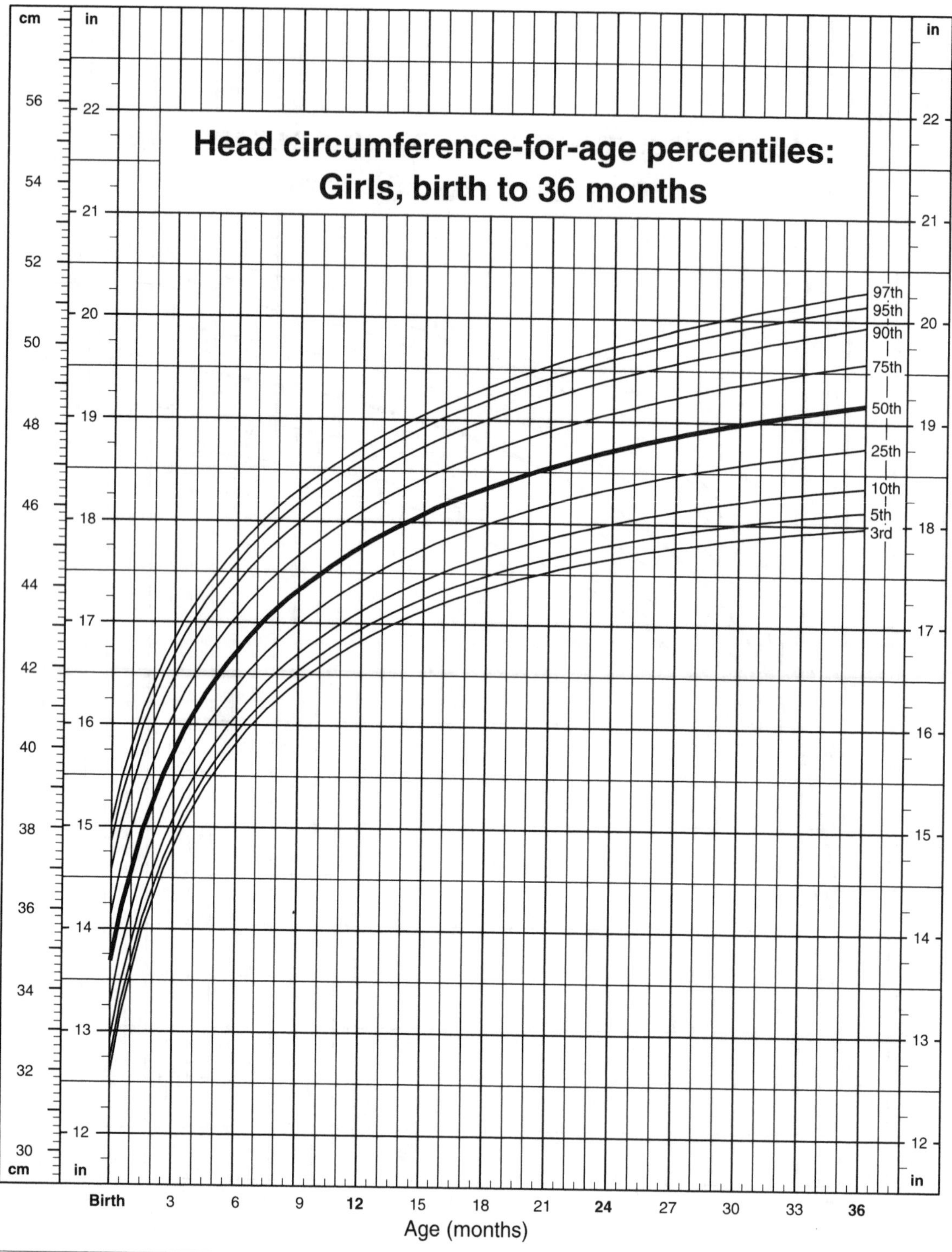

Head circumference-for-age percentiles, girls, birth to 36 months, CDC growth charts: United States. *(Source: Developed by the National Center for Health Statistics in collaboration with the National Center for Chronic Disease Prevention and Health Promotion (2000). From Kuczmarski RJ, Ogden CL, and Gummer-Strawn LM et al.: CDC growth charts: United States. Advanced data from vital and health statistics, no. 314, Hyattsville, Maryland, 2000, National Center for Health Statistics.)*

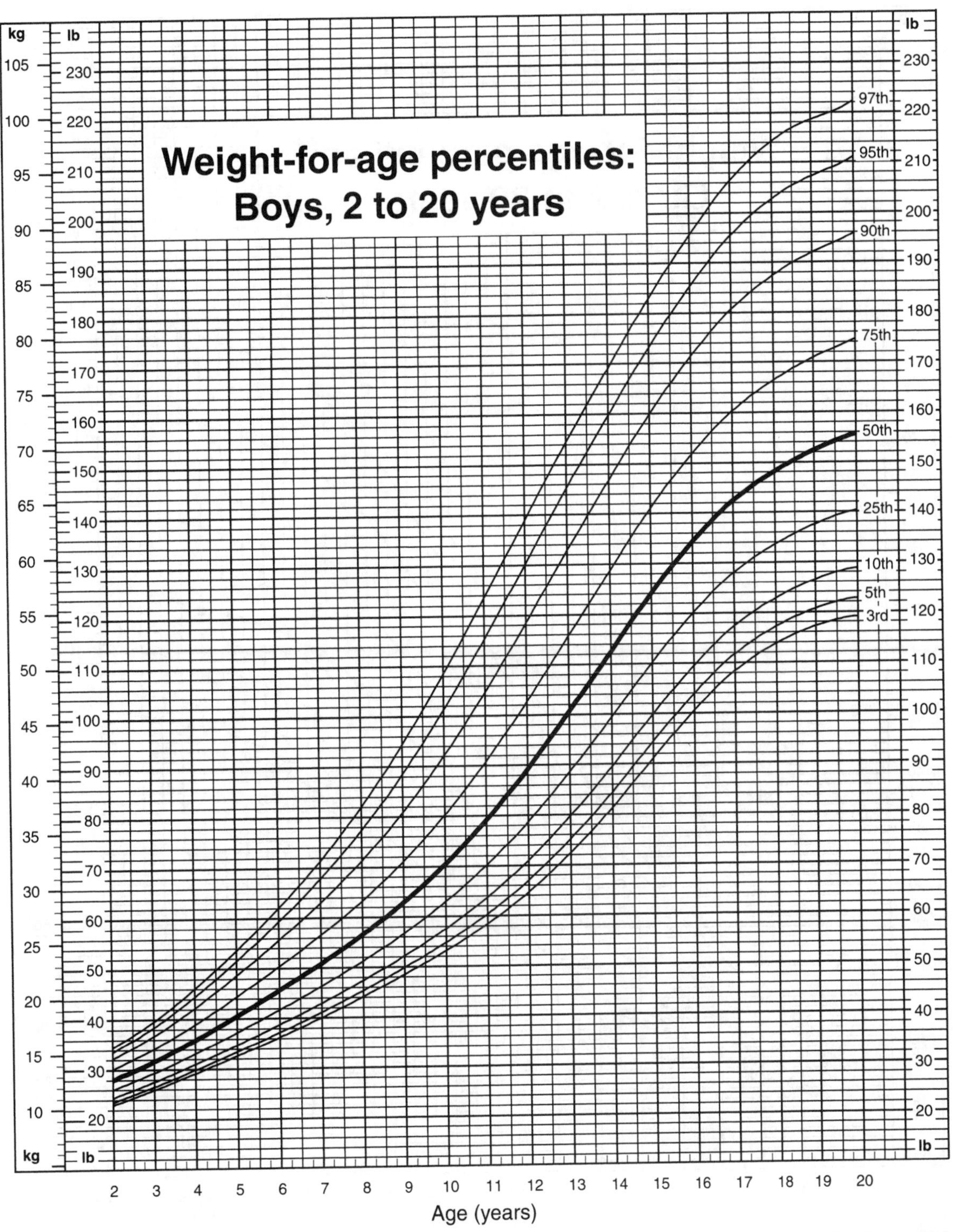

Weight-for-age percentiles, boys, 2 to 20 years, CDC growth charts: United States. *(Source: Developed by the National Center for Health Statistics in collaboration with the National Center for Chronic Disease Prevention and Health Promotion (2000). From Kuczmarski RJ, Ogden CL, and Gummer-Strawn LM et al.: CDC growth charts: United States. Advanced data from vital and health statistics, no. 314, Hyattsville, Maryland, 2000, National Center for Health Statistics.)*

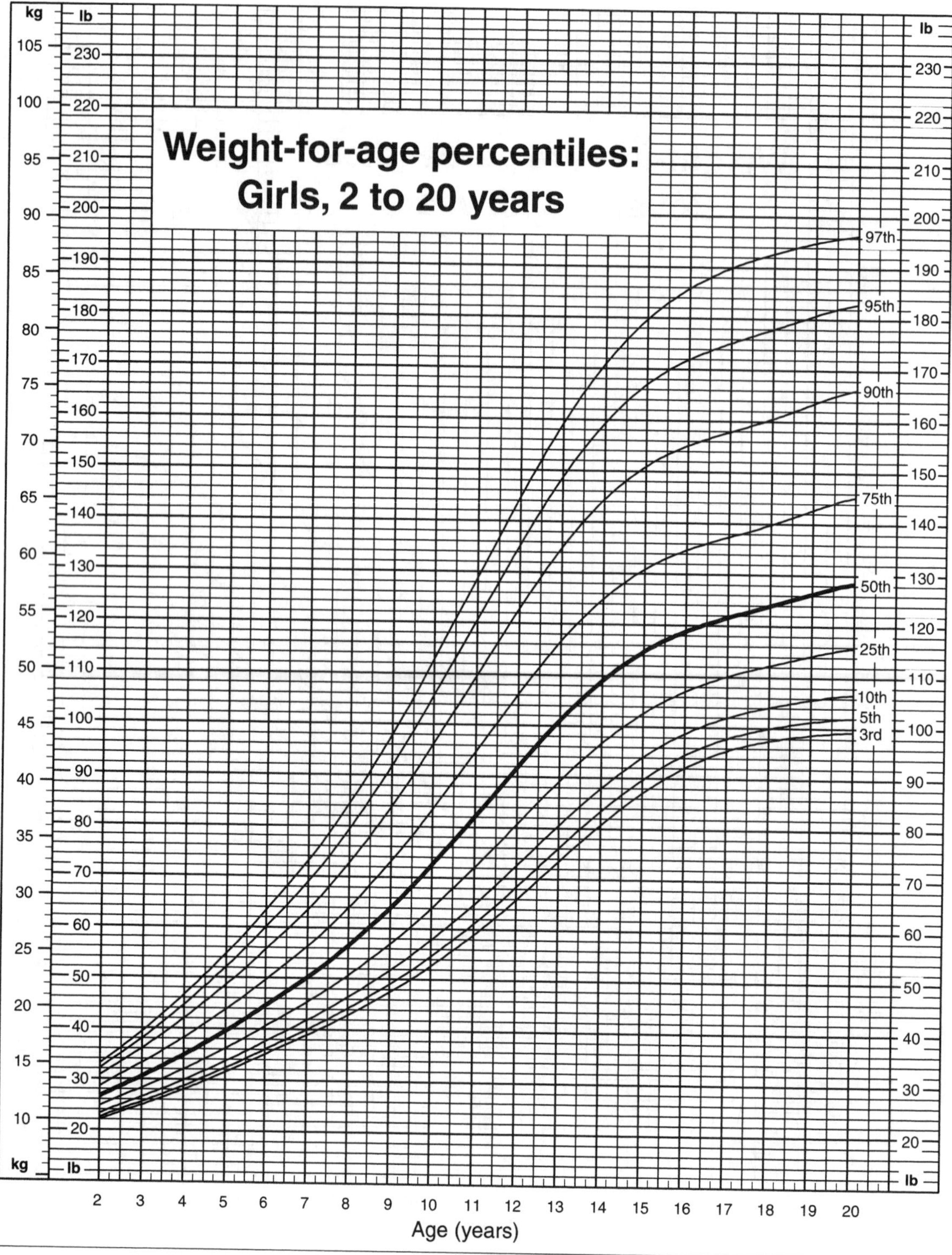

Weight-for-age percentiles, girls, 2 to 20 years, CDC growth charts: United States. *(Source: Developed by the National Center for Health Statistics in collaboration with the National Center for Chronic Disease Prevention and Health Promotion (2000). From Kuczmarski RJ, Ogden CL, and Gummer-Strawn LM et al.: CDC growth charts: United States. Advanced data from vital and health statistics, no. 314, Hyattsville, Maryland, 2000, National Center for Health Statistics.)*

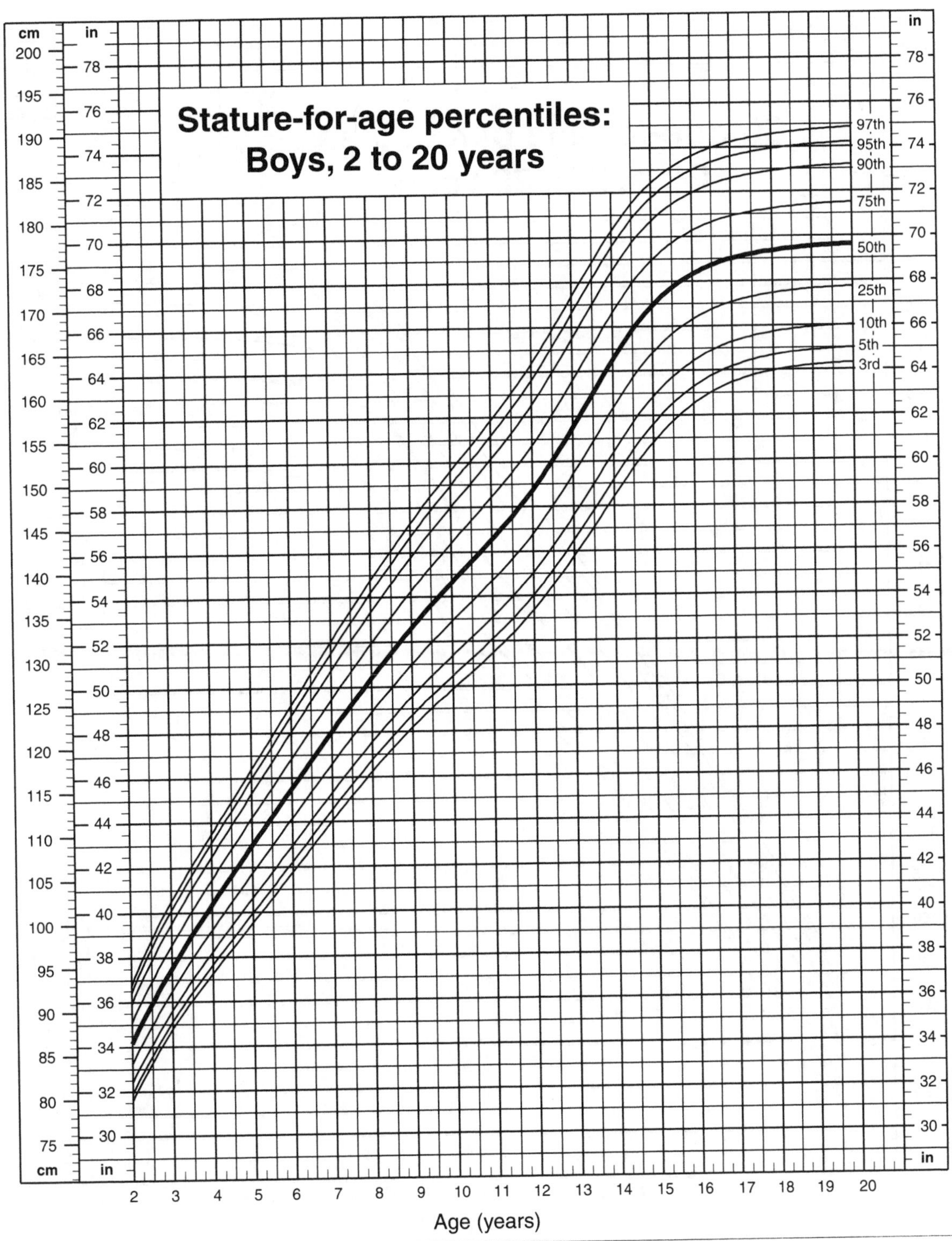

Stature-for-age percentiles, boys, 2 to 20 years, CDC growth charts: United States. *(Source: Developed by the National Center for Health Statistics in collaboration with the National Center for Chronic Disease Prevention and Health Promotion (2000). From Kuczmarski RJ, Ogden CL, and Gummer-Strawn LM et al.: CDC growth charts: United States. Advanced data from vital and health statistics, no. 314, Hyattsville, Maryland, 2000, National Center for Health Statistics.)*

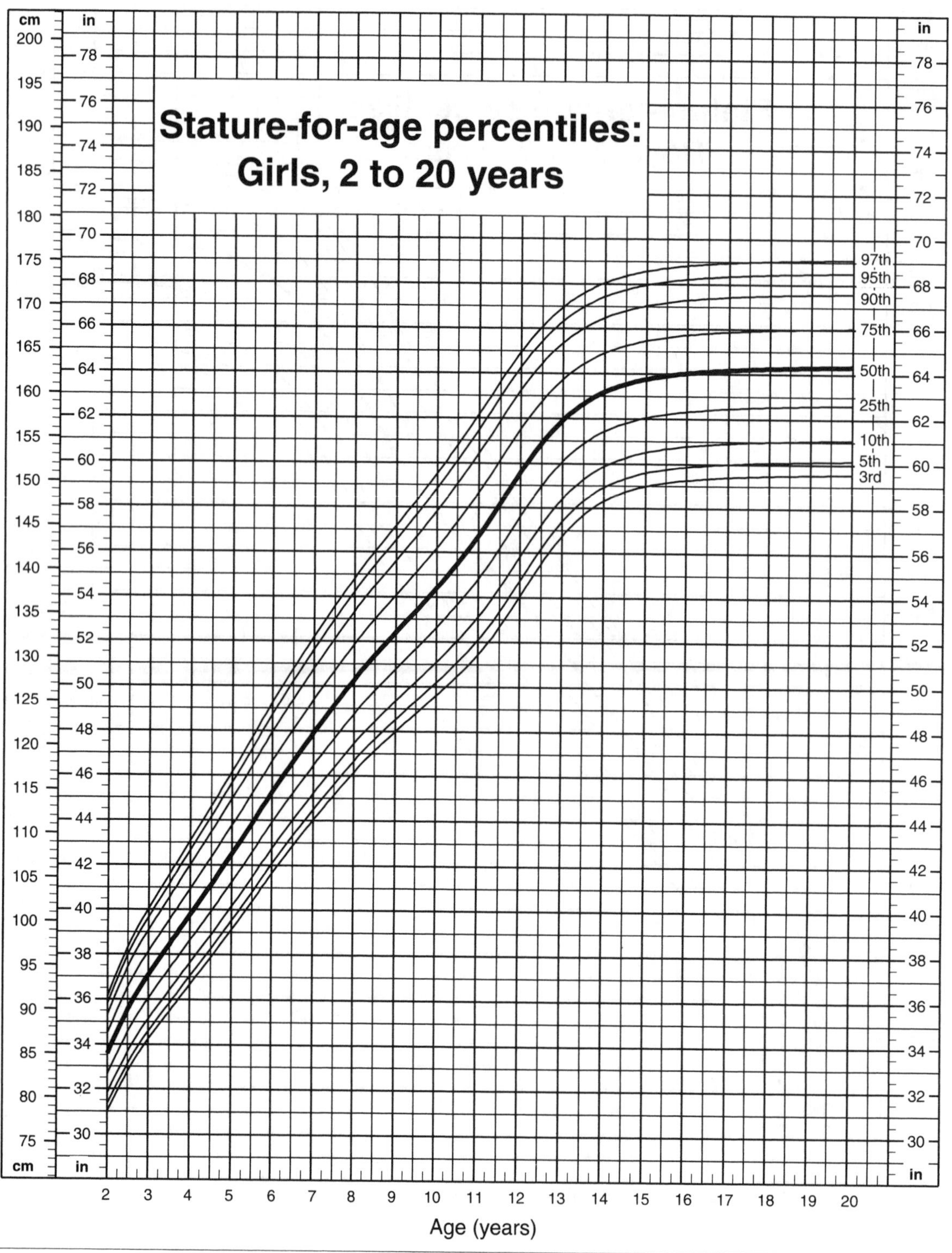

Stature-for-age percentiles, girls, 2 to 20 years, CDC growth charts: United States. *(Source: Developed by the National Center for Health Statistics in collaboration with the National Center for Chronic Disease Prevention and Health Promotion (2000). From Kuczmarski RJ, Ogden CL, and Gummer-Strawn LM et al.: CDC growth charts: United States. Advanced data from vital and health statistics, no. 314, Hyattsville, Maryland, 2000, National Center for Health Statistics.)*

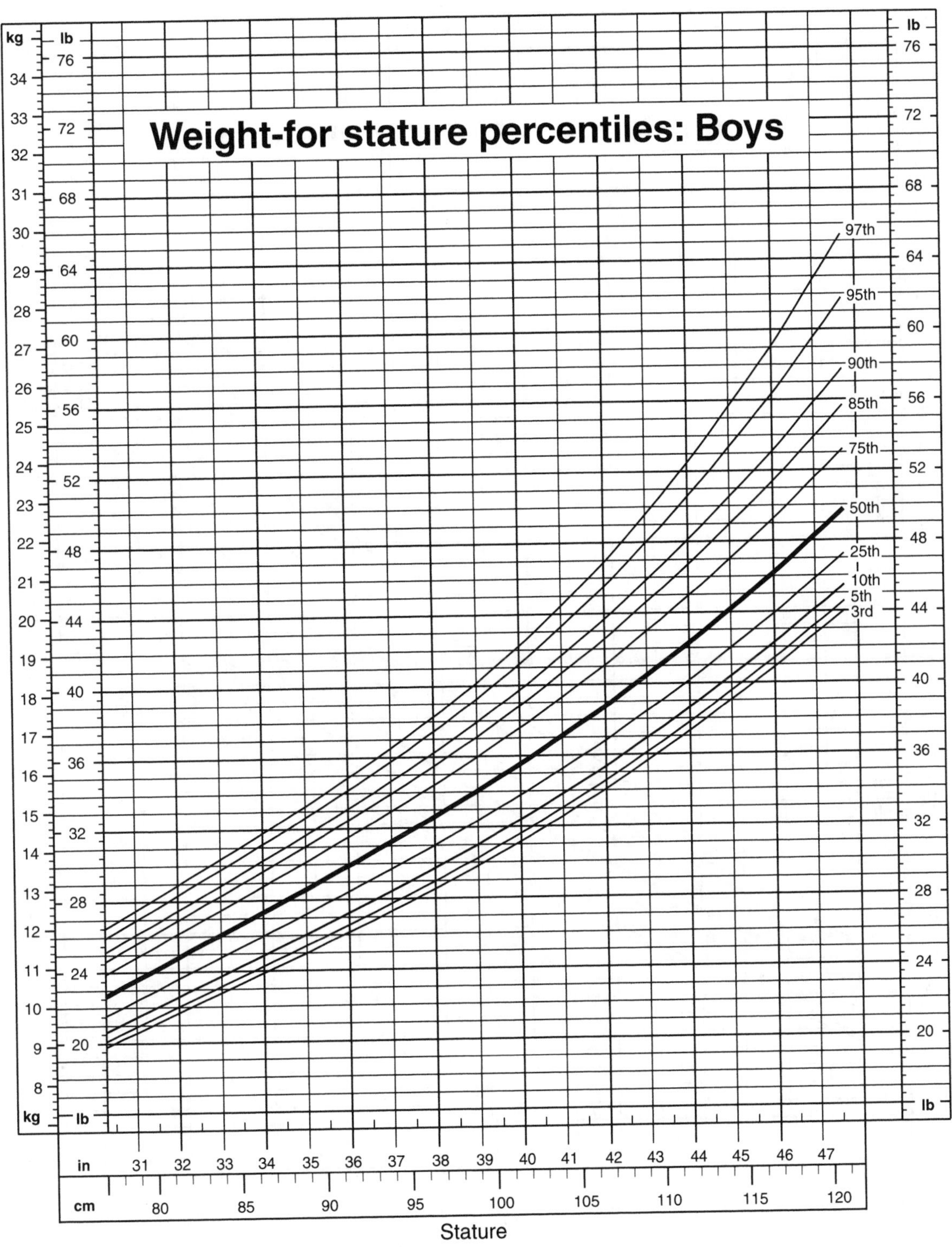

Weight-for-stature percentiles, boys, CDC growth charts: United States. *(Source: Developed by the National Center for Health Statistics in collaboration with the National Center for Chronic Disease Prevention and Health Promotion (2000). From Kuczmarski RJ, Ogden CL, and Gummer-Strawn LM et al.: CDC growth charts: United States. Advanced data from vital and health statistics, no. 314, Hyattsville, Maryland, 2000, National Center for Health Statistics.)*

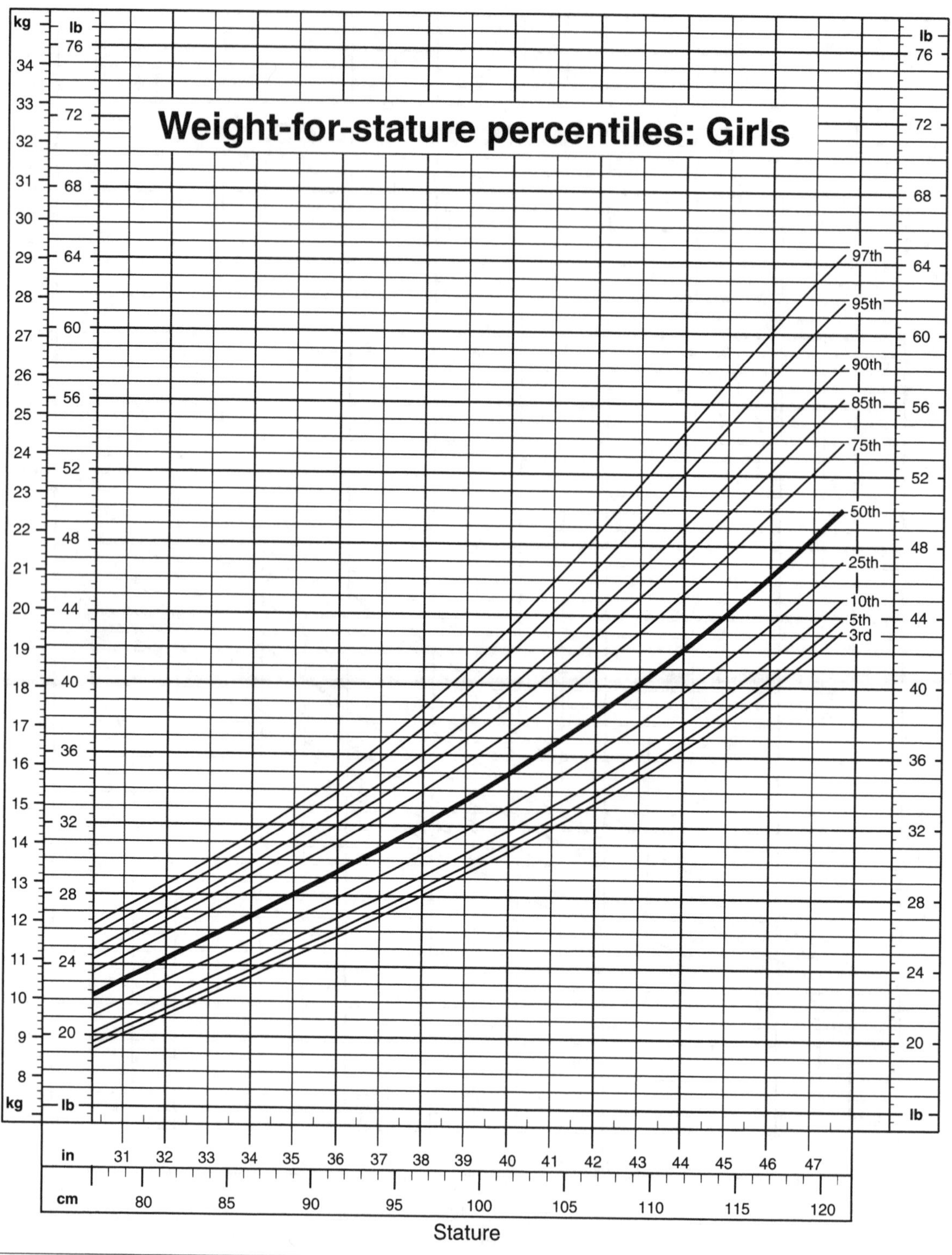

Weight-for-stature percentiles, girls, CDC growth charts: United States. *(Source: Developed by the National Center for Health Statistics in collaboration with the National Center for Chronic Disease Prevention and Health Promotion (2000). From Kuczmarski RJ, Ogden CL, and Gummer-Strawn LM et al.: CDC growth charts: United States. Advanced data from vital and health statistics, no. 314, Hyattsville, Maryland, 2000, National Center for Health Statistics.)*

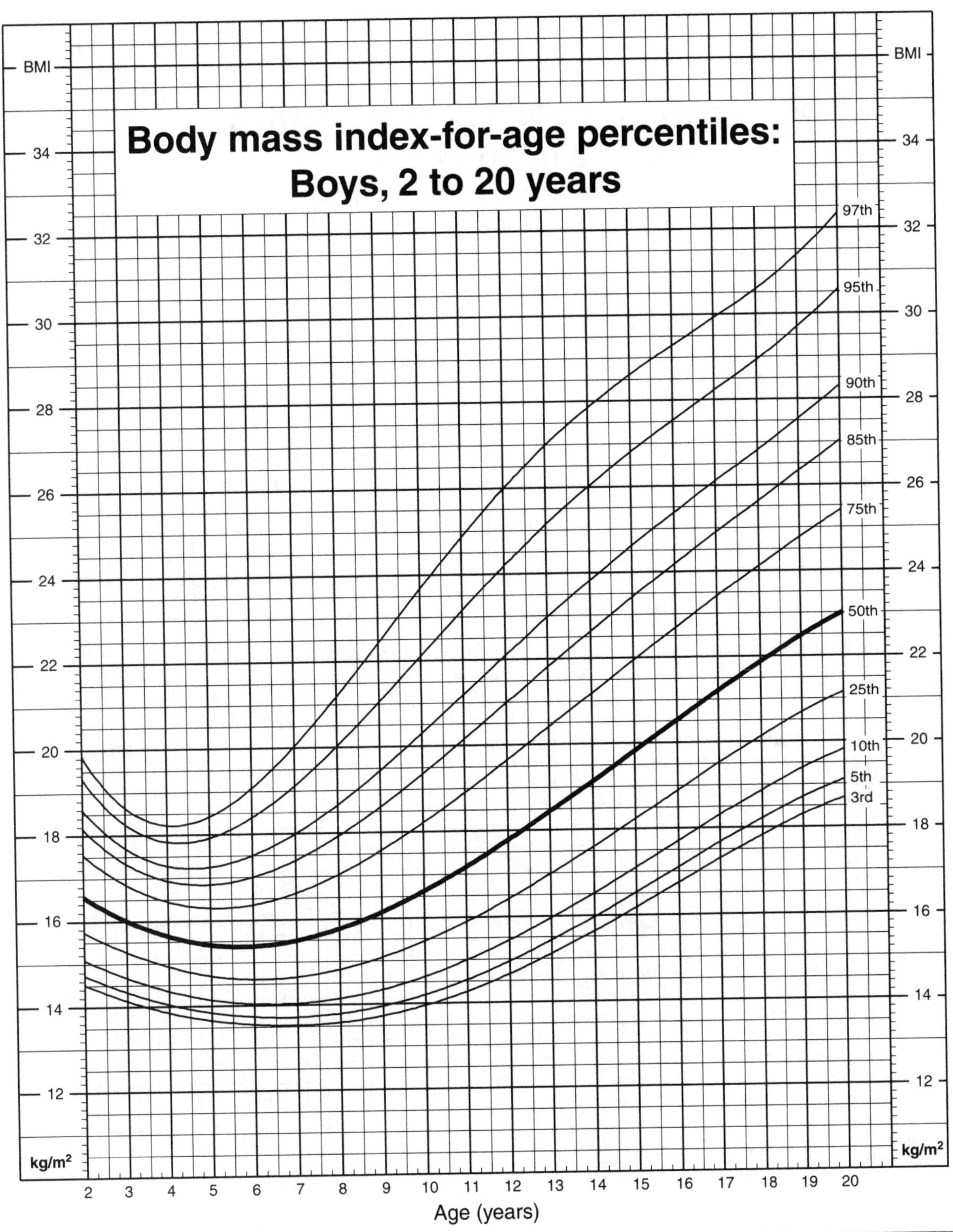

Body mass index-for-age percentiles, boys, 2 to 20 years, CDC growth charts: United States. *(Source: Developed by the National Center for Health Statistics in collaboration with the National Center for Chronic Disease Prevention and Health Promotion (2000). From Kuczmarski RJ, Ogden CL, and Gummer-Strawn LM et al.: CDC growth charts: United States. Advanced data from vital and health statistics, no. 314, Hyattsville, Maryland, 2000, National Center for Health Statistics.)*

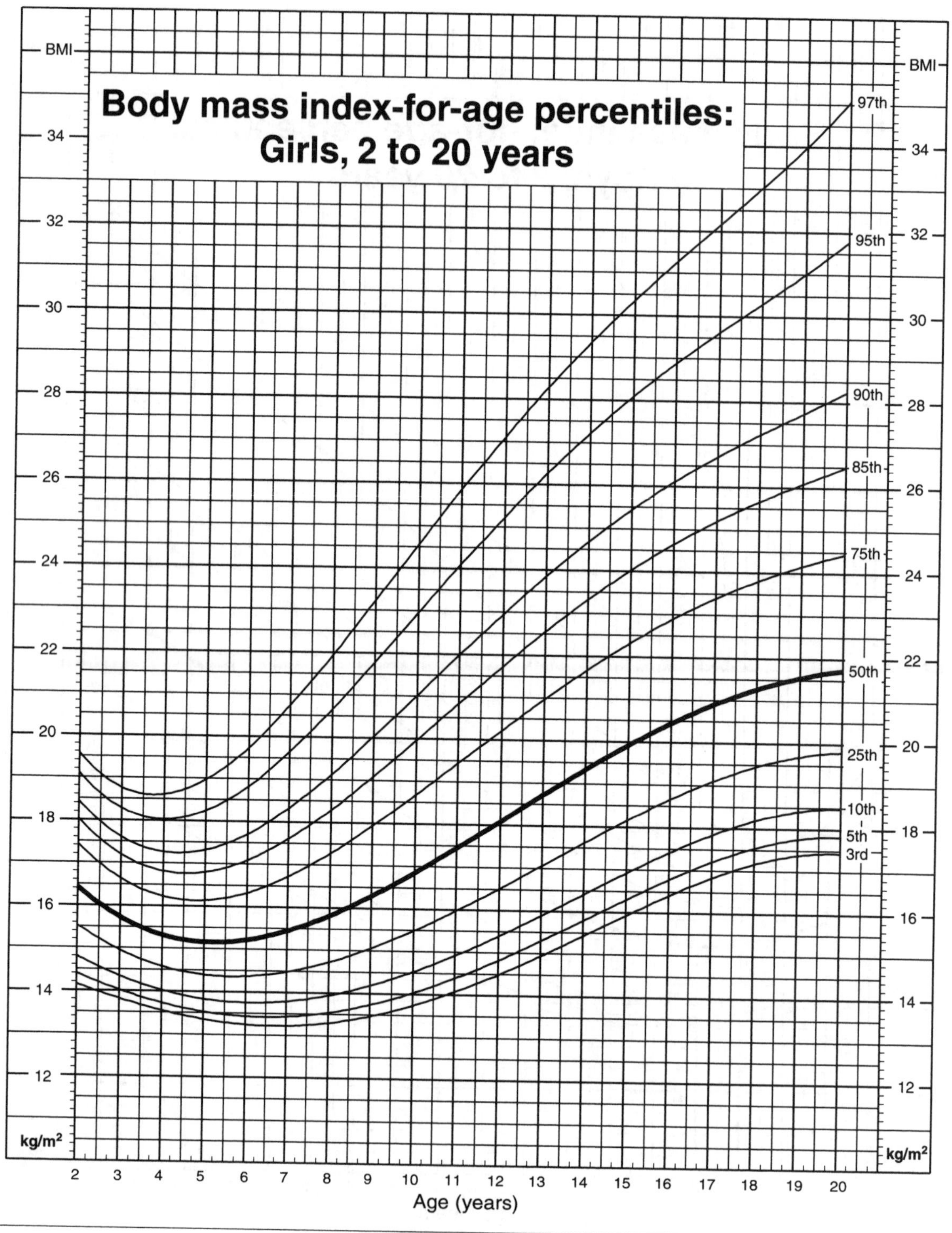

Body mass index-for-age percentiles, girls, 2 to 20 years, CDC growth charts: United States. *(Source: Developed by the National Center for Health Statistics in collaboration with the National Center for Chronic Disease Prevention and Health Promotion (2000). From Kuczmarski RJ, Ogden CL, and Gummer-Strawn LM et al.: CDC growth charts: United States. Advanced data from vital and health statistics, no. 314, Hyattsville, Maryland, 2000, National Center for Health Statistics.)*

APPENDIX F

EQUATIONS FOR ESTIMATING STATURE FROM KNEE HEIGHT FOR VARIOUS GROUPS

Age*	Equation†	Error‡
BLACK FEMALES		
>60	S = 58.72 + (1.96 KH)	8.26 cm
19-60	S = 68.10 + (1.86 KH) − (0.06 A)	7.60 cm
6-18	S = 46.59 + (2.02 KH)	8.78 cm
WHITE FEMALES		
>60	S = 75.00 + (1.91 KH) − (0.17 A)	8.82 cm
19-60	S = 70.25 + (1.87 KH) − (0.06 A)	7.20 cm
6-18	S = 43.21 + (2.14 KH)	7.80 cm
BLACK MALES		
>60	S = 95.79 + (1.37 KH)	8.44 cm
19-60	S = 73.42 + (1.79 KH)	7.20 cm
6-18	S = 39.60 + (2.18 KH)	9.16 cm
WHITE MALES		
>60	S = 59.01 + (2.08 KH)	7.84 cm
19-60	S = 71.85 + (1.88 KH)	7.94 cm
6-18	S = 40.54 + (2.22 KH)	8.42 cm

Adapted from Chumlea WC, Guo SS, and Steinbaugh ML: Predication of stature from knee height for black and white adults and children with application to mobility-impaired or handicapped persons, J Am Diet Assoc 94:1385, 1994. Copyright The American Dietetic Association.

*Age in years rounded to the nearest year.

†S = stature; KH = knee height; A = age in years

‡Estimated stature will be within this value for 95% of persons within each age, sex, race group.

APPENDIX G

ANTHROPOMETRIC REFERENCE DATA FOR AMERICANS 50 YEARS AND OLDER. NATIONAL HEALTH AND NUTRITION EXAMINATION SURVEY (NHANES III)

Weight for Men and Women Examined in the Third National Health and Nutrition Examination Survey (1988-1994) by Race/Ethnicity and Age

Characteristic	n	Mean ± Standard Error	Percentile 15th	Percentile 50th	Percentile 85th
		kg			
MEN					
All ethnicities					
50-59 y	855	86.0 ± 0.80	72.0	84.1	100.7
60-69 y	1175	83.1 ± 0.65	67.7	82.4	98.4
70-79 y	875	79.0 ± 0.71	64.2	77.9	93.5
80+ y	700	71.8 ± 0.74	58.4	70.8	84.1
Non-Hispanic white					
50-59 y	418	87.1 ± 0.82	73.6	85.1	102.1
60-69 y	510	84.3 ± 0.71[vw]	69.0	83.6	98.8
70-79 y	524	79.6 ± 0.66[v]	65.5	78.5	93.6
80+ y	560	72.3 ± 0.59[v]	59.8	71.5	84.5
Non-Hispanic black					
50-59 y	217	84.6 ± 1.41	65.8	82.9	101.6
60-69 y	295	80.4 ± 1.02[w]	64.3	78.3	98.3
70-79 y	187	77.2 ± 1.19	60.0	76.2	91.9
80+ y	59	70.7 ± 2.04	57.1[a]	71.8	84.5[a]
Mexican-American					
50-59 y	178	82.8 ± 1.40	68.2	81.5	97.1
60-69 y	337	78.3 ± 0.87[v]	64.6	77.3	92.0
70-79 y	149	73.1 ± 1.31[v]	59.9	74.7	84.9
80+ y	63	66.3 ± 1.62[v]	57.6[a]	66.8	74.5[a]
WOMEN					
All ethnicities					
50-59 y	1006	74.4 ± 0.84	57.2	71.5	91.6
60-69 y	1172	70.9 ± 0.71	55.4	68.8	86.9
70-79 y	988	67.4 ± 0.75	52.9	64.7	82.1
80+ y	790	60.5 ± 0.68	47.9	59.7	72.3
Non-Hispanic white					
50-59 y	484	74.3 ± 0.99	57.2	71.4	91.1
60-69 y	501	70.7 ± 0.87[x]	55.5	68.9	86.8
70-79 y	644	66.8 ± 0.74[x]	52.9	64.4	81.1
80+ y	621	60.4 ± 0.63[y]	47.9	59.7	72.2
Non-Hispanic black					
50-59 y	275	80.8 ± 1.34	62.5	79.3	100.1
60-69 y	300	78.8 ± 1.29[xz]	61.5	76.4	95.1
70-79 y	182	75.5 ± 1.57[xz]	58.0	72.6	93.3
80+ y	93	63.1 ± 1.66[z]	50.4	61.8	80.2
Mexican-American					
50-59 y	193	70.9 ± 1.20	56.1	70.0	83.1
60-69 y	321	70.2 ± 0.99[z]	56.8	67.5	82.3
70-79 y	127	63.7 ± 1.38[z]	51.7	61.6	74.5
80+ y	59	53.8 ± 1.74[yz]	40.8[a]	52.7	64.6[a]

From Kuczmarski MF et al.: Descriptive anthropometric data for older adults, J Am Diet Assoc 272:1335, 2000.

[a]Figure does not meet standard of reliability or precision.

[v-z]Within age category, mean weights with the same superscript are significantly different ($P < .05$).

Weight by Height for All Men Aged 50 Years and Older Examined in the Third National Health and Nutrition Examination Survey (1988-1994)

Height (in) by Age Group	n	Percentile 15th	50th	85th
		← lb →		
50-59 Y				
Total n	855	158.4	184.7	221.6
<65	78	140.8[a]	159.5	177.5[a]
65	58	123.6[a]	170.1	215.0[a]
66	92	146.3	173.4	198.5
67	116	156.4	177.6	207.0
68	100	166.2	191.7	225.5
69	127	164.1	184.1	223.0
70	115	166.4	196.3	229.1
71	66	168.0[a]	190.0	224.5[a]
72 and over	103	175.5	205.8	251.6
60-69 Y				
Total n	1175	148.8	181.1	216.4
<65	184	133.8	155.9	177.9
65	112	139.1	157.8	185.0
66	145	146.4	170.6	197.1
67	142	139.5	172.7	197.7
68	173	151.7	183.4	212.7
69	135	159.6	192.2	222.0
70	126	167.4	195.0	229.0
71	73	167.5[a]	205.3	232.7[a]
72 and over	85	178.0	203.0	240.1
70-79 Y				
Total n	875	141.2	171.3	205.7
<65	169	129.4	153.3	181.7
65	88	133.5	162.3	189.1
66	125	136.1	159.3	193.2
67	111	150.2	172.1	194.7
68	120	146.7	170.9	211.2
69	93	151.5	181.9	211.2
70 and over	169	160.8	186.8	220.3
80-89 Y				
Total n	699	128.4	155.9	185.2
<65	188	119.2	140.8	159.2
65	83	126.5[a]	151.8	170.7[a]
66	110	139.7	161.0	189.1
67	99	133.1	160.2	183.7
68	84	145.8	167.7	189.9
69	54	146.5[a]	172.4	200.2[a]
70 and over	81	141.6	171.5	203.5
60-89 Y				
Total n	2749	143.0	174.3	209.4
<65	541	124.5	151.7	174.2
65	283	134.5	157.0	186.2
66	380	142.0	165.5	195.3
67	352	141.9	170.9	194.7
68	377	149.4	176.2	210.6
69	282	154.2	187.4	215.8
70	249	160.7	184.8	223.0
71	235	165.8	200.1	232.6
72 and over	150	166.7	199.7	236.5

From Kuczmarski MF et al.: Descriptive anthropometric data for older adults, J Am Diet Assoc 272:1335, 2000.

[a]Figure does not meet standard of reliability or precision because of small sample size.

Weight by Height for All Women Aged 50 Years and Older Examined in the Third National Health and Nutrition Examination Survey (1988-1994)

Height (in) by Age Group	n	Percentile 15th	50th	85th
		← lb →		
50-59 Y				
Total n	1007	125.7	157.2	201.6
<60	98	112.2	147.2	181.1
60	71	112.5[a]	143.5	187.0[a]
61	133	123.2	153.6	194.1
62	136	120.0	145.7	191.3
63	148	130.2	155.1	211.0
64	149	134.1	165.0	203.2
65	100	126.1	158.1	182.5
66	74	142.0[a]	182.0	200.4[a]
67 and over	98	137.9	171.1	226.5
60-69 Y				
Total n	1172	121.9	151.4	191.1
<60	195	115.4	135.0	165.9
60	128	114.3	140.7	178.2
61	174	117.2	142.0	179.2
62	164	119.9	147.4	193.6
63	158	116.0	153.9	189.5
64	124	129.9	158.4	193.9
65	105	134.6	159.2	209.7
66	48	129.7[a]	160.9	202.1[a]
67 and over	76	142.7[a]	171.3	207.8[a]
70-79 Y				
Total n	985	116.3	142.4	180.5
<60	203	97.4	125.8	163.2
60	128	107.4	133.4	164.1
61	157	116.3	140.4	179.5
62	157	117.5	141.2	180.4
63	110	125.8	152.9	183.1
64	103	131.3	159.2	192.4
65 and over	127	130.8	154.5	189.5
80-89 Y				
Total n	788	105.4	131.4	159.1
<60	274	96.1	119.0	147.1
60	126	106.5	132.9	155.0
61	120	112.3	138.8	159.7
62	106	110.3	132.0	155.9
63	72	120.0[a]	140.8	170.7[a]
64	45	121.3[a]	139.7	170.4[a]
65 and over	45	112.6[a]	155.7	201.8[a]
60-89 Y				
Total n	2945	115.9	144.6	182.5
<60	672	101.0	126.1	158.9
60	382	110.2	134.7	169.1
61	451	116.2	140.7	172.6
62	427	117.1	141.6	184.3
63	314	121.4	152.0	186.1
64	272	129.6	156.0	191.7
65	206	130.8	157.5	200.1
66	92	131.0	160.9	198.4
67 and over	103	142.5	168.1	206.4

From Kuczmarski MF et al.: Descriptive anthropometric data for older adults, J Am Diet Assoc 272:1335, 2000.

[a]Figure does not meet standard of reliability or precision because of small sample size.

Body Mass Index, Mid Upper Arm Circumference, Triceps Skinfold Thickness, and Arm Muscle Circumference for Men 50 Years of Age and Older Examined in the Third National Health and Nutrition Examination Survey (1988-1994)

Variable and Age Group[a]	n	Mean ± SE[b]	Selected Percentile						
			10th	15th	25th	50th	75th	85th	90th
BODY MASS INDEX[c]									
50-59 y	855	27.8 ± 0.23	22.6	23.5	24.7	27.2	30.7	32.1	33.5
60-69 y	1175	27.3 ± 0.18	21.9	23.1	24.4	27.1	30.0	31.7	32.8
70-79 y	875	26.7 ± 0.21	21.5	22.3	23.8	26.1	29.3	30.7	31.7
80+ y	699	25.0 ± 0.22	19.8	21.1	22.4	25.0	27.1	28.7	29.5
MID UPPER ARM CIRCUMFERENCE (CM)									
50-59 y	824	33.7 ± 0.18	29.2	30.0	31.1	33.7	35.6	37.2	37.9
60-69 y	1126	32.8 ± 0.15	28.4	29.2	30.6	32.7	35.2	36.2	37.0
70-79 y	832	31.5 ± 0.17	27.5	28.2	29.3	31.3	33.4	35.1	36.1
80+ y	642	29.5 ± 0.19	25.5	26.2	27.3	29.5	31.5	32.6	33.3
TRICEPS SKINFOLD THICKNESS (MM)									
50-59 y	813	13.7 ± 0.29	7.5	8.0	9.4	12.6	16.0	18.7	21.8
60-69 y	1122	14.2 ± 0.25	7.7	8.5	10.1	12.7	17.1	20.2	23.1
70-79 y	825	13.4 ± 0.28	7.3	7.9	9.0	12.4	16.0	18.8	20.6
80+ y	641	12.0 ± 0.28	6.6	7.6	8.7	11.2	13.8	16.2	18.0
ARM MUSCLE CIRCUMFERENCE (CM)[d]									
50-59 y	811	29.2 ± 0.15	25.6	26.2	27.4	29.2	31.1	32.1	33.0
60-69 y	1119	28.3 ± 0.13	24.9	25.6	26.7	28.4	30.0	30.9	31.4
70-79 y	824	27.3 ± 0.14	24.4	24.8	25.6	27.2	28.9	30.0	30.5
80+ y	639	25.7 ± 0.16	22.6	23.2	24.0	25.7	27.5	28.2	28.8

From Kuczmarski MF et al.: Descriptive anthropometric data for older adults, J Am Diet Assoc 272:1335, 2000.
[a]All racial/ethnic groups included.
[b]SE = standard error.
[c]Calculated as kg/m^2.
[d]Arm muscle circumference = midarm circumference (cm) − π × triceps skinfold thickness (cm).

Body Mass Index, Mid Upper Arm Circumference, Triceps Skinfold Thickness, and Arm Muscle Circumference for Women 50 Years of Age and Older Examined in the Third National Health and Nutrition Examination Survey (1988-1994)

Variable and Age Group[a]	n	Mean ± SE[b]	Selected Percentile						
			10th	15th	25th	50th	75th	85th	90th
BODY MASS INDEX[c]									
50-59 y	1006	28.4 ± 0.31	21.0	22.2	23.6	27.2	32.1	35.1	37.1
60-69 y	1172	27.6 ± 0.27	20.9	21.8	23.5	26.6	30.8	33.6	35.7
70-79 y	985	26.9 ± 0.28	20.7	21.4	22.6	25.9	29.9	32.1	34.5
80+ y	788	25.2 ± 0.26	19.3	20.3	21.7	25.0	28.4	30.0	31.4
MID UPPER ARM CIRCUMFERENCE (CM)									
50-59 y	970	32.5 ± 0.25	26.6	27.5	28.7	32.0	35.3	37.5	39.2
60-69 y	1122	31.7 ± 0.21	26.2	26.9	28.3	31.2	34.3	36.5	38.3
70-79 y	914	30.5 ± 0.23	25.4	26.1	27.4	30.1	33.1	35.1	36.7
80+ y	712	28.5 ± 0.25	23.0	23.8	25.5	28.4	31.5	33.2	34.0
TRICEPS SKINFOLD THICKNESS (MM)									
50-59 y	929	26.7 ± 0.40	16.4	18.3	20.6	26.7	32.1	35.2	37.0
60-69 y	1090	24.2 ± 0.37	14.5	15.9	18.2	24.1	29.7	32.9	34.9
70-79 y	902	22.3 ± 0.39	12.5	14.0	16.4	21.8	27.7	30.6	32.1
80+ y	705	18.6 ± 0.42	9.3	11.1	13.1	18.1	23.3	26.4	28.9
ARM MUSCLE CIRCUMFERENCE (CM)[d]									
50-59 y	927	23.8 ± 0.15	20.4	20.9	21.5	23.3	25.4	26.5	27.8
60-69 y	1090	23.8 ± 0.12	20.6	21.1	21.9	23.5	25.4	26.6	27.4
70-79 y	898	23.4 ± 0.14	20.3	20.8	21.6	23.0	24.8	26.3	27.0
80+ y	703	22.7 ± 0.16	19.3	20.0	20.9	22.6	24.5	25.4	26.0

From Kuczmarski MF et al.: Descriptive anthropometric data for older adults, J Am Diet Assoc 272:1335, 2000.

[a]All racial/ethnic groups included.

[b]SE = standard error.

[c]Calculated as kg/m^2.

[d]Arm muscle circumference = midarm circumference (cm) − π × triceps skinfold thickness (cm).

APPENDIX H

CULTURAL DIETARY PATTERNS

Only foods that are specifically associated with these cultural groups are noted. Individuals may also consume typical American foods as well; assumptions of dietary patterns cannot be made, but knowledge of these unique foods provides a common understanding of the range of possible food choices.

NATIVE AMERICAN

Each tribe may have specific foods; listed here are commonly consumed foods.

1. Bread, Cereal, Rice, and Pasta Group

Blue corn flour (ground dried blue corn kernels) used to make cornbread, mush dumplings; fruit dumplings (walakshi); fry bread (biscuit dough deep fried); ground sweet acorn; tortillas; wheat or rye used to make cornmeal and flours

2. Vegetable Group

Cabbage, carrots, cassava, dandelion greens, eggplant, milkweed, onions, pumpkin, squash (all varieties), sweet and white potatoes, turnips, wild tullies (a tuber), yellow corn

3. Fruit Group

Dried wild cherries and grapes; wild banana, berries, yucca

4. Milk, Yogurt, and Cheese Group

None

5. Meat, Poultry, Fish, Dry Beans, Eggs, and Nuts Group

Duck, eggs, fish eggs (roe), geese, groundhog, kidney beans, lentils, peanuts, pinenuts, pinto beans, all nuts, venison, wild rabbit

6. Fats, Oils, and Sweets

None

AFRICAN-AMERICAN

1. Bread, Cereal, Rice, and Pasta Group

Biscuits, cornbread as spoon bread, cornpone or hush puppies, grits

2. Vegetable Group

Leafy greens including dandelion greens, kale, mustard greens, collard greens, turnips

3. Fruit Group

None

4. Milk, Yogurt, and Cheese Group

Buttermilk

5. Meat, Poultry, Fish, Dry Beans, Eggs, and Nuts Group

Pork and pork products, scrapple (cornmeal and pork), chitterlings (pork intestines), bacon, pig's feet, pig ears, souse, pork neck bones, fried meats and poultry, organ meats (kidney, liver, tongue, tripe), venison, rabbit, catfish, buffalo fish, mackerel, legumes (black-eyed peas, kidney, navy, chickpeas)

6. Fats, Oils, and Sweets

Lard

JAPANESE

1. Bread, Cereal, Rice, and Pasta Group

Rice and rice products, rice flour (mochiko), noodles (comen/soba), seaweed around rice with or without fish (sushi)

2. Vegetable Group

Bamboo shoots (takenoko), burdock (gobo), cabbage (nappa), dried mushrooms (shiitake), eggplant, horseradish (wasabi), Japanese parsley (seri), lotus root (renkon), mustard greens, pickled cabbage (kimchee), pickled vegetables, seaweed (laver, nori, wakame, kombu), vegetable soup (mizutaki), white radish (daikon)

3. Fruit Group

Pear-like apple (nasi), persimmons

4. Milk, Yogurt, and Cheese Group

None

5. Meat, Poultry, Fish, Dry Beans, Eggs, and Nuts Group

Fish and shellfish including dried fish with bones, raw fish (sashimi), and fish cake (kamaboko); soybeans as soybean curd (tofu), fermented soy bean paste (miso), and sprouts; red beans (azuki)

6. Fats, Oils, and Sweets

Soy and rice oil

CHINESE

1. Bread, Cereal, Rice, and Pasta Group

Rice and related products (flour, cakes, and noodles); noodles made from barley, corn, and millet; wheat and related products (breads, noodles, spaghetti, stuffed noodles [won ton] and filled buns [bow])

2. Vegetable Group

Bamboo shoots; cabbage (napa); Chinese celery; Chinese parsley (coriander); Chinese turnips (lo bok); dried day lillies; dry fungus (Black Juda's ear); leafy green vegetables including kale, Chinese cress, Chinese mustard greens (gai choy), Chinese chard (bok choy), amaranth greens (yin choy), wolfberry leaves (gou gay), and Chinese broccoli (gai lan); lotus tubers; okra; snow peas; stir-fried vegetables (chow yuk); taro roots, white radish (daikon)

3. Fruit Group

Kumquat

4. Milk, Yogurt, and Cheese Group

None

5. Meat, Poultry, Fish, Dry Beans, Eggs, and Nuts Group

Fish and seafood (all kinds, dried and fresh), hen, legumes, nuts, organ meats, pigeon eggs, pork and pork products, soybean curd (tofu), steamed stuffed dumplings (dim sum)

6. Fats, Oils, and Sweets

Peanut, soy, sesame and rice oil; lard

FILIPINO

1. Bread, Cereal, Rice, and Pasta Group

Noodles, rice, rice flour (mochiko), stuffed noodles (won ton), white bread (pan de sal)

2. Vegetable Group

Bamboo shoots, dark green leafy vegetables (malunggay and salvyot), eggplant, sweet potatoes (camotes), okra, palm, peppers, turnips, root crop (gabi)

Continued

3. Fruit Group

Avocado, bitter melon (ampalaya), guavas, jackfruit, limes, mangoes, papaya, pod fruit (tamarind), pomelos, tangelo (naranghita)

4. Milk, Yogurt, and Cheese Group

Custards

5. Meat, Poultry, Fish, Dry Beans, Eggs, and Nuts Group

Fish in all forms; dried fish (dilis); egg roll (lumpia); fish sauce (alamang and bagoong); legumes such as mung beans, bean sprouts, chickpeas, organ meats (liver, heart, intestines); pork with chicken in soy sauce (adobo); pork sausage; soybean curd (tofu)

6. Fats, Oils, and Sweets

None

SOUTHEASTERN ASIANS: (LAOS, CAMBODIA, THAILAND, VIETNAM, THE HMONG, AND THE MIEN)

1. Bread, Cereal, Rice, and Pasta Group

Rice (long and short grain) and related products such as noodles; Hmong cornbread or cake

2. Vegetable Group

Bamboo shoots, broccoli, Chinese parsley (coriander), mustard greens, pickled vegetables, water chestnuts, Thai chili peppers

3. Fruit Group

Apple pear (Asian pear), bitter melon, coconut cream and milk, guava, jackfruit, mango

4. Milk, Yogurt, and Cheese Group

Sweetened condensed milk

5. Meat, Poultry, Fish, Dry Beans, Eggs, and Nuts Group

Beef; chicken; deer; eggs; fish and shellfish (all kinds of freshwater and saltwater); legumes including black-eyed peas, peanuts, kidney beans, and soybeans; organ meats (liver, stomach); pork; rabbit; soybean curd (tofu)

6. Fats, Oils, and Sweets

Lard, peanut oil

MEXICAN

1. Bread, Cereal, Rice, and Pasta Group

Corn and related products; taco shells (fried corn tortillas); tortillas (corn and flour); white bread

2. Vegetable Group

Cactus (nopoles), chili peppers, salsa, tomatoes, yambean root (jicama), yucca root (cassava or manioc)

3. Fruit Group

Avocado, guacamole (mashed avocado, onion, cilantro [coriander], and chilis), papaya

4. Milk, Yogurt, and Cheese Group

Cheese, flan, sour cream

5. Meat, Poultry, Fish, Dry Beans, Eggs, and Nuts Group

Black or pinto beans (reijoles); refried beans (frijoles refritos); flour tortilla stuffed with beef, chicken, eggs, or beans (burrito); corn tortilla stuffed with chicken, cheese, or beef topped with chili sauce (enchilada); Mexican sausage (chorizo)

6. Fats, Oils, and Sweets

Bacon fat, lard (manteca), salt pork

PUERTO RICAN AND CUBAN

1. Bread, Cereal, Rice, and Pasta Group

Rice; starchy green bananas, usually fried (plantain)

2. Vegetable Group

Beets; eggplant; tubers (yucca); white yams (boniato)

3. Fruit Group

Coconuts, guava, mango, oranges (sweet and sour), prune and mango paste

4. Milk, Yogurt, and Cheese Group

Flan, hard cheese (queso de mano)

5. Meat, Poultry, Fish, Dry Beans, Eggs, and Nuts Group

Chicken, fish (all kinds and preparations including smoked, salted, canned, and fresh), legumes (all kinds especially black beans), pork (fried), sausage (chorizo)

6. Fats, Oils, and Sweets

Olive and peanut oil, lard

JEWISH

The foods below reflect both religious and cultural customs of Jewish people. Adherence to religious dietary patterns by followers of the different forms of Judaism (Orthodox, Conservative, Reform, and Reconstructionist) vary. Generally, Orthodox Jews and many Conservative Jews follow kosher dietary rules both at home and when out. Others may only observe when in their own homes. These rules of "keeping kosher" are reviewed in the next section on religious dietary patterns.

1. Bread, Cereal, Rice, and Pasta Group

Bagel, buckwheat groats (kasha), dumplings made with matzoh meal (matzoh balls or knaidelach), egg bread (challah), noodle or potato pudding (kugel), crepe filled with farmer cheese and/or fruit (blintz), unleavened bread or large cracker made with wheat flour and water (matzoh)

2. Vegetable Group

Potato pancakes (latkes); a vegetable stew made with sweet potatoes, carrots, prunes, and sometimes brisket (tzimmes); beet soup (borscht)

3. Fruit Group

None

4. Milk, Yogurt, and Cheese Group

None

5. Meat, Poultry, Fish, Dry Beans, Eggs, and Nuts Group

A mixture of fish formed into balls and poached (gefilte fish); smoked salmon (lox)

6. Fats, Oils, and Sweets

Chicken fat

RELIGIOUS DIETARY PATTERNS

Beliefs of several major religions include practices that affect or prescribe specific dietary patterns or prohibit consumption of certain types of foods. Individuals practicing these religions may or may not adhere to all of the prescribed customs. Following is a brief review of some of these practices.

Moslem

Pork and pork-related products are not eaten. Meats that are consumed must be slaughtered by prescribed rituals; these procedures are similar to the Judaic kosher slaughtering of animals, so Moslems may eat kosher meats. Coffee, tea, and alcohol are not consumed. During the month of Ramadan, Muslims fast during the day from dawn to sunset.

Continued

Christianity

Some sects may not eat meat on holy days; others prohibit alcohol consumption.

Hinduism

Animal foods of beef, pork, lamb, and poultry are not eaten. Followers are lacto-vegetarians or vegans.

Judaism

Food consumption is guided by religious doctrines; no pork or pork-related products nor seafood or fish without scales and fins are eaten. Dairy foods are not consumed with meat or animal-related foods (excludes fish). If meat or dairy is eaten, 6 hours must past for the other to be acceptable for consumption. Animals are slaughtered according to a ritual in which blood is drained and the carcass is salted and rinsed; meat prepared in this manner is "kosher." The preparation of all processed foods eaten must also adhere to these guidelines. Because meat and dairy must not mix, two sets of dishes and utensils are used at home and in kosher restaurants. Foods that are neither meat nor dairy are called parve and are often so labeled by food manufacturers. Additional customs affect food consumption on Saturday, the Sabbath, during which no cooking occurs. Special foods are associated with each religious holiday. Fasting (no water or food) for 24 hours occurs during Yom Kippur (Day of Atonement). During Passover, an 8-day holiday, no leavened bread is consumed, only matzoh (made from flour and water) and products made from matzoh flour; other symbolic food restrictions are also observed.

Seventh Day Adventist

General restrictions of pork and pork-related products, shellfish, alcohol, coffee, and tea are followed. Some followers are ovo-lacto-vegetarians, whereas others are vegans.

From Grodner M, Anderson SL, and DeYoung S: Foundations and clinical applications of nutrition: A nursing approach, ed. 2, St. Louis, 2000, Mosby.

INDEX

C

I